C0-FLN-512

COMPARATIVE HEALTH SYSTEMS

Descriptive Analyses of Fourteen National Health Systems

Edited by

Marshall W. Raffel

Wingate College Library

THE PENNSYLVANIA STATE UNIVERSITY PRESS
UNIVERSITY PARK AND LONDON

099492

Second printing, 1985

Library of Congress Cataloging in Publication Data

Main entry under title:

Comparative health systems.

1. Medicine, State. 2. Insurance, Health.
3. Medical care, Cost of. I. Raffel, Marshall W.
[DNLM: 1. National health programs. 2. Health services. WA 540.1 C737]
RA411.C66 1984 362.1 83-43032
ISBN 0-271-00363-4

Copyright © 1984 The Pennsylvania State University
All rights reserved
Printed in the United States of America

Rittenhouse
10-14-85
$ 29.95

Comparative Health Systems

Contents

Introduction

Marshall W. Raffel

Medical science is making great strides, coming forth with new knowledge and, in turn, both new technology and new therapies. Along with this, peoples' expectations rise, as do health care costs, all over the world. In all countries, these rising costs impose new pressures on the allocation of limited, and indeed sometimes scarce, resources.

Attempts to restrict rising health costs cover a broad spectrum—slowing down hospital construction, freezing hospital and physician charges, modifying hospital and physician reimbursement mechanisms, requiring the patient to bear an increasing share of the costs, restricting the acquisition of new technology, encouraging alternative delivery systems, introducing drug formularies, and increasing the emphasis on the importance of prevention. These and other attempts to deal with the cost issue typically translate into rationing of care—by price, by quality, or by availability. For some would-be patients the cost of care is beyond their ability to pay; for others there is simply no access, due to the absence of appropriate facilities or services; other patients are forced to queue for long periods of time. The costs still rise.

The problem of rising costs is both elusive and intractable. Some of the more critical variables are frequently not identified. Seemingly sound approaches, on the other hand, are commonly undercut by the pincers of new health opportunities and public demand.

There is a growing interest in what other countries are doing with respect to the problems of costs, quality, and access. How do different countries organize, deliver, and finance their health services? What problems have they encountered, and how have they dealt with them? How successful or unsuccessful have they been, and why? Can we learn from them, and adopt, adapt, or avoid certain approaches?

These questions are not unreasonable, for—despite political, cultural, economic, and other differences—there are in reality more similarities than differences among health systems. In seeing and emphasizing the differences, we often overlook the similarities.

One problem faced by those who wonder about other health systems is the paucity of readily accessible literature. While the body of literature appearing in English is growing, it is still relatively small, and what does exist is often limited by its having been written for a domestic audience or with a focus on special issues, from which it is difficult to draw parallels across national boundaries. It was the felt need to make more available descriptive analyses of national health systems, which could serve for comparative studies, that led to this book.

The idea was to ask scholars in a number of countries to write an account of their respective health systems, following a common outline and providing common statistical data. Each author was asked to bear in mind that he was writing for the edification of people in other countries. It was hoped that the final product would be insightful for those who want to know how others have dealt with problems and would open up lines of inquiry for the readers to pursue. It was also hoped that the accounts would prove useful to university teachers in courses on comparative health systems.

There are fourteen countries covered, with native authors from twelve. I was not able to secure native authors from the Soviet Union and the People's Republic of China. All authors were asked to submit their chapters in English; as editor, I have tried not to alter the flavor of each author's rhetoric.

As the manuscript was going to the publisher, attention was drawn to an excellent account of the Danish health system, which came fairly close to the prescribed outline. It was decided to include it in this book with minor editorial adjustments. The account lacked a discussion of the system's problems, but we were able to enlist the help of a member of the Danish Hospital Institute to write the analytical addendum and provide additional statistical data. Because of the short time frame available to the Danish author, collecting all of the desired statistical data was not feasible. Most of the tabular data for Denmark is taken from *Health Statistics in the Nordic Countries 1980,* published by the Nordic Medical Statistical Commission. The data covers the five Nordic countries (Denmark, Finland, Iceland, Norway, and Sweden), and it was decided to retain the data on all of the countries. The tables in the Swedish chapter are thus incorporated at the end of the Danish narrative.

One problem arose with regard to the statistical data. Not all countries collect their data in the same way. Twenty tables with 1980, or the latest available, data were requested from each country. Some later U.S. data is reported in the text, but for the tables it was decided to standardize the data for 1980 to facilitate comparisons among countries. Changes from year to year are, of course, generally not significant. In a few instances where tabular data is lacking, some of the data may be found in the text. In some cases certain tables would not be relevant due to the nature of the health system. In some instances the data were simply not available. In still other instances the data were collected in a somewhat different manner. One common variation is that not all countries analyse *personal* health services expenditure data on a per capita and percentage basis as distinct from the more inclusive figures for national health expenditure data. A common table numbering system is used; thus, the data that appears for each country may not always be exactly comparable but should describe basically the same universe—more or less. An exception to this is China: data was not readily available, so its tables do not conform to the format of the others and are thus numbered by a letter system. Our success with the Soviet Union stems from the fact that the author accompanied the editor to the Soviet Union in the Spring of 1982; in anticipation of our inability to secure a Soviet author, she made efforts to gather most of the relevant data while there.

The table numbering system used, except in the China chapter, is as follows:

Table 1 Population by age, race, sex, and—where relevant—by national origin or language groups.
Table 2 Live births, birth rates, and fertility rate.
Table 3 Infant mortality by age and race (or other special population groups) for se-

lected years and broken down as follows: under 1 year, 28 days to 11 months, under 28 days.

Table 4 Infant mortality rates by 6 most common causes.

Table 5 Estimated death rates for 100,000 population for the 15 leading causes of death.

Table 6 Selected operative (surgical) procedures: number in thousands and average length of stay when performed in hospital.

Table 7 Most frequent medical (nonsurgical) reasons for admission to hospital: number in thousands and average length of stay in hospital.

Table 8 Estimated number and rate per 100,000 population of persons active in the major health field occupations.

Table 9 Number of operational medical schools, medical students enrolled by sex, and medical school graduates by sex for the year.

Table 10 Total number of physicians, and physicians per 100,000 population for selected years.

Table 11 Breakdown of physicians by place of practice: office-based patient care, hospital-based patient care, hospital-based *in specialty training* (supervised) patient care, medical teaching, administration, research, other. Indicate which specialties, if any, are considered primary care specialties.

Table 12 Average net income of physicians by specialty before taxes, but excluding business- or practice-associated expenses.

Table 13 Number of hospitals broken down by type and size of hospital, number of beds in thousands, admissions per year in thousands, average daily census in thousands, percentage occupancy.

Table 14 Of the total hospitals, indicate the number by type of ownership or sponsorship—i.e., public, church, or other nonprofit, or for-profit—and number of beds in each category.

Table 15 Number of long-term care or nursing homes, and number of beds. (Exclude long-term-care hospitals and institutions that do not provide a significant amount of nursing care.)

Table 16 Average cost of inpatient care per day in acute care (general) hospitals. Indicate any differences between cities and rural areas.

Table 17 National health expenditures: amount and per capita amount by major source of funds and percentage of Gross National Product, in selected calendar years.

Table 18 National health expenditures by type of expenditure and source of funds, per capita amounts, and percentage distribution.

Table 19 Personal health care expenditures by selected third-party payers and type of expenditure, amount, per capita amount, and percentage distribution.

Table 20 Percentage of population covered by private health insurance for selected calendar years.

Each author was free to include, in addition to these tables, other data and tables as part of their text.

A number of authors refer in their chapters to dollars ($). The dollar ($) currency base is common to Australia, Canada, New Zealand, and the United States. When used in those chapters, the value relates to local currency values. To convert to other currencies, the reader should refer to the conversion table that appears at the end of this Introduction. Where reference is made to dollars ($) in other chapters, the reference is to the U.S. dollar.

Languages are replete with ambiguities and peculiarities, and they are forever changing.

The same words are used in different ways by different countries. The word "physician" in the United States, for example, describes all medically qualified practitioners, whereas in other countries—most notably England, Australia, and New Zealand—it applies to a more narrow range of practitioners, that is, the specialist or consultant in internal medicine. So it is, also, with the male pronoun "he." While some authors have begun to modify their use of the pronoun, recognizing that females are fulfilling a growing professional role in the health field, others still use the pronoun in a generic sense to mean both the male and female. Where "he" appears in the text, it should generally be so viewed.

A final note on language relates to spelling. I have tended to retain the English or American spellings as the respective authors chose them. Because we read each other's books and articles, we are, of course, influenced not only by ideas but also by manners of expression and of spelling. None of us is completely consistent. Consequently, within a chapter one may find some words spelled the American way, and other words—including the same words—spelled the English way. Whichever way the word appears, the meaning is the same.

The editor's task was simplified by the ease of international direct dialing telephone service. But more importantly his task was eased by the excellent cooperation from each of the authors. Working with them was a most gratifying experience.

Foreign Exchange Rates

	Value Per Unit of Foreign Currency in U.S. $		Units of Currency Per Each U.S. Dollar	
	12/31/80	9/15/82	12/31/80	9/15/82
Australia (dollar)	1.182	.9576	.8460	1.0443
Belgium (franc)	.0317	.0209	31.50	47.90
Canada (dollar)	.8379	.8100	1.1934	1.2346
China (renminba or yuan)	—	.5150	—	1.9417
Denmark (krone)	.1661	.1131	6.01	8.84
England (pound)	2.392	1.7070	.4181	.5854
Finland (mark)	.2603	.2083	3.8415	4.81
France (franc)	.2214	.1411	4.5175	7.0850
Germany (mark)	.5092	.3979	1.9640	2.5130
Japan (yen)	.004936	.003797	202.60	263.40
Netherlands (guilder)	.4725	.3650	2.1160	2.7395
New Zealand (dollar)	.9635	.7242	1.038	1.3808
Norway (krone)	.1932	.1442	5.1750	6.9335
Sweden (krona)	.2288	1.607	4.37	6.2230
USSR (ruble)	—	1.395	—	.7168

The Authors

AUSTRALIA

John Dewdney, BA, MD, BS (Melb), SM (Harv), DPH (Lond), FRACMA, FHA, is on the staff of the School of Health Administration, University of New South Wales, Australia. His major research and teaching interests are epidemiology and the planning of health services. He is the author or co-author of ten books and more than fifty published papers. He has worked in Southeast Asia, Europe, and North America, his most recent major assignment being WHO consultant and programme coordinator in the Republic of Korea.

BELGIUM

Herman Nys studied law at the Universities of Leuven (Belgium) and Nijmegen (the Netherlands). He obtained his PhD in law at Leuven University (1980) with a thesis on health care planning in different European countries. He co-authored *National Health Insurance and Health Resources* (Harvard University Press, 1978). He is presently the principal investigator at the Law School of Leuven University, with a special interest in the field of health care law.

Paul Quaethoven has a PhD in Political Science from Leuven University, Belgium. He is an associate professor at the School of Public Health, Leuven University, and is general secretary of the Hospital Committee of the European Economic Community.

CANADA

Gordon Hollett Hatcher, MD, DPH, FRCP(C), studied medicine at McGill University and public health at the University of Toronto. He is a Fellow of the Royal College of Physicians and Surgeons of Canada and of the American Public Health Association. He taught public health and medical care administration at the graduate schools of public health in Toronto and Montreal; was head of the Department of Preventive Medicine at Dalhousie University in Halifax; and was a visiting research professor at the Fogarty International Center, National Institutes of Health, United States Public Health Service, Bethesda, Maryland. He has conducted research and served as a consultant to various government departments in Canada, the United States, and the Caribbean, and to private hospital consulting firms in the United States. He is author of a number of research reports and scholarly publications. He is president of the Hatcher Research Associates Corporation.

Peter Robert Hatcher, BA, DHA, studied political science at McGill University and hospital administration at the University of Toronto. He has held administrative positions of increasing responsibility in several teaching and regional hospitals in Ontario. His research includes studies of primary care in a teaching hospital medical group practice, of hospital capital and operating cost controls in Ontario, and of long-term care and extra billing by physicians under Canadian health insurance. He is vice president for Hospital Management Studies with the Hatcher Research Associates Corporation.

Eleanor Clair Hatcher has studied architecture at Carleton University in Ottawa. Her research activities include assistance in preparation of a monograph on utilization review and quality assurance under Canadian health insurance, graphic arts for a cancer research study, a survey of hospices in America and Northern Europe, and data collection for this study of the Canadian health care system. She is a research associate with the Hatcher Research Associates Corporation.

China, People's Republic

Teh-wei Hu, professor of economics at The Pennsylvania State University, received his PhD from the University of Wisconsin. His major interests are in the application of economics to the field of human resources. He teaches and publishes in health economics and applied econometrics. He spent one year at the National Institutes of Health as a visiting research professor. He has served as consultant to numerous public and private institutions, including the Institute of Medicine of the National Academy of Sciences, National Institute of Mental Health, National Institutes of Health, and Urban Institute.

Denmark

Willy Søndergaard, MD, is chief of anesthesiology at Tawam Hospital, Al Ain, Abu Dhabi, United Arab Emirates. From 1977 to 1980 he was project manager at the Danish Hospital Institute, where he authored the descriptive account of health services in Denmark. He received his degree in medicine from the University of Copenhagen in 1959 and was recognized in the specialty of anesthesiology in 1968. He headed the anesthesiology department at the Danish Teaching Hospital in Kinshasa, Zaire from 1969 to 1977 and the county hospital in Frederikssund, Denmark from 1972 to 1977.

Allan Krasnik, MD, MPH, PhD, is presently research coordinator at the Danish Hospital Institute, co-editor of the Danish Medical Journal, and a member of the board of the Danish Association of Social Medicine. He graduated in medicine from the University of Copenhagen (1971), and received a Master of Public Health from the Hebrew University, Hadassah Medical School, Jerusalem (1973) and a PhD at the University of Copenhagen (1976). From 1972 he was engaged in research and teaching activities at the Department of Social Medicine, University of Copenhagen, in the fields of community medicine, epidemiology, preventive medicine, and health services administration, especially focusing on the development of primary health care.

England

David Allen, PhD, is senior lecturer at Manchester University and director of studies at the Health Services Management Unit of the university. Educated at Birmingham, Yale, and Manchester universities, he has worked for the RAND Corporation, Santa Monica, and has taught at the European Institute of Advanced Studies in Management in Brussels and Manchester University and New York University business schools. He is a member of his local community health council, and his research interests are in resource allocation and decision making, on which he has published several books.

FRANCE

Jean-François Lacronique, MD, born in 1943, is a professor of public health at the University of Paris. A radiologist by training, he underwent a one-year teaching program at IBM-France in 1968. This experience led him to work as a consultant for the use of computers in the field of health for the French ministry of health until 1973. He was then appointed Science Attaché at the Embassy of France in the United States. He graduated from M.I.T. in 1977 in the MS program at the Sloan School of Management and returned to France to become medical editor of the newspaper *Le Monde.* He went back to academia in 1980 and was appointed deputy director for Health and Hospitals at the French ministry of health for two years. He is currently medical directeur at Institut Pasteur Production, a leading pharmaceutical unit in sera and vaccines in France.

GERMANY, FEDERAL REPUBLIC

Siegfried Eichhorn, Dr. rer. pol. habil., Dipl.-Kfm, studied the science of business management at the University of Cologne. He is currently executive director of the German Hospital Institute, which is affiliated with the University of Duesseldorf. He is also professor of health and hospital economics on the medical faculty of Duesseldorf and a lecturer at the Universities of Cologne, Berlin, and Duesseldorf. An advisor to WHO and OECD, and a member of numerous national and international associations, he has more than 250 publications in books and magazines about health and hospital economics.

JAPAN

Masami Hashimoto, professor emeritus of the National Institute of Public Health in Tokyo, has been rector of the Saitama Prefectural College of Health since July 1982. He received MD and Dr. Med. Sci. degrees from the Osaka University in 1940 and 1948, respectively. He served in health administrative positions at municipal, regional, and national levels before joining the institute in 1957. With a specialty in health administration and planning, he served on many occasions in international health supported by WHO and other agencies. He has been editor of the Japanese *Journal of Public Health* since 1958, and he is the author of some 150 articles and 8 monographs related to public health.

NETHERLANDS

Harmen A. Tiddens, MD, began his medical career as a paediatrician, became head of a district hospital and then professor of paediatrics and associate director of the university children's hospital at Utrecht, where he participated in the reorganization of the hospital, developed paediatric nephrology, and headed the development of medical education at Utrecht University. He was later founding dean of the medical faculty at the University of Limburg, and later rector of that university. Since 1979 he has been professor and chairman of the Department of Health Care Organization at Tilburg University, director of the National Hospital Management Course, and board member of the Institute for Health Services Research. From July 1982 through August 1983 he served temporarily as chief scientist, Health Manpower Development at WHO in Geneva.

Joep (P) Heesters studied economics and business administration at Tilburg University. After five years' experience as a financial staff member of a joint venture of a number of sickness funds, he started as a lecturer at the Economic Faculty of Tilburg University, Department of Health Care Organization. He is also doing research in the field of doctors' remunerations, on which he is writing a dissertation.

Joost (M) van de Zande finished his study of economics at Tilburg University in 1982. He is currently working as a staff member of a joint venture of the Dutch Hospital Organization and the Dutch Organization for Ambulatory Mental Health Care. This venture seeks to realize full integration of all mental health institutions per region.

New Zealand

B. Joan Mackay, BSc, MB, BCh (Wales), DPH (London), FFCM (UK), MPP (Vict), and MCCM (NZ), is currently senior lecturer in the Department of Community Health at the Wellington Clinical School of Medicine, New Zealand. She was formerly medical officer of health for the Wellington and Hutt health districts, and for a number of years was assistant director in charge of family health for New Zealand. Her areas of interest are in policy making, planning, and management of health services.

Sweden

Edgar Borgenhammar since 1978 has been professor of health services management at the Nordic School of Public Health in Gothenburg. He holds a PhD from the Stockholm School of Economics, a Master of Business Administration degree from the University of California at Berkeley, and a diploma from the School of Social Work at Lund. He was administrative director at the South District of the Health Services Board, the County Council of Stockholm from 1971 to 1978, and was hospital director at Danderyd Hospital in Stockholm in 1969–70. He served as a planning expert for the city of Stockholm in 1968–69, and as a teacher and researcher at the Stockholm School of Economics from 1962 to 1968.

Union of Soviet Socialist Republics

Norma K. Raffel received a Master of Science and a Doctor of Philosophy from the University of Maryland. After completing her studies, she worked in the Department of Medicine at the University of Maryland School of Medicine. She has taught biological sciences at Goucher College and The Pennsylvania State University, and has served as a consultant to state education agencies and universities on educational policy. Her international activities include professional travel in the People's Republic of China, the Middle East, Latin America, eastern Europe, and the Soviet Union, studying health services and the position of women. Currently, Dr. Raffel is writing a history of hospitals.

United States of America

Marshall W. Raffel, PhD, professor of health planning and administration at The Pennsylvania State University, is a graduate of the University of Illinois and has a doctorate in political science from Victoria University of Wellington, New Zealand, where he also taught. He has worked in health insurance and industrial health and safety as well as in government at the state and federal levels. He has served as a WHO consultant in Asia and traveled extensively in western and eastern Europe, studying various health systems.

Health Services in Australia

John Dewdney

INTRODUCTION

Big Country, Small Population

With a land area of nearly three million square miles (7.68 million square kilometers), Australia ranks sixth among the world's largest countries. Much of the country is inhospitable desert, and nearly 40% of the total area lies north of the Tropic of Capricorn.

Since World War II the population has almost doubled, rising from 7.6 million in 1947 to 15 million in 1982. Compared with most other developed countries, Australia's current rate of population growth—more than 1.6 percent in 1980–81—is high. In common with all developed countries, Australia has an ageing population, but the proportion of the population aged 65 years or over is markedly less than in many other affluent countries. One in five of the population was born overseas, with settlers from the United Kingdom, Eire, and continental Europe making up about 15% of the total population. Among recent immigrants, people born in Asia have constituted the largest group, but the Asian-born population still makes up less than 2% of Australia's population. People claiming descent from the dark-skinned indigenous occupants of the country prior to European settlement—the Australian Aborigines—now number around 1.2% of the population.

The most striking feature of Australia's population distribution is the very high concentration in the temperate coastal plains in the east, southeast, and southwest, with some 80% of the population contained in 1.6% of the total land area. Also, Australia is one of the most highly urbanized countries in the world, having two-thirds of its population congregated in major urban centres, with nearly 90% of all major city dwellers living in the five mainland state capitals.

The Commonwealth Constitution

In 1901, by an Act of the British Parliament, the six separate British colonies in Australia were federated into one nation, the Commonwealth of Australia. The three-tier structure

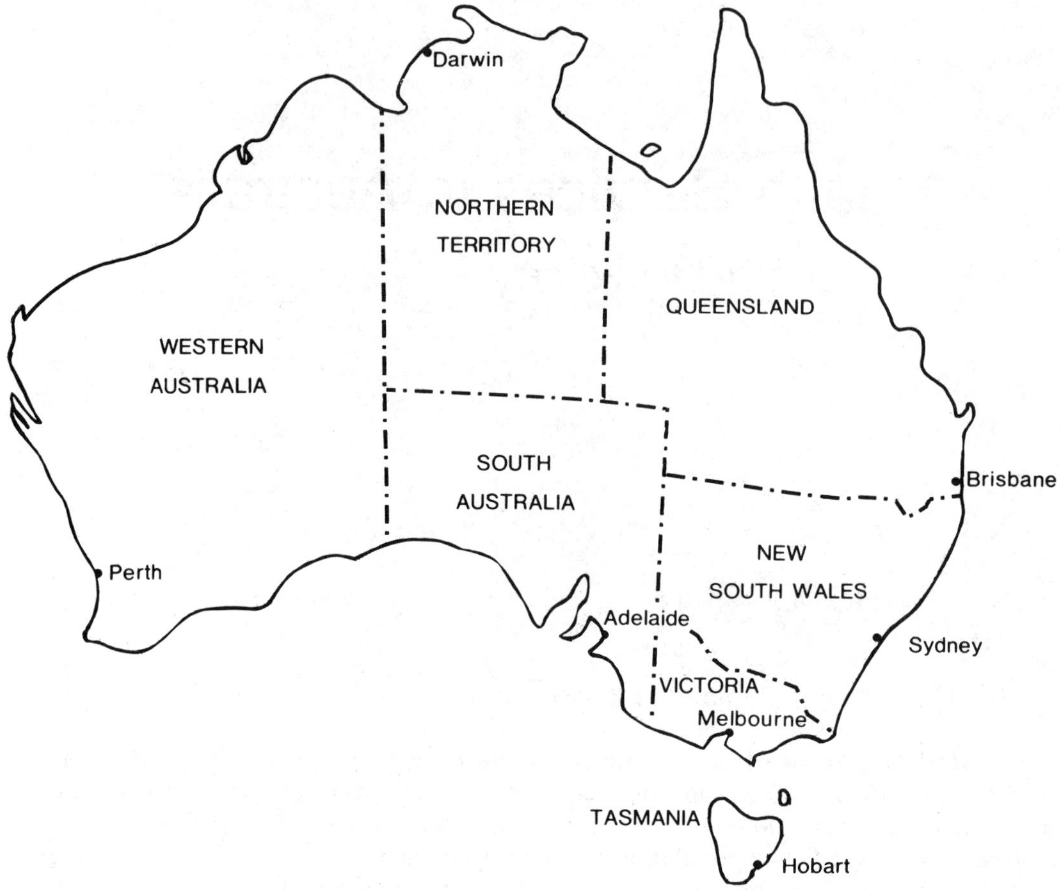

of government has at the highest level the Commonwealth Government, also sometimes referred to as the Australian Government or the Federal Government. Next come the governments of the six states and one territory, and at the third level are about 900 local government bodies. The tiny Australian Capital Territory, within which lies the national capital, Canberra, is administered by Commonwealth Government agencies, including the ACT Health Commission. Throughout this chapter, unless stated otherwise, the term *states* includes the territories.

At the federal level, in each of the states, and in the Northern Territory there is an elected parliament that largely follows the Westminster model of responsible government but is constrained by the limitations imposed by written constitutions. The Commonwealth Constitution enumerates the exclusive powers and powers held concurrently with the state governments. The undefined residue of powers belongs to the states. Responsibility for deciding the constitutional validity of Commonwealth and state legislation rests with the High Court of Australia. Within the specified limits of federal jurisdiction, Commonwealth legislation overrides any state law that is inconsistent with it. By the use of a number of powers the Commonwealth has established a monopoly of income taxation and has made the states dependent for their solvency upon Commonwealth grants. This enables the Commonwealth to exercise very considerable influence upon many matters where it has no specified powers or relatively small ones.

The Commonwealth Constitution Act of 1900 made little mention of health matters—the only one specified in the Commonwealth's enumerated powers was the provision of quarantine services. At that time it was thought that health and health care were predominantly of personal and local concern and thus were appropriately left to state governments and nongovernment enterprise. Problems arising during the First World War (1914–18)—the high rate of rejection from the armed forces of young men found to be unfit; Australia's vulnerability because of reliance upon distant overseas sources of vaccines and other pharmaceuticals; difficulties in effective control of sexually transmitted diseases; the dangers of introduction of exotic diseases from the theatres of war to Australia's tropical zone; the need to provide continuing care for sick and disabled war veterans together with the disastrous postwar influenza pandemic—led to calls for a more vigorous national policy on health. The Commonwealth Government in the succeeding two decades developed a comprehensive health care service for war veterans, established a Commonwealth Department of Health headed by a minister of health, and set up a number of consultative, coordinating, and research agencies, but still the major responsibility for health care provision rested with the states and nongovernment providers.

The Political Scene

Three political groups dominate the political scene at all levels of government. Two parties stand on the right: the "Liberals" (not to be confused with "small 'l' liberals"), representing essentially conservative interests of commerce and industry, and "Country Party" organizations committed to protecting and furthering the interests of agriculture and the rural population. In the parliaments these two factions almost invariably work in coalition to defeat opposition from the left. To the left, but only mildly socialist by European standards, the Labor parties are closely linked with the trade union movement. Particularly at the state level, the "Labor" parties have relied heavily on the support of Roman Catholics, who comprise a quarter of Australia's population and maintain a nationwide school system alongside the state education system. This church lobby within the Labor parties has exerted considerable influence on health policies, particularly on such issues as abortion and family planning. Although all parties have from time to time changed their stands on health policy, the rightwing parties' basic philosophy supports notions of individual responsibility for health care and of private medicine, while Labor favours services that are free at the point of service from a salaried staff, and sees the health care system as one mechanism for the redistribution of wealth.

Powers and Responsibilities in Health Care

Shortly after the outbreak of World War II (1939) a Labor government took office at the national level. The party's platform included the provision of "free health care." The first move in this direction, legislation to make available without charge a range of pharmaceuticals, was challenged in the High Court and held invalid. The government then sought, by referendum, to amend the Constitution. This resulted in an extension of the Commonwealth's legislative powers in 1946 to include the provision of ". . . pharmaceutical, sickness, and hospital benefits, medical and dental services (but not so as to authorize any form of civil conscription) . . ." (Placetum xxiiiA, Section 51, Constitution of the Commonwealth of Australia). On several occasions the High Court has attempted to interpret the exact meaning of this placetum, and it remains a major source of debate among constitutional lawyers. Whatever its precise meaning, however, this addition to the Constitution permitted an enormous increase in the involvement of the Commonwealth Government and its agencies in health matters. Thus, the Commonwealth now provides more than half of all health service funding and exercises tight control over the operations of the health insurance organizations. Although the financial nexus places considerable power in the Commonwealth's hands, much of the regulation of health service activity is the responsibility of state governments. Most of the provision of health care facilities and of the operation of health services is shared between the state governments and the private sector. Local authorities have limited powers and responsibilities for the protection and promotion of public health—mainly in areas of environmental control.

Health Ministers and Departments

Within each of the federal and state parliaments one minister is primarily responsible for health matters. Health ministers rank low in the order of ministerial precedence. While ministers come and go, as the exigencies of parliamentary government demand, the permanent heads of the health departments, who are career public servants (and not necessarily medically qualified), stay on, usually, until they reach retirement age or reach the end of some statutory term of office.

Several ministries other than health play important parts in health policy and administration, for example, those concerned with social security, industry and commerce, migration and transport, and particularly the treasuries, as keepers of the public purse. It is now the pattern for governments to have a separate ministry of the environment. The Commonwealth Minister for Veterans' Affairs is responsible for the care, including comprehensive free health care, of ex-service personnel and their dependents through his department, which was formerly named the Repatriation Department and is still commonly called "Repat."

The 1970s witnessed several changes in state health authority administrative organisation, but the basic pattern of three major administrative divisions remains: one concerned with the provision and regulation of hospitals and nursing homes, the second providing services for the mentally ill and intellectually handicapped, and the third covering the broad field of public health.

The activities of public health committees of the elected local government councils and their salaried public health personnel are supervised and assisted by the state departments of health and of local government.

Mixed Health Care Provision

Complementing the government-provided services are those of the very extensive private providers. Among these, the profit-seeking hospitals and nursing homes, the private practitioners of medicine, and the pharmaceutical industry loom largest. All of these, however, rely very heavily on government subsidies, as we shall see later. Not-for-profit nongovernment agencies range from large hospitals and nursing homes run by religious and other benevolent organizations to the thousands of small groups that contribute to the health of the community by provision of services, by augmenting services provided by government, by conducting public education campaigns, by lobbying for particular interest groups, and by maintaining channels through which well-intentioned citizens can assist their less fortunate fellows. Some of these nonprofit agencies receive government subvention; most of them do not. The registered health insurance agencies are required by law to operate on a not-for-profit basis.

The National Health

On all the commonly used indicators of community health, Australia ranks high among the nations of the world. As in other relatively healthy countries, this partly reflects the adequacy and wide availability of the health services—but also, and more importantly, it reflects the general well-being that comes from widely distributed prosperity and a favourable environment. For many Australians immoderate self-indulgence and foolhardy behavior pose the biggest threats to life and health.

One group in Australia stands out as singularly unhealthy—those who identify themselves as descendants of this country's precolonial population, the dark-skinned Australian Aborigines. Those living in squalor in Australia's few urban slums and in shantytowns at the edge of rural settlements, supported principally by social service pensions, have morbidity and mortality rates far higher—though now declining—than those for the great majority of Australians. Although numerically small, this minority group presents a persistent and perplexing challenge to the would-be social meliorist.

MEDICAL PRACTICE

Faced with a health problem, an Australian may decide to do nothing about it, seek the advice of family or friends, or resort to self-medication. For many trivial conditions and for most serious ones professional advice will be sought, most commonly from a medical practitioner. In the majority of cases, the doctor of first contact is a general practitioner. Much less often contact will be made first with a doctor employed in the casualty department of a hospital; these departments usually function both as emergency departments and, to a limited extent, as general practice clinics. The primacy of the general practitioner is hallowed by tradition, buttressed by both social security and health insurance arrangements which impose financial penalities upon direct access to specialists, and founded on the very sound premise that the general practitioner shall be the triage agent, dealing with the wide range of problems within his own sphere of professional competence and referring the others to specialists, hospitals, and nursing homes or other agencies.

The Medical Workforce

The vagaries of the medical practitioner registration system in Australia—each state has its own system—make it impossible to know exactly how many doctors are in active practice. Probably the most accurate indicator is a nationwide mailing list maintained, with frequent updates, by a commercial firm supported by the pharmaceutical industry. As of late 1982, an estimated 29,000 to 30,000 doctors were practising, of whom one in five is a woman.

The medical workforce is divisible into four major groups, the largest being general practitioners in private practice who represent more than 40% of the total. The second largest group contains specialist practitioners in private practice, though many of them also hold one or more part-time salaried posts in public hospitals and some have honorary (unpaid) public hospital appointments. These specialists make up nearly one-third of the medical workforce. A third, much smaller group is composed of salaried doctors, mostly with specialist status, employed on the staff of government health departments, medical schools, research institutes; together these salaried practitioners represent perhaps 3% of all practitioners. The fourth large group of doctors, employed by hospitals as full-time salaried staff, make up about 22% of the workforce and are subdividable into interns, residents, and others. These others are mostly specialists or specialists-in-training (generally ranked as registrars). Overall, then, the medical workforce is comprised of general practitioners, over 40%; specialists (including trainee specialists), about 50%; and the rest, less than 10%, junior house (hospital) staff. Of all doctors in active practice, only one in four is in full-time salaried employment.

General Practice

The metamorphosis of the traditional general practitioner—a sort of general medical factotum—to a primary care physician, resulting from the growth of medical specialisation, has been fostered in Australia by Commonwealth legislation. General practitioners are remunerated on a fee-for-service basis and are free to charge whatever fees they wish. However, the fees they charge are in fact closely tied to the level of government benefit (reimbursement) to patients covered wholly or in part by social service and health insurance arrangements. The schedule of insurance benefits provides for a flat rate reimbursement of fees paid by the patient for primary care items, but services appropriately provided by specialists carry two levels of benefit—a lower level if the service is provided by a general practitioner, a higher level if the doctor is a specialist. The patient can claim the higher rate of reimbursement only if referred to the specialist by a general practitioner. Thus, the general practitioner is encouraged to concentrate on primary care with referral to specialists when appropriate. Nevertheless, some general practitioners—particularly in rural areas where ready access to specialist care is limited—do undertake some work that goes beyond primary care. Recent moves towards delineation of hospital roles and of medical privileges within hospitals also serve to focus the activities of general practitioners on primary care. However, many general practitioners do at present have hospital appointments, and many country hospitals would be unable to function without them.

General practitioners quite commonly work within some sort of partnership arrangement whereby accommodation, office staff, and ancilliary staff are shared, but each general practitioner tends to operate as a solo practitioner with his or her "own" list of regular patients; similarly, patients tend to identify one practitioner as "their own" doctor. Some years ago there was a trend towards mixed group practice in which general practitioners and specialists worked together, the specialists sharing responsibility for out-of-hours calls with the general practitioners and undertaking some general work. This pattern seems to be much less common now, partly because of the "two-level" benefits arrangement and partly because of the widespread use of deputising services to cover out-of-hours calls.

Another noticeable recent change in the field of general practice has been the increasing attraction of young graduates to general practice, partly attributable to an increasing emphasis upon "family medicine" in medical schools, partly because of government sponsorship of a formal training program for general practice under the Family Medicine Program, and partly perhaps due to the growth of deputising, which both provides young graduates with medical practice experience while they moonlight during their hospital residency and makes the life of a general practitioner less onerous. Whereas a few years ago some of the less-affluent urban areas and rural communities did not attract general practitioners, this deficit is now less apparent.

Specialist Practice

The introduction of the "two level" medical benefit schedule has led to a clearer differentiation between general and specialist practice and, through the work of a national committee on specialist qualifications, has produced a clearer delineation of specialities. The third of the medical workforce in specialist private practice can be enumerated as follows:

	Percentage of Specialist Workforce
Surgeons	15
Physicians (internists in U.S. terminology)	15
Anaesthetists	11
Psychiatrists	11
Obstetricians	9
Pathologists	7
Radiologists	7
Paediatricians	5
Ophthalmologists	5
Orthopaedic surgeons	4
Oto-rhino-laryngologists	3
Dermatologists	2
Urologists	2
Neurologists, neurosurgeons, chest physicians, etc.	each 1 or less

In addition to maintaining their own consulting rooms, most specialists, unlike general practitioners, must have access to hospital beds. Private hospitals provide an important source of beds and other facilities for specialists, and indeed many private hospitals are owned wholly or in part by doctors and their nominees. Still, more than four-fifths of all hospital beds in Australia are in public hospitals, and these are accessible to doctors holding hospital appointments. Until a few years ago doctors were appointed to the honorary medical staff of most public hospitals with the obligation to treat public patients without any remuneration from either patients or hospital. By way of *quid pro quo* the honoraries were entitled to admit their own patients to the hospital and charge them fees for services rendered. During the 1970s a federal Labor government abolished the honorary system as anachronistic and ideologically unacceptable. Initially, there was vociferous opposition from many doctors who thought this presaged the introduction of "socialized medicine." Quite soon, however, offers of visiting medical staff positions with paid sessional appointments or modified fee-for-service agreements were accepted; boycotts lapsed; and now one hears few demands for a return to the honorary system—though there are still some doctors who, on ideological grounds, serve as honorary medical officers. For most specialists a public hospital appointment is now doubly attractive: not only does he have access to beds in which to treat his private, paying patients, but he is now also paid for treating "public" patients. This change has undeniably increased the public hospital authorities' control over visiting medical staff, with greater accountability of doctors to hospital management bodies and growing use of peer review and utilization review as a means of ensuring proper standards of patient care and efficient use of hospital resources.

Before the virtual abolition of the honorary system, public hospitals had been moving towards the employment of a full-time specialist staff as medical administrators and as heads of clinical departments, particularly the anaesthetics, radiology, and pathology departments. This trend continues. In addition to their hospital salaries, clinical specialists are generally permitted limited rights of practice. Terms of appointment vary, but typically a salaried specialist may be permitted to augment his income by private practice fees of up to 20% of his hospital salary, any additional earnings being paid into a medical staff fund that is used to finance the staff's research projects, overseas study tours, and other professional activities. Specialists on the staff of medical schools are in a similar position to full-time hospital specialists, but they may be paid through university funding instead of from hospital sources.

Doctors' Remuneration

The salaries of doctors employed full time in public hospitals and other government agencies are fixed through Commonwealth and state wage-fixing tribunals, as are the wages, salaries, and allowances of most people employed in Australia. The tribunals' decisions, known as "awards," are frequently reviewed in adversary proceedings with legal representation of both employees and employers. Because of present inflationary pressures the figures appearing in the awards tend rapidly to lose any meaning; but some notion of the doctors' salaries in late 1982 is conveyed by noting that the average male weekly earnings then were $320, while the award salary for junior residents was around $400 weekly and that for senior specialists was around $1,000 per week.* These salaries may be augmented by various additional awards such as on-call allowances, overtime payments, and holiday pay loadings, while staff with permanent tenure enjoy generous superannuation benefits with premiums paid largely by the employer. The payments to visiting staff in public hospitals are determined on the basis of half-day sessions and tied to the awards for full-time staff.

*All dollar references for Australia are Australian dollars. See conversion table in the Introduction.—Ed.

The income of general practitioners is, for the most part, derived from payments through the health insurance arrangements and social service benefit schemes. Because both systems of payment are under Commonwealth Government control, the monetary rewards of general practice are not, in most cases, very different from those of senior, full-time salaried staff, when account is taken of the superannuation, leave entitlements and other fringe benefits of salaried employment. However, the taxation laws do favour the self-employed doctor as against the salaried specialist in respect to expense allowances and some other items.

Since a substantial part of the income of specialists in private practice is derived from sessional payments for hospital work and from fees largely covered by health insurance, the government exercises considerable control. In general, the private specialist's income is not much different from a practitioner's; indeed, a young general practitioner may be making considerably more than his confreres at medical school who are struggling to establish a specialist practice. Recently changes have been made in the medical benefits arrangments to curb the extremely high incomes received by some radiologists and pathologists. The leading specialists in most of the procedural specialties can earn very large incomes, which, of course, are heavily taxed.

Medical practitioners rank as the highest paid sizeable professional group in Australia. The great majority of them, whether in private practice or in salaried posts, have professional incomes within the top 1% of the national income distribution scale. This high earned-income level permits doctors to secure additional income, often very substantial in amount, from investment and speculation in real estate and other business ventures, including private hospitals and nursing homes.

Patient Satisfaction with Doctors' Services

A national survey (1978–79) of patient satisfaction with their most recent doctor consultation among persons who had consulted a doctor within the previous three months reported that 93% of patients were satisfied (67%) or very satisfied (26%) while only 7% expressed dissatisfaction. When responses were divided into three groups according to the type of doctor consulted, the dissatisfaction level was lowest for general practitioner consultations, highest for hospital doctor consultations (10%), and for specialist consultations the percentage of reported dissatisfaction was seven.

The Medical Colleges and Associations

Each major specialty has its own college or society which exercises control over entry to the specialty through conditions for membership, demands of curriculum, difficulty of examination, and influence over the numbers of trainee posts available. These bodies also provide spokesmen for the professional interests of their members on many committees convened by government and other agencies concerned with health care. Some of the smaller specialties, sub-specialties, and many special professional interest groups have professional associations that play an important part in furthering the educational and other professional interests of their members; however, membership to any of these groups does not confer any legally recognised specialty status. Some of these professional bodies are affiliated with the Australian Medical Association (AMA). With a membership of more than half of all doctors, the AMA is the most powerful medical lobby in Australia. Vehement proponent of private practice and fee-for-service payment, the AMA has repeatedly fought against and defeated governmental attempts to introduce compulsory health insurance and "free" pharmaceuticals. Like it or not, governments have had to negotiate with the AMA on virtually every major matter affecting medical practice and medical finance, often through the parliamentary and departmental committee system, sometimes through more informal channels.

In the past few years the AMA has attempted to present a public face which shows concern for health issues such as quality of patient care and reduction of cigarette smoking rather than concentrating exclusively on the sectional political and economic interests of its members. This partial volte-face resulted from a declining public image of the medical profession, the declining membership of the AMA (particularly among younger doctors), and a genuine concern among some of the Association's leaders for those broader issues.

Closely linked with the development of organised medical consumerism in the 1970s, the Doctors' Reform Society has become something of a second public voice from the medical profession, well informed, socially concerned, and articulate, and nurtured by a media grateful for having a youthful telegenic opposition to the AMA establishment.

INSTITUTIONAL CARE

The Australian institutions which provide inpatient care fall conveniently into three major categories: hospitals, mental health institutions, and nursing homes. It is necessary to consider them together because in the course of a single episode of illness a patient may move between institutions in two or even three of these groups, and in some cases it may be local circumstance or chance which determine to which type of institution a particular patient is admitted. There are significant differences between these categories in terms of function; legal status under Commonwealth and state legislation; ownership; administrative supervision and control; internal management; arrangements for capital and operating finance; staffing; patient classification; and admission procedures. In 1982 there were about 1,150 hospitals, some 1,400 nursing homes, and 35 major mental health institutions. Overall, there were approximately 6.4 hospital beds, 4.7 beds in nursing homes, and less than two mental institution beds per 1,000 population.

There are also numbers of hostels, halfway houses, live-in rehabilitation centres, and other facilities to provide accommodation and care for persons with health problems which do not demand the level of medical and nursing services available in institutions covered by the threefold classification described in this section.

The Role of Hospitals

The great majority of institutions in this category are short-stay general hospitals, short-stay in the sense that the average length of stay is less than two weeks (though some patients stay much longer) and general in the sense that at least general medical and surgical care is provided; in most of these hospitals obstetric, gynaecologic, and paediatric care is also available. The range and sophistication of services and facilities increases as one moves from small rural hospitals with less than fifty beds, through rural district hospitals with 50 to 150 beds, to rural regional or base and urban district hospitals with 200 to 300 beds, to the large teaching hospitals with upwards of 400 beds and covering the gamut of up-to-the-minute diagnostic and treatment services. There are a few special hospitals: women's hospitals, children's hospitals, cancer institutes, eye hospitals, and hospitals for the treatment of tuberculosis. Australia's relatively high hospital bed: population ratio means that waiting lists for admission are generally short or are nonexistent, a notable current (1982) exception being renal transplantation where the number of donors falls seriously short of the number of would-be recipients.

Public hospitals are important centres for care of the ambulatory, to be discussed later. They also provide the venue for teaching health personnel of many categories, and some are world-recognised centres of medical research. Most private hospitals concentrate on the rapid throughput of an uncomplicated case load, preferably with a high procedural content and do not carry the high overhead expenses of teaching and research. However, very recently some private hospitals have begun to exploit the earning potential of high technology, for example, by installing CAT scanners and developing cardiac surgery units. Government attitudes to these innovations appear ambivalent, somewhat apprehensive about the cost implications for the health insurance arrangements coupled with relief that public funds will not have to be found for very expensive capital items.

Classification and Legal Status of Hospitals

The great majority of institutions in the "Hospitals" category are designated as either *public* or *private* hospitals under state legislation. The definitions of public and private hospitals vary from state to state, but the essential difference is that a public hospital is open to anyone in need of inpatient care of the type provided by that institution, whereas a private hospital has a restrictive admission policy and is therefore not open to the public at large. Any hospital seeking to show a profit on its activities cannot be classified as a public hospital under either Commonwealth or state law. Although the majority of private hospitals are conducted on a profit-seeking basis, some private hospitals, particularly those run by religious bodies, are nonprofit enterprises. A third and smaller group of government hospitals is not covered by the public and private hospital legislation of the states. Among these are the hospitals conducted by the Commonwealth Department of Veterans' Affairs—known generally as Repatriation hospitals—and the Armed Services hospitals.

Ownership of Hospitals

With few exceptions, public hospitals are either government property or are vested by the government in a statutorily constituted board of management, and thus held in trust for the community. The exceptions are hospitals owned by religious or other philanthropic bodies, and operated in compliance with Commonwealth and state legislation covering public hospitals. Owners of private hospitals include religious and philanthropic bodies, individual investors, business partnerships, registered companies, and cooperatives.

Control and Management of Hospitals

In each state the health authority is responsible for the administration of the public hospital system. Those public hospitals operated directly by health authorities are subject to very close supervision by those authorities. Where the administration of one or more of these institutions is vested in a board of management, the central authority retains considerable control over finance, staffing, and operating policies, but at least until recently this control has not been strongly exercised. The degree of autonomy exercised by a hospital board depends upon a number of factors, including the powers conferred upon it by the state's hospital legislation; the policy of the central health authority; the constitution, method of appointment, and length of tenure of board members; the energy, competence, and political influence of board members; and the wishes and power of the hospital staff. The very considerable autonomy that public hospital boards have enjoyed is now being curbed by much stricter government control over hospital finance. Private hospital proprietors are licensed by the state health authority, which sets minimum standards for accommodation, staffing, facilities, and records; but the degree of the authority's supervision of and interference with the conduct of private hospitals is relatively small.

Hospital Funding

State governments provide the major share of capital funds for public hospitals. Individual hospitals may be permitted to raise bank loans guaranteed by the state health authority and to conduct public appeals, and a relatively small amount of capital funding is received by way of bequests. Capital finance for private hospitals is obtained from the sources available to commercial enterprise generally; private hospitals conducted as religious and philanthropic agencies obtain capital funding from the bodies under whose auspices they operate and from donations and bequests.

Public hospitals derive funds for recurrent (operating) expenditure principally from both Commonwealth and state governments and from charges to patients. Charges to patients constitute the major source of income for recurrent expenditure by private hospitals, which also receive a per diem payment from the Commonwealth Government for each insured patient.

Staffing of Hospitals

Small public hospitals may have no full-time medical staff, the medical care of patients being in the hands of visiting medical staff who are paid partly by the hospital on a sessional basis and partly by patients through fee-for-service arrangements. Larger public hospitals employ some full-time salaried medical staff, who may have a limited right of private practice on a fee-for-service basis, and a visiting medical staff who, again, is paid partly by the hospital on a sessional basis and partly by patients through fee-for-service arrangements. In the largest public teaching hospitals one finds: a full-time salaried group of medically qualified administrators; a full-time staff of salaried specialists and a group of teaching clinicians who hold conjoint appointments from the hospital and its associated university medical school (members of both groups may have limited rights to private

practice on a fee-for-service basis); a full-time salaried house staff of interns, residents, and registrars; and a visiting staff working both on a sessional and on a fee-for-service basis. It is extremely unusual for a private hospital to have any salaried medical staff. Of course, a doctor or a group of doctors who own or have shares in a private hospital will treat their patients at the hospitals, on a fee-for-service basis. Other doctors wishing to admit and treat a patient in a private hospital will seek permission to do so from the hospital management. The patient will be charged by the hospital for accommodation and services it provides, and the doctor will bill the patient for his services on a fee-for-service basis.

The staff, including the medical staff, employed in public hospitals may be employees either of the government or of a hospital board of management where there is one. A hospital board is required to seek the state health authority's confirmation before making an appointment to senior positions such as chief executive officer, director of medical services, director of nursing services, and director of administrative services. In a private hospital the staff are employees of the hospital proprietor, but, as mentioned above, doctors are very rarely employees of private hospitals.

Admission and Classification of Patients

Admission to a public hospital is usually arranged by the general practitioner or specialist attending the patient. Some admissions, particularly those of urgent cases, are through hospital casualty or outpatient departments. The classification of a patient in a public hospital reflects the type of accommodation to which he or she is admitted and the method by which the attending doctor or doctors are to be paid for their services. Public hospital accommodation is available at two levels, the "shared ward" and the "private ward" (single room). However, the number of single-bed rooms in a particular hospital may be less than the demand, and also a "shared ward" patient may be treated in a single room (at no extra cost to the patient) if the patient's medical condition makes this desirable or necessary. Consequently, a patient who is prepared to pay the additional charge for admission to private accommodation may have to accept shared ward accommodation.

A person admitted as a shared accommodation patient in a public hospital may elect to be treated as either a "hospital" patient or a "private" patient. A "hospital" patient is treated by doctors employed and paid by the hospital, the patient having no say as to the particular attending doctors. Many of these patients are social service beneficiaries provided with accommodation and medical care in public hospitals free of charge under Commonwealth or state government health benefits arrangements. The majority of "hospital" patients, however, are charged a flat rate per diem accommodation charge and a flat rate per diem medical service charge, both of these charges being payable to the hospital. A basic hospital insurance package covering both of these charges is available.

Patients who elect to be treated as "private" patients in either a shared or single room are admitted to the care of a particular doctor or group of doctors chosen by the patient from among the doctors on the hospital staff having the right of private practice. Private patients pay the hospital for their accommodation and nursing and ancillary care; they are billed separately by their chosen doctors on a fee-for-service basis. Insurance packages covering all or most charges and fees to private patients are available.

Private hospital charges are not regulated by government, so proprietors may set room tariffs at whatever level they think the market will stand. They are, however, constrained by the "private hospital" benefit rates payable through the registered health insurance funds; these benefits are controlled by the Commonwealth and geared to the private accommodation rates charged in public hospitals. Although the basic daily accommodation charges of private hospitals are similar to those for private accommodation in public hospitals, private hospitals commonly levy additional charges for the use of facilities such as labour wards, delivery rooms, and operating theatres. Attendance to private hospital patients by doctors is charged on a fee-for-service basis.

Repatriation hospitals provide completely free care to Repatriation beneficiaries and care to other members of the public on the same basis as public hospitals.

Hospital Accreditation—Abuse of Hospital Facilities

Talk of hospital accreditation in Australia began soon after, and was no doubt inspired by, the establishment of the American College of Surgeons' hospital standardization program more than sixty years ago. This talk reached fruition with the setting up of the Australian Council on Hospital Standards in 1974 as a nongovernment, not-for-profit body. The Council's constitution, manual of standards, survey, and accreditation procedures are remarkably similar to those of its U.S. exemplar. As yet, a hospital's accreditation status is not linked in any way to arrangements for government subsidy or health insurance schemes.

Again copying predecessors overseas, Australian consumer activists, reformist health economists, and some doctors have focussed attention on high rates of surgical intervention, inappropriate length of patient stay, and general inefficiency in hospital management. Abuse and incompetence undoubtedly occur; their nature and dimensions have not been fully assessed. The present climate of financial stringency is giving added impetus to the closer scrutiny and improvement of hospital practice through such devices as peer review of patient care and hospital management audits.

Mental Health Institutions

Disturbances by mentally ill detainees in the gaols that housed most of Australia's first colonists led the authorities to open a lunatic asylum on a farm outside of Sydney Town. The tradition of government provision is carried on today, with most psychiatric inpatient care (and residential care of the mentally handicapped) and much outpatient care being provided by state government institutions—usually without charge. A few public and private hospitals have short-stay psychiatric inpatient units.

Voluntary patients make up the greatest number of inpatients in Australian mental health institutions. Some are admitted and detained involuntarily under legislation relating to mental health, alcoholism, and drug addiction. A small number of detainees have been committed to the institutions for criminal behavior while of unsound mind or, having been charged with a criminal offence, they were found to be mentally unfit to plead. Current philosophy regarding mental health care, underlined by financial considerations, has dictated an "admit reluctantly and discharge early" policy. This has produced some problems for nursing homes that are not appropriately staffed and equipped to care for senile psychiatric cases, and has fostered the growth of low-standard boardinghouses catering to low-income, chronically mentally handicapped social service beneficiaries. These difficulties are recognised, but remedial action is slow to occur, partly because mental health institutions are financed from state coffers while the Commonwealth shoulders most of the burden of financing nursing homes and provides social service pensions.

The Nursing Homes

The first example of government joining with private charity to provide health care was the establishment of a nursing home in Sydney. In 1820 the government relinquished a building to the New South Wales Benevolent Society to be used as an asylum for the "Poor, Blind, Aged, and Infirm." Although this institution was governed by the Benevolent Society, the wages of the matron and master were paid by the government. Today, the nursing home industry is heavily dependent upon private profit-making providers of nursing home services, but the Commonwealth and state governments and religious and charitable organisations are all heavily involved.

With 1,400 nursing homes providing more than 75,000 beds, there were in 1982 approximately 4.7 such beds per thousand population. Nursing home bed to population ratios vary somewhat from state to state, reflecting to some degree interstate differences in the availability of long-term-care beds in hospitals and psychiatric institutions.

The Commonwealth provides about two-thirds of the current revenue of nursing homes and has control over the number of nursing home beds, the target being 50 beds per 1,000 persons aged 65 and over. The Commonwealth also fixed the fees charged by individual homes. Approved fees are based on costs of running the homes, and then the Commonwealth nursing home benefits paid to patients are set on a state-by-state basis so that the benefit plus the statutory patient contribution (approximately 90% of the single rate social service pension) will cover fully the fees charged for 70% of the beds in nongovernmental nursing homes.

Nursing homes are licensed under state legislation, with considerable variations between states in standards for accommodation and staffing. Thus, their costs vary from state to state; and since Commonwealth benefits are related to costs, the benefit paid in one state is $150 per week per patient, whereas it is $300 per week per patient in another state.

For funding purposes the Commonwealth classifies nursing homes as "government," "deficit-funded," or "other nursing homes." The government category includes homes operated by state health authorities; these institutions receive both Commonwealth and state finance. Under the Commonwealth Nursing Homes Assistance Act, voluntary, non-profit-seeking nursing homes may enter into an agreement whereby approved operating deficits are met by the Commonwealth—these are deficit-financed homes. Both the government and the deficit-financed categories cover about 23% of the total bed provision. "Other nursing homes," which are mostly private, for-profit institutions, provide more than half the total number of nursing home beds in Australia; their patients are eligible for Commonwealth nursing home benefit coverage.

The nursing home patient population is predominantly aged (more than 85% are aged 65 or over) and female (more than 70%), and the majority are social service pensioners. Pensioners are required to contribute about 90% of their weekly social service entitlement towards the payment of nursing home fees. The official estimate (1981) showed that between 10 and 15% of all nursing home patients (pensioners and nonpensioners) had to contribute more than the statutory contribution towards the payment of nursing home fees. Health insurance arrangements through the registered funds do not cover nursing home fees. Veterans are provided with nursing home care free of charge.

The standards of accommodation and care provided in nursing homes vary widely. Generally, the standards set for state licensing and Commonwealth approval for benefit purposes represent bare minima. Many nursing home proprietors complain that the return on their investment is low, that the government fixed fees do not include provision for capital replacement, and that at present levels of funding there is little hope of improving services. The Commonwealth in October 1982 set up a committee of officials to inquire into problems of caring for the aged, particularly the problems of providing nursing home care. Also, the Australian Council on Hospital Standards is working to introduce a voluntary program of nursing home accreditation.

MEDICAL EDUCATION

The Continuum of Medical Education

The typical entrant to an Australian medical school is eighteen or nineteen years of age and has had six years of high school education. After successfully completing the five or six years of the undergraduate medical school course, the student is awarded the combined Bachelor of Medicine, Bachelor of Surgery (MB, BS) degree and proceeds to a one-year hospital internship. By custom, holders of this degree may use the title "Doctor." At the end of that "preregistration" year, application is made to a state or territory medical registration board for registration as a medical practitioner; there is no federal registration board. The registration boards do not conduct their own examinations of the medical skill and knowledge of applicants for registration; their function is to examine documentary and, if necessary, other evidence that the applicant meets the statutory requirements to practise medicine. Upon registration, the fledgling doctor may set up an independent private practice, but one or more years of hospital residency is more common after an internship. Residency may serve either as a means of gaining wider experience before entering general practice without specialist qualifications or as a part of the four to six years of postgraduate training that leads to a specialist diploma or a university higher qualification. A variety of continuing education programs provides opportunities for updating and extending the professional knowledge and skills of the practising doctor. Thus, undergraduate medical schools, internships, postgraduate training, and continuing education programs provide a continuum of medical education extending over the span of the medical practitioner's professional life.

Undergraduate Medical Education

Ten university-based medical schools, together with their affiliated teaching hospitals, provide undergraduate medical education in Australia. The medical schools are financed by the Commonwealth Government through its Tertiary Education Commission; most of the funding of teaching hospitals is derived from federal and state government sources.

The faculty in each medical school, with an elected or appointed dean as its executive head, is responsible to its university council. The provision of training courses and the conduct of research is subject to the approval of the professorial board composed of all professors on the university staff. The medical school itself is divided into departments (sometimes called "schools" or "divisions" or "units"), usually according to discipline, with each department answerable to the medical faculty for its own training and research programs. Part of the medical student's course may be provided by faculties outside the medical school, particularly for basic science subjects and general studies electives.

Much of the clinical sciences teaching is conducted within the teaching hospitals that are public institutions, generally not under the control of the medical school or the university, although it is usual for the university to have representation on the governing boards of these hospitals. Professorial units, staffed by members of the medical faculty and sometimes including clinicians appointed by both the university and the teaching hospital conjointly, provide clinical teaching and some of the patient care within the major teaching hospitals.

In order to obtain sufficient quantity and range of clinical teaching material, a medical school will be affiliated with one or more major teaching hospital and also with other hospitals, sometimes called associated hospitals, to which faculty members may hold visiting appointments and where nonfaculty clinicians and other staff participate in undergraduate training programs. The two exceptions to this pattern are Flinders University's Medical Centre and Sydney University's Westmead Centre, where there is close integration of medical school and teaching hospital.

Selection for admission to medical schools is based primarily upon performance in the final year examination at high school—the Higher School Certificate examination. Some medical schools make special provision for a very limited number of mature-age students and students from overseas. One school selects half of its intake on criteria of academic achievement and the other half on the basis of a series of tests and structured interviews.

In general, medical school entrants are drawn from the top 3% of high school graduates. Medical students pay no tuition fees for their training. Under the Federal Government's Tertiary Education Assistance Scheme, financial assistance by way of a living allowance is available to medical students (and all other students in tertiary education programs) on a noncompetitive basis, subject to means tests. Annual intake to medical schools of recent years has totalled about 1,500, of whom around one-third have been females. Attrition rates in medical schools are relatively low, with some 1,250 students graduating every year.

The traditional British medical undergraduate course structure—basic, paraclinical, and clinical sciences taught sequentially—provided the pattern for Australia's system. Australian schools are now making some efforts to integrate teaching programs both vertically and horizontally, and to introduce some student-patient interaction quite early in the course. Two schools have moved quite a distance from the traditional programs. Teaching at Newcastle University's medical school is centred around a sequence of progressively more complex clinical problems; the medical curriculum at Flinders has been structured around organ systems rather than observing the traditional boundaries of disciplines.

With the exception of the three medical schools in New South Wales, which conduct a five-year course, undergraduate education is of six years' duration.

In the late 1960s the federal and state health ministers considered the necessity to establish a national body to provide advice on medical school standards and accreditation. In October 1970 the inaugural meeting of an Advisory Medical Council of Australia was held. Partly because of the refusal of the Victorian health authorities to participate, this council lapsed. Although establishment of a General Medical Council of Australia has since been proposed on several occasions, no positive action has been taken. At the present time Australia's medical schools are accredited by the General Medical Council of Great Britain.

Recurring matters of concern about the criticism of undergraduate medical education in this country will be familiar to observers of medical education in many countries: (1) relative degrees of control to be examined by governments, the universities, their medical faculties, and the teaching hospitals respectively; (2) relationships between preclinical and clinical disciplines and departments within medical schools, and employment of nonmedical graduates in preclinical departments; (3) organizational separation of university medical schools from teaching hospitals, as well as conflict between teaching, research, and patient care activities within teaching hospitals; (4) training of medical practitioners largely in isolation from the training of other health professionals; (5) structure, content, and length of medical school programs, and appropriate emphasis upon primary care in the undergraduate curriculum; (6) method of selection and size of the medical school student intake.

Hospital Internship—The Preregistration Year

The basic requirements for registration as a legally qualified medical practitioner by a state or territory medical registration board are possession of a medical degree recognised by that board and completion of a twelve-month internship (six months in medicine and its branch specialties and six months in surgery and its branches) with a certification of approval from the employing hospital. Unless an intern is unusually incompetent, the hospital's certification and thence registration are virtually assured.

Medical school graduates are permitted to express preferences as to the hospitals in which they will serve as interns, but the final allocation is made by the hospital authorities in consultation with the medical schools. An intern is a salaried employee of the hospital to which she or he is appointed, is paid from hospital funds, and is accountable to the hospital's medical superintendent and chief executive officer.

The level, range, training, and experience provided for interns varies considerably from hospital to hospital. Each institution organizes its own internship program. The training and supervision of interns is carried out by the hospital's salaried and visiting specialist staff, registrars, and residents. One argument advanced for reducing the length of the medical school curriculum in New South Wales from six to five years was that this would enable the medical schools to play a larger part in the internship phase of medical education; it was proposed that the term of internship be extended to two years. Neither of these proposals has been implemented.

Postgraduate Specialist Education

Following registration, the doctor may elect to enter general practice with no further formal training or hospital experience. However, most entrants to general practice complete one or two years of hospital residency, sometimes more. Since 1973 the Royal

Australian College of General Practitioners (RACGP), with federal funding, has provided training in general practice for recent medical graduates through the Family Medicine Program (FMP). The training usually consists of two years of hospital experience, followed by nine months of supervised training in general practice, then a further fifteen months under supervision in a College-accredited general practice, together with attendance at College-sponsored educational programs. By 1982 about 2,000 doctors had passed through the FMP. Among the aims of the program were the encouragement of doctors to enter general practice and to practice in rural areas. The Commonwealth Government, which has provided several million dollars annually to the FMP, established in February 1982 a committee of review to make recommendations regarding the future operation of the program.

Formal training for specialist practice is conducted under the aegis of "learned colleges," among which the largest are the Royal Australian College of Physicians (RACP) and the Royal Australasian College of Surgeons (RACS). Each of the major specialties and a growing number of minor specialties and subspecialties have their own colleges or societies incorporated either by Royal (British) Charter—hence the Royal Colleges—or under state legislation. These bodies determine the length and content of training programs, approve training posts, and examine and certify the competence of candidates as specialist practitioners. Certification usually takes the form of admission to fellowship of the college; thus, for example, a specialist physician becomes a Fellow of the RACP (FRACP), while a specialist surgeon is named a Fellow of the RACS (FRACS).

The general pattern of specialist training consists of two years of basic training as a hospital resident medical officer, aimed at developing a broad knowledge of medicine and acquiring some technical skills. Completion of basic training is marked by the "Part 1" examination. The successful candidate then proceeds to three or four years of advanced training and is designated "Registrar." In most specialties, comprehensive examinations are contested in the final year of advanced training, but admission to fellowship in the RACP is contingent upon obtaining satisfactory reports from training supervisors. There is no final examination.

Specialty training posts are provided by public hospitals, subject to approval of the appropriate learned colleges and with the concurrence of the state hospital authority. Trainees are selected by the individual hospitals, employed by them, and paid from hospital funds as members of the hospital medical staff. Each hospital organises the training of its residents and registrars within guidelines provided by the colleges. Colleges may designate supervisors in the hospitals to monitor trainees' progress and ensure that college standards are met. University medical schools contribute to specialty training programs by providing courses in basic and paraclinical sciences and, to some extent, in clinical practice—particularly in hospitals where professorial units are located—and through the involvement of medical school clinical teachers in the affairs of the learned colleges to which they belong. Still, the conduct of specialty training is regarded as primarily a college responsibility, rather than as a major function of university medical schools.

The universities do provide some formal programs of academic training and research leading to higher degrees such as the Doctorate of Medicine (MD), Doctorate of Philosophy (PhD), and Masters Degree in Surgery (MS). These university awards are most likely to be sought by doctors pursuing academic and research careers; teachers and researchers in fields of clinical practice may acquire a university higher degree in addition to their specialist certification by a learned college. The Commonwealth Institute of Health, a federal agency with academic links to the University of Sydney, offers postgraduate training in various branches of public health, including occupational health. The University of New South Wales provides formal training for medical graduates in health services administration.

Although there is some consultation between the learned colleges, federal and state health authorities, and hospitals, there is no national standing body charged with continuing oversight and regulation of postgraduate medical education.

Continuing Medical Education

In 1974 a federally sponsored committee defined continuing medical education as "training which an individual doctor undertakes with the object of maintaining or extending professional competence after the end of undergraduate education, including intern training, and where applicable, after the end of any traditional education leading to a further qualification or to the completion of a step in specialist training." Medical practitioners are under no legal or other formal obligation to participate in continuing education activities.

The learned colleges, professional societies and associations, teaching hospitals, pharmaceutical companies, and universities, through their postgraduate medical education committees, are among the many organizations providing continuing medical education. The postgraduate committees are associated with the Australian Medical Association, the universities, and the professional societies in an incorporated body, the Australian Postgraduate Federation in Medicine, which attempts to coordinate the activities of the postgraduate committees. However, continuing medical education is inadequately financed and there is a lack of coherent organization or policy.

Medical Graduates from Overseas

Considering that the Australian medical education system is an offshoot of the British system and is still linked to it through the General Medical Council, it is not surprising that medical degrees and postgraduate qualifications awarded in the United Kingdom (and New Zealand) rank equally with Australian qualifications for purposes of registration and specialist recognition by the Australian authorities.

Since 1978 the position regarding medical graduates from other countries has changed quite drastically. Up to that time graduates from most medical schools where the language of instruction was English and the curriculum was modelled on the British pattern could obtain registration in Australia with little or no difficulty. Graduates from elsewhere, depending upon such factors as language and the international reputation of their medical schools, would be required to undergo a period of hospital training or complete part of the undergraduate program in an Australian medical school, perhaps even to serve as medical officer in an isolated community for a period of years or contest a special examination before being registered to practise in Australia. The requirements varied over time and from state to state. Then, in 1978, at a time of increasing concern about the possible oversupply of doctors, the Australian Medical Examining Council was established by the Federal Government as a national body to examine the fitness of holders of medical qualifications obtained overseas for registration by Australian state medical boards. The advent of the AMEC has been followed by a significant fall in the numbers of registrations of holders of overseas qualifications.

Reduce Student Intake, Cut Immigration—Or Not?

With Australia's doctor:population ratio approaching 1:500, fears are being expressed that an imminent oversupply of medical practitioners will escalate health costs, lead to doctors being unemployed and force specialists to turn to general practice for which they have not been appropriately trained. But no one body has responsibility for controlling the input to the medical workforce from medical schools and via doctor immigration. In 1980 an official committee was convened with representation from the university authorities and the federal departments of health, education, employment, and immigration. Although the implications of oversupply were canvassed, only the Commonwealth Health Department, in a minority report, recommended that student intake into medical schools be reduced. Certainly stringent examination standards are limiting the registration of immigrant doctors, but there is no proper planning for an appropriately sized medical workforce. At present, that is nobody's job.

NURSES AND OTHER HEALTH PERSONNEL

The Nursing Workforce—Composition and Training

Constituting more than two-thirds of the health workforce in Australia, the nursing staff can be grouped into three major categories reflecting their levels of training and their role in the health care system. At the highest level in this three-tiered classification are the professional (registered) nurses and student nurses, together forming about three-fourths of the nursing workforce. Next come the nursing aides and nursing aides in training, followed by nursing assistants. These latter two groups are similar in size.

All registered nurses have completed a minimum of three years of nursing training, qualifying them for certificates in general nursing or psychiatric nursing awarded by state examination boards and thus for admission to the state nurses' register. "Postbasic students" are registered nurses currently being trained in some specialist nursing field; these further education programs vary in length from a few weeks to one year, and generally lead to additional certification in, for example, midwifery, maternal and child health, and intensive-care nursing. The range of available postbasic training programs is very wide, and many registered nurses hold one or more postbasic certificates in addition to their basic registrable certificates in general or psychiatric nursing. "Student nurses" are currently preparing for one or another of the basic certificates. The great majority of student nurses are paid employees, members of the hospital nursing workforce, in hospitals that offer three-year apprenticeship-type training programs.

For many years some members of the nursing profession have been arguing for the closure of hospital-based nurse training programs with removal of nurse-trainees from the hospital workforce and their replacement by registered nurses. Since 1974 some colleges of advanced education have offered campus-based programs that include some periods of hospital attachment and lead to the award of a diploma and registration as a nurse. In 1977 and 1978 a committee appointed by the Commonwealth Tertiary Education Commission inquired into nurse training. The committee recommended a small scale, cautious, exploratory expansion of college-based nurse education. Since the appearance of that report there has been little change apparent in the pattern and system of nurse education.

No Australian university offers degrees in nursing, and less than 1% of registered nurses have a university degree of any type. Several colleges of advanced education provide courses leading to a bachelor's degree with a nursing major; only registered nurses are admitted to these courses. The annual output of graduates from these courses is very small. The CAEs also offer postbasic diploma courses, usually one year long, leading to a Diploma in Nursing Administration (DNA), a Diploma in Nurse Education (DNE), and a Diploma in Community Nursing (DCN). The University of New South Wales plans to offer a Master of Nursing Administration degree in 1983.

At the second level, the nursing aide category includes nursing staff who have completed or are undertaking a training program that is usually one year long and largely spent in supervised employment in hospitals, but includes a formal instruction component which varies from nearly 600 hours in one state to less than 100 in another. Once trained the student nursing aide is eligible for registration or enrollment by the state registration body with the titles of enrolled nursing aide (NSW), registered nursing aide (Victoria), enrolled nurse (Queensland, South Australia, Western Australia), and auxiliary nurse (Tasmania).

At the third level in this workforce are nursing personnel having no statutory training, not subject to regulation by the nurses' registration boards, and variously known as assistants-in-nursing, nursing attendants, or noncertified nursing personnel.

In addition to the three major classes of personnel described above, the nursing workforce includes a small number of mothercraft nurses and mothercraft nursing trainees whose training, in apprenticeships, qualifies them for employment only in the care of nursing mothers, infants, and very young children.

Role and Deployment of Nursing Personnel

A 1978 national survey of nursing personnel indicated that probably 75% of all professional (registered) nurses were employed in settings, mainly hospitals and nursing homes, where they worked in close association with doctors—the doctors being responsible for the medical aspects of patient care, including diagnosis, prescription of therapy, and performance of all but minor procedures. The role of the professional nurse here embraces observation of patients; planning and evaluation of nursing care; administration of drugs under medical prescription; performance of nursing procedures; intervention in emergencies and assistance to doctors in performance of other procedures; and supervision of the patients' environment. In addition, these professional nurses may perform a considerable range of administrative tasks relating to ward management and may be involved in the supervision and education of student nurses and other nursing personnel.

Around 10% of the professional nurses were in posts carrying predominantly administrative responsibilities, and about 3% were employed principally as nurse educators.

Relatively, only very small numbers are employed in settings such as community health centres or nursing posts in remote areas where they usually have more responsibility for screening patients and providing medical care than hospital nurses. "Nurse practitioners" and "nurse anaesthetists" are virtually unknown in Australia. Although more than 40% of all registered nurses hold a midwifery certificate, confinements are almost always attended by a doctor assisted by a nurse-midwife rather than by a midwife as the sole *accoucheuse*.

Nurse aides assist professional nurses in meeting the nursing and personal needs of hospital and nursing home patients, and they carry out some of the domestic work of the wards; the assistants in nursing perform similar duties to those of the aides. The overlapping of roles and responsibilities within the three-tier system has prompted suggestion that a firmer distinction be made between nursing and non-nursing aspects of patient care, with possible restructuring of the staffing pattern into a two-tier system with clerical and domestic work placed more appropriately in the hands of non-nursing personnel.

Other Health Personnel

Doctors and dentists aside, the professionals most commonly consulted by people with health problems are the following in approximate order of frequency of consultation: pharmacist; chiropractor, naturopath, or osteopath; optician or optometrist; physiotherapist; chiropodist; social worker or welfare officer. The pharmacist provides advice gratis, and the social worker or welfare officer, being invariably a salaried employee of a health or welfare agency, also provides counsel free of charge. Physiotherapists—who are ethically bound to provide treatment only upon doctors' orders—and chiropodists may be employees of hospitals or other agencies, but many are in private practice, charging fees-for-service, as do those individuals in the other categories of health personnel listed here. These fees may be covered in part by health insurance ancillary benefit packages.

Completion of at least three years of training at a university or college of advanced education is required for registration as a practitioner in most of these professions. The number of types of professional groups for which registration is mandatory varies from state to state.

Associations and Unions

Most of the health professions have their own associations that are concerned with professional ethics, codes of practice, and continuing education. The larger professional groups also have their own trade unions, registered under Commonwealth or state conciliation and arbitration legislation as representing their members before tribunals that determine nationwide or statewide wage awards. Other health professionals and nonprofessional employees belong to registered unions that cover a variety of occupational groups, not necessarily only health service personnel. An award specifies wage rates, allowances, conditions of work, and fringe benefits for a particular category and level of employee. Although it is enforceable only in the case of an employed person, an award exercises a very strong influence on the income of similar workers who are "self-employed."

CARE OF THE AMBULATORY

General and specialist medical practitioners in private practice make up the largest source of medical care for the ambulatory. Pharmacists, too, from their ubiquitous retail pharmacies, offer advice and a wide range of over-the-counter medicaments in addition to dispensing scripts for prescriptions written by doctors. The outpatient and casualty departments of public hospitals also provide a very wide range of care for ambulant patients. Early in the history of colonial Australia, charitable individuals and some of the friendly societies established "dispensaries" and "clinics" that provided free or low-cost care to the ambulant, and a few of these establishments still exist today. Beginning early this century, government and charitable associations have built up a nationwide coverage of "baby health centres" providing antenatal, postnatal, and infant health care free of charge. Much of the work of these centres is carried on by nurses with medical supervision and support. Following the movement to deinstitutionalize mental health care in the 1950s and 1960s, outpatient mental health services expanded somewhat.

In 1973 the federal Labor government established its Community Health Program to provide grants towards both capital and operating costs for the establishment or improvement of a wide range of community-based health and health-related welfare services. The emphasis of the program was to be upon preventive activities, health education, health maintenance, and rehabilitation and domiciliary services as an alternative to institutional care, with particular attention to the coordination and development of services in areas with a health service scarcity. Initially, the Commonwealth offered 90% funding for new projects; the remainder was to come from the states.

Under the aegis of the Community Health Program, more than 300 community health centres were established, offering varying ranges of services, including domiciliary nursing, counselling for drug abusers and the mentally ill, health promotion activities, and, in less than 100 of the centres, primary medical care. Noteworthy achievements of the program were the expansion of day care centres, the establishment of about 100 women's refuges (providing accommodation and care for women and children from homes broken by marital discord or violence), and the development of the Family Medicine Program, which provided training in general practice. Since 1978, in line with the federal Liberal government's "New Federalism" policy, Commonwealth funding of the Community Health Program has been reduced and the states have moved to curtail their commitments to the program. In May 1981 the Commonwealth announced that separate funding of community health services was to cease, thus virtually abolishing the program. Some services will be maintained by state and local authorities, particularly those that have been integrated into public hospital outreach schemes. At its peak of activity the Community Health Program accounted for less than 1.5% of all current health service expenditure.

Dental Care

"There is a significant degree of under-employment in dentistry . . . [and] accumulating evidence of a growing trend throughout Australia of unemployment among dentists. . . ." Those statements from top officials of the Australian Dental Association in 1981 point to an overproduction of graduates from dental schools and a decreasing demand for dental services.

The level of dental health in this country has risen markedly over the past two decades, the most important contributory factor being the extension of fluoridated water supplies to cover more than two-thirds of the population. The reduced incidence of dental disease has undoubtedly had an impact on dental workload, and this has been further reduced by a contracting economy and recent abolition of specific taxation deductability for dental services. In 1975 the introduction of dental insurance as an auxiliary benefit by the registered health insurance funds produced a utilization peak, but this has now tailed off, as much of the backlog of need has been dealt with.

Social service beneficiaries may be eligible for free dental care through the public hospital system, while the dental care of Repatriation beneficiaries is paid for by the Commonwealth. The School Dental Scheme, established in 1973 by cooperation between the Commonwealth and state governments, trains and employs dental therapists who, working under the supervision of dentists, provide free dental care to primary school children. This service covers about one-third of all primary school children. Expenditure on dental care amounts to slightly more than 4% of total current health expenditure in Australia, accountable mostly in direct payments to dentists in private practice and to dental technicians for dental prostheses, and in payments through dental insurance arrangements.

Domiciliary Care

General practitioners and nurses are the most frequent providers of care in patients' own homes. In the early 1970s one in eight GP-patient contacts occurred in the home. Towards the end of that decade the Australian Health Survey found that home visits constituted one in every fourteen GP consultations. In addition, the growing use of deputising services means that fewer home calls, particularly out-of-hours calls, are made by the patients' "own" general practitioner.

Nearly 200 nonprofit home nursing services receive government financial assistance to employ some 2,000 domiciliary nurses who each made (in 1982), on the average, between 50 and 60 home calls per week. Governments provide funding for approved paramedical and speech therapy for aged persons in their homes. Subvention is also available for the provision of housekeeping and other domestic assistance and of delivered meals ("meals on wheels") to the elderly living at home. Someone caring at home for an aged or disabled person who would otherwise require institutional care may apply for a Commonwealth domiciliary nursing benefit or a handicapped children's benefit.

Ambulance and Other Patient Transportation Services

Statewide organizations—of which four are government agencies and two are voluntary bodies—provide most of the patient transportation services in Australia. Finance is provided from state and local government grants, local fund-raising activities, subscriptions to insurance funds operated by the ambulance services themselves, and charges for service. Free services are provided to social service and Repatriation beneficiaries. These services, which include air ambulances for rural areas, cater to emergency cases and a much larger nonurgent, mainly nonstretcher case load. These "official" services are augmented for the transportation of nonurgent cases by vehicles and a staff supplied by individual public and private hospitals and many voluntary associations, together with taxicabs and other cars hired by hospitals for patients entitled to free transport.

Volunteers play a significant part in patient transportation services, but each of the major statewide services employs ambulance officers on a full-time basis. The majority of these officers receive formal training in first aid and patient care. Recently, small groups of more intensively trained officers—the "paramedics"—have been established to man intensive care ambulances. Also, a third tier of officers has emerged to man vehicles for ambulant patients. This stratification of ambulance officers has led to some hostility and industrial unrest within the workforce.

Aerial ambulances are available throughout Australia for the evacuation of patients from remote and otherwise inaccessible areas, but difficulties have been experienced in coordinating these services with road transport services and between states. Helicopters operated by the armed services or the police, or sponsored by television stations and other commercial interests, are occasionally used for patient evacuation.

Patient transport services are beset with problems such as a lack of organization and coordination; dissatisfaction among paid staff regarding status and remuneration; inappropriate vehicles; lack of uniform standards of training; and funding arrangements that are both complicated and inadequate. Describing nonemergency transport services several years ago, a government inquiry reported: "In short, [the nonemergency services] are fragmented, and may also be inaccessible, undignified, uncomfortable, inefficient, or expensive both to the patient and the community." A number of more recent reports echo that conclusion.

Aerial Medical Services

Pioneered by the now-legendary doctor-priest John Flynn, aerial medical services have spread "a mantle of safety" over the small population scattered over Australia's vast outback regions. The largest single organization is the Royal Flying Doctor Service (RFDS), which, from thirteen bases, links together a network of more than 5,500 transceivers in station homesteads, bush nursing centres, outback hospitals, aboriginal settlements, mission stations, survey camps, and police posts. Base doctors conduct daily clinics over the radio network, taking case histories and progress reports from patients and, where appropriate, instructing callers in the use of supplies from the medicine chests issued by the service at the Commonwealth expense. In more serious cases a plane, carrying a doctor or nurse if needed, is dispatched from the base to collect and take the patient to the nearest suitable hospital. Medical, dental, and nursing staff are also flown to conduct regular clinics at remote settlements.

The RFDS is an independent, nonprofit organization, subsidized by the federal and state governments. Income is also derived from a voluntary contributory scheme, donations, legacies, and, commissions paid for radiograms transmitted over the RFDS radio network. This network is also used for School-of-the-Air broadcasts and social and business purposes, but emergency medical calls take top priority over all other communications.

The Northern Territory Government operates its own fleet of aircraft for emergency and routine clinic purposes; the Queensland Government has a Flying Surgeon Service, which flies a specialist surgeon and an anaesthetist on a regular round of the remote hospitals in that state.

HEALTH COSTS AND FUNDING

Exponential Escalation or Rational Incrementation?

Echoing their overseas mentors, Australian prophets of doom have been uttering doleful warnings that health costs, escalating exponentially, will by the year 2000 consume the whole and more of Australia's Gross National Product. It certainly is true that in the ten-year span from 1967 to 1976 the national Consumer Price Index doubled while health expenditures, similarly indexed, rose by a factor of four. But it is also true that since 1976 the rate of growth of health expenditure has slowed down both absolutely and in relation to the CPI. Furthermore, although health expenditure as a percentage of Gross Domestic Produce rose from 5.0 in 1966 to 7.7 in 1976, it has since remained relatively stable at around 8%. To account for these changes and make some reasonable predictions of future trends one needs to examine the sources of health care funding, the arrangements to provide cover of health care costs, and the pattern of health expenditure.

The Sources of Health Care Finance

When in 1788 the first colonists settled unwillingly in Australia, they brought with them their own "nationalised" health service. The doctors were government officers—the medicines they dispensed were supplied by the government, the simple hospital and clinic facilities were provided by the government and what nursing was available was provided by those involuntary servants of the government, the transported convicts. With an increasing influx in the first half of the nineteenth century of free settlers and a growing number of freed convicts, people able to pay for medical care and indeed to contribute to the care of poorer members of the community by way of charity, the colonial authorities, chronically underfunded, were no doubt pleased to see the development of private medical practice on a fee-for-service basis and the establishment of outpatient clinics and inpatient institutions supported by private benevolence. Although the biblical tenet that "charity never faileth" was strongly held in nineteenth-century Australia, charity was found to be an inadequate means of providing care for all those who needed it. Consequently, very early in the nineteenth century a system of government subvention was established to support private philanthropy in providing health care, particularly institutional care, for the less affluent members of the community.

Also in the nineteenth century, following the pattern of mutual aid organizations established in Britain, "friendly societies" were set up by groups of artisans and others with some common interest. In return for small weekly contributions society members and sometimes their families were entitled to financial benefits covering such exigencies as unemployment, sickness, and death; to the services of doctors empanelled by the society and paid on a per capita basis; and to "free" medicines prescribed by the "panel" doctors. At the turn of the century about one in four of Australia's population was covered by one or other of these friendly society health insurance schemes.

The five major categories of health service financing—charity, direct personal payment for goods and services, private investment, health insurance, and government funding—well established by the turn of the century, still persist today. The relative contributions of these five sources to current expenditure and to capital expenditure have varied considerably over the past eight decades.

Now, in the early 1980s, the government sector provides about 60% of all health service funding. Within the government sector, the Commonwealth carries a somewhat heavier share of the funding of current operations, while the states provide the lion's share of capital finance. Local government contributes a relatively small share of current funding, a very small amount to capital investment. Overall, the government provides 76% of the funds for capital works and equipment.

Within the private sector, the principal contributors to current funding are the health insurance schemes, to be discussed in some detail below, and direct out-of-pocket payments by the recipients of health care. Charity and other local fund-raising activities, such as lotteries and fetes organized by individual hospitals, make a very minor contribution to current funds. Of the 40% of current funding from the private sector, health insurance furnishes slightly more than half, direct payments slightly less. Private investment provides capital for private hospitals and nursing homes, the pharmaceutical industry and other enterprises providing health service supplies and equipment. Some government health authorities require public hospitals to raise a substantial share of funds required for capital projects before being granted government subsidy; some private not-for-profit hospitals and nursing homes have raised substantial sums for capital works through public appeals and other fund-raising activities. Because these local initiatives commonly lead to sometimes embarassing demands for government to provide the recurrent funding necessary to staff and maintain the capital projects, the authorities tend to view them with mixed feelings.

Health Cost Cover—Without Insurance

A very substantial range of health services and benefits are available either at no charge or at a price far below the cost of provision, quite irrespective of the health insurance status of the user. The gap between the price, or no price, and the cost of goods and services is met by government funding. For example, pharmaceuticals, if prescribed by a doctor from an extremely comprehensive list of "pharmaceutical benefits" scheduled for Commonwealth subvention, are supplied to eligible social service and Repatriation beneficiaries without charge and to the rest of the population upon payment of $3.50 per item, irrespective of the cost of the item. The schedule includes virtually every drug required in medical practice, but medicaments that are more expensive alternatives to listed items and preparations sold over-the-counter without prescription in pharmacists' shops are not listed.

The Commonwealth social security arrangments provide, generally subject to a means (income) test, a weekly income and in many cases other allowances to specified disadvantaged persons and their dependents, including the aged (females aged 60 years and over, males 65 years and over); persons unable to support themselves because of illness or infirmity; sole parents having children in their care; and recently arrived immigrants. Repatriation beneficiaries are generally ex-members of the armed forces who served in a theatre of war and certain categories of their dependents. Something like 15% of Australia's population are social service or Repatriation beneficiaries. Persons covered by the Repatriation scheme are entitled to virtually all forms of health care without charge; social service beneficiaries receive most of their health care either entirely without charge or at greatly reduced rates, depending upon eligibility related to the amount of income they receive in addition to their social service pensions. For the remaining 85% of the population many health care services—including public hospitals, nursing home care, ambulance services and, as we have seen above, pharmaceuticals—are available at much less than cost because of government subvention. The Commonwealth meets part of private hospital costs. Services completely "free" to all comers include most of the psychiatric care provided through state mental health agencies; some services provided through community health centres; maternal and child health clinic services; the provision of certain prescribed prostheses, appliances, and equipment; and school dental services. The cost of health care to the recipient may be further reduced if that person takes out voluntary health insurance which attracts Commonwealth government assistance in meeting doctors' bills and additional government subsidy of public hospital costs. Some 70% of the population have this voluntary coverage. Another 15% are covered very extensively by social service and Repatriation arrangements as mentioned. This leaves 15% of Australia's people, mostly young adults and their children, who, if they are unfortunate enough to suffer illness or injury, may be faced with large bills from doctors and hospitals but have no insurance or other cover to assist in paying those bills.

Health Insurance—Voluntary but Government Supported

Much enamoured of the American Blue Cross-Blue Shield system, a right-wing federal minister of health during the 1950s established a nationwide scheme of voluntary health insurance, carried by nongovernment, nonprofit-seeking medical and hospital benefits organizations registered under the National Health Act and subsidized by the Commonwealth Government. Despite many modifications of administrative details and revisions of the schedules of contributions and benefits, that voluntary, private but government-supported scheme remains the basis of the present health insurance arrangements.

The Present Arrangements

Although the National Health Act requires separate registration of medical benefit and hospital benefit organizations, any one carrier usually has dual registration and is popularly known as a "health insurance fund." Members are enrolled as either single or family contributors, the family contributions (premiums) being double that of the single, irrespective of family size. The funds operate on a community rating basis, and contribution rates, although varying from fund to fund and state to state for a given benefit package, must be approved by the federal authorities. A contributor may enrol for either or both of medical and hospital benefits, and some funds offer ancilliary benefits such as coverage for dental treatment, supply of spectacles, chiropody, and ambulance charges.

Medical Benefits

Under the arrangements in force in fiscal 1982–83, registered medical benefits organizations are required to offer a basic medical benefit which, together with the Commonwealth benefit, covers 85% of the Commonwealth Schedule fee for each medical service, with a maximum patient payment of $10 for any one service where the Schedule fee is charged. In addition, many of the registered organizations offer supplementary benefits up to the maximum of the Schedule fee level and ancilliary benefit tables. Premiums for the basic component of medical insurance qualify for a rebate from income tax.

Hospital Benefits

Registered hospital benefit organizations are required to provide a basic hospital benefit covering both the standard fee for shared ward accommodation in public hospitals for patients who choose to be treated by the doctor of their choice and charged for professional services rendered to inpatients and for outpatient services. Additionally, many organizations offer supplementary benefits covering charges raised for single-bed ward accommodation in public hospitals and benefits to wholly or substantially defray private hospital charges. Basic hospital insurance premiums qualify for a taxation rebate.

The hospital benefit arrangements ensure complete coverage of fees charged to a "standard ward" patient in a public hospital and most charged to a "private" patient, but the fees charged represent only a fraction of the actual costs of providing public hospital care—the balance of the cost is met by Commonwealth and state government sources. The fees charged by private hospitals reflect much more closely the costs of providing care; these account for more than 75% of private hospital revenue, the remainder coming from Commonwealth subsidy paid directly to the hospitals on a per patient-diem basis.

Similar Benefits—Different Premiums

Within any one state all the funds must, by law, offer the same basic benefits package; there is therefore relatively little difference between the various supplementary packages available, but contribution rates vary considerably between funds. In 1982 in the state of New South Wales, for example, the weekly family contribution rates for basic medical and hospital coverage ranged from $11 to $15. Few employers pay voluntary health insurance premiums for their employees, and so the decisions of whether or not to insure, with which fund, and for which benefit package are essentially personal choices. Having joined one of the registered funds—and the decision to join was made decades ago by many contributors—members tend to stay with that fund rather than move to another that offers a more favourable contribution rate. Although some of the larger funds regard themselves as highly competitive industries, the Australian public appears somewhat unaware of or indifferent to their blandishments.

Other Health Insurance Schemes

Commercial firms are permitted to operate health insurance schemes outside government subvention. Because their packages require members to meet large "front end deductibles" before claiming any benefits, the premiums are low. Very few people have joined these unregistered schemes.

While no individual is required by law to insure self or dependants against health costs, employers are required by law to carry workers' compensation insurance to protect their employees in work-related accident or illness. Also, all motor vehicle owners are required to carry third-party insurance to cover costs arising from traffic accidents.

The Medibank Experiment

Committed to a policy of providing basic health care free at the point of delivery, a left-wing (Labor) federal government sought in the early 1970s to oust the voluntary system by introducing a compulsory health insurance scheme financed by a levy on taxable income and administered by a government agency—"Medibank." After bitter parliamentary battles resulting in the financing of the scheme from government general revenue, not by levy, what became known as "Medibank Mark I" commenced operation in 1975. The registered benefit organizations, however, continued in existence, offering ancilliary benefits; the government established its own "private" registered fund to compete against them. A few months later a conservative government took office, determined to cut federal government spending and reduce the budget deficit. The compulsory arrangement was abandoned and a succession of legislative amendments was passed that aimed to reduce the rate at which federal expenditure on health was growing, to increase the state government share of health expenditure, and to encourage membership of the voluntary health insurance funds. The only present remnant of the Labor party's attempt to provide universal health coverage is the Commonwealth Government's registered voluntary insurance fund—"Medibank Private."

Now completely dismantled, Medibank Mark I did enjoy very wide public support during its brief period of operation, 1975 and 1976. It did not last long enough to demonstrate its possible value as a means of restraint on the supply of services; however, it did point up some administrative problems that could have been resolved with time. Privatization of hospital and medical financing since 1976 has certainly shifted a very substantial fraction of total health expenditure from the federal budget to the private sector, but this has reinstated the inequity of health insurance premiums unrelated to income. The federal Labor party's policy now includes the reintroduction of universal health cover, financed by a levy on taxable income. Currently, psephologists are predicting a return to power of a federal Labor government in the near future; therefore, Australia may quite soon again see its health insurance arrangements very radically revamped.*

The Pattern of Health Care Expenditure

Capital expenditure—building new facilities, major works at health care institutions, and purchase of major equipment—accounts for about 6 to 7% of total health expenditure each year. Because it is generally easier to delay capital spending than to curtail existing services, and because vote-seeking politicians recognise that bigger and newer hospitals have a popular appeal, capital expenditure programs have a tendency to reflect concern for budgetary balancing and political expediency rather than community health needs.

*The Labor party was returned to power in the elections of March 1983.—ED.

Expenditure on current, day-to-day activities may be broken down under five major headings, although two of these will embrace most of the expenditure. In round figures, institutional services expend 55% of all health service finance and noninstitutional services nearly 40%; the other 5% is divided between preventive services and research, with each having less than 1% of total funds, the other few percentage points representing expenditure on administration by government agencies and the voluntary insurance funds.

Institutional services, the largest area of expenditure, is divisible into hospital expenditure, taking nearly half of all the national current spending on health services; nursing home expenditure, requiring one-fourteenth of all current spending; and ambulance services, demanding about one-sixtieth of the total. The largest item under the noninstitutional services heading is expenditure on medical services—that is, expenditure on fee-for-service care for medical practitioners both outside and within hospitals—which accounts for about one-sixth of all current expenditure. This understates actual expenditure on doctors' services because the significant quantity of patient care provided in hospitals by salaried and sessional medical staff is included under the institutional services heading. The second largest noninstitutional expenditure is on pharmaceuticals; this amounts to nearly one-tenth of all current expenditure—again, this is an understatement because institutional service expenditure includes the cost of drugs supplied to patients by public hospitals. Spending on dental services, one twenty-fifth of all health expenditure, is mainly composed of payments to dentists in private practice, but also includes the cost of government-provided dental services for school children and Repatriation beneficiaries. Other noninstitutional service expenditure covers provison of some ambulatory and domiciliary care through government agencies and expenditure upon appliances and prostheses.

Controlling Health Care Costs

Hospitals, medical services, nursing homes, and the pharmaceutical benefits scheme, in that order, are the four biggest items of health expenditure in Australia. In the public hospital field, the main cost containment strategy used by governments has been simply to make across-the-board cuts in the annual allocation of government funds to hospitals. Public hospital boards and their executive officers are becoming aware that deficit financing by government—called by one health minister the "money-tree" philosophy—has ceased and that their responsibilities include proper planning and budgetary control. Also, governments have made some moves towards the closing of inappropriately located and underutilized hospitals, the delineation of hospital roles, and development of systems of certification of need for new facilities and equipment, the encouragement of utilization review, and peer evaluation of performance. Attempts have been made to confine the development of high technology services to selected public hospitals, thus keeping them out of the private sector where their control would be more difficult. Statewide systems of recording utilization of all institutional facilities are being developed so that performance may be more accurately monitored. However, a major problem in hospital cost control arises from the Australian system of nationwide and statewide wage fixing by independent tribunals. Thus, the major item of hospital budgets, wages and salaries, is placed beyond the control of hospitals and hospital authorities.

The major means of control of medical service costs is the Commonwealth Government's medical benefits schedule. The items listed and the scheduled fee for each item of service are under constant review by the government and a series of independent quasi-judicial tribunals. An indicator of the success of this method of control is the recent failure of medical practitioners' income to keep pace with increases in the cost of living index. Until recently, however, accurate information regarding practitioners' income was notoriously difficult to obtain. With the advent of the Medibank Mark I computerized information system, it became possible to draw a reasonably accurate picture of an individual doctor's practice. It soon became apparent that some doctors' workloads were markedly different from those of most of their peers. Clearly a significant degree of overservicing was occurring and some doctors' claims for payment of social service beneficiaries were fraudulent. Little official action was taken for several years; then in 1982 the matter became a public scandal, dubbed "Medifraud" by the media. Senior spokesmen of the AMA admitted that deception of a large scale had been practised by some doctors. It has been suggested that 10% or more of total payments of medical services per year may have been claimed fraudulently. Legislation has now been introduced in an attempt to stamp out Medifraud. Proponents of the compulsory universal health coverage arrangements, along the lines of Medibank Mark I, assert that its highly centralized information system offers much greater power to detect irregularities in medical practitioner behaviour than the fragmented and incomplete coverage afforded by a multiplicity of voluntary funds.

The Commonwealth Government's attempts to control nursing home costs by fee-fixing and restrictions upon admission eligibility have had limited success. The attempt to limit provision of nursing home beds using an arbitrary bed-population ratio as a target figure has underlined the inadequacy of present provision for care of the aged. An official inquiry was being conducted in 1982 to investigate, again, the alternatives to institutional care of the aged, with the implicit assumption that cheaper alternatives must exist.

Australia's pharmaceutical-manufacturing industry, dominated by supranational firms, maintains a constant barrage of criticism and propaganda against the Commonwealth Government's Pharmaceutical Benefits Scheme. This reflects the industry's chagrin at the success of the Commonwealth as a monopsonist in keeping prices paid for scheduled pharmaceuticals at what are, by world price standards, a very low level. Commentators from outside the pharmaceutical industry generally agree that the government's policy has benefited the patients and the Australian taxpayer at large.

In summary, then, in the 1960s there was a growing awareness of the enormous and ever-increasing costs of providing health care in Australia; the 1970s saw the emergence of means whereby control might be exercised; and in the 1980s those means are being further developed and strictly applied.

PUBLIC HEALTH SERVICES

State and Local Public Health Authorities

The gold-fever epidemic that hit Australia in the 1850s—with a sudden influx of wealth seekers, the hasty erection of squalid camps and shantytowns, a lack of sanitation, and an overcrowding of urban settlements—precipitated the very speedy adoption of public health legislation that was virtually a verbatim copy of English law. That legislation set the pattern for the development of the present public health administration: a central authority in each state shares responsibility with local health authorities—the 900 elected municipal and shire local government councils. At the state level, the public health authority was, until very recently, one of the three major arms of health service administration, the other two being concerned principally with public hospital services and the care of the mentally ill. Each of these three arms in any one state operated largely independently of the other two, although all three were subject to the control of the state health minister and the permanent head of the ministry of health.

It became fashionable in Australia during the 1960s to talk about rationalization and regionalization of government activities. It was then becoming increasingly clear that the hospital arm of state health administrations had been taking a larger and larger share of the available health care resources. With much repetition of words and phrases—such as "coordination," "integration," "appropriate allocation of resources," "total health care," and so on—three states made drastic changes in their health service administrative structures. In each of these states the three arms—hospitals, mental health, and public health services—were brought together under a health commission. The first commission was established in 1972 with five full-time commissioners. Under the health commission, public health services deteriorated rather than improved, probably because the commission was overwhelmingly concerned with administering the public hospital system. The commission was abolished in 1982, and the state health services were placed under a single permanent head. The other two state health commissions have not been operating long enough to gauge their success at giving proper attention to public health activities.

Prominent among the preventive and health promotive activities that make up the workload of state and local public health authorities are environmental control, including food hygiene, water, and air quality surveillance; enforcement of sanitation standards and radiation control; and the provision of a limited range of personal services, including immunization and clinics for mothers and babies. Other activities include communicable disease control, operation of public health and forensic medicine laboratories, and pathology services. Environmental control work is largely performed by sanitarians known as health inspectors or health surveyors. Most local health authorities employ one or more health inspectors, who commonly double as building inspectors, enforcing building construction legislation. This duality of function is sometimes criticised on the grounds that the building inspector role tends to overshadow that of health inspector.

A very considerable body of occupational health legislation exists in all states, with responsibility for its enforcement divided between state public health authorities and other ministries concerned with industrial matters. Much of this legislation is inadequate, carrying very low penalties and barely enforced due to underfunding and understaffing of inspectorates. Generally, occupational health and safety services are poorly developed, one important factor being the emphasis given by Australian trade unions to increasing the contents of members' pay packets with little concern for other aspects of their welfare. Within the past few years signs of change have appeared, with some worker organizations setting up their own occupational health and safety services, and with the drafting of new legislation providing greater worker involvement in its implementation and enforcement.

Expenditure on public health service activities calls for about 2% of the total expenditure on all local government activities. Public health activities absorb less than 2% of all state government expenditure on health. It must be noted that most of the widely used systems of classifying public and private expenditure upon health care present a somewhat misleading picture, in that huge sums of money are spent on water supply and sewerage systems, on meeting environmental control and safety standards, on satisfying food production and food processing regulations and so on, but this enormous commitment of resources to health preservation and advancement is omitted from the health service financial statement. These expenditures in fact contribute more to the public's health in Australia, and in other countries, than do all the hospitals and medical services.

The Federal Government's Role in Public Health

Before the Commonwealth Department of Health was established the only major public health responsibility of the Federal Government was a national quarantine service. The government's role has been expanded to include formulation, largely through the multifarious committees of the National Health and Medical Research Council, of national standards and codes of procedures covering many areas of public health promotion and protection. But its role in such matters is advisory and, because the adoption and implementation of these standards and codes rests with the states, it is in fact rather unusual to find nationwide uniformity in any area of public health, except where other countries are involved, and consequently the Commonwealth is the responsible authority—for example, in the import and export standards of foodstuffs and drugs, and in the medical examination of immigrants. The Commonwealth Department of Health provides the official link with the World Health Organization.

The department also operates several standard setting, testing, and research laboratories concerned with biologicals, dental materials, ultrasonics, and radiation control. The Commonwealth Serum Laboratories produce a limited range of biologicals, including antibiotics and insulin, in competition with commercial producers. The Commonwealth has contributed much of the funding for joint federal-state mass vaccination campaigns, such as the highly successful antipoliomyelitis campaign and the antituberculosis campaign—both diseases are now rarely seen in Australia.

The Commonwealth and state health departments each have responsibilities for the collection and distribution of a limited range of communicable and chronic disease data, but the major part of the epidemiological and vital statistics collecting and processing is done through the Australian Bureau of Statistics, in cooperation with federal and state agencies. Relying heavily upon state agencies for raw data input the bureau has, in many areas of concern to health service administrators, been unable to produce national statistics that are comprehensive in coverage and comparable on an interstate basis. Nevertheless, the material produced by the Bureau is of very high standard.

Constitutionally and administratively, the Commonwealth Government can have a very strong influence and control over hospital, medical, and pharmaceutical services; however, it is in a weak position vis-à-vis public health, where, except in international health matters, it must proceed by encouragement and persuasion rather than through the power of the purse. Its efforts to encourage and persuade have not been very noteworthy for either their volume or their success, and insofar as a high standard of health in a population depends upon public health service activity, then credit must go to the state and local government authorities rather than to the Commonwealth.

CONCLUSION

The Modified Clone

Clones of Britain's health care system, the services in the Australian colonies at the end of the nineteenth century were indeed true to type. In the first forty-five years of federation little real change occurred. From the end of World War II, however, Australian federalism and concepts imported principally from the United States of America have produced significant, sometimes rapid changes, exacerbating old problems, generating new ones, and at least suggesting the way to some improvements.

The "health and welfare" amendment of the Commonwealth Constitution and the emergence of the Commonwealth as the indisputably dominant controller of government funds during the 1940s have helped to erode the autonomy of the medical profession and of the boards of individual hospitals and state hospital authorities. It is somewhat ironic that a voluntary health insurance system imported from the United States with a view to preserving private enterprise in health care delivery has, with local modification, been the mechanism for this erosion. Though short-lived or now emasculated, the schemes for federal-state cooperation introduced by the Australian Labor government from 1972 to 1975 illustrated the willingness of the states to respond to federal hegemony in the improvement of health service planning and health care delivery. The Commonwealth Government's Pharmaceutical Benefits Scheme has shown the ability of government to regulate that industry's activities. All of these federal initiatives, together with an extension of social service beneficiary entitlements, have undoubtedly improved consumer access to health care and made for greater equity in health service provision.

As to quality of care provided, only recently have serious attempts been made to evaluate service in a detailed and systematic fashion. Here, too, the concepts and procedures have been, for the most part, imported from the United States, as have notions of health consumer activism. The developing systems of resource allocation and utilization review are derived from North American and, to a lesser extent, British examples. The salutary impact of these systems is being shown at present mainly in efforts to improve data collection and processing, but some greater rationality in planning and deployment of resources is beginning to be seen.

Complexity and Inadequacy, But Mostly . . .

The catalogue of outstanding and impending problems facing the Australian health care system is large. It reflects in greater or lesser degree the difficulties confronting most of the relatively affluent countries that attempt to ensure comprehensive and high quality care to an entire population within a health delivery system having a large public sector and a great number of private providers operating within a federal system of government. It would be merely tedious to present the catalogue here. Despite the complexity of the system and the admitted inadequacies of some services, we can say that the majority of Australians enjoy a high standard of health most of the time, and that when health services are required, for most people they are readily available and mostly of good standard.

For Further Study

Dewdney, J.C.H. *Australian Health Services.* Sydney: John Wiley and Sons, 1972.

Grant, C. and H. Lapsley. *The Australian Health Care System, 1982.* Kensington: University of New South Wales, 1982.

Hawker, J., J.C.H. Dewdney, and C. Grant, eds. *Hospitals and Health Services Yearbook, Australia* (annual). Melbourne: Isaacson Publications, annual.

Health Research Project. Research reports and monographs, and technical papers. Australian National University, P.O. Box 4, Canberra, A.C.T. 2600, Australia.

Sax, S. *Medicine in the 80's: Can We Afford It? An Australian Perspective.* Kensington: University of New South Wales, 1981.

Table 1 Australian population by sex and age, 1980

Age	Males	Females	Persons	% Males	% Females	% Persons
All ages	7,335,497	7,356,687	14,692,184	100.0%	100.0%	100.0%
Under 5	579,542	551,309	1,130,851	7.9	7.5	7.7
5 to 13	1,192,448	1,140,263	2,332,711	16.3	15.5	15.9
14 to 17	522,517	499,973	1,022,490	7.1	6.8	7.0
18 to 24	913,966	887,503	1,801,469	12.5	12.1	12.3
25 to 34	1,208,137	1,180,482	2,388,619	16.5	16.1	16.3
35 to 44	899,896	861,231	1,761,127	12.3	11.7	12.0
45 to 54	774,660	738,598	1,513,258	10.6	10.0	10.3
55 to 64	648,858	679,612	1,328,470	8.9	9.2	9.0
65 and over	595,473	817,716	1,413,189	8.1	11.1	9.6
Median age	27.8	29.0	28.4	—	—	—

SOURCE: Australian Bureau of Statistics, *Estimated Resident Population by Sex and Age: States and Territories of Australia, June 1971 to June 1981* (Canberra: ABS, 1982).

NOTE: Data are estimates of resident population as at 30 June 1980. Minor discrepancies are due to rounding off.

Table 2 Live births, birth rates, and fertility rates, Australia

	Live Births	Birth Rate	Fertility Rate
1979	223,129	15.4	68.9
1980	225,527	15.3	68.2
1981	235,842	15.8	69.6

SOURCE: Australian Bureau of Statistics, *Births, Australia, 1981* (Canberra: ABS, 1982).

NOTE: Rates are on an annual basis. Birth rates per 1,000 population and fertility rates per 1,000 women aged 15–44 years.

Table 3 Neonatal and infant mortality rates, Australia

Years	Infant Mortality Rates[a] Males	Females	Persons	Neonatal Mortality Rates[b]	Postneonatal Mortality Rates[c]
1946–50	30.1	23.7	27.0[d]	19.3	7.6[d]
1951–55	26.0	20.6	23.3[d]	16.5	6.9[d]
1956–60	23.3	18.7	21.1[d]	15.1	6.0[d]
1961–65	21.7	17.0	19.4[d]	14.0	5.4[d]
1966–70	20.4	15.7	18.1[d]	13.1	5.0[d]
1971	19.0	15.5	17.3	12.2	5.0[d]
1972	18.9	14.4	16.7	12.0	4.7[e]
1973	18.6	14.3	16.5	11.8	4.7[e]
1974	18.4	13.7	16.1	11.6	4.6[e]
1975	16.3	12.1	14.3	10.0	4.3[e]
1976	15.1	12.4	13.8	9.9	3.9[e]
1977	14.1	10.9	12.5	8.7	3.8[e]
1978	13.7	10.6	12.2	8.1	4.1[e]
1979	12.6	10.1	11.4	7.6	3.8[e]
1980	11.9	9.4	10.7	7.1	3.6[e]

SOURCE: Commonwealth Department of Health, *Annual Report of the Director-General of Health* (Canberra: Australian Gov. Publishing Service, selected years). This is the source of all statistics in this table unless a different source is indicated.

NOTE: The postneonatal mortality rate showed a great change between 1921 and 1946, decreasing rapidy from 28.0 to 7.6. (1921–25 : 28.0; 1926–30 : 23.0; 1931–35 : 14.0; 1936–40 : 12.6; 1941–45 : 11.1.). During the same period, the neonatal mortality rate decreased from 29.9 in 1921–25 to 19.3 in 1946–50.

[a]Number of deaths of live-born children *within one year of birth* per 1,000 live births.
[b]Number of deaths of live-born children *within 28 days of birth* per 1,000 live births.
[c]Number of deaths of live-born children *from 28 days to 11 months* per 1,000 live births.
[d]Australian Bureau of Statistics, *Demography Bulletin,* No. 85, Australian Government Printer, Canberra 1970.
[e]Calculated by subtraction.

Table 4 Infant mortality rates by most common causes, selected years, Australia

	Death Rates in Under 1 Year Age Group[b]							
	1968		1971		1975		1978	
Cause of Death[a]	M	F	M	F	M	F	M	F
Other causes of perinatal mortality	7.2	5.6	7.0	5.6	6.1	4.6	4.2	3.1
Congenital anomalies	3.5	3.4	3.3	3.4	3.5	2.9	3.5	2.8
Birth injury, difficult labour, and other anoxic and hypoxic conditions	4.0	2.7	3.4	2.5	2.2	1.4	1.9	1.4
Pneumonia	1.7	1.3	1.5	1.0	0.6	0.4	0.4	0.4
All other accidents	0.7	0.4	0.6	0.4	0.4	0.3	0.2	0.2
Enteritis and diarrhoea	0.4	0.4	0.5	0.5	0.3	0.2	0.2	0.2
All causes	19.8	15.6	19.0	15.5	16.3	12.1	13.7	10.6

SOURCE: Australian Bureau of Statistics, *Causes of Death: Age Specific Death Rates Australia, 1968 to 1978* (Canberra: ABS, 1982).

[a]Cause of death was classified according to the Abbreviated List of 50 Causes of Death, Eighth Revision (1965) of WHO International Classification of Diseases.
[b]Rates per 1,000 live births.

Table 5 Death rates for leading causes of death, Australia

Cause of Death	Deaths per 100,000 Mean Population 1976 (ICD 8th Revision)	1980 (ICD 9th Revision)
Diseases of the circulatory system	432.6	381.5
Ischaemic heart disease	243.2	210.2
Other heart/hypertensive disease	50.5	51.3
Cerebrovascular disease	109.7	93.9
Atherosclerosis	14.9	12.1
Other	14.3	14.0
Malignant neoplasms	151.0	159.6
Digestive organs and peritoneum	48.8	49.2
Lung	30.3	34.2
Other	71.9	76.2
Diseases of the respiratory system	63.2	50.8
Bronchitis, emphysema and asthma	34.2	15.4
Pneumonia	18.4	12.1
Influenza	4.7	0.9
Other	5.8	22.4
Motor vehicle accidents	26.0	24.3
All other accidents	21.1	18.5
Diseases of the genito-urinary system	11.6	11.3
Diabetes mellitus	12.4	11.2
Suicide and self-inflicted injuries	10.8	11.0
Chronic liver disease and cirrhosis	8.1	8.4
Perinatal conditions	11.0	7.4
Congenital anomalies	8.4	6.2
Alcohol dependence syndrome	3.0	1.2
Intestinal infectious diseases	1.4	0.5
Tuberculosis	0.9	0.4
All other causes	48.2	51.2
All causes	809.5	743.6

SOURCE: Commonwealth Director General of Health, *Annual Report, 1981–82* (Canberra: AGPS, 1982).

NOTE: Due to rounding, numbers do not add exactly to totals.

Table 6 Information not available—no nationwide collection of hospital morbidity and procedural statistics. Limited information is available for some states; see, for example, Table 7.

Table 7 Hospital separations (discharges) classified by principal diagnosis (morbidity list), New South Wales, 1980

ICD Code Number	Principal Diagnosis	Separations	Proportion of Total Percentage
140–208	Malignant neoplasms	40,556	3.9
290–319	Mental disorders	47,528	4.6
390–459	Diseases of the circulatory system	84,660	8.1
580–599	Diseases of the urinary system	27,692	2.7
640–646, 651–670	Direct obstetric conditions	60,830	5.8
650	Normal delivery	31,479	3.0
710–739	Diseases of the musculo-skeletal system and connective tissue	59,557	5.7
800–999	Injury and poisoning	100,678	9.7
V01–V82	Other reasons for contact with health services	97,904	9.4
	All other separations	491,787	47.1
	Totals	1,042,671	100.0

SOURCE: Australian Bureau of Statistics, *Hospital and Nursing Home Inpatients, New South Wales, 1980* (Sydney: ABS, 1982).

Table 8 Health professional personnel in Australia

	1976		1981	
Occupation	Number	Rate Per 100,000	Number	Rate Per 100,000
Medical practitioners	20,480	145.9	27,128	181.7
Dentists	4,630	33.0	5,585	37.4
Nurses, certificated	79,787	568.6	106,566	713.9
Nurses, not certificated	15,480	110.3	14,412	96.6
Nurses, trainee	22,295	158.9	18,456	123.6
Total (nurses)	117,562	837.7	139,434	934.1
Pharmacists	9,154	65.2	9,839	65.9
Physiotherapists	2,971	21.2	4,478	30.0
Radiographers	1,979	14.1	3,018	20.2
Occupational Therapists	1,787	12.7	2,528	16.9
Optometrists	973	6.9	1,277	8.6
Speech Therapists	523	3.7	1,076	7.2
Chiropractors	592	4.2	956	6.4
Chiropodists	804	5.7	911	6.1
Dieticians	359	2.6	684	4.6
Other professional health workers	1,004	7.2	1,637	11.0
Total	162,818	1160.3	198,551	1330.2

SOURCE: Data from the Australian Bureau of Census and Statistics

NOTE: These figures represent readily identifiable health professional full-time and part-time workers—unofficial estimates of the numbers of all persons employed in the health care system in 1981 suggest a total health care workforce in excess of 300,000. The 1981 figures are preliminary counts and subject to revision.

Table 9 Medical schools and medical school graduates in Australia

	Operational Medical Schools	Medical Schools with Graduating Students	Medical School Graduates (MBBS)[a]
1977	10	8	1198
1978	10	8	1264
1979	10	8	1593[b]
1980	10	9	1341[c]
1981	10	9	1311[c]
1986	10	10	1374[c]
1991	10	10	1378[c]

SOURCE: *Medical Manpower Supply: Report of the Committee of Officials* (Canberra: AGPS, 1980).

[a]MBBS refers to the registrable qualification Bachelor of Medicine and Bachelor of Surgery.
[b]This large figure results from a "double graduation" from New South Wales medical schools following the change from a 6-year to a 5-year medical course in 1974.
[c]Estimated numbers of graduates if entry policies remain unchanged.

Table 10 Medical practitioners and the Australian population

Census Year		Medical Practitioners[a]	Population	Practitioners Per 100,000 Population	Practitioners: Population Ratio
1961	F	1,309			
	M	10,595[b]			
		11,904	10,508,186	113	883
1966	F	1,488			
	M	12,209			
		13,697	11,550,462	119	843
1971	F	2,104			
	M	14,003			
		16,107	13,067,265	123	811
1976	F	3,269			
	M	17,211			
		20,480	14,033,083	146	685
1981	F	5,133			
	M	21,995			
		27,128	14,926,786	182	550

SOURCES: Commonwealth Statistician, reports upon the *Commonwealth Census of Population and Housing.*

[a]The practitioners enumerated are registered medical practitioners who regard themselves as being actively engaged in their profession either full- or part-time.
[b]F and M refer to female and male medical practitioners respectively.

Table 11 Medical practitioners by specialty and sex, Australia, mid-1982

	Practitioners		
	Female	Male	Total
General practice	2,416	10,266	12,682
Full-time salaried practice (mostly specialist)	195	613	808
Specialties			
Surgery (general)	15	1,353	1,368
Internal medicine	70	1,280	1,350
Anaesthetics	143	905	1,048
Psychiatry	169	838	1,007
Obstetrics and gynaecology	74	808	882
Pathology	104	536	640
Radiology	49	580	629
Ophthalmology	30	456	486
Paediatrics	62	377	439
Orthopaedics	2	390	392
ENT	3	270	273
Dermatology	31	154	185
Urology	4	178	182
Cardiology	6	171	177
TB and chest diseases	9	107	116
Neurology	7	90	97
Rheumatology	12	65	77
Neurosurgery	1	67	68
Allergy	5	38	43
Hospital doctors (junior and senior)	1,535	5,091	6,626[a]
Grand Total			29,575

SOURCE: Permail Pty. Ltd. listing—although unofficial, this is the most up-to-date and comprehensive source available.

[a]The distribution of hospital doctors is approximately 1,901 juniors and 4,725 seniors for a total of 6,626.

Table 12 Remuneration of medical practitioners in Australia

Private Practice Incomes: Information regarding private practice incomes is notoriously difficult to obtain. In 1982 the Australian Association of Surgeons publicly stated that the average net income for a specialist surgeon in full-time private practice was $A54,574 after deduction of costs and before tax. The average hours worked per week was 56.5.

Visiting (private) Medical Officer (VMO) Payments: One state award in 1981 fixed the following hourly rates for VMOs

General practitioner	$A22–24.50–30 depending on years of experience
Specialist	$A35
Senior Specialist (at least seven years practice in his specialty)	$A38

Contracts permit a maximum of 70 hours of practice as a VMO per four-week period.

Salaried Medical Staff Awards: A typical award made in 1982 fixed annual salaries for full-time medical staff employed in public hospitals as follows:

Junior resident	$A14,850
Resident medical officers	$A18,420–25,560
Senior registrars	$A32,278–33,423
Specialists	$A33,110–45,061
Senior specialists-in-charge	$A47,506

Additional payments of up to $5,000 per annum were provided to cover on-call duty.

SOURCES: *AMA Gazette,* May and September 1982; *Health Commission Circular,* 12 October 1981.

Table 13 Hospitals, beds, and occupancy data, Australia

	Hospitals		Beds		Beds Per 1,000 Population		Occupied Bed Days (in Thousands)		Bed Days Per 100,000 Population		Occupancy Rate (%)	
	1971	1981	1971	1981	1971	1981	1971	1981	1971	1981	1971	1981
Public hospitals	776	302	63,631	74,975	5.0	5.0	16,422	17,963	1,297	1,220	71	69
Private hospitals	325	340	13,914	19,956	1.1	1.3	3,279	4,252	259	290	70	59
Total	1,101	1,142	77,545	94,931	6.1	6.4	19,701	22,215	1,556	1,510	70	66

SOURCES: Commonwealth Director General of Health, *Annual Report* for 1972–73 and 1980–81 (Canberra: AGPS, 1973 and 1981).

NOTES: Hospitals and beds shown in this table are those approved by the Commonwealth for hospital benefit purposes. Consequently, a small number of hospital beds, mostly used for long-stay patients, are not shown here.

Numbers of inpatients treated in 1970–71 were 1.7 million for public hospitals and 0.51 million for private hospitals, giving numbers of inpatients treated per 1,000 population as 400 and 135.3 for public and private hospitals, respectively. This information is not available for 1980–81.

In 1970–71 the average patient stay in public hospitals was 9.6 days, in private hospitals 6.5 days. This information is not available for 1981, but there has been some decrease in the average length of stay over the past decade.

Table 14 Information not available.

Table 15 Nursing homes and nursing home beds in Australia

	1973	1977	1981
Approved nursing homes			
Deficit financed[a]	—	260	340
Government[b]	84	101	148
Other[c]	1,152	799	856
Total	1,236	1,160	1,344
Beds			
Deficit financed	—	11,439	15,414
Government	10,833	13,080	14,758
Other	42,583	31,993	37,740
Total	53,416	56,512	67,912
Beds per 1,000 population	4.1	4.0	4.6

SOURCES: Commonwealth Director General of Health, *Annual Report* for 1976–77 and 1980–81 (Canberra: AGPS, 1977 and 1981).

[a]Deficit financed homes approved under the Nursing Homes Assistance Act for the payment of their approved operating deficits. Under the Act the Commonwealth Government meets the approved operating deficits of certain voluntary nonprofit nursing homes that enter into an agreement with the government for this purpose.

[b]Government homes approved under the National Health Act for the payment of nursing home benefits.

[c]Private profit and voluntary nonprofit homes approved under the National Health Act for the payment of nursing home benefits.

Table 16 Average costs per occupied hospital bed day in Australia

Year Ending 30 June	Public Hospitals[a]		Private Hospitals	
	Cost	Index	Cost	Index
1967	19.6	100	10.9	100
1970	27.5	140	—	—
1973	42.4	216	—	—
1976	94.2	481	53.7	493
1977	118.0	602	67.2	616
1978	137.5	701	74.1	680
1979	153.0	781	—	—

SOURCE: J.S. Deeble, "Financing Health Care in a Static Economy," *Social Science and Medicine* 16, no. 6 (1982): 713–24.

[a]Includes Repatriation and Defence Forces hospitals.

Table 17 National health expenditures: amount and per capita amount by major source of funds and percentage of Gross Domestic Product, selected fiscal years, Australia

	1960–61[a]	1969–70[a]	1974–75	1978–79	1979–80
National expenditure on health services (in millions of dollars)	668	1,537	4,149	7,921	8,631
Health service expenditure as percentage of Gross Domestic Product	4.6	5.2	6.7	7.8	7.5
Sources of funds					
Private expenditure	322	696	1,537	2,998	3,283
Public expenditure	346	841	2,612	4,923	5,347
Federal	187	457	1,266	2,887	3,140
State/local	159	384	1,346	2,036	2,207
Per capita expenditures	64	124	303	549	591
Sources of funds					
Private expenditure	31	56	112	208	225
Public expenditure	33	68	191	341	366
Federal	18	37	92	200	215
State/local	15	31	99	141	151
Percentage distribution of funds					
Private funds	48.2	45.3	37.0	37.8	38.0
Public funds	51.8	54.7	63.0	62.2	62.0
Federal	28.0	29.7	30.5	36.4	36.4
State/local	23.8	25.0	32.5	25.7	25.6
Gross Domestic Product (in billions)	14.6	30.3	59.0	101.1	114.3
Mid-fiscal year population (estimated in thousands)	10,392	12,446	13,849	14,517	14,727

SOURCE: Commonwealth Director General of Health, *Annual Report* for 1972–73 and 1981–82 (Canberra: AGPS, 1973 and 1982).

[a]Statistics for 1960–61 and 1969–70 do not include capital expenditure, which, in those years, was about 7% of current expenditure.

Table 18a National health expenditure in million dollars (Aust.) by type of expenditure and source of funds, Australia, fiscal year 1978–79

Source of Funds	Government			Private				
	Commonwealth	Other	Total Government	Health Insurance Funds	Individuals	Other	Total Private	Grand Total
Current expenditure								
Institutional services								
Public hospitals	1,134	1,058	2,193	311	..[a]	160	471	2,664
Private hospitals	86	—[b]	86	203	67	6	276	362
Other hospitals								
Repatriation	126	—	126	—	—	—	—	126
Mental	10	325	335	—	39	—	39	374
Total (hospitals)	1,356	1,384	2,740	515	106	166	786	3,526
Nursing homes								
Government and other	247	36	283	60	107	..	168	451
Deficit financed	73	—	73	—	32	—	32	106
Total (nursing homes)	320	36	356	60	140	..	200	556
Ambulances	12	28	39	3	71	7	81	120
Other services	6	..	6	—	—	—	—	6
Total institutional	1,695	1,447	3,142	578	316	173	1,067	4,208
Noninstitutional services								
Medical services	565	—	565	483	161	68	712	1,277
Dental services	18	10	27	108	185	1	294	321
Other professional services	12	—	12	31	99	8	138	151
Community health services								
Community health (incl. Aboriginal health)	71	39	109	—	—	—	—	109
Domiciliary care benefit	11	—	11	—	—	—	—	11
Home nursing	12	14	26	2	—	—	2	27
Maternal and child care	1	28	29	—	—	—	—	29
Pharmaceuticals								
Benefits paid items	307	—	307	—	130	—	130	436
All other items	—	—	—	8	263	2	273	273
Appliances	18	—	18	15	91	..	106	124
Other services	6	36	43	1	—	—	1	44
Total noninstitutional	1,021	127	1,147	648	929	80	1,656	2,803

Preventive services	6	41	47	—	—	—	—	47
Administration								
Hospital insurance	30	—	30	56	—	—	56	183
Medical insurance				97			97	
Other	83	82	165	—	—	—	—	165
Total administration	113	82	195	153	—	—	153	348
Research	17	4	21	—	31	—	31	52
Total current	2,851	1,701	4,552	1,378	1,276	252	2,907	7,459
Capital expenditure	71	323	395	—	—	128	128	523
Total expenditure	2,922	2,024	4,947	1,378	1,276	380	3,035	7,982

SOURCE: Commonwealth Department of Health, *Australian Health Expenditure 1974–75 to 1978–79: An Analysis* (Canberra: The Department, 1981).

NOTE: Minor errors due to rounding off.

[a]The symbol .. indicates very minor expenditure.
[b]The symbol — indicates no expenditure.

Table 18b National health expenditure by type of expenditure and source of funds, per capita amount, Australia, fiscal year 1978–79

Source of Funds	Government			Private				
	Commonwealth	Other	Total Government	Health Insurance Funds	Individuals	Other	Total Private	Grand Total
Current Expenditure								
Institutional Services								
Public hospitals	78.1	72.9	151.1	21.4	..[a]	11.0	32.4	183.5
Private hospitals	5.9	—	5.9	14.0	4.6	0.4	19.0	24.9
Other hospitals								
Repatriation	8.7	—	8.7	—	—	—	—	8.7
Mental	0.7	22.4	23.1	—	2.7	—	2.7	25.8
Total (hospitals)	93.4	95.3	188.7	35.5	7.3	11.4	54.1	242.9
Nursing homes								
Government and other	17.0	2.5	19.5	4.1	7.3	..	11.6	31.1
Deficit financed	5.0	—	5.0	—	2.2	—	2.2	7.3
Total (nursing homes)	22.0	2.5	24.5	4.1	9.6	..	13.8	38.3
Ambulances	0.8		2.7	0.2	4.9	0.5	5.6	8.3
Other services	0.4		0.4		—	—	—	0.4
Total institutional	116.8	99.7	216.4	39.8	21.8	11.9	73.5	289.9
Noninstitutional services								
Medical services	38.9	—	38.9	33.3	11.1	4.7	49.0	88.0
Dental services	1.2	0.7	1.9	7.4	12.7	0.1	20.3	22.1
Other professional services	0.8	—	0.8	2.1	6.8	0.6	9.5	10.4
Community health services								
Community health (incl. Aboriginal health)	4.9	2.7	7.5	—	—	—	—	7.5
Domiciliary care benefit	0.8	—	0.8	—	—	—	—	0.8
Home nursing	0.8	1.0	1.8	2	—	—	0.1	1.9
Maternal and child care	0.1	2.0	2.0	—	—	—	—	2.0
Pharmaceuticals								
Benefits paid items	21.2	—	21.2	—	9.0	—	9.0	30.0
All other items	—	—	—	0.6	18.1	0.1	18.8	18.8
Appliances	1.2	—	1.2	1.0	6.3	..	7.3	8.5
Other services	0.4	2.5	3.0	0.1	—	—	0.1	3.0
Total noninstitutional	70.3	8.8	79.0	44.6	64.0	5.5	114.1	193.1

Preventive services	0.4	2.8	3.2	—	—	—	—	3.2
Administration								
Hospital insurance	2.1	—	2.1	3.9	—	—	3.9	12.6
Medical insurance				6.7			6.7	
Other	5.7	5.7	11.4	—	—			11.4
Total administration	7.8	5.7	13.4	10.5	—	—	10.5	24.0
Research	1.2	0.3	1.5	—	2.1	—	2.1	3.6
Total current	196.4	117.2	313.5	94.9	87.9	17.4	200.2	513.8
Capital expenditure	4.9	22.3	27.2	—	—	8.8	8.8	36.0
Total expenditure	201.3	139.4	340.8	94.9	87.9	26.1	209.0	549.8

SOURCE: Adapted from Commonwealth Department of Health statistics.

[a]See Table 18A for explanation of symbols.

Table 18c National health expenditure by type of expenditure, source of funds and percentage distribution, Australia, fiscal year 1978–79

	Government			Private				
Source of Funds	Commonwealth	Other	Total Government	Health Insurance Funds	Individuals	Other	Total Private	Grand Total
Current expenditure								
Institutional services								
Public hospitals	14.2	13.3	27.5	3.9	..[a]	2.0	5.9	33.4
Private hospitals	1.1	—	1.1	2.5	0.8	0.1	3.5	4.5
Other hospitals								
Repatriation	1.6	—	1.6	—	—	—	—	1.6
Mental	0.1	4.1	4.2	—	0.5	—	0.5	4.7
Total (hospitals)	17.0	17.3	34.3	6.5	1.3	2.1	9.9	44.2
Nursing homes								
Government and other	3.1	0.5	3.6	0.8	1.3	..	2.1	5.7
Deficit financed	0.9	—	0.9	—	0.4	—	0.4	1.3
Total (nursing homes)	4.0	0.5	4.5	0.8	1.8	..	2.5	7.0
Ambulances	0.2	0.4	0.5	..	0.9	0.1	1.0	1.5
Other services	0.1	..	0.1	—	—	—	—	0.1
Total institutional	21.2	18.1	39.4	7.2	4.0	2.2	13.4	52.7
Noninstitutional services								
Medical services	7.1	—	7.1	6.1	2.0	0.9	8.9	16.0
Dental services	0.2	0.1	0.3	1.4	2.3	..	3.7	4.0
Other professional services	0.2	—	0.2	0.4	1.2	0.1	1.7	1.7
Community health services								
Community health (incl. Aboriginal health)	0.9	0.5	1.4	—	—	—	—	1.4
Domiciliary care benefit	0.1	—	0.1	—	—	—	—	0.1
Home nursing	0.2	0.2	0.3	..	—	—	..	0.3
Maternal and child care	..	0.4	0.4	—	—	—	—	0.4
Pharmaceuticals								
Benefits paid items	3.9	—	3.9	—	1.6	—	1.6	5.5
All other items	—	—	—	0.1	3.3	..	3.4	3.4
Appliances	0.2	—	0.2	0.2	1.1	..	1.3	1.6
Other services	0.1	—	0.5	0.6	..	—	..	0.6
Total noninstitutional	12.8	1.6	14.4	8.1	11.6	1.0	20.8	35.1

Preventive services	0.1	0.5	0.6	—	—	—	—	0.6
Administration								
Hospital insurance	0.4	—	0.4	0.7	—	—	0.7	2.3
Medical insurance				1.2			1.2	
Other	1.0	1.0	2.0	—	—	—	—	2.0
Total administration	1.4	1.0	2.4	1.9	—	—	1.9	4.4
Research	0.2	0.1	0.3	—	0.4	—	0.4	0.7
Total current	35.7	21.3	57.0	17.3	16.0	3.2	36.4	93.5
Capital expenditure	0.9	4.1	5.0	—	—	1.6	1.6	6.6
Total expenditure	36.6	25.4	62.0	17.3	16.0	4.8	38.8	100.0

SOURCE: Adapted from Commonwealth Department of Health statistics.

[a]See Table 18A for explanation of symbols.

Table 19 Information not available.

Table 20 Proportion of Australian population covered by private health insurance

	Percentage of Population Covered	
At 30 June	Hospital Benefits	Medical Benefits
1953	39[a]	—
1954	51	39[a]
1955	56	45
1960	72	72
1965	77	75
1970	79	75
1975	79	78
1980	58[b]	56[b]

SOURCES: Commonwealth Department of Health and Department of Social Security, *Annual Reports.*

[a]First years of operation of the Commonwealth-subsidised voluntary health insurance schemes.
[b]These figures reflect changes in voluntary health insurance following the introduction in 1975 and subsequent dismantling of the Medibank universal health cover schemes financed from general revenue.

Health Services in Belgium

Herman Nys and
Paul Quaethoven

INTRODUCTION

The kingdom of Belgium has been, since its birth in 1830, a hereditary, representative, and constitutional monarchy. Its 11,782 square miles (30,515 square kilometres) hosts a population of over 9,800,000. Culturally and geographically, Belgium is a heterogenous nation, divided between Flemings, a Dutch-speaking people, and Walloons, a French-speaking group.

The king shares legislative power with the Chamber of Representatives and Senate, the members of these two bodies being elected for four-year terms. Since the constitutional revision of 1980, the Flemish and Walloon communities have legislative (regional council) and administrative (regional government) responsibilities; the provision of health care is one of them. The nine provinces—which are divided into administrative districts—and their communes are each under the authority of a governor, with some legislative power exercised by the provincial council.

The central and regional authorities have only financial and supervisory responsibilities in health care. As a rule they do not provide health services themselves, this being left to municipal and private initiative.

MEDICAL PRACTICE IN BELGIUM

Medical practice in Belgium is the legal monopoly of the "doctor of medicine, surgery, and obstetrics." Only this title gives the right to practice medicine, although dental practitioners and midwives have a limited qualification. In 1980 there were 24,536 doctors of medicine, surgery, and obstetrics (physicians) in Belgium. About 16% of them were women. The ratio of physicians to population has grown steadily over the years: in 1940 there were 78 physicians per 100,000 population; in 1950, 94 physicians per 100,000; in

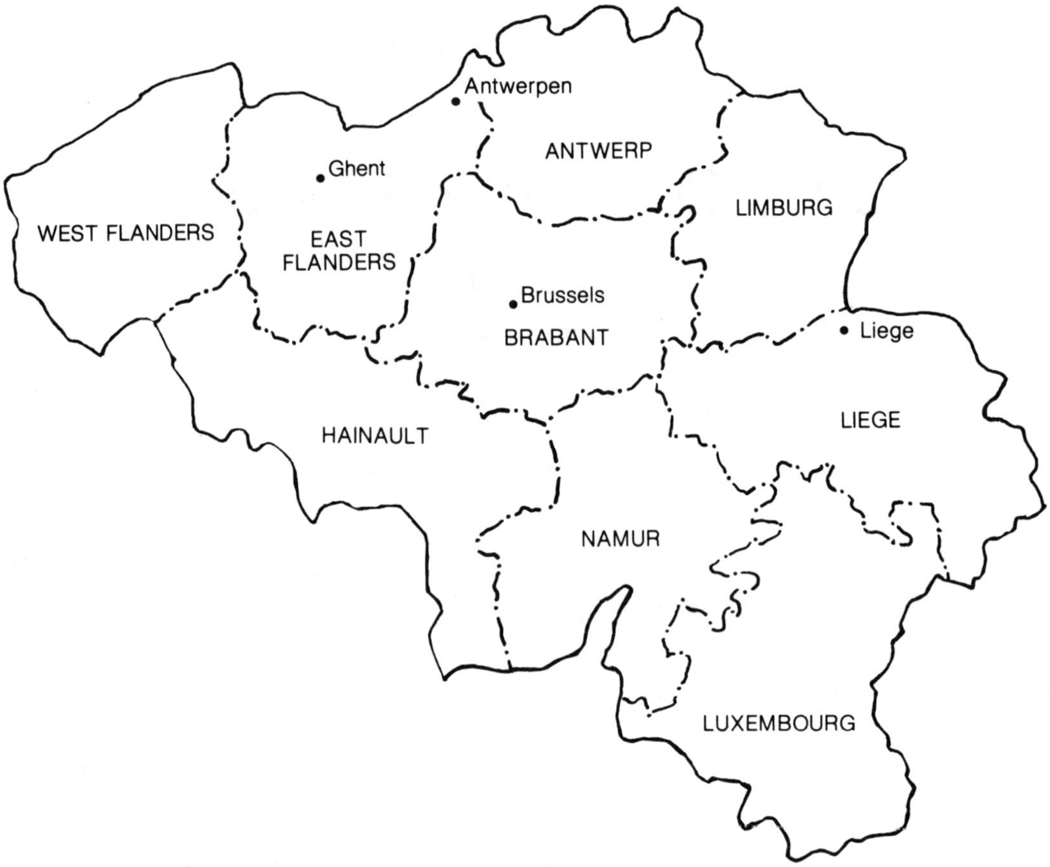

1980, 248 physicians per 100,000. It is estimated that in 1985 the supply of physicians will be about 291 for every 100,000 inhabitants, or one physician to 342 people. About 5% of Belgium's physicians are inactive.

The diploma of doctor of medicine, surgery, and obstetrics qualifies one to practice medicine and surgery in all cases. Actually, there is a distinction between a "general practitioner" and a "medical specialist." Of all the doctors in Belgium in 1980, 10,234 were licensed as medical specialists by the minister of health. The remaining group includes 2,174 candidate-specialists and 12,486 general practitioners. On 1 July 1980 the medical specialists numbered as follows:

Specialty	
General Internal Medicine	1,298
General Surgery	1,085
Neuro-psychiatry	1,039
Radiology	864
Paediatrics	830
Obstetrics/Gynaecology	699
Anaesthesiology	618

Ophthalmology	597
Clinical Biology	589
Physical Medicine	350
ENT	345
Orthopaedics	336
Dermatology	326
Cardiology	325
Stomatology	266
Pneumonology	181
Urology	160
Rheumatology	153
Gastro-enterology	138
Neuro-surgery	55

Both general practitioners and medical specialists are mainly engaged in private individual practice—that is, they practice independently. Most medical specialists also have staff appointments in hospitals, but only a small number have "full-time" status. The average general practitioner spends virtually all of his or her time in private office service (the office usually located in the doctor's home) or on house calls. House calls constitute two-thirds of a general practitioner's practice, office consultations about one-third. A general practitioner is seldom assisted by nursing or paramedical personnel.

The fee-for-service is the dominant payment system for general practitioners and medical specialists outside the Belgian hospitals. Even specialists who work full-time in hospitals earn their incomes from individual patient fees rather than from salaries. Methods of payment to hospital specialists often employ a mixture of different compensation forms, arranged by the physicians themselves. By pooling the patient fees they receive a lump sum plus a variable amount per service, after a deduction of hospital costs that cover the use or hiring of equipment and facilities.

Though a number of different payment systems exist, little is known of them because they are negotiated in each case between the medical staff and the hospital. Capitation payments do not exist. The amount of the fee is decided upon between physician and patient; however, this freedom has been limited through the health insurance system. Fees for general practitioners and specialists are calculated on the basis of a schedule of medical services (nomenclature).

Private group practice is rare in Belgium, though there is an increasing number of partnerships among general practitioners in which each practitioner serves his or her own patients individually and receives a fee for that service. In addition, there are about forty group practices with pooling of fees and shared ancillary personnel. Collaboration between general practitioners and other health personnel is hindered by the legal prohibition of splitting fees (called "dichotomy"). With the exception of France, Belgium is probably the only western European country where the legal position of physicians has been regulated in detail by the legislature. In 1967, after years of tenacious relations between the Belgian government and the medical associations, the physicians succeeded in forcing the government to enact a law on the practice of medicine. This law contains a number of prescriptions that in other countries are part of medical ethics, such as the prohibition of fee splitting and the abuse of the diagnostic and therapeutic freedom of the physician vis-à-vis the patient. It reflects the liberal and individualistic ideas that were predominant at the time, and it is essential for an understanding of the main characteristics of medical practice in Belgium.

Also present to impede group practice is the health insurance system, which gives no special encouragement to this idea. No additional support is given for the larger number of ancillary personnel required to realize the efficiencies of medical grouping. According to Roemer, "One of the reasons for group practice—the coverage of a doctor's patients by his colleagues during times that he is away—is obviated through arrangments by the Order of Physicians for such coverage among individual practitioners in a community" (Roemer 1977, 8). Private grouping and sharing of certain facilities applies only to general practitioners. Medical specialists work together in providing ambulatory care in outpatient departments of hospitals or in the polyclinics of the sick funds, but not on a private basis.

General practitioners have no access to hospitals, although some minor exceptions do exist. Normal childbirths in a hospital may be attended by general practitioners; when surgery is required, the referring general practitioner may assist in the operating room.

Each practicing physician must enroll in the Order of Physicians. This organisation, established by law in 1938, exercises a considerable influence on Belgian medical practice because disenrollment bans a physician from practice. Its disciplinary boards—ten provincial councils and two councils of appeal—are composed totally (partially for the council of appeal) of physicians elected by their colleagues. The Order drafts a code of medical ethics that has to be approved by a royal decree to be binding. The draft produced in 1975 by the National Council of the Order was a reflection of the liberal and individual characteristics of medical practice in Belgium, focusing on the general duties of physicians, relations between physicians and third parties, the doctor in the service of the patient (quality of care, medical records, confidentiality, fees, and so on), and the doctor in the service of the community. Approval by royal decree was hard to obtain because of severe criticism from physicians, sick funds, and organizations of hospitals and patients. Important criticisms of the draft are that it inhibits the introduction of new methods of paying the doctor (salary and capitation payment), neglects preventive medicine, and obstructs group practice. Nevertheless, the Belgian Supreme Court has already accepted the binding force of different articles of the draft.

Apart from and along with the Order of Physicians exist a number of medical associations with voluntary membership. Some are more unionlike; others are scientific organisations, such as the Association of Belgian Specialists and the Scientific Association of Flemish General Practitioners. The scientific associations have an important function in the licensure of medical specialists. (See "Medical Education" below). The "medical unions" influence medical practice because of their powerful position in the health insurance system. The agreements they conclude with the sickness funds do not only deal with the tariffs of medical care: they also cover the administrative formalities; the beginning and the duration, the notice and the renewal of agreements; limitations on the application of the agreed tariffs, supervision of compliance, and sanctions against breaches. The most important medical union is the Federation of Medical Unions, which, according to Glaser, behaves like a real union, "defending the economic interests of their members, influencing legislation about the economics and organisation of practice, and negotiating agreements with the sick funds and other public authorities" (Glaser 1978, 59). Membership figures are kept secret but are estimated at 6,000. Another, smaller association is the Generale Syndicate of Belgian Physicians. This body favors new forms of organisation to facilitate medical teamwork and promote comprehensive care. Many of its members are Flemish and are general practitioners, whereas French-speaking specialists are particularly numerous in the Federation. Membership figures of the Generale Syndicate are estimated at 2,000.

Through the election of members to the Order of Physicians' disciplinary councils, the

Federation has gained considerable influence in its professional field. In a number of cases physicians have been sanctioned by the Order because of their hostile attitude toward the Federation. Recently this abuse of public power by a private organisation has been severely criticized in Parliament.

In 1971 and 1972 the average Belgian physician worked 60 hours per week. Female physicians put in 49 hours per week; male physicians, 61 hours. Candidate specialists and general practitioners, with 65 and 62 hours respectively, had longer working weeks than did specialists with 58 hours. There was little variation of amount of working hours between the different specialties. However, only 71% of the working time, or 39 hours per week, was used directly for medical services, the rest being devoted to administrative and secretarial tasks (Deliège-Rott 1976, 63).

Different sources offer a variety of estimations of the average remuneration of physicians in Belgium. Based on data from the Christian Sick Fund, Deliège-Rott and other investigators have projected the annual income of physicians in 1972 to be between $38,100 and $40,600. For general practitioners the average gross remuneration was estimated at $24,000; for medical specialists, at $58,000. General practitioners earned substantially less than specialists, from 37% to 62%, according to various sources. Amount of extra income—that income above the basic level of fees from health insurance—is largely unknown. The net income usually amounts to 67% of the total gross.

The lack of a clear division of tasks and duties between general practitioners and medical specialists is characteristic of medical practice in Belgium. As a rule, general practitioners have no access to hospitals; nor is primary care their monopoly. There are no financial restraints against the direct access of patients to medical specialists. An act was passed in 1971 permitting the government to set rules for health insurance to promote cooperation among general practitioners and specialists for better organization; this act, however, has not been implemented. Referral from a general practitioner is not required in having the specialist's fee reimbursed by health insurance. As a result, general practitioners *and* medical specialists—especially paediatricians, gynaecologists, and ophthalmologists, working in what is known as the "popular specialties"—provide primary care. The government's attempt in 1979 to introduce an obligatory referral from a general practitioner to a specialist provoked a "medical strike." The principle of free choice of physician by the patient, be it a general practitioner or a medical specialist, still prevails.

Due to the high ratio of physicians to population there are no widespread practitioner shortages—geographical or functional. Physicians are entirely free to choose where they practice. There are no restrictions or financial or other incentives to establish in certain regions. This is not to say, however, that there are no problems. The unequal geographical distribution of physicians around the country is related to socio-cultural and demographical variables, as well as to economic factors. For instance, in 1979 there was one medical specialist to 4,414 population in the arrondissement of Maaseik (a province of Limburg), while in Ghent there was one to a 1,065 population. In the suburbs of Brussels, where more than 60% of the population are immigrants (Maroccans, Turks, etc.) there does exist a severe shortage of general practitioners and "popular specialists."

A person in Belgium in need of some kind of health care either goes to a physician's office or calls a physician. The majority of general practitioners do not have an appointment system; they do more home visits than office consultations. A patient's waiting time is seldom more than a few hours. Emergency care can also be received immediately. A single telephone number (900) is established throughout Belgium for summoning an ambulance, the police, the fire brigade, or other forms of emergency service. There is a tendency to go directly to hospital emergency services during the night and weekends.

Access to hospital care is closely related to the health insurance system. To gain admission into a hospital, a "prior authorization" of the health insurance physician is required except in emergencies. In practice this is given automatically.

BELGIAN HOSPITALS

General

A distinction is usually made between five categories of hospitals: acute general hospitals, geriatric hospitals, special hospitals, psychiatric hospitals, and sanatoriums. University hospitals, or teaching hospitals, are accredited as such; they differ from general hospitals in that they do medical research and are responsible for both basic and specialist training of doctors.

Access to hospital care is basically similar for all hospitals; the sponsors are the same and in all cases payment is the responsibility of health insurance, government, and patient. In all there are 92,000 beds, of which 53,500 are in acute general hospitals. (All figures refer to the 1980 year, unless stated otherwise.) Per 1,000 population there are 9.3 and 5.4 beds respectively. The beds are unevenly distributed over the country; Brussels, for example, has 7.2 acute general beds per 1,000 population, whereas Wallonia has only 4.9.

The average Belgian hospital has only 179 beds. Acute general hospitals are a bit larger, having 186 beds on the average, while psychiatric hospitals are much larger, with an average of 322 beds. Very few hospitals actually have over 1,000 beds. The large majority of hospital beds are found in private, nonprofit hospitals (63% of all beds), mainly belonging to religious orders. With only a few exceptions, public hospitals are municipal establishments.

Legislation on hospitals was first passed by Parliament in 1963. Several specific laws have been voted on since then, all aiming at four objectives: (1) improved quality of hospital equipment; (2) free treatment for patients who benefit from health insurance, provided they are treated in a common room (over two beds); (3) a solution to the troubled financial situation of both private and public hospitals; and (4) the introduction of adequate hospital planning. Not all of these objectives have been realised. Although provisions have been made to remedy the financial situation and to plan hospitals in a much more restrictive way, it seems fair to say that only the first objective was met—and perhaps that too well.

Accreditation

Each of the eighteen departments in hospitals must be accredited by the health minister upon advice from the National Hospital Council. Belgium is presently divided into three regions (Flanders, Wallonia, and Brussels), which leads to a division of powers; therefore, accreditation has become a regional matter, based upon norms of an architectural, organisational, and functional nature. Norms differ according to the "level" at which hospitals function: "common" hospital departments, those that adhere to specific higher norms, or university hospital departments. Thus far, hospitals function at either a first (common) or a third (university) level.

Departments are accredited for six years. Those that are not accredited are closed, either immediately or after some time, definitely or temporarily. However, this seldom happens if it happens at all. As indicated, accreditation is, amongst other things, based upon architectural norms. Consequently, there is a rather strict control on patient accommodation in hospitals. The norms are very detailed, prescribing the full accommodation and equipment of rooms and wards. It is now common to construct or reconstruct hospital floors that consist of private, two-bed, and four-bed rooms (sometimes rooms are built to hold six beds). Larger wards do not exist anymore. Any patient can ask to be hospitalised in a private room, though availability and added cost come into play here.

Financing

Each hospital is responsible for its own management and financial administration. A uniform accounting system, which must show the costs of each hospital department, is imposed on all establishments.

Investments

The national government will finance up to 60% of construction or reconstruction costs, as well as the expense of medical equipment, on condition that the hospital is either a public or private *nonprofit* institution and that construction or reconstruction fits the hospital plan. The remainder must be paid by the hospital, and this is usually accomplished by loans. The government's financial contribution is provided through a special government fund, which was created in 1973 for just this purpose. The fund is now said to be the motor for excessive construction programs.

Operating Costs

Operating costs are split into three groups: day costs; medical and paramedical fees; and costs of pharmaceuticals—drugs not manufactured by the hospital itself.

The day price is fixed for each hospital department and according to each level (see "Accreditation" above). It is a lump sum, covering all day costs in a ward (more than two beds). However, any day price is composed of the same elements: depreciation; financial charges; general expenses; maintenance, heating, administrative, laundry, and catering costs; and some drug costs.

Because it is fixed for treatment in a ward, the day cost does not fully cover costs accrued in a private room (unless the doctor requires such a room for medical reasons) or in a two-bed room. Free treatment, therefore, is only guaranteed under specific conditions. However, the hospital bill does not include medical and paramedical fees nor the costs for all drugs, and these payments must all be met separately. For a number of years now it has also been government policy to have patients pay part of the so-called hotel costs.

The large majority of the Belgian population is covered by health insurance. Consequently, sickness funds pay the hospitals directly on behalf of their patients, leaving it to the patient to cover the extras (private room, medical and paramedical fees, drugs). The costs for drugs and fees, however, are also partially reimbursed, which means that the patient pays only a small percentage of total costs.

To facilitate payment by sickness funds, the day price per department is transformed into a price per hospital, based upon the number of bed days per department. This individual hospital day price can be modified in light of special situations (costs) of a particular hospital. Decisions are made by the national minister of health. University hospitals in general benefit from a higher day price. Under the limitations detailed above, 75% of the day price is covered by health insurance and 25% by the health minister.

Planning

Since 1973 no hospital or department can be constructed or reconstructed, nor can the number of beds be changed, unless this fits the hospital plan. One national and three regional hospital planning commissions advise the minister of health on matters like planning criteria, infrastructure and equipment of hospitals, and construction, reconstruction, and expansion of hospitals, as well as their role within the hospital plan. The health minister sets the criteria for planning and in so doing takes into account population needs, demography, morbidity, geographical distribution, sound management needs, the existence of other health care provisions, and the ratio of beds in public and private hospitals. As a result of planning, the law fixes the number of beds in academic and nonacademic hospitals, as well as dealing with matters relating to the proliferation of heavy medical equipment.

The National Hospital Council represents hospital owners, doctors, and nurses and advises the minister of health in most decisions concerning the organisation, management, planning, financing, and equipment of hospitals.

Access to Hospital Care

The patient may go to his or her family doctor, to a private specialist, to an outpatient department, or to an emergency service for hospital admission. Generally, it is the family doctor or the private specialist who makes the decision to send the patient to a hospital. A large number of patients enter the hospital through the emergency service. As a rule it is the hospital doctor who makes the decision to admit, in both public and private institutions. The Belgian health care system is thus structured in such a way that a patient (or a doctor) can request admission at any acute general, university, special, public, or private hospital. Legally and structurally, there is nothing to prevent a patient from going to the hospital of his or her choice.

In fact, a number of patients do profit from this possibility and go, for example, to an expensive teaching hospital when an acute general hospital would have been at least as appropriate. The majority of doctors and patients, though, select hospitals on the basis of distance. Also, many patients do not take into account whether or not the hospital they choose is public or private.

Most patients do not have to wait before admission; Belgian hospitals, generally speaking, do not operate on the basis of long waiting lists. However, some categories of patients (for example, those involved in renal dialysis and heart surgery) have problems in being immediately admitted to the hospital. Moreover, only a small number of hospitals provide highly specialised services, and patients, therefore, may not be able to go to the nearest hospital. Indeed, important barriers to hospital care are the unequal distribution of facilities throughout the country and the lack of adequate information, which, obviously, is more difficult to overcome for the less developed strata of the population.

Cost Containment

Several reasons for rising hospital costs can be identified. The first is of a general nature and no doubt applies to most if not all the industrialised countries: overall costs (maintenance, electricity, and heating, for example) are going up all the time. Wages in Belgium are among the highest in the world, and this, together with the growing cohort of highly qualified personnel, causes enormous financial problems for the health care sector. Rising costs are also linked to the overall health care system: social insurance and sick insurance in particular are in critical financial states. It has become clear that the Belgian health insurance scheme is unable to bear the costs. This situation has at least two consequences: first, reimbursement is kept at a lower level than real costs and, second, hospitals are reimbursed too late, which forces them to borrow or rent money under very unattractive conditions.

Yet another reason for rising costs is found in the development of medicine and in the doctor's behavior. On one hand, treatment is now available in a number of cases where a few years ago hospital care was useless; the cases being treated now often cause extra costs. On the other hand, Belgian doctors seem to prescribe more drugs than doctors in many other countries. In addition, it is commonly believed that medical examinations, either in private practice or in another hospital, cannot be trusted the first time and therefore must be carried out again. One consequence is an overproduction of technical and laboratory examinations; another is the purchase of extra medical equipment.

Demographic and medical factors also figure into rising costs. Belgium's constantly growing population of elderly people means that more demand will be made for access to hospital care. The growing demand has created a larger supply of beds and equipment. The average length of stay has dropped and the average occupancy rate has improved (although not enough), but the result is still more beds.

To correct this situation the government intends to tackle at least some of the problems. Within the Belgian health care system it seems that two factors can be "manipulated": financing and planning.

Efforts have been made to change the health insurance system and to replace it with a scheme less favorable to the patient. Possible solutions are to raise the overall income of the scheme (for example, through taxation) and/or to raise the personal contribution of the patient. It seems that the system will be unable to cover all or even most of the expenses of the patients: more selective procedures, such as taking into account the financial status of the patient, seem to be indicated.

The direct financing of the hospitals should also be questioned. Because of existing legislation, hospitals can claim a higher reimbursement when they can prove that receipts and expenditures are unbalanced. Although there is rather strict control (at least officially), the situation seems to have deteriorated: higher reimbursement has become a reward for bad mangement. To solve this problem modifications of the system should be far-reaching. We cannot help but question the fact that in one hospital the average length of stay is more than twice as long as in another hospital, yet, nothing prevents health insurance from paying the costs on both scenes.

Planning, of course, enters the picture as a second major vehicle for rationalization and cost-containment. Too many of Belgium's overabundant supply of hospital beds are not occupied. This is an area for possible cutdown in investment and running costs. If this was actually done—if the supply or offer was reduced—and if this was accompanied by better control on medical care patterns (introduction of medical audit) and by a stricter control of money spending, costs could be contained.

Another possibility is often seen as the magic solution: a shift from inpatient to outpatient care. An important shift like this, however, is likely to increase the costs of hospital care. It remains to be seen whether the overall health care costs would be contained.

The present situation clearly provides an opportunity for fewer medical and technical examinations (the latter being more severely controlled) and fewer drug prescriptions, without hindering the overall health care status of the population.

Conclusion

As with many other hospital schemes in the Western world, the Belgian system is a mixture of autonomy and control. Hospital policies are set by the national and regional governments, but trustees have sufficient autonomy and freedom to innovate. Any innovations, however, must be approved by the government simply because any innovation will be paid for by that body; still, even if no costs are involved, innovation must fit the hospital plan.

We should not conclude that such an approach would end competition among hospitals; an upward spiral can be seen pushing one hospital's trustees to offer the same services as the hospital next door. Central and regional administrations are often not strong enough to resist pressure, and good relations seem as important as good dossiers. Unneccessary admissions, procedures, and medications are known to exist and have at least partially been identified. However, real control, let alone real punishment, is absent.

MEDICAL EDUCATION

The history of medical education in Belgium is comparable to that of other Western European countries. In the 17th century and after, medical practice was mainly exercised by two professional groups: the physicians, trained at a university and competent in internal medicine, and the surgeons, less respected and trained by practice. During the French Revolution all universities, including the medical schools, were abolished. By decrees of 2 and 17 March 1781 the freedom for anyone to practice medicine was proclaimed. Supervision of medical practice was abolished, and a new type of practitioner, the officer of health, replaced the prerevolutionary physician. The resulting chaotic situation, however, did not last for long, and the medical schools soon reopened their doors. In 1816 three state universities with medical schools were established in Ghent, Leuven, and Liège. A decree in 1818 abolished the health officers and created a number of paramedical rolls, apart from the medical profession; it also restricted the simultaneous practice of medicine, surgery, obstetrics, and pharmacy. The 1835 law on higher education required a university diploma for the practice of medicine, surgery, and obstetrics. However, these three branches remained separate. It was not until 1849 that a law created the unified diploma for doctors that remains unchanged today. This unification has been influenced more by external than internal pressures. As Glaser (1978, 58) states: "Belgium has had professional associations and scientific societies in medicine, but the customs of localism and the doctors' antipathy to dues have prevented the organizations from acquiring the large nationwide scale and the multiple functions common in other countries." It was not until 1863 that a national organisation of Belgian physicians, the General Physicians' Association, was formed. It has never become a strong organisation, internal conflicts dividing it from the first years onwards.

Undergraduate Education

In Belgium the normal course of medical studies lasts seven years. These studies are divided into two cycles: the first, lasting three years, comprises basic scientific education ("candidature"); the second, spanning four years, includes three years of clinical studies and one of practical training in a hospital ("doctorat"). There are presently seven medical schools and four university institutions for the basic training cycle. Two of the medical schools, Ghent and Liège, are part of a state university; the others are privately owned, except Antwerp and Diepenbeek, which are mixed in character. During the academic year 1976–77 there were 19,606 medical students, of whom 3,443 were foreigners. That same year, 3,939 students began medical studies; 901 were foreign students, the large majority (725) of whom studied at one of the French-speaking universities.

The only condition required for admisson to a medical school is the possession of the "maturity diploma," the diploma of completion of secondary studies. This is usually obtained at the age of 18 years. All medical schools have open enrollments—all applicants who meet the requirements are admitted. According to Roemer (1977, 33), "the rationale for the Belgian system of open medical school admission is the view that everyone has a right to study medicine." Another reason for the open admission, however, is the impossibility of reaching agreement on the practical modalities of a "numerus clausus"; for instance, the competition between the different medical schools inhibits an agreement on the number of students each faculty may admit. Moreover, state subsidy is determined according to the number of students enrolled. There is, therefore, no incentive for a self-imposed restriction of students. Finally, politicians are unwilling or unable to alter the existing situation. In late 1980 a bill was introduced to limit subsidies for medical schools to 80% of the students enrolled in previous years. Clearly, the government hoped this action would indirectly limit the number of medical students; however, the bill has never been approved by the Belgian Parliament.

The pursuit of medical studies from the first year onward is only limited by failures in successive examinations. Actually, there is a fairly high attrition rate at the start—as many as 50% at the end of the first year and 25% a year later—but few failures in subsequent years.

Students are legally permitted to sit as many times as they want; however, the university does not receive subsidy for students who failed more than twice in the same year. Private medical schools, Leuven, for example, refuse these students. State medical schools are obliged by law to accept them.

The exam for the grade of candidate in medical sciences covers nine different branches of study: experimental physics, chemistry, biology, embryology, anatomy, dermatology, physiology, biochemistry, and psychology. These nine must be spread over at least three school years. The medical schools have a certain autonomy in programming the different branches, and may add other subjects, such as logic and medical sociology. During these 3 years, there is no contact with patients.

Graduate Education

The exam for the grade of doctor in medicine, surgery, and obstetrics covers fifteen different subjects, spread over at least four years of study. During the last year (the seventh year of study) practical hospital work must be done. This is the "internship," normally served in smaller, regional hospitals (CREMEL, or complementary regional medical centers). The medical schools have a certain autonomy in programming the different subjects; for instance, the internship for the Leuven medical school is not in the seventh but in the sixth year. In the seventh year the possibility exists to specialise. There are four options of specialised training: family medicine, medical specialties, research, and social medicine. The option in family medicine consists of a two-month preceptorship with a general practitioner, one week's experience in a group practice, sixty hours of seminars on problems related to group practice, and rotating activities in a few hospital departments. About 40% of the students choose the family medicine option. Other Belgian universities (Brussels, Antwerp, and Ghent) are promoting the teaching of general practice. It can be questioned, however, whether this university training adequately equips a general practitioner for cooperation in work concerning the early detection and the prevention of disease, the supervision of the chronically sick, and other problems.

Moreover, since the general practitioner is on the lowest payment level for visits and consultations, there is little time and money to spare for his or her continuing education. Therefore, it is recognized that the training of these physicians should be reorganised. In the future this may become a legal obligation for Belgium, following a directive of the European Economic Community (EEC).

Postgraduate and Continuing Education

In Belgium there exists no legal obligation for specialisation or continuing medical education. The diploma of doctor in medicine, surgery, and obstetrics entitles a physician to practice medicine during his or her total professional career. However, the health insurance system, through the payment of higher fees, promotes specialisation.

The licensing process is difficult to describe because it is partly based on legislation and partly on practical experience. Three different parties are involved: the minister of health, the scientific organisation of specialists, and the medical schools.

In 1978 the process of specialisation underwent a fundamental revision to bring it into line with a directive of the EEC. It now resembles the Dutch system—that is, it is entirely privately initiated. Since 1978 specialisation has been restricted to a very limited number of candidates. To be eligible for specialisation an individual has to submit a training plan indicating the name of a trainer with whom one wants to specialise and the training center where one wants to work, together with the agreement of the trainer and the training center named. This plan must be approved by a specialisation committee, because without approval one cannot be licensed as a specialist. There are twenty-five specialisation committees, one for every medical specialty. Each committee has two chambers: a Flemish- and a French-speaking one. The chambers consist of eight members: four representatives of the medical schools and four of the professional societies. Thus, the decision whether someone may specialise is completely up to the medical specialists, who ultimately decide on the total number of specialists. The government does not interfere.

Also since 1978 specialty training has been a privilege of trainers and training centers, licensed for this purpose by the health ministry. In general, only university hospitals and professors are licensed as trainers and training centers, although there are exceptions. The minister of health is advised by the High Council of Medical Specialists. For each specialty the minister also determines the training criteria, for example, the length of the specialty training.

For purposes of reimbursement under the insurance system there exist postgraduate training opportunities for general practitioners. Those general practitioners who obtain 200 hours of credit are entitled to charge higher insurance fees. The training courses must be applicable to general practice; a syllabus is required for each course; and there has to be opportunity for discussion. Courses organised by professional societies must be offered in collaboration with one or more medical schools.

Foreign Medical Graduates

In June 1975 the ministers of health of the EEC member states agreed on a directive that clearly states the mutual recognition of the medical doctor's diploma. Further, the specialist's certificates or titles are recognized in those countries where the specialty exists. Member states are bound to accept foreign diplomas and certificates as right of access to medical activities without any further check of knowledge. The right to free establishment for physicians in the member states of the EEC entered into force on 1 January 1977. Graduates of medical schools of non-European Economic Community countries may be authorized to practice in Belgium under agreements for reciprocity.

NURSES, PHYSICIAN ASSISTANTS, AND HEALTH PRACTITIONERS

Nurses

Since the 1974 act on nursing, the profession of and the diploma for nursing are legally protected: no one is permitted to practice who is not properly qualified and registered.

Before enactment of this legislation, only the title of "nurse" was protected. Registration is handled by the provincial medical commissions (see "Public Helath" below). Neither these commissions nor any other comparable body have disciplinary powers over nurses. There is a variety of qualifications that entitle one to practice nursing: the diploma of graduated nurse, or higher level nurse; the diploma of certificated nurse, or second level nurse; and the certificate of hospital assistant.

The diploma of graduated, or higher level, nurse takes three years after secondary school. There are four specialties in this classification: hospital, pediatric, and psychiatric nurse, and social nurse. For social nursing an additional year of training is required. The first two years of study are the same for all specialties. In 1977 fifty schools in Belgium awarded the diploma of graduated nurse. During the 1977–78 school year, 4,362 were enrolled for the first year of study, 3,441 females and 921 males; in that same year 2,896 followed the courses of the second year, 2,329 females and 567 males. Almost two thousand students had chosen the hospital nurse option. In 1976–77, 1,477 students obtained the diploma of graduated nurse, 1,240 female and 237 males.

The educational program for the second level, or certificated, nurse consists of two years of training which leads to the certificate of hospital assistant. At the end of these two years the students may begin to work or may continue for an additional year with theoretical and practical studies, after which the diploma of certificated nurse can be obtained. There are two specialties: the general hospital nurse and the psychiatric nurse. In 1977 there were sixty-seven schools for training certificated nurses and hospital assistants. That same year about 4,500 nursing diplomas or certificates were awarded.

Professional organisations pay great attention to postgraduate and continuing education for nurses. The Center for Postgraduate Education for Nurses organises courses for learning to become a head nurse or a nursing teacher. These courses are conducted on a part-time basis, three days a month covering two years while the students are employed full time. Every year the professional association of Catholic nurses organises a "Nursing Week," with a separate program for every specialty in nursing. The program is financed through fees paid by each participant and a subsidy from the ministry of health.

The training of nurses and the practice of nursing are now in transition. The relations between the medical and the nursing professions have to be defined more clearly. In hospitals, nurses are performing functions that actually are medical functions—such as immunizations, injections, and blood pressure readings—though they are not legally permitted to do this. The Act on Nursing of 1974 had been intended to define medical practice and nursing. By giving a definition of nursing, and through the implementation of long lists of medical services that can be performed by nurses under certain conditions, the legislature had hoped to give nurses a professional status. These lists of medical services must be approved by a royal decree, after advice of a commission that is equally composed of physicians and nurses. In 1977 unanimous advice was given by this commission, but royal approval is still lacking. Therefore, nurses are now working under illegal conditions in Belgium and still are an "extension of the arm" of the physicians.

The total number of nurses is, of course, not known. Statistics tell that in 1977 there would have been 17,480 graduated and certificated nurses and 5,025 hospital assistants. These figures only include nurses working in hospitals.

A directive of the Council of Ministers of the European Economic Community has proclaimed the freedom of establishment for nurses responsible for general care throughout the member states. Hospital assistants, however, cannot profit from this emancipation.

Allied Health Personnel

In Belgium a distinction is made between the paramedical professions, which are authorized to provide supportive services linked to diagnosis or treatment, and the medical auxiliaries, who are authorized to perform, under the control of the doctor, certain acts preparatory to diagnosis or related to the application of treatment. At his or her own responsibility a physician may authorise a paramedical to execute acts that involve technical innovation and require no separate judgment but rather precise execution. Enumeration of these acts must meet approval by royal decree—which has not happened up to now. As a result, these paramedical professions work, as do nurses, mostly in illegal circumstances. Ancillary services, which do not relate to medical practice, can be performed by paramedicals on their own responsibility. Clinical laboratory technology, physical, occupational, and speech therapy, audiology, and dietetics are all examples of paramedical professions.

Medical auxiliaries, such as dental and pharmaceutical assistants, are viewed as an extension of the physician. Actually, the difference between paramedical professions and medical auxiliaries is very difficult to define. The most important paramedical professionals are the physical, or rehabilitation, therapists. There exist two different diplomas: the first is obtained through a three-year program after secondary school, the second after a four-year university program. Until now internal conflicts between those two groups have impeded the development of a clear legal status for physical therapists. Their number has been growing very fast in recent years. In 1970 they totalled 4,683; in 1977 this count had almost doubled to 8,987.

NURSING HOMES AND COMMUNITY HEALTH AGENCIES

A distinction can be made between home care and long-term-care facilities. Nursing homes in the common sense of the terms do not exist.

Home Care

Home care in Belgium remains underdeveloped despite all kinds of efforts for change. For over thirty years organisations providing home care have profited from government allowances and patients cared for at home by nurses or nursing aides have been reimbursed by sickness funds. (Doctors' fees are always partially reimbursed, as has been indicated.) Home care is provided mainly through municipal services, sickness funds, and a large private, nonprofit home-care organisation; it is either community-based or hospital-based. For over two years now home care legislation has been advocated as a means for reducing overall health care costs. This drive has not been more successful, though, because of the large offer (supply) of doctors and of inpatient care, almost always within a few miles or minutes of the patient's residence.

Long-Term-Care Facilities

In addition to geriatric hospitals, long-term-care facilities consist of departments within the general hospitals, rest homes, day or night centres, and service centres.

The legislation and all regulations that apply to hospitals in general also apply to the special departments within the institutions. Geriatric departments for long-term care (which are open to all patients, not only to the older ones) are planned to provide 1.5 beds per 1,000 population.

Rest homes provide lodging, including full or partial family care, to people over sixty years of age. In theory rest homes are meant for healthy elderly people; in practice the majority of the inmates are sick. This was recognized in 1971 when a bill was passed to modify the conditions for subsidies, and since 1978 rest homes can be reimbursed by the sickness funds. Like hospitals, rest homes must be accredited by the minister of health; accreditation is based upon specific criteria concerning the building, the personnel, and the overall care of the "patient." However, almost 50% of all rest homes are not accredited, perhaps because of the severe rules for fire security.

Day or night centres are still in an experimental stage. Financial problems are of paramount importance, since these centres are neither subsidised nor reimbursed in any way.

Service centres offer provisions of a material, social, hygienic, cultural, and recreational nature to elderly people. Construction, reconstruction, and the equipment of such centres can be subsidised only when they fit the appropriate planning.

HEALTH INSURANCE

Health insurance undoubtedly is one of the key factors of the Belgian health care scene. Sickness and invalidity insurance is compulsory and, as such, is the major financial element in the provision of health care.

Beneficiaries

A distinction should be made between different classes of beneficiaries. "Beneficiaries of health benefits and cash benefits" are employed persons, apprentices, handicapped persons, domestic servants, and some persons in public service. "Beneficiaries of the sole health benefits" are mostly members of the clergy and of religious communities, most public servants, some handicapped persons, and students of the higher education. "Beneficiaries of cash benefits and of some health benefits" (considered heavy risks) are usually self-employed persons and former colonists. "Beneficiaries of some health benefits" (also considered heavy risks) are some self-employed persons and some members of religious communities.

Health Benefits Insurance

The aim of the health benefits insurance is to ensure payment for medical care, dental treatment, hospital and sanatorium treatment, and maternity assistance. Health benefits include preventive as well as curative care and comprehend: ordinary medical care (visits by, and consultations of, general practitioners and specialists; care provided by nurses, attendants, and sick nurses; care provided by physiotherapists; technical assistance for diagnosis and treatment not requiring the qualification of a specialist; dental care, preventive as well as corrective, including dental prostheses); confinements; benefits requiring a special recognized qualification of specialist, chemist or bachelor of science; supply of glasses and other prostheses for the eyes, hearing aides, orthopaedic appliances, and other prostheses; supply of pharmaceutical products, including magistral preparations (drugs compounded by the pharmacist) and pharmaceutical specialties; treatment of mental illnesses, tuberculosis, cancer, poliomyelitis, and congenital ailments and malformations; hospitalization for observation and treatment; benefits for functional and vocational rehabilitation; admission as a preventive measure against tuberculosis, in preventoriums and in homes for weak children, and as, specifically, childrens' protection against tuberculosis, in day nurseries, in protection homes, or in families; travelling expenses of those patients admitted into a pulmonary tuberculosis sanatorium or treated as ambulatory patients in anticancer centres.

The insurance refund for ordinary medical care amounts to 75% of the fees (100% for entitled widows, orphans, pensioners, and invalids with income not exceeding an annual ceiling amount, and for their dependants). For most of the benefits referred to above the refund equals 100% of the fees; however, part of the costs for pharmaceuticals is always charged to the beneficiary; hospitalization for observation and treatment is paid for by health insurance, government, and the patient; and admission (as described) and travelling expenses are refunded as the minister for social affairs determines.

Self-employed persons do not enjoy the same benefits; they are reimbursed for what are usually called "heavy risks." The following risks are covered: treatment of mental illnesses, tuberculosis, cancer, poliomyelitis, and congenital ailments and malformations; medical and obstetrical care relating to confinement; hospitalization for observation and treatment; drugs administered during a stay in a hospital; surgery of a given financial value; anaesthetics relating to the surgery; reanimation as enumerated under article 13 of the above-mentioned royal regulation of 16 November 1973; general special care enumerated under article 11 of the same royal regulation; radiodiagnostics; radio- and radiumtherapy; internal medicine; clinical biology; surveillance of entitled inpatients; supplementary fees for urgent technical care, administered during the night or the weekend or on a holiday; hemodialysis at home; some functional and vocational rehabilitation benefits. The amount of the reimbursement is equal to that for the insured under the general scheme described above.

Cash Benefits Insurance

The initial incapacity insurance protects the workers against the pecuniary consequences of accidents and sickness, pregnancy, and confinement; however, accidents at work, those involving the liability of a third party, and those resulting from a serious fault committed by the insured person are excluded. In the case of incapacity for work, the beneficiary is entitled to an allowance amounting to as much as 60% of the limited daily remuneration. Employers often pay the difference between 60% and the normal salary. Allowances are paid for a maximum period of one year. In the case of pregnancy and confinement, the allowance equals 60% of the limited daily remuneration, during fourteen weeks.

The invalidity insurance ensures the employed person against the pecuniary consequence of a long-term incapacity to work. The right to an invalidity allowance is obtained when the initial incapacity for work has reached one year. Allowances amount to 65% of the daily (ceiled) remuneration for persons with, and to 43.5% for persons without, dependants.

Conditions to Qualify for Benefits

To receive the benefits of the sickness and invalidity insurance for oneself and one's dependants, the insured person must fulfill three general and essential conditions: (1) join an insurance body—the person must join one of the recognized sickness funds; (2) regularly submit contribution vouchers—to be entitled to benefit, the insured is required to pay, in due time, a sufficient contribution; (3) fulfill the qualifying period—the insured person must have worked during a set period for a minimum number of days and submit, for this period, contribution vouchers that reach a minimum value (if necessary, through additional personal contributions).

Financing

There are six national sickness funds in Belgium which are supervised by, and get their funds from, the National Institute for Sickness and Invalidity Insurance (INAMI). The INAMI, though a government agency, is controlled by a board of directors broadly representative of Belgian society. Its funds come from: (1) contributions from employers and employees, paid for "health benefits" as well as for "cash benefits," including the payments due employees who are victims of an accident at work or of an occupational disease; (2) personal contributions paid by some entitled persons (mainly the self-employed); (3) the proceeds of the deduction of 1.5% from the retirement and survivors' pensions in the public branch; (4) state subsidies; (5) gifts and legacies; and (6) the proceeds of a supplementary contribution or premium of the compulsory insurance for civil liability for motor cars.

Relations with Health Benefits Suppliers

Relations with suppliers of health benefits are settled through conventions and agreements.

The conventions concern the hospitals and nursing homes, and the chemists, midwives, nurses, physiotherapists, suppliers of prostheses and appliances, and all persons providing benefits to the insured persons, with the exception of physicians and dentists. The conventions rule the financial and administrative relations between the beneficiaries and the insurance bodies, and those between the beneficiaries and the above-mentioned suppliers of health benefits. They are concluded on a national level, after negotiation within the Department for Health, by standing commissions in which all sides are equally represented. When national conventions do not exist, regional conventions can be concluded. The terms of the conventions vary according to the category of insurance auxiliaries concerned.

(1) For midwives, nurses, physiotherapists, and suppliers of prostheses and appliances, the conventions determine the amounts of the fees and prices and of the travelling expenses for visits or benefits provided at the home of the patient; they may contain clauses dealing with straight payment (third paying party) of fees and prices for expensive supplies, and lay down special conditions for persons with high incomes as well as for those persons who may obtain a partial dispensation of the payment of the cost of the benefit.

(2) The convention with the hospitals recapitulates and explains the applicable provisions of the Hospital Act: it sets the rate of the daily maintenance cost for the establishments not referred to in the Act and outlines matters relating to the required notice to the insurance bodies of hospitalization and length of stay, as well as of the obligations of the insurance bodies, such as the prompt payment of bills and the sanctions if the terms of the Act have not been respected.

The convention sets the charge for a private room in the hospitals to which the Hospitals Act does not apply. The convention contains the commitment of these establishments to adhere, for the beneficiaries of the insurance, to the daily maintenance cost rate fixed for each of them.

(3) The convention with the pharmacists sets the amount of the fee for magistral preparations and lays down the rules concerning the "responsibility fees" for supply of pharmaceutical specialties, the terms and conditions of the third payer scheme, the lump sum payment for drugs supplied to hospitalized patients, the preferential fees for magistral prescriptions for the privileged categories (widows, orphans, and disabled and retired persons), and the special conditions for benefits supplied to persons with high incomes.

The agreements concern the physicians and the dentists. They rule the relations between the professional organisations and the insurance bodies; they also usually direct the financial and administrative relations between physicians and dentists on the one hand, and the beneficiaries on the other. The agreements are negotiated on a national level, respectively, by a national commission of doctors and the representatives of the mutual insurance funds, and by a national commission of dentists and the representatives of the mutual insurance funds. Meetings are held in the Department of Health, and each commission is composed of an equal number of representatives from both sides.

The agreements lay down the fees applicable to the insurance beneficiaries, which the doctors and dentists are supposed to adhere to, as well as the circumstances under which the amount of these fees may be exceeded. For visits to or benefits supplied at the home of the patient, a lump sum is fixed for the travelling allowance the suppliers are allowed to charge to the beneficiaries. However, when a specialist or a dentist is called to the home of the patient by the practicing doctor, the agreement may provide for a kilometric allowance. Of course agreements do not, in any way, condition the freedom of care.

When conventions and agreements do not exist, the minister for social affairs may determine the maximum fees and prices.

HEALTH COSTS

The percentage distribution of health costs among the providers in 1978 was: hospital care 23%, doctors' fees 18%, drugs 19%, special care 22%, minor surgery 5%, dental care 3%, physiotherapy 4%, and all other costs 6%. The principal factors that make up health care costs and that are responsible for the increases are numerous. In 1976 and again in 1980, the Royal Commission for the reform of the health insurance indicated twelve key factors, which can be grouped into five categories.

Demography. The Belgian population as a whole is rapidly ageing—15% of the population is over 65—and older people are heavy consumers of health care. At the same time, the population has, in some aspects, dramatically changed its life style. This results in some new disease patterns and requires constant adaptation of the services offered. Such adaptations are often expensive.

Extension of health insurance. Between 1945 and 1974 the number of insured persons increased from 3.7 to 9.8 million. The increase, however, is not spread equally over all categories of the insured; the nonactive population has been growing more rapidly than the active population (63% versus 37%), which spawns some important financial problems. More people now seek more care, and they very often utilize more expensive care. Research has given ample indication that a higher standard of living leads to a demand for more specialized and more expensive care. Because almost the entire population is covered by health insurance, the cost of health care in Belgium has increased. A new trend recently emerged whereby people would go initially to their family doctor instead of to a specialist. It is not unlikely, though, that lower income groups, when their incomes increase, will still prefer a specialist and will only after some time "discover" the new trend. Meanwhile, the present health insurance scheme is being questioned: it has become common knowledge that more extensive insurance coverage opens the door for not necessarily more effective and efficient care, but certainly more expensive care. Awareness of this cause and effect situation might lead to an alternative and less comprehensive health insurance scheme.

Medical development. Medicine and technology have been developing rapidly, with the introduction of new techniques, new services, and new equipment. These developments have not been counterbalanced by a dramatic fall in the number of doctors' consultations, or hospital days, nor have they caused a similar drop in the length of hospital stays. The health status of the Belgian population—if one looks at it in terms of the number of visits and hospital days—has not improved over the last two decades.

The number of medical and paramedical personnel, as well as of hospital beds, has been increasing. The resulting higher costs of construction, and operating are primarily taken care of by the government. Some statistical data may illustrate this growth: (1) Between 1969 and 1979 the number of beds in acute general hospitals increased by 8,390 units; beds in geriatric hospitals increased from 2,100 to 9,900 in the same period. (2) Between 1970 and 1978 reimbursed hospital days increased by almost 3.5 million, the number of patients by over 330,000; the average length of stay decreased from 15 to 14 days; the total population remained almost stable. (3) Allowances from the minister of health amounted to 2.5 billion BF (Belgian franc) in 1970 and 11 billion BF in 1979; total hospital costs went from 10.7 billion BF in 1970 to 43.5 billion BF in 1979.

Observing this evolution, we cannot help but wonder how much longer this trend can go on.

Consumption of medical care. The above figures give a clear indication of some developments in consumption of care. Research has indicated that hospital care—which is among the most expensive care—is influenced by age, sex, morbidity, and social factors such as civil status, family size, nationality, and comprehensiveness of health insurance. Many of these factors are difficult, if not impossible, to influence; some, however, can be influenced either indirectly (size of family, for example) or directly (health insurance). Noting that the average length of stay is dramatically influenced by the particular hospital, we see an opportunity for direct action. Medical (but also hospital) behavior is important in this respect. Within a system that allows the patient to choose freely his or her doctor (either general practitioner or specialist) and hospital, and that permits the doctor to decide what kind of and how much care is appropriate, the doctor becomes the key factor in the distribution and consumption of care. The wisdom of maintaining the fee-for-service system might therefore be questioned. Overconsumption should be searched out, difficult as it is to identify. However, the consumption of at least some parts of the overall health care do raise questions about the behavior of both doctors and the populace. One will note, for example, that the expenses for drugs went from 4.6 billion BF in 1966, to 15.8 billion BF in 1975, and to more than 20 billion BF in 1979.

Price development. The development of prices highly influences the cost of health care: wages (which are so important in the hospital sector), construction, medical equipment, doctors' fees, and drugs are caught in an almost constant increase of the price per unit. The average price for a hospital day came to 340 BF in 1966 and to 2,440 BF in 1980 (4,200 in academic hospitals). Inflation reached 8% in 1981. As a result of the Royal Commission's work, some steps are now being taken to contain rising health care costs.

Hospital care being so expensive, it seems logical to reduce the number of admissions. This could be done by dropping the number of hospital beds to such a minimum that long waiting lists would replace normal admissions, leaving the hospital doctor to decide on prompt admissions. Such a dramatic operation has not yet been introduced and is unlikely to be adopted in the near future. The government has taken a different course.

In 1977 a bill was passed that promoted appropriate nonhospital care for the elderly and the chronically ill, either at home or in special institutions. Services for home care and institutions for the elderly were entitled to give complete care in order to reduce or prevent hospital stays. So far, there is no evidence that the provisions of the bill have had any real impact on hospital care.

Unless formal patterns of patient referral are imposed on doctors and hospitals, a shift from hospital care to outpatient or less expensive care in general is unlikely. It seems, therefore, necessary to tackle directly the average length of stay and the average occupancy. The government acts very slowly in this respect and seems to temporize a great deal.

Private medical care, both at the general practitioner and the specialist levels, is another important field of action. The National Institute for Sickness and Invalidity Insurance has introduced medical and nursing profiles, enabling it to identify or at least question possible overconsumption of care. The mechanism is rather simple: medical and nursing services (the latter only within outpatient care) require a document that is sent to the health insurance supplier, enabling the patient to be reimbursed. These documents state the name of the care provider, which allows the Institute to see what happens in a given medical practice. From the same source, the Institute can learn whether there is drug abuse or overconsumption of laboratory tests.

If offer (supply) and demand do influence one another, it becomes necessary to control the offer. Legislation has introduced coercive planning of hospital beds and expensive hospital equipment: the health minister must approve both any modification in the number of beds and the purchase of heavy expensive medical equipment.

Legislation has also produced an imposed regional distribution of pharmacists, and discussions on a similar approach for doctors have started. There is, however, no proof that control of the offer has in any way cut the expenses; for example, too many hospital owners have been able to get around the difficulties.

It appears that the easiest way to contain costs (or to increase income) is to have the insured person contribute to the expense of medical care. The principle of free hospital care, as explained above, has been abandoned; the government has decided that all patients must pay part of the fee from the first day of hospitalization. In addition, patients must also contribute to the costs of drugs and dental and medical care, inside and outside of the hospital. A real cut in the consumption of care cannot yet be seen; however, a serious increase of personal contributions is likely to be followed by a decrease in the consumption of care, particularly by the less-privileged groups in society. This mechanism must therefore be used with care, for it can easily lead to serious problems for the poor.

PUBLIC HEALTH

Administrative Organisation

National

The major administrative responsibility for health services in Belgium is carried by the ministry of public health and environmental hygiene, established in 1936. The functions of the ministry are, principally, the establishment of health standards for environmental hygiene, research, administration of subsidies, and the control of health services delivered by hospitals and other health care institutions. The direct provision of health services is only one limited task of the ministry, which also has responsibility for four psychiatric institutions.

The most important functions of the ministry are carried out by the office of the secretary-general and eight directorates. The office supervises and coordinates the different directorates and has direct responsibility for international relations; one part of it is the institute for hygiene and epidemiology; therefore, its duties include epidemiological research and technical supervision of the quality of drugs and alimentation.

The directorate of general services is concerned with personnel, financial accounts, legal affairs, statistics, and other administrative functions. The office of medical practice is responsible for the implementation of laws and regulations on the medical, nursing, and paramedical professions.

The directorate of public health supervises all aspects of environmental sanitation and the control of communicable diseases through inspections by officers of the ministry of health. It also performs the pharmaceutical inspection and is responsible for sanitary help and protection of civilians during calamities.

The directorate of social medicine assumes a wide range of preventive responsibilities, including health education, school and physical education, and medico-legal matters. The National Foundation for Child Welfare and the Belgian Red Cross are supervised by this directorate.

The important directorate of health care institutions is responsible for the licensure and planning of hospitals, nursing homes, and other medical institutions. It supervises both schools that train paramedical personnel and all mental health services. The hospital council, the national and regional hospital planning committees, and the fund for the building of hospitals fall within this directorate.

The directorate of social wellbeing supervises the institutions for handicapped and nursing homes. The three other directorates are of relatively minor importance.

Apart from the ministry of health, other national ministries having responsibilities for public health are: the ministry of labour, regarding occupational health; the ministry of social security, regarding health insurance; the ministry of economic affairs, for the price of drugs and pharmaceuticals; and the ministry of education, for the training of physicians.

Regional

In 1980 the Belgian constitutional structure underwent considerable change. Important functions were delegated by the national government toward the Dutch- and French-speaking communities. Ambulatory services and health care in institutions were transferred to newly created administrations at the regional level. However, there were important exceptions. Financing of overhead costs, health insurance, the rules concerning the planning of health services and the financing of hospital building and heavy medical equipment, national licensure criteria, and the establishment of criteria for the licensure of academic hospitals remain duties of the national ministry of health. Health education and preventive health care have also been delegated to the regional communities. The newly created administrations do not employ their own personnel; these employees are appointed by the national ministry of health, and have responsibility for implementing the regional functions. However, there are ministries for health care in each region.

Provincial

Each of the nine provinces has a provincial health officer, who represents the minister of health in the field of public hygiene and whose responsibilities include receiving reports and taking necessary actions in cases of acute communicable diseases, and registering births and deaths. He is also responsible for the administrative work of the provincial medical council.

A provincial pharmaceutical inspector conducts the inspection and approval of pharmacies and is responsible directly to the directorate of public health of the ministry. For inspection of alimentation, there is a provincial veterinarian.

In the principal town of every province exists a provincial medical council. This statutory agency has a general advisory function, and it may take any measure necessary to deal with contagious diseases. Its specific duties include controlling the authenticity of the diplomas of physicians, pharmacists, nurses, and the paramedical professions; supervising the practice of medicine, nursing, and paramedics; determining the need for arrangements to replace physicians during the nights and weekends; and supervising the results of these arrangements. In the event of a "medical strike" this task is of great importance. Each provincial medical council is composed of one president and one vice president (both physicians), two representatives each of the medical, dental, pharmaceutical, and veterinarial professions, two midwives, two nurses, and one representative of each paramedical profession.

Municipal

Local government has some responsibilities in health care. Besides performing traditional duties relating to environmental hygiene, the municipalities, especially the larger ones, may initiate health care services such as health centres in which maternal and child health clinics are conducted; they also administer medical examinations to school children, help run hospitals, and are responsible for nursing homes and schools for the training of nurses and paramedical personnel. Also at the municipal level are public centres for social wellbeing (OCMW) which are responsible for public hospitals and for emergency medical services in their communities.

Public Control of Health Care

The government (national, regional, provincial, and local) was a primary donor of all monies spent for health in 1975 (200 billion BF, or 5 billion US dollars); it was the source for 40% of it, the private sector contributed 37%, and the national institute for health insurance (RIZIV, a public but independent body) provided 23%. The national government subsidises 60% of building costs of hospitals and other health care institutions. The investment costs for "heavy medical" equipment—for example, CAT scanners—are even subsidised for 100%. The health insurance act obliges the national government to finance 27% of the health insurance budget; however, the government actually pays about 40%. These examples illustrate the important financial contribution of the state to the cost of health care provision.

There exists in Belgium a close relationship between the financing of services by the state, and the control it exercises on these services. The right of the state to plan the health care system could be regarded as a logical consequence of its obligation to provide health care to its citizens. This reasoning, however, is not accepted. In hospital planning, for example, the state had to pay, and still is paying, for the "privilege" of planning the hospital system, an opportunity granted by the private hospitals and the local governments, yielded only in exchange for large financial compensation. It is as though the autonomy of the hospital boards and the governors to decide on their own the location, capacity, and function of hospitals had been expropriated by the state and, therefore, large indemnities must be paid. Since 1973 there has been a certificate-of-need system for hospital building. Once the certificate is obtained, its owner is entitled to a guaranteed subsidy of 60% for the building costs. The operation of this subsidy fund is not subjected to the normal budgetary control of Parliament, meaning that there is very little parliamentary supervision of hospital planning even though the state had to grant large financial concessions to gain acceptance of the principle of compulsory hospital planning. The example of hospital planning is somewhat illustrative of the sometimes ambiguous role of the national government in health care.

The Belgian constitution, dating from 1831, does not contain any stipulation on the provision of health services. Social economic rights, such as the right to health care, are not incorporated into the constitution, although various attempts have been made in this direction. Nevertheless, the amount of legislation concerning the delivery of health services has been growing steadily in Belgium since the Second World War. Legislative authority is exercised collectively by the king, the Chamber of Representatives, and the Senate. Broadly speaking, the parliamentary legislative process falls into three stages: in the first, a bill is drafted and introduced in one of the chambers; in the second, a standing, or *ad hoc,* parliamentary committee discusses the bill extensively; finally, the bill is debated, passed or defeated, and sent to the other chamber in the third stage. Although members of parliament have the right to initiate legislation, there is a common trend towards minimizing parliament's legislative functions and increasing ministerial involvement in the originating of bills. Parliamentary legislation tends to take the form of a general framework, to be filled in with statutory regulations by the government. Since the state reform of 1980, the regional communities also have a decision-making capacity towards the delivery of health services. Each community has a community council, with directly elected members. These councils may issue decrees having the same force as an act adopted by the national parliament.

Public Health Agencies, Activities, and Services

The Belgian health care system is highly pluralistic. The provision of health services is not a privilege of private or public initiative, although most services have been privately initiated. As already mentioned, the national and provincial authorities do not provide services themselves, apart from some minor exceptions; at the municipal level, however, there have been public initiatives.

Historically, public health problems have been in the hands of local authorities. Today, it is still the mayor's responsibility to cope with most of the health questions—environmental hygiene and the like. However, as it became evident that the small municipalities were unable to cope with the health problems, due to lack of finances and technical ability, the central government took over most of them, such as the control of communicable diseases. Most of the traditional public health problems (water distribution, sewage, waste disposal, food and drug control), although still under local authorities, were taken over technically and financially by the ministry of interior and other ministries such as those of public works and agriculture and justice.

After the French Revolution, local authorities became responsible for hospital care. The twentieth century saw considerable development of private hospitals, mainly belonging to religious congregations, while municipal hospitals were transferred to the local public assistance boards. These boards are now known as public centres for social wellbeing. The legal task of the public centres for social wellbeing is very large. Each centre is governed by a council composed of representatives of every political party represented on the municipal council, and is free to take any initiative regarding health care it thinks fit.

Actually, very few public centers for social wellbeing have used their broad authority to establish health services other than hospitals. The lack of money and an ideological preference for private initiative can explain this.

The most important public health activities regarding preventive care are mother and child health care and school health. Preventive care for mother and child is delivered by local services that are licensed, subsidised, and, in some cases, initiated by the National Foundation for Child Wellfare. Founded as a statutory body in 1919, and with hundreds of local councils throughout Belgium, the Foundation operates several types of clinics and services for children and expectant mothers: sessions for routine preventive services to childen up to 3 years of age and infant welfare clinics where children in their first months of life are vaccinated; 1,200 clinics for more comprehensive care of children 3 to 6 years of age; and 344 prenatal clinics providing medico-social and obstretic supervision for expectant mothers and preparation for childbirth. The Foundation is 90% subsidized by the ministry of health.

In 1921 school health became a legal concern of the local community officials, who were obliged to establish a service for school health attendance that was available to school children at no cost. Apart from some minor exceptions, the results were disappointing, and in 1949 school health centres were integrated into "health centres," units that provide solely preventive services. School health centres are not located within the schools, but in separate buildings belonging to the municipality, the ministry of health, or the Catholic schools. These centres provide examinations of school children four times between ages 6 and 12, two times between age 12 and 18. The examinations are executed by a team consisting of a physician and various nursing and social personnel. For each examination, the team receives a fixed fee from the ministry of health. About 90% of the physicians who do the school examinations are general practitioners.

The main public health activities regarding curative health care are home care services and mental health centres. Organised care at the patient's home has existed since 1937 and is almost a monopoly of a voluntary organisation, the Yellow and White Cross. In 1976, 220 home care service organisations of the Yellow and White Cross, with about 2,000 personnel, served virtually every community of Belgium. There were also at that time 23 home care service organisations belonging to the socialist sick funds, with about 200 personnel. The health insurance pays for 80% of the fees for nursing visits, sent directly to the Yellow and White Cross. In addition, this organisation receives a small subsidy for each nurse ($40 per year) from the ministry of health.

In the past mental health centres only offered preventive services; however, since 1975 they also have an important function in ambulatory psychiatric care. A royal decree of 25 March 1975 introduced a totally new licensing, planning, and subsidising system for these centres. Most of the centres have been privately initiated. Of the fifty-four licensed mental health centres in Flanders, only three were public: two of these depended on a public centre for social wellbeing, and another has been established by a local community. Mental health centres are organised around a team consisting of a psychiatrist, a psychologist, a social worker, and a secretary. Overhead costs and salaries are entirely subsidised by the ministry of health. The psychiatrist's fee, however, is paid by health insurance.

CONCLUSION

Several characteristics can be identified and several remarks can be made of the overall health system: (1) It is a mixture of public and private initiative; (2) It is basically financed through health insurance and direct governmental support; (3) It has gradually been brought under the increasing control of national and regional authorities—health care planning, although not always very efficient and successful, has been a major vehicle in this respect; (4) There is a perceptible shift from national to regional (Flemish, Walloon) organisation and management (not including finances) of health care; (5) At present an enormous effort is being expended to contain costs: both health insurance and a number of health institutions are confronted with important deficits, and a reorganisation toward a smaller offer of health care provisions follows; (6) Over-medicalisation of society *and* traditional medicine, as well as many aspects of the health care organisation, are being questioned more than ever; (7) Despite the publicity given to all kinds of outpatient care and to preventive medicine, it seems that specialist inpatient care and curative care remain most attractive.

Bibliography

Deliege-Rott, D. 1975. Medical doctors in the nine countries of the common market. Systems of payment and levels of remuneration. Brussels: Department of medical demography and health economics.

Deliege-Rott, D., and X. Leroy. 1976. *L'exercise de la médecine.* Brussels: Nauwelaerts.

Glaser, W. 1978. *Health Insurance Bargaining: Foreign Lessons for Americans.* New York: Gardner Press.

Hospital Committee of the European Economic Community.

1975. First costs and day costs in the hospitals of the E.E.C. Acco: Leuven.

1977. Access to general hospital care within the European Economic Community. Acco: Leuven.

1978. Methods of cost containment in hospitals. Acco: Leuven.

Huyghe, B. 1981. The consumption of medicines in Belgium between 1970 and 1978. In *Health and Economy,* pp. 118–53. Antwerpen: Van Loghum-Slaterus.

Koninkrijk België. 1981. Ministerie van Volksgezondheid. Eerste en voornaamste statistische uitkomsten van de enquête in de verzorgingsinstellingen. Toestand op 1 januari 1980. Brussels: Ministerie van Volksgezondheid.

National Institute for Sickness and Invalidity Insurance. 1978. Outline of the Belgian Compulsory Sickness and Invalidity Insurance. Brussels: NISII.

Nys, H. 1979. Rights and duties of the state in the field of health care: the example of Belgian health care planning. Reports of the fifth World Congress on Medical Law, II, pp. 313–16. Gent.

Prims, A. 1979. De organisatie van de gezondheidszorg in België: een schematisch overzicht. *Belgisch Tijdschrift voor Sociale Zekerheid,* vol. 21, nos. 4–5, pp. 249–301.

Quaethoven, P.

1978. Quality and cost of health services. *World Hospitals* 14, no. 4: 232–33.

1981. Morfologie van het ziekenhuis. In *Welzijnszorg.* Antwerpen: Van Loghum-Slaterus.

Quaethoven, P., and A. Colla. 1980. Consumptie van ziekenhuiszorgen. *Belgisch Tijdschrift voor Sociale Zekerheid,* vol. 22, nos. 11–12: 939–1063.

Roemer, R., and M. Roemer. 1977. *Health Manpower Policies in the Belgian Health Care System.* Washington, D.C.: U.S. Department of Health, Education, and Welfare.

Van Langendonck, J. 1975. Prelude to harmony on a community theme. In *Health Insurance Policies in the Six and Britain.* London: Oxford University Press.

Verslag over de ziekteverzekering (Verslag Petit). 1976. Brussels: Kamer van Volksvertegenwoordigers.

Table 1 Belgian population by age and sex in 1980

Age	Male	Female
Under 1 year	62,813	59,006
1–4	243,540	233,197
5–9	340,781	325,906
10–14	373,853	359,747
15–19	406,568	390,739
20–24	403,956	386,711
25–29	390,573	367,607
30–34	370,138	351,374
35–39	284,193	275,207
40–44	296,440	295,188
45–49	313,174	316,748
50–54	303,353	313,898
55–59	294,451	315,547
60–64	172,839	197,448
65–69	205,449	258,966
70–74	160,731	233,103
75–79	110,678	183,188
80–84	56,464	109,107
85 and over	28,950	63,479
Total	4,818,944	5,036,166

Table 2 Birth data for 1980, Belgium

Births	Births − Deaths	Births Per 10,000 Women
124,794	+ 10,430	16,912[a]

[a]This figure is for 1978.

Table 3 Infant mortality by age, Belgium

	Age	
Year	Less Than 1 Year	Less Than 28 Days
1950	7,786	4,144[a]
1960	4,824	3,153
1965	3,684	2,494
1970	2,999	2,022
1975	1,932	1,404
1980	1,516	952

[a]One month.

Table 4 Infant mortality by six most common causes, 1980, Belgium

Cause	Total
Perinatal death	678
Congenital abnormalities	384
Symptoms and not well-defined morbidity	215
Accidents, poisonings, and traumas	90
Infectious and parasitic diseases	40
Respiratory diseases	35

Table 5 Death rates for sixteen causes of death, 1981, Belgium

Cause	Per 100,000 Population
Diseases of the tractus circulatorius	501
Neoplasms	274
External causes of lesion and poisoning	83
Diseases of the tractus respiratorius	77
Symptoms and inadequately defined syndromes	60
Diseases of the tractus digestivus	42
Endocrine, nutritional, and metabolic diseases and immunity disorders	30
Diseases of the tractus urogenitalis	20
Diseases of the nervous system and the senses	16
Psychic disorders	12
Infectious and parasitic diseases	8
Affections from the perinatal period	7
Congenital anomalies	5
Diseases of the blood and bloodmanufacturing organs	3
Diseases of the skin and the subcutis	2
Diseases of muscles, bones, and connective tissue	2

Table 6 Information not available.

Table 7 Information not available.

Tables 8 and 10 Persons active in the major health field occupations per 100,000 population, Belgium

	Number			Rate		
Occupation	1960	1969	1980	1960	1969	1980
Physicians	11,703	14,991	24,536	127.5	155.2	248.8
Pharmacists	5,383	6,735	9,682	58.7	69.7	98.2
Dentists	1,092	1,758	3,896	11.9	18.2	39.5
Veterinarians	1,012	1,303	2,398	11.0	13.5	24.3
Midwives	—	1,370	1,666	—	14.2	16.9
Physical therapists	—	3,547	10,658[a]	—	36.8	108.2[a]

SOURCE: Ministère de la Santé Publique et de la Famille, *Annuaire Statistique de la Santé Publique, 1980,* 1981, p. 242.

[a]Figure for 1979.

Table 9 Operational medical schools, students enrolled (by sex), and graduates by sex, 1980, Belgium

Medical schools	11
Total entering medical students	3,906
Women medical students	916 (23.4%)
Total medical graduates	2,458
Women medical graduates	698 (28.4%)

SOURCE: Ministère de la Santé Publique et de la Famille, *Annuaire Statistique de la Santé Publique, 1980,* 1981, p. 293.

Table 10 See Table 8.

Table 11 Information not available.

Table 12 Average income of Belgian physicians before taxes

	1966	1969	1972
General practitioners	579,000[a]	714,000	963,000
Specialists	1,415,000	1,700,000	2,316,000

SOURCE: Deliege-Rott, D., e.o.. Medical doctors in the nine countries of the common market. Systems of payment and levels of remuneration, 1975, p. I.21.

[a]Figures represent number of Belgian francs.

Table 13a Belgian hospitals in 1980

Type of Hospital	Hospitals	Beds	Beds Per 100,000 Population	Average Length of Stay (Days)	% Occupancy
Acute general	288	55,880	5.43	11.86	81.32
Psychiatric	76	26,248	2.49	138.93	91.28
Geriatric	123	11,328	1.12	73.26	95.98
Special	18	2,100	0.21	—	—
Sanatoria	9	763	0.08	122.71	49.62
Total	514	96,319	9.32	19.46	85.70

Table 13b Total beds by type and size of hospitals in 1980, Belgium

Size (in Beds)	Acute General	Psychiatric	Geriatric	Special	Sanatoria	Total
Less than 20	4	3	—	2	—	9
20–49	22	9	39	3	—	73
50–99	60	10	49	5	6	130
100–149	57	12	23	3	3	98
150–199	49	6	5	2	—	62
200–299	55	8	3	2	—	68
300–499	28	7	2	1	—	38
Over 500	13	21	2	—	—	36
Total	288	76	123	18	9	514

Table 14 Belgian hospitals by type of ownership and beds in each category in 1980

Type of Hospital	Public		Private		Total	
	Hospitals	Beds	Hospitals	Beds	Hospitals	Beds
Acute general	101	21,617	187	31,860	288	53,477
Psychiatric	14	5,396	62	19,110	76	24,506
Geriatric	62	7,099	61	3,937	123	11,072
Special	1	16	17	2,055	18	2,071
Sanatoria	2	127	7	636	9	763
Total	180	34,255	334	57,634	514	91,889

Table 15 Information not available.

Table 16 Average cost of inpatient care per day in acute general hospitals, Belgium

Year	Average Cost
1975	1,598
1978	2,166

NOTE: Average costs are unknown. Figures indicate average prices in Belgian francs, as refunded by health insurance. These prices cover between 50% and 70% of average costs; the remainder is paid by patients or doctors, or is not paid and is seen as a debt.

Table 17 Expenditures by national health insurance: amount and per capita amount by major source of funds and percentage of Gross National Product, Belgium

Year	Amount (BF)	Per Capita (BF)	% of GNP
1960	11,655,500,000	2,248	1.11
1965	28,950,900,000	3,256	2.22
1970	50,639,700,000	5,342	2.70
1975	123,684,500,000	12,604	3.48
1977	163,446,200,000	16,615	3.74

Table 18 Information not available.

Table 19 Information not available.

Table 20 Population covered by health insurance, Belgium

Year	% of Population
1960	54.5
1965	77.5
1970	96.0
1975	99.5
1980	99.5

Health Services in Canada

Gordon H. Hatcher,
Peter R. Hatcher, and
Eleanor C. Hatcher

INTRODUCTION

Canada is a federal state with a parliamentary form of government. Ten provinces, from Newfoundland off the east coast to British Columbia on the Pacific, share sovereign powers with the government of Canada, which directly administers the Yukon and the North West Territories. The Canadian Parliament resembles the British rather than the Australian, in that the Upper House, the Senate, has power only to delay temporarily legislation that the House of Commons has passed. Senators are appointed for life on nomination by the government that has control of the House. The prime minister appoints the cabinet almost exclusively from members of his party elected to the House of Commons. Occasionally he names a senator to a minor portfolio. The governor general is appointed by the queen on nomination by the prime minister, and he can similarly be dismissed. His power is largely ceremonial. Standing aside from party politics, he can represent the nation as a whole and relieve the prime minister of the burden of entertaining visiting heads of state and other social functions. Parliament is dissolved and new federal elections are called whenever the prime minister so requests, or when the government is defeated on a vote in the House of Commons on a major issue or money bill. The Supreme Court of Canada probably has less power than that of the United States, both because the House of Commons combines legislative and executive powers, and because there has not been the tradition of the Supreme Court ruling on the constitutionality or interpreting the intent of every major law—as was early established in the United States by Chief Justice Marshall.

Most of Canada's written constitution is embodied in the British North America Act, an Act of the British Parliament in 1867 that defined the separate powers of the provinces and of the Government of Canada. Recently, the power to amend that Act was transferred to Canada, together with an amendment that includes a Bill of Rights, but, except for the division of governmental powers, most of the democratic procedures and civil rights are established by tradition and precedent, and are not embodied in a written constitution.

The British North America Act is, in a sense, the obverse of the U.S. Constitution in

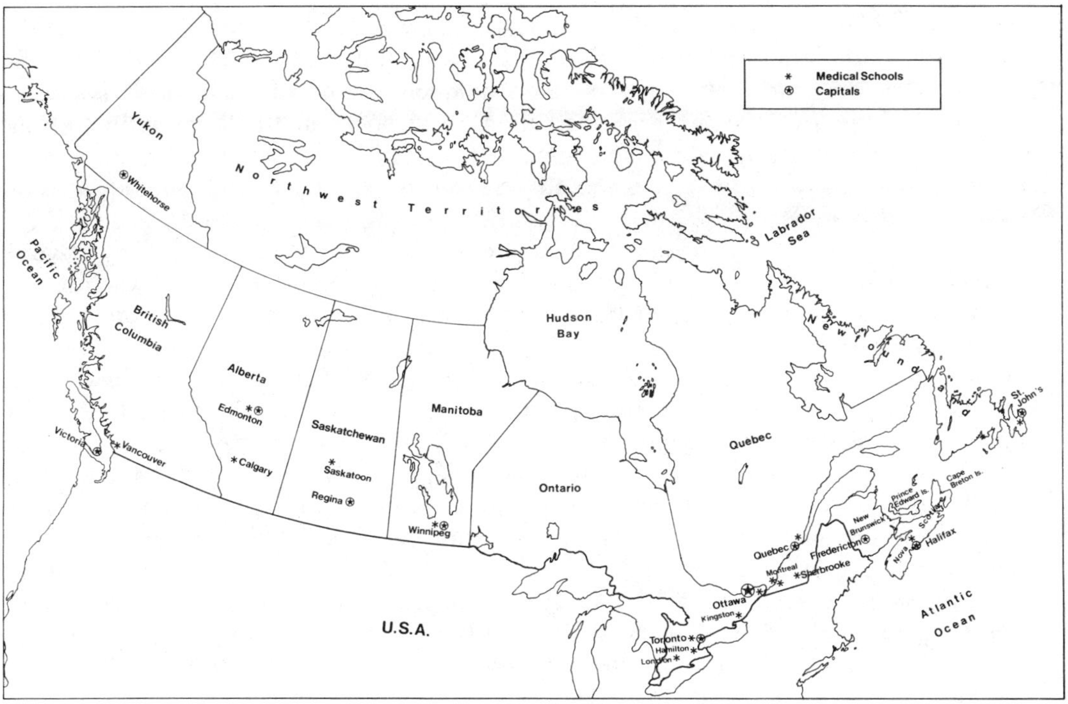

that it assigns to the provinces only limited and defined powers, and reserves for the Government of Canada all residual powers, including a general grant of authority for the "peace, order, and good government" of the people of Canada. Later interpretations, and the absence of public health or medical care services of any significance a century ago, led to the assumption of most health responsibilities by provincial governments. Given the vast distances, scattered population, and rudimentary transportation of nineteenth-century Canada, and the strong executive powers of provincial governments whose democratic organization parallels that of Canada, both health and welfare services evolved as provincial activities primarily. It was not until after the First World War that the federal government introduced pensions for the aged and the blind, supplemented by public assistance during the depression of the 1930s.

The low health status of many recruits in the 1914–18 war stimulated the Liberal party in 1921 to recommend a national health insurance program, inspired by the British example of 1911 and Bismarck's original model in 1884. Earlier, in 1912, Ontario, the most industrialized province, had pioneered a unique design of Workmen's Compensation as a provincial responsibility.[1] Private insurance companies and the law courts are excluded from the system; a case is never closed; benefits are established for the lifetime of the worker or his dependents; and lump sum payments are discouraged. The board is essentially both an administrative court and the executive for the program; it is appointed by the provincial government, and usually consists of one physician, one former employer, and one former union leader. The objective is to keep injured workmen and their dependents off the welfare rolls. By the 1920s comprehensive medical care and rehabilitation services were added, and by the 1940s, quality control of surgical and medical care. Other provinces followed this example.

The influence of Wisconsin's early social legislation and the rehabilitation movements in the United States after the two world wars is apparent, but the Ontario Workmen's Compensation program is perhaps the first uniquely Canadian health care system. It foreshadowed the inventiveness and adaptation of European and U.S. concepts to Canadian conditions and ideals, which later emerged as universal hospital and medical insurance programs in several provinces, notably Saskatchewan and Newfoundland, after the Second World War.

Local governments in Canada are "the creatures of the Provinces." They have no independent constitutional status, but are established by provincial law. It was not until the 1941 census that a majority of Canadians lived in urban municipalities, and "urban" was defined as a population of five thousand or more. Most of the Canadian population lives within one hundred miles of the U.S. border. Many of the northern municipalities developed as isolated lumbering, fishing, mining, electric power, or transportation communities. Organizing health care services was a major problem for such communities, as it was for the wheat farmers of the great western plains that stretch over 1,000 miles from the Lake of the Woods district of Western Ontario to the towering eastern escarpment of the Rocky Mountains on the Alberta-British Columbia border. In the province of Quebec religious orders organized and still own most of the hospitals. In northern "company towns" the major industry usually established a nonprofit voluntary hospital—which is the dominant pattern of hospital ownership in most of Canada, although a few cities still operate a municipal hospital. In Newfoundland, with its isolated fishing villages, the British-appointed government that preceded its becoming a province in 1949 set up the first publicly owned regional hospital and medical care system in this hemisphere, modeled after the Scottish Highlands and Islands system.[2] Nurse practitioners provide much of the care in this program. Map #2 shows the boundaries of the Newfoundland Cottage Hospital districts, and of the medical and nursing practices within them, in about 1950. Religious groups operated similar services in Twillingate, St. Anthony, and other areas, and the base hospital was in St. John's. Pulp and paper and mining industries helped supply physicians in Corner Brook, Buchans, and Grand Falls; private practitioners were available mainly in the remaining coastal areas near St. John's and Bonavista.

In the three prairie provinces—Manitoba, Saskatchewan, and Alberta—the principal unit of local government was the rural municipality, about eighteen miles square, which numbered its population in the hundreds. There are no counties west of Ontario, except as judicial districts.

From about 1910 to 1940 many rural municipalities in the midwest built their own small municipal hospitals, erected houses beside them for the doctors, advertised for doctors in eastern medical journals, and hired on salaries "municipal doctors" to care for their citizens.[3] They paid for these services by imposing a local land tax—in some cases even before the provincial government knew about it and passed a law to authorize it. In the 1930s almost one-third of all doctors in the midwest were thus employed, as were half of the doctors in Newfoundland. After the 1939–45 war, most of the returning doctors resumed their fee-for-service practices in the west, but local governments there still operate most of the small rural hospitals.

The subsequent introduction of universal hospital insurance by the Saskatchewan government in 1947, and its pilot program of universal medical insurance in the southwest Swift Current region of Saskatchewan at the same time, had its roots in this local government experience.[4] This compromise guaranteed universal access to care, but left hospitals and doctors as relatively independent agents who contracted with the state to provide universal insured health care services under the Provincial Health Insurance programs.

Voluntary and commerical health insurance developed alongside public programs in Canada in the 1940s and 1950s. When the national health insurance program extended the Saskatchewan pattern to the whole country, some provinces made a single voluntary plan the sole carrier for the provincial program. Ontario Blue Cross thus became a department of government, while Nova Scotia's Maritime Medical Services is a private, nonprofit corporation that pays all doctors' bills.

By 1960 all the Canadian provinces had introduced universal hospital insurance programs, encouraged by federal grants-in-aid of about 50% of the cost, and subject to federal requirements of universal access, comprehensiveness of benefit, public administration, and portability between provinces.[5] By 1971 all Canadian provinces had introduced

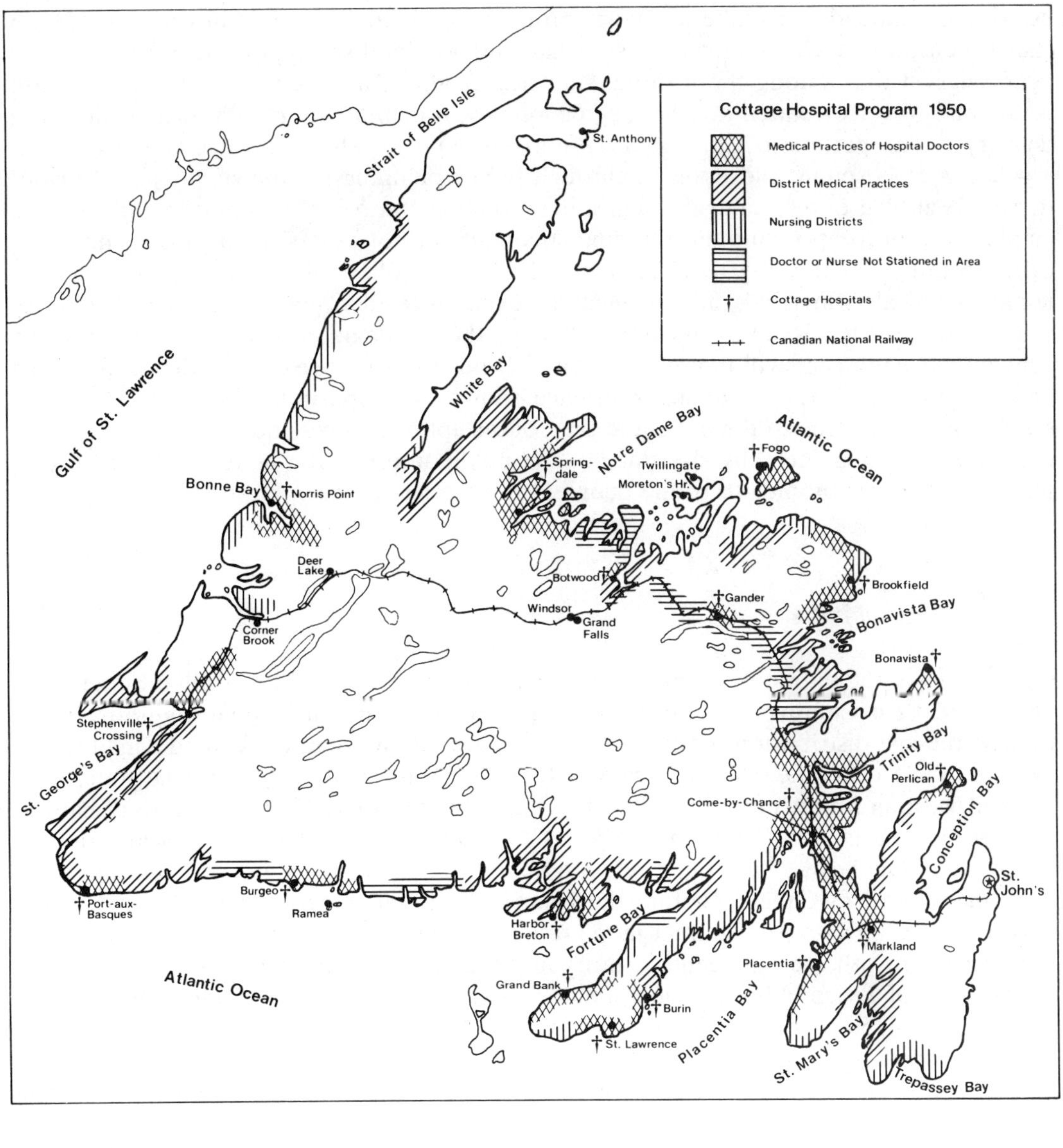

parallel universal medical insurance programs.[6] In 1977 the federal government vacated some federal tax fields in part, permitting provinces to raise the funds themselves to extend health insurance benefits to include long-term care, drugs, appliances, and prostheses, and dental care for children.[7] It also allowed the federal government to set a limit on federal health care expenditures incurred by the provincial health insurance plans. In 1982 the federal-provincial health care programs were subject to their periodic (five year) review. Two recent reports suggest that these insurance programs are to be extended and perhaps even made more cost-effective.[8,9]

Despite the universality, equality, and generosity of benefits under its health insurance programs, Canada is one of the few countries that has held the cost of all health care to a constant proportion of the Gross National Product for nearly ten years. Total health care expenditures in Canada are only half those of the United States, yet in both countries most hospitals are privately owned and most doctors are in independent private practice. In Britain, with greater control over medical practice under the National Health Service, health care expenditures take a smaller proportion of the GNP than in Canada. Health status measures, such as mortality statistics and availability of physicians and hospital beds, suggest that among these three countries, health is inversely related to health care costs, but directly related to the degree of governmental intervention in health care delivery.[10] The pattern of that intervention—through standards enforcement by public regulation of hospitals and doctors, through public planning for the supply and distribution of health resources, and through universal state-controlled reimbursement methods emphasizing prevention and encouraging adequate but not excessive diagnostic and surgical procedures—is the key to effective public health policy. There is no historical economic, medical, statistical, or management experience in Canada over the past thirty years to support the Reagan/Stockman ideology that deregulation and competition in the delivery of health care will improve the public's health or reduce costs, either in the short or thc long run. The Canadian experience shows the opposite to be true. The more services are made free to the patient at time of receipt of service, and the more the system is planned and regulated by the state in the public interest, the better is the quality of service, the better the health of the people—and the less it costs.

Population

Canada has a population of nearly 25 million, about one-tenth of the United States, or a little more than California. With 9.5% over sixty-five years, and about one-third under twenty, the age distribution is young when compared to Sweden, the United Kingdom, or even the United States. The birth rate of 15.5 is high for a western industrial state, and, coupled with an infant mortality rate of 7.2 per thousand live births, the rate of natural increase is substantial. The "baby boom" of the post-Second World War era was tempered in Quebec by "the quiet revolution," where the birth rate dropped in ten years from the highest in Canada (before the fecund Newfoundlanders joined Canada) to the lowest. There was also substantial immigration during the postwar era, although modest in comparison with the nineteenth century and the first decades of the twentieth. There is a suggestion of a second baby boom impending, with the birth rate starting up again as the babies of the 1950s become the parents of the 1980s.

Population data by race has not been collected since 1941. There is both a myth and a message in this failure, in a country where accurate statistics are almost a way of life: the myth is that there are only "two founding races"; the message is that at least one of these "races" is not too keen to be reminded of the many later immigrants who have enriched Canada's cultural life without claiming a sovereign right to a separate identity. The first "race" is descended largely from the early French colonists, mostly from Normandy, Brittany, and the Isle de France, who numbered perhaps ten thousand at the time of the British conquest in 1760. Their gene pool was already enlarged from the native Indian populations, and, particularly in Montreal and Quebec City, the survivors of the Irish potato famine made a substantial later contribution. In the predominantly rural countryside, however, the French Canadians retained a separate identity, fostered by the new civil rights accorded them by the British. Freedom of religion, retention of their pre-Napoleonic French civil law that ensured they would not lose their land titles, and the right to use the French language in education, law courts, and government, were initially a blessing, though later a burden. The separateness that preserved their culture left them out of the mainstream of scientific development and economic progress until the Second World War.

The second "founding race" is supposedly English Canadian, whose first wave consisted of Tories driven north after the American Revolution. Many of them settled in the eastern townships of Quebec, north of Vermont. Others built "York" boats from green lumber on the shores of Lake Champlain and rowed north to the St. Lawrence, coasted the northern shore of Lake Ontario, and founded York—the present-day Toronto (renamed after the Americans burnt the city to the ground in 1812). In Canada the "Tories" are honored as "United Empire Loyalists." Scottish highland regiments sometimes were settled in Canada at strategic locations, such as the Stormont Dundas and Glengarry Highlanders at the confluence of the St. Lawrence and the Ottawa rivers. Other Scots fled after the Battle of Culloden to the Maritime Provinces, where to this day nearly everyone in Cape Breton is either a Macdonald or a McLeod. More Irish immigrants joined the "English Canadian" gene pool than the French in Quebec and Ontario. Newfoundlanders still speak with a touch of Irish brogue. The Canadian coat-of-arms and a patriotic song proclaim that "the thistle, shamrock, and rose entwine, the maple leaf forever."

The cosmopolitan natures of Montreal for half a century and of Toronto today, where one finds thriving subcultures of Hungarians, Italians, Greeks, Ukrainians, Rumanians, Armenians, Lebanese, and many other "races," greatly enrich Canadian life.

The flood of European immigrants who settled the western plains were neither of French or British origin. As recently as 1950, less than an hour's drive from Winnipeg, the capital of Manitoba, one entered German-speaking Gruenwald, Russian-speaking Komarno, and Icelandic-speaking Inwald. It is said that more Icelanders live in the district between Lakes Winnipeg and Manitoba than in Iceland, and that more Icelandic poetry has been written there than in the home island. The Scandinavian sod-buster, the Chinese laborer who built the transcontinental railroad, and the Japanese salmon fisherman on the Pacific belie the quaint notion of "two founding races."

Western Canada has many islands of British stock, and a rich Indian heritage laced with mixed French "metis," but it is dominantly a confident "Canadian" population that has not rejected its multinational European heritage in an American-style melting pot.

Ontario has over 9 million people, and Toronto is now the major banking and cultural center of Canada. Quebec is the next largest province, with a population of over 6 million. Nova Scotia has about three-quarters of a million people, New Brunswick and Newfoundland each about half a million, and little Prince Edward Island only one hundred thousand. Manitoba and Saskatchewan each with over 1 million inhabitants, and Alberta and British Columbia with about 2 million each make up the balance. Alberta has most of the Canadian oil reserves, while British Columbia, with a coastal climate like Seattle, is the "Florida" to which many Canadians retire. It also has great mineral, agricultural, and commerical resources, and Vancouver is now the third-largest Canadian city.

THE MEDICAL PROFESSION AND MEDICAL EDUCATION

The first Canadian medical schools were founded on the Scottish model in Edinburgh, as was Johns Hopkins in Baltimore. Many teaching hospitals, such as the Royal Victoria in Montreal and the Albany Medical College Hospital in New York, were similarly replicas of the Edinburgh Infirmary. Since the Flexner reform of U.S. medical schools, before World War I, all Canadian medical schools have been accredited by the same agencies that accredit U.S. medical schools. Most offer four years of medical education, two in basic sciences and two in clinical, after a four-year science degree. Some also have a six-year biomedical accelerated program for exceptional students. McMaster University in Hamilton, Ontario, and Calgary in Alberta, like Western Reserve in Ohio, offer a three-year medical course, heavy in clinical training, to students required to complete more of their basic sciences in the premedical education. There are five medical schools in Ontario, eleven in the rest of the country. All are university based and subsidized substantially by the provincial governments, so fees are less than a quarter of the U.S. average. Postgraduate medical specialty training is also similar to that in the United States, but the specialty "Boards" for all specialties except Family Practice are concentrated in a single body—the Royal College of Physicians of Canada. No teaching hospital may offer residency training in a medical specialty unless it is part of the residency of a department of a medical school. In this, Canada differs from the United States. This both ensures the quality of specialty training and enables provincial governments to control the relative proportions of generalists and specialists. The goal has been to have at least 50% family or general practitioners, in contrast to only 20% in the United States, and residency training positions reflect this.

There are slightly more medical than surgical subspecialists in Canada, and about one doctor in nine is a "support specialist" in anesthesia, pathology, and radiology.

The physician population ratio is about one doctor to 550 people nationwide, including interns and residents, or about one to 630 persons if they are excluded. In addition to interns and residents, almost an equal number of doctors are engaged in hospital-based patient care, administration, or research, including about 1,500 in medical education. From this it may be said that between 25% and 30% of Canadian doctors are essentially hospital based, although not government employees, and nearly all the rest are in office-based private practice. However, as in the United States, nearly all office-based doctors, both generalists and specialists, have hospital privileges, admit their patients to hospitals, and care for them there.

Fee-for-service is the dominant method of physician payment, both for hospital and office practice, except, of course, for interns and residents, researchers and administrators, who are paid salaries. In some provinces support specialists are paid salaries by hospitals, while in others they are reimbursed by fee-for-service or by a proportion of the patient care charges for laboratory or x-ray services.

Data on average physician incomes are probably less reliable than other kinds of data. The Hall Commission reported data from income tax indicating a net income average of about $55,000 in 1978, or four times the average weekly wages and salaries of all Canadians.* In 1971 doctors reported net (after practice expenses) incomes of about five times the average wages, and negotiations with provincial health insurance plans over doctors' fee schedules have used such data.

Reported physician incomes by specialty are even less reliable than averages for all specialties together. Further, they are greatly influenced by the experience of Ontario, both because about 40% of doctors practice in Ontario, and because the Ontario fee schedule has been the model for some of the other provinces. However, many provincial medical care insurance plans publish data on payments to physicians by specialty under the universal health insurance plan, which represents nearly all the income of most doctors. Generally, surgical specialists earn more than general or family practitioners, while the highest incomes go to support specialists in areas such as pathology, radiology, or anesthesia. This is a function both of market forces and of "medical politics" in the negotiations between the medical associations and the government health insurance plan in each province.

Physician income is a multiple of fees and utilization. Each year or two, all the doctors in a province, through negotiations conducted by their medical associations, agree to accept a set fee provincewide for each medical service or procedure, such as an office visit, operation, interpretation of an electrocardiogram, and so on. In some provinces, some doctors may charge patients more if the patient agrees to it in advance, but this is the exception. The relative incomes of specialists are determined in major part by the prices set for services of one specialty as opposed to others.

Historically, surgical services and procedures have been more highly paid than nonoperative services. Because general practitioners perform many surgical procedures in Canada, this differential has persisted. Another factor influencing income is the supply of a given specialty in relation to demand. Specialization and subspecialization evolved from general practice; small numbers of many subspecialists are therefore found in the more sparsely settled areas. They tend to be concentrated in small cities and towns with a hinterland served by general practitioners, who refer problem cases to them for consultation. In larger cities, such as in Ontario and Quebec, many of these specialists are in competition with general practitioners and with the newer family practice specialists for general primary-care patients. In some cases hospitals employ a few subspecialists to head departments, supervise a neonatal ward, read electrocardiograms, etc., usually on a part-time salaried basis. The larger hospitals in larger cities usually restrict general practitioners' privileges when they have available enough specialists, so the active general practitioner surgeon who also delivers babies and provides care for children is found mainly in the small towns, or in more sparsely populated provinces.

A common fee schedule provincewide and, to a lesser extent, similar fee schedules between provinces (because they tend to pay more in wealthier provinces) use market forces to redistribute physicians from overdoctored to underdoctored areas. The zero price feature of Canadian medical insurance, with universal coverage and virtually no out-of-pocket payment to a doctor, means that a poor farmer or a blue collar worker in an industrial area is just as good a source of income as a wealthy suburbanite. Going into practice in a poor area with twice as many patients per doctor is more lucrative than in a

*All dollar references for Canada are Canadian dollars. See conversion table in the Introduction.—ED.

wealthy area with a higher physician population ratio. However, very sparsely populated areas can only support a doctor if fee-for-service income is supplemented.

Universal medical insurance in Canada began with a serious maldistribution of doctors. They were concentrated in areas where patients had money and/or private health insurance coverage through a common industrial employer; this was particularly true for specialists. Since 1971 these differentials between over- and underdoctored areas have been decreasing.[11] Most provinces have identified a few sparsely settled or undesirable areas and have used various methods to recruit doctors for them, such as guaranteeing an income above the returns from health insurance fees. Many more doctors have been attracted by health insurance fees to provinces and areas previously underdoctored. In the far north, air transport and nurse practitioners or frontier nurses have been used. Some medical schools rotate residents to outpost hospitals in the Arctic, and the Newfoundland Cottage Hospital system has evolved into a regional health care system with specialist as well as generalist services.

In every Canadian province for over a decade the medical care insurance program has been collecting and analyzing computerized data on virtually all medical care activities of every physician, including his earnings from these activities. The provinces have population bases as denominators that enable them to develop indices of utilization of services. From this experience, many administrators and physicians have been convinced that a good general physician engaged mainly in primary care can be the family doctor for as many as two thousand patients a year without working more than forty hours a week. Even in Newfoundland and New Brunswick by 1975 there were fewer than two thousand patients for each general or family practitioner. Needed ratios of various specialists to population are harder to estimate and are subject to more rapid changes as technology advances. In 1975 an extensive nationwide study of medical manpower needs developed such ratios, compared them to current supply, and calculated the annual supply of each type of specialist and family physician needed to achieve the proposed ratios by 1981.[12] They recommended one general or family practitioner for every 2,300 people, one internist (in six subspecialties) for every 8,200, one neurologist for every 90,000, one psychiatrist and one general surgeon for every 11,000, and so on. This indicated that Canada needed to have completing their specialty training each year 452 additional full-time equivalent, family practice specialists, 182 general internists, 96 general surgeons, 4 or 5 neurosurgeons, 63 obstetric/gynecological specialists, 105 anesthesiologists, and so on. It may not be entirely coincidental that the required number of new physicians each year was estimated at close to the nearly 1,800 graduates of Canada's sixteen medical schools in 1980. The report, developed with substantial medical school input, called on medical schools to adjust the supply of various specialists to the estimated needs, through both adjustments in the numbers of specialty training positions offered and influence on medical students' career preferences in favor of needed specialties and geographic locations.

Two years earlier the two largest provinces, perceiving a doctor surplus, had already persuaded the federal immigration authorities to cut off immigration of foreign doctors, unless these newcomers contracted to serve in underdoctored areas.

If the data used by these medical manpower planners are correct, it seems probable that the Canadian physicians' work week is substantially less than forty hours. For example, they estimated that the 16,937 fee-for-service general or family practitioners represented only the full-time equivalent of 10,755 doctors, using health insurance data on the number of doctors earning $20,000 a year or more as an indication of full-time activity. With women constituting over one-third of the medical students in Canada, one can expect doctors to take more time off for family life than in the past, when less than 10% were woman.

HOSPITALS

The Canadian hospital system evolved from a collection of separate units of various kinds developed by local communities to meet perceived needs for care. Public authorities established provincewide hospital systems for tuberculosis and for mental illness, and for a time operated provincewide clinical laboratory services and provided free supplies of immunizing agents for the use of doctors in private practice. These public programs were most extensive in the 1930s, and in many provinces hospital care for tuberculosis and mental illness was a public service without a means test or charge to the patient. With the advent of greater herd immunity and/or less exposure to tuberculosis, and with the antituberculosis and psychotropic drugs, there was less and less need for separate services of this kind. After the Second World War the mental hospital system was further reduced by deinstitutionalization; the tuberculosis sanitaria were closed, except for one special facility for aboriginal people.

By 1980 there remained only twenty-three mental hospitals in Canada, with a resident population of about nine thousand. An additional sixteen smaller psychiatric institutions, including those for alcoholism, accommodated another two thousand patients. Only about three hundred patients were in proprietary institutions.

The dominant hospital "system" in Canada—if it can yet really be called a system—is made up of over 1,000 nonfederal hospitals with about 164,000 beds. Only 3,300 beds are in proprietary institutions. An additional 3,300 beds are in federal hospitals, and about 10,000 in the remaining provincial mental hospitals.

The federal hospitals include only two veterans hospitals, most of the rest having been transferred to other nonprofit agencies, with care being purchased by the Department of Veterans Affairs. For example, Sunnybrook Veterans Hospital in Toronto was sold to the University of Toronto for one dollar shortly after it was built. The National Health and Welfare Department hospitals include marine hospitals, which provide care to foreign merchant seamen under the international convention, and some facilities for aborigines.

Most of the hospitals in Canada are called "public" hospitals, but 125,000 out of 175,000 beds are owned and operated by private organizations, and about another 5,000 of the provincial hospital beds are in hospitals managed by provincial medical schools. Most of the hospitals owned and operated by municipal governments are really community hospitals very similar to those owned by a lay corporation consisting of local citizens. Although all nonfederal public hospitals and some proprietary ones derive most of their income from the provincial hospital insurance programs, and all are regulated by the provincial health authorities, they perceive their constituencies as local and they serve the entire local community.

Even before the Great Depression of the 1930s, Canada had rejected the principle of separate hospitals for the poor. In some of the leading institutions as recently as the early 1940s, the Board of Governors passed around a checkbook at their annual meeting and wrote off the deficit. Even though provincial and local governments contributed to the cost of hospital care for those who could not pay, before universal hospital insurance many local banks carried a hospital overdraft of a million dollars or more in large cities like Toronto. In conscience and in law, every "public" hospital must be open to everyone who needs care.

The principle of a two-class system of health care, one for the rich and another for the poor, is alien to the dominant Canadian political philosophy. Democracy in Canada includes not only political equality but equality in providing for common human needs as a public service "on the same terms and conditions" for all, without a demeaning test of income or need. This is the language of the legislation, whereby the federal government pays about one-half the cost of hospital and medical care provided under provincial health insurance. The principle was reaffirmed in the First Hall Commission Report in 1964, and again in the Second in 1980, that there would not be a two-class system of medical care in Canada.[13] There was hardly a dissenting vote when the health insurance legislation was passed in the federal parliament, and the hospital insurance legislation was introduced by a conservative government.

This is not to say there was no objection to establishing equal access to an essentially free hospital and medical care service, both at the onset and again in the 1970s with the economic recessions. Some patients seeking doctors' services may be more equal than others, depending on their educational and social status. There are extra charges for private rooms in hospitals, and in some provinces some doctors may charge patients in excess to the established fees. Finally, long-term care outside of hospitals was not included in the early hospital insurance program of the late 1950s. Universal physicians' services insurance came a decade later and long-term institutional care was only added in the 1970s. By 1982 Quebec and the five provinces west of it included most nursing home and home care services in universal health insurance. Almost all of these programs impose daily charges on patients of eight to fourteen dollars a day. The Atlantic provinces also set standards and rates for nursing homes, but patients are subjected to a means test and the payment schedules are related to income. These charges are still very modest by U.S. standards because the costs of long-term-care institutions are subsidized by provincial governments, assisted by an earmarked federal allocation since 1977.[7]

There are sixty-two teaching hospitals affiliated with university medical schools in Canada, eight of which are children's hospitals. All of the patients in teaching hospitals are offered the opportunity to assist in the training of physicians. Medical students, interns, and residents take medical histories and perform physical examinations, and may perform other procedures under the supervision of the full-time or part-time medical faculty. Most patients are willing to be admitted to a teaching hospital because of the special competence of the medical staff and agree to be subjects at group teaching sessions such as ward rounds or class presentations. They can refuse, although patients would usually not go to a teaching hospital if they were unwilling to be teaching patients. The choice of a doctor who is a faculty member of a teaching hospital or of an outpatient department no longer need be made in Canada because one is poor and cannot pay. With universal health insurance, access to medical care is no longer dependent on income. Canadian medical educators and the classes they teach have learned that nearly all patients in teaching hospitals, when approached with respect for their feelings and needs, willingly assist in medical education, and that society has no need of an impoverished underclass to supply "teaching material" to be "used" to teach medicine.

Some of the teaching hospitals are owned and operated by the universities, but most are not. Some are owned by the provincial government that also supports the university and its medical school. Most have independent Boards of Governors and operate under provincial regulations, and are financed mainly by the National Provincial Health Insurance Program, just like any other public hospital.

Special federal assistance for the capital costs of medical schools and teaching hospitals was made available in the 1960s through a Health Resources Fund. Federal grants for clinical research through the Medical Research Council operate in much the same way as research grants from the National Institutes of Health in the United States. One difference is that in Canada, except for a limited number of research scholars who are awarded stipends for full-time work, medical research grants do not include payment for the time of the principal investigator or for overhead costs to the medical school or hospital. It is assumed that the university supports the researcher and agrees to the allocation of his time to the research project, and that the province pays enough of the university costs for overhead to be covered. As a result, research grants in Canada tend to be smaller than in the United States, and are not used to subsidize teaching or patient care.

There are 18 rehabilitation or convalescent care hospitals and 132 chronic or extended care hospitals in Canada. In addition, over 300 acute general hospitals in Canada have specifically designated long-term-care, psychiatric, or rehabilitation beds.[14] Many small rural hospitals have a higher proportion of chronic, or long-term-care, patients than will be found in a larger urban hospital. As a result, the average length of stay of patients in Canadian hospitals is approximately two days longer than in the United States.

Federal Hospital Survey and Construction grants were made to hospitals in Canada, commencing in 1949, much as was done in the United States under the Hill-Burton Hospital Survey and Construction Act. These grants were based on a required prior Provincial Hospital Survey, with both standards-setting for facilities and regionalization of high technology services in mind. In the next two decades most Canadian hospitals were rebuilt or upgraded, but regionalization was resisted by local communities and by the medical staff of hospitals not designated as regional or central referral hospitals. Many provinces entered the universal hospital insurance program anticipating a flood of demand for care (that failed to materialize), so, with federal encouragement, they built too many acute hospital beds. In some provinces over seven acute hospital beds per thousand population were available, in contrast to the four or five now believed necessary.[15] This change also militated against regionalization of hospital services, except for rehabilitation and long-term-care services. By the 1970s, under fiscal pressures, provinces were more effective in hospital regionalization, using the leverage of control established over hospital expenditures through universal hospital insurance.

In Ontario, for example, the designation of regional hospital centers for rehabilitation and psychiatric care was effected with input from community health councils, set up somewhat along the lines of U.S. health systems agencies. In Quebec, an edict of the provincial government required all large hospitals to convert a fraction of their beds to long-term care. University teaching hospitals emerged as the major central referral hospitals.

By the end of the 1970s most provinces were successful in limiting the acquisition of new high technology services, such as computerized axial tomography, to designated central or regional referral hospitals. The money to extend universal health insurance to include long-term care without increasing the percentage of the GNP spent on health care was obtained in part by the cost savings from the more efficient—and higher quality—regionalized services.

The provincial governments set standards for hospital facilities and staffing through their procedures for approving new capital construction grants and their annual review of each hospital's operating budget under hospital insurance. In addition, however, Canadian hospitals typically seek voluntary accreditation—originally through the Joint Commission on Accreditation of Hospitals, which was established in the United States with Canadian participation (as was done also for medical school accreditation jointly in the United States and Canada), and later through its own Canadian Commission on Accreditation of Hospitals (CCAH), with a program similar to that in the United States. Both the provincial authorities and the Board of Governors of a hospital consider accreditation important and encourage the hospital medical staffs to take seriously the medical audit evaluations required by the CCAH.

The operating expenses of acute care hospitals in Canada in 1980–81 were highest in children's hospitals—at $433.77 a day—and lowest in hospitals under 50 beds with long-term-care units, which averaged $157.17 a day. Nonteaching hospitals over 300 beds with no long-term units averaged $196.20 a day, while all teaching hospitals (other than pediatric) averaged $271.04 a day.

Some provinces are more stringent than others in their controls over hospital operating costs. Most began universal health insurance by requiring line-by-line reporting of all hospital operating costs, using an adaptation of the Canadian Hospital Accounting Manual developed by the Hospital Association and elaborated by the Saskatchewan Hospital Services Plan. Hospitals of similar size and characteristics are grouped together, and a hospital had to justify any deviation from the average. Later, the provinces often moved to a "global budget" approval, derived from the earlier line-by-line review but allowing the hospital administration more discretion in how it used the money as long as it did not exceed the total or reduce standards or services. Statistics Canada assists in compiling statistics from each hospital on a vast array of hospital indicators, and the Department of National Health and Welfare has issued standards for a number of hospital departments and units that have gained general acceptance. The principal controlling authority, however, is provincial.

Saskatchewan's method of developing each hospital's budget and daily rate for reimbursement under hospital insurance is the model most provinces have tried to follow.[16,17] First, capital costs and depreciation are excluded from the operating budget; most of these replacement costs are either contributed to the hospital by government or raised in public subscription. Hospitals are allowed to collect extra charges for private and, in some cases, semiprivate rooms, so they may be able to finance some additional services if approved by the provincial health authority; however, they could rarely finance major construction alone. Exclusion of capital costs gives the province the economic power to regionalize hospital services—in theory at least. Politically, it is not always so easy. The unanticipated advantage of letting hospitals keep the private room cost differential has seen a trend away from large public wards to private and semiprivate rooms.

In the second step of the Saskatchewan method, a hospital utilization study is completed, using place of residence, age, and race (Indian versus white) of patients admitted during the previous year. These facts are derived from the computerized hospital discharge data under universal hospital insurance. The population served by each hospital is thus defined geographically, and, using census data, age-adjusted and race-adjusted hospital utilization rates are calculated. It is assumed that the hospital should have the same hospital utilization rates as the provincial averages for patients of the same ages and race. The application of these utilization rates to the total population in the area served by the hospital, multiplied by the proportion who actually went to that hospital (rather than another in the previous year), results in an "approved" number of patient days of hospital care projected for the coming year.

Using initially a line-by-line review of each budget item in an approved hospital accounting manual, the hospital's annual budget for the coming year is approved by the Provincial Hospital Rate Board. The rate-setting body in each province is usually appointed by the minister of health, and the senior official in the Hospital Insurance Plan or his designee has a major role. Dividing the approved budget by the approved patient days of care gives the approved hospital rate.

Provinces usually pay hospitals one twenty-fourth of their approved budget twice a month. As each patient is discharged, a discharge form is sent in to the hospital insurance plan; therefore, the Provincial Health Department or Health Insurance Commission can monitor utilization. If the hospital is running over its approved utilization, the province may analyze length of stay by diagnosis, age, and race, to see if the budget should be increased or if the hospital should tighten its utilization review process. If hospital utilization is down, the province will usually still reimburse the hospital according to the budget for its fixed costs, but may withhold the variable costs (food, supplies, and perhaps some staff if they are laid off or are not replaced).

Hospital costs per capita in Canada have risen at a fairly steady rate for the past two decades. The main reason for this rise has been the increase in both the wages paid hospital workers and in their numbers, which accompanied advancing technology.[18] Hospital care is labor intensive. In the 1970s most provinces began to attempt the substitution of physician's office or outpatient and nursing home care for hospital inpatient care. This began with universal medical insurance adopted by all provinces, except Saskatchewan, between 1969 and 1971 (Saskatchewan's program began in 1962). The trend accelerated with the 1977 revision of federal financing of health insurance, placing responsibility on each province for expenditures beyond certain limits and making the first specific federal allocation for the first time for long-term care. Stringent hospital cost containment efforts in the larger and more cost-demanding provinces were introduced in the late 1970s, resulting in a trend to fewer hospital beds per thousand population and a shorter length of stay.[19] Whether this recent cost containment was due mainly to specific hospital utilization and operating budget controls, or to overall constraints on supply of physician specialists and acute hospital beds, is not certain. We believe the evidence favors the overall provincial health system control structures as the cause of cost containment in Canada, rather than any specific measures directed only at hospitals. It might be argued that hospital costs in Canada have been harder to control than other health expenditures. The jury is still out on whether the inclusion of long-term care under health insurance will be a substitute for more costly hospital care or an added expense. There are some early indications that it has been both: the percentage of the GNP spent on health care in Canada may rise above 8% in the 1980s, and many aged and disabled persons previously receiving long-term-care services in hospitals now do so in more appropriate settings. Only patients in the old provincial mental hospital systems were excluded from federal support for universal hospital insurance, on the grounds that they were already a provincial responsibility.

In May 1982 the federal minister of health proposed including all institutional mental health services on the same basis as physical health.[20] Some provinces already do so, using provincial funds, and all ambulatory psychiatric care by private practitioners and short-term psychiatric care in general hospitals are already universally insured benefits. Controls over overutilization and access of patients to care are discussed in "Health Costs and Health Insurance."

NURSING HOME AND COMMUNITY HEALTH AGENCIES

Data on long-term institutional care in Canada have only been collected systematically, on a comparable basis, nationwide for about a decade. However, different provinces have used somewhat different categories to classify nursing home patients by levels of care. Thus, data corresponding to intermediate and skilled nursing care levels in the United

States are not reliable. The term *Special Care Facilities* is used in Canada to describe nursing homes—homes for the aged, mentally retarded, and others needing special care at a nursing home or domiciliary care level.

The number of beds in such facilities in 1980 exceeded the number of approved hospital beds in Canada, numbering about 200,000, or about 7.5 beds per thousand population. Of these, only about 60,000 beds were in institutions classified as nursing homes.

A number of midwestern provinces have relatively high acute hospital beds to population ratios, and most have a substantial number of patients in long-term-care units of general or allied special hospitals. Initially, the national health insurance program in Canada inadvertently provided economic incentives for some provinces to care for long-term-care patients in hospitals, where part of the cost was borne by hospital insurance; after 1977, however, nursing home care could be a universally insured service with federal support. The total number of institutional-care beds for the elderly is estimated at about 80 per 100,000 population; this number has about kept pace with the elderly population for the last decade. However, the 1970s have seen a substantial improvement in the quality of institutional care and means of access of the chronically sick and the frail elderly to such services outside of hospitals.

Alberta as early as 1962, and Manitoba, Ontario, and British Columbia in the 1970s, established a pattern of assessment of long-term-care needs, improved standards-setting and surveillance, rate-setting at levels that permitted adequate care, and fixed daily charges to patients related to the amount of the old age pension but reduced in cases of economic need. These charges ranged from eight to fourteen dollars a day in 1982 for the highest (chronic hospital) level of care. Quebec and Saskatchewan, on the other hand, adopted a system of standard charges and publicly insured long-term-care programs. Only the four (poorer) Atlantic provinces retained the public assistance approach to long-term care by 1982, and even there, under the Canada Assistance Plan, federal funds enabled them to improve services. Total expenditures on long-term care in Canada have more than doubled in the past five years. William Mennie, in a presentation in 1982, provided the most up-to-date analysis of long-term-care developments in Canada.[21]

Community health agencies—other than health planning councils or public health departments, which are sponsored by provincial, or local, governments—are largely voluntary. Blue Cross programs sell insurance to cover the private-public hospital cost difference and have substantial coverage in some provinces. In contrast, private medical insurance is largely excluded from the medical care program, except for items like cosmetic surgery, since the public programs must be comprehensive to qualify for federal financing.

Visiting nursing agencies—notably, the Victorian Order of Nurses, providing bedside nursing in the home—are among the most competent private health agencies. A full range of home-care services, including drugs, dressings, and visiting homemakers, are universally insured benefits in Manitoba and Quebec, with no charges to the patients. More limited home-care programs are operated under "national" health insurance in the other four provinces west of Quebec. Home care in the four Atlantic provinces is more limited, provided by public health departments or the Victorian Order of Nurses, usually for a subsidized fee related to income.

There is also a large number of voluntary health agencies, related to specific diseases—such as the Cancer Society, the Heart Association, and the Arthritis and Rheumatism Association—or to specific target populations, for example, the crippled children. Most of these agencies have provincial and local chapters. With so many health care services generally financed by many provincial governments in Canada—including dental care for children, drugs, hearing aids, prosthetic services, and long-term care—the scope of the private health promotion agencies is narrowed, but perhaps is more effective. They concentrate on three types of activity: research, health promotion through prevention and life style changes, and supplementation of services not fully covered by public programs.

OTHER HEALTH PRACTITIONERS

A review of data on the steady increase in the supply of most health practitioners suggests both the success of the Canadian health care system and a major problem:

Health care is an appealing professional and/or technical occupation. Educational standards in Canada are high, in part because of the strength of the Canadian high school and university system, in part because of the perceived value of education to immigrants and to pioneers widely dispersed across a vast land mass. But as each new category of health professionals establishes high standards for training and certification or licensure, its professional domain becomes more rigidly defined and crossing career ladders from one to another becomes more difficult. Salary negotiations with hospital employees or those in other institutions financed largely through public health insurance increasingly are province-wide. Although most of these workers are not civil servants, the knowledge that government is present at or is behind the bargaining table tends to drive salaries up and to harden the job descriptions and career ladders even more.

The very generous supply of nurses in Canada has attracted attention abroad, although some Canadian hospitals still must recruit actively. The Roemers in 1977 reported on the training of nurses as well as other health personnel, comparing the experience in five countries. Canada had by far the most nurses in relation to population.[22]

There are two basic training programs for becoming a registered nurse in Canada: hospital-based diploma programs or university-based baccalaureate degree programs. About four times as many RNs took the three-year hospital-based route, where expense is almost nil and training is more practical. Some special training programs have been developed that offer two years of training and one of practice under supervision, somewhat like the three-year medical curriculum. Other programs offer master's degrees in nursing, with specialization usually in administration or education. Public health nursing is usually a one-year master's degree program added to a four-year baccalaureate program. Frontier nurses have a preparation similar to that of primary-care nurse practitioners in the United States, enabling them to diagnose and treat illness as a physician extender in isolated areas. The Newfoundland Cottage Hospital program recruited British-trained nurse-midwives for decades before such nurses were trained in Canada.

It is interesting that physician assistants have never been approved as practitioners in Canada, and that nurse practitioners have been restricted mainly to the far north despite promising beginnings in urban Ontario at the new medical school in Hamilton. The perception of an oversupply of physicians as a major cause of health care cost escalation is the principal reason for this failure to follow the U.S. example. Despite evidence that the primary care given for most common ailments by such practitioners was at least as good as that by physicians, it seems unlikely that their role or supply will be substantially increased.

In contrast, nursing assistants—similar to licensed practical nurses in the United States—are the second largest category of health workers in Canada and are about one-half as numerous as registered nurses. Their training takes one year or less. In the past they were employed more for long-term care, but increasingly general hospitals are employing them to work alongside registered nurses on the wards and in special care units.

The supply of dentists in Canada is not nearly as generous as in the United States, in contrast to the nursing supply or even to the pool of physicians. This may be due in part to the lower average income in Canada and to the failure to include dental care as a health insurance benefit except for dental surgery under general anesthesia in the hospital.

When several Canadian provinces—notably Saskatchewan, Quebec, and Nova Scotia—first initiated free dental care programs for children, they followed the New Zealand pattern of training "school dental nurses" to fill cavities under the supervision of a dentist. Other provinces, such as Ontario, permitted a new category of "denturists" to take impressions and prepare dentures without requiring them to become doctors of dental surgery.

HEALTH COSTS AND HEALTH INSURANCE

Between 1960 and 1979 Canadian total expenditures on health services, public and private, increased from about $120 to about $800 per person. As percentage of the Gross National Product, the increase was from about 5.6% to 7.3%, from 1960 to 1970, when only hospital insurance—not medical insurance—was universally available and subsidized through general taxation. For the next decade, after universal physicians' services were available at almost zero cost to the patient—in home and office as well as at a hospital—total health care costs as percentage of the GNP remained virtually constant. However, estimates of the GNP are often corrected after several years, so the figures from 1977 on are still tentative. With the advent of Reaganomics and the worst depression since the 1930s, Canada's economy has been much harder hit than the United States'. Some economists believe that Canada cannot constrain its planned regular increases in health care expenditures sufficiently to keep the percentage of the GNP from rising above 8% in the early 1980s, because the GNP will be so much less than expected.

About one-quarter of all Canadian health expenditures are still from private sources—largely payments by individuals for dental care, private hospital accommodations, payments of daily charges for nursing home care, and contributions to capital construction costs of health care institutions. More than half of all dental care costs are now publicly financed, due to public programs of care for the aged as well as children.

There has been some unrest in the last few years among doctors, who exercise the option available to them in most provinces of charging some patients in addition to the established fees; however, this private expenditure is surprisingly small—less than 5% Public funds pay for 95% of all physicians' services.

Hospitals take the lion's share of Canadian health care expenditures—over 40%. Physicians absorb another 15%. Homes for special care take almost 12%, and the next largest category, drugs and appliances, account for over 10%. Notable is the small amount spent on prepayment and administration costs—only about 1.5%. This is despite separate hospital and medical insurance programs, and a number of smaller dental, drug, and appliance programs—in twelve different provinces or territories, all government-operated—plus a federal administrative and statistical oversight. Those who believe that government administration of health insurance is always more expensive than private enterprise should compare this 1.5% to the administrative costs of a U.S. Blue Cross, Blue Shield, or commerical health insurance plan. Even in individual provinces, where administrative costs are divided only by the money paid out to hospitals or doctors, administrative costs are often less than 2%.[4]

Economies of scale alone do not explain this remarkable efficiency, for some of the provinces are quite small. Rather, the universality of coverage and the comprehensiveness of the benefits are largely responsible. There is no doubt whether a patient is covered or whether the service will be paid for in the vast majority of cases. Further, only three provinces still collect part of the cost in premiums or health insurance taxes. Most of the costs are collected more efficiently, from taxes people pay anyway—income or sales taxes.

Since 1977 the provinces have been paying slightly more than half of the public costs for capital investment in hospitals or special care homes and for public health services, and more than half the public expenditures for special care homes. Provinces and the private sector each contributed about one-fifth of health research costs, while the Government of Canada provided three-fifths.

There has been some criticism in Canada of meager government spending on health research—just over 1% of nearly 20 billion dollars. It is hard to say whether this is justified or to know what yardstick to use. It seems probable that research on prevention of disease and accidents, if it paid off, would be a better investment than is high technology research, such as on heart transplants.

The gaps in health insurance coverage in Canada are principally for long-term nursing care in the four Atlantic provinces for the middle and upper income groups, for dental care and drugs for the working populations in most provinces, and for private and semi-private room extra charges by hospitals where privacy is not medically necessary. Outside of Canada, health insurance usually pays to travelers only what would have been paid within the nation's boundaries, and only for emergency care while traveling, or if referred out for specialized care.

Portability of benefits between provinces is one of the four conditions of federal financial assistance for health insurance, along with universal access, comprehensive benefits, and public administration. This presents some problems in a country where the population tends to move from low-cost to high-cost provinces to seek employment or specialized services. These problems were addressed by the ministers of health in meetings initiated in 1982 by the federal minister, and discussions are continuing.

Health care costs have been contained in Canada by a combination of measures, beginning with constraints on hospital bed supply and on the pool of physician specialists. Controls were later placed on hospital rates and physician fees—that is, on prices—and on utilization of hospitals and physicians' services; these probably would not have been effective in the absense of constraints on supply. Deterrent charges to sick patients were tried on a limited scale in Canada, but were found ineffective as cost constraints and were politically unpopular.[23] It soon became apparent that physician behaviour, not patient behaviour, is the main determinant of health care costs. Hospital wage and salary increases are a second major factor, and are equally difficult to control.

Figure 1 depicts the control structures Canadian provinces have evolved, with federal assistance. These have been successful in keeping Canadian health cost escalation in line with the growth of the GNP for a decade. Mention has already been made of methods of controlling physician supply, hospital capital investment, and operating costs of hospitals. Physicians' provincewide fee schedules have also been described, and the data base derived from each physician's fee-for-service billings discussed in medical manpower projections.

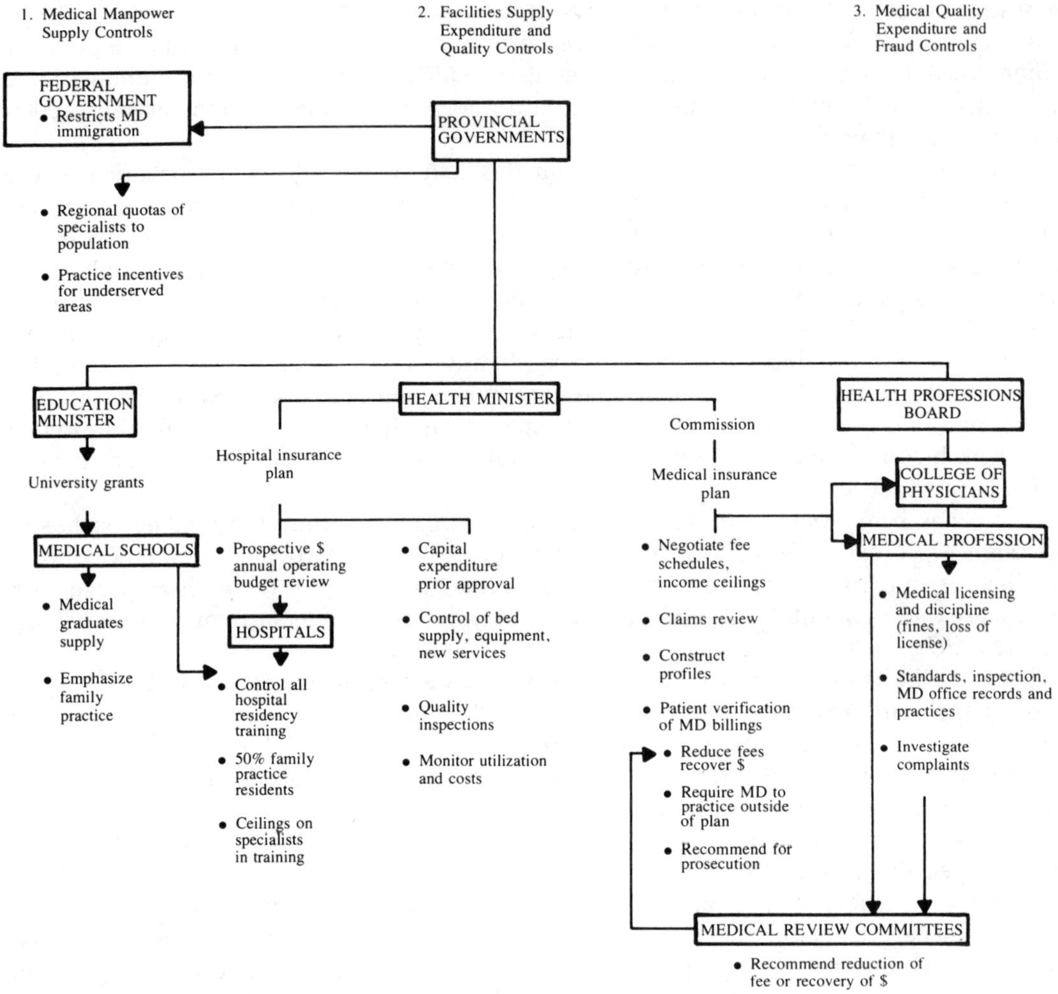

Figure 1 Canadian health care system control structures

In Figure 1 there are references to computerized physician profiles (construct profiles) and to the review of exceptions to group averages by peer (medical) review committees. Figure 2 shows an example of one of the early physician profiles used in Nova Scotia in the early 1970s. More elaborate versions are in computer memory in most provincial medical insurance programs and are too voluminous to print here. The exceptions to group averages are made available regularly to the medical review committees variously constituted in different provinces. The medical licensing body in most provinces has emerged as a major element in the utilization and quality control program, with power to remove a physician's license and impose fines, or lesser sanctions, for fraud, incompetence, or serious malpractice. This is further elaborated in a monograph published by the U.S. National Institutes of Health in 1981.[15]

The profile in figure 2 is that of a general practitioner who also did some obstetrics and surgery. A few of the hundreds of medical fee schedule services he performed in a year are listed in the center. In the left columns we see the actual volume of each service, the

Figure 2 Medical profile used in Nova Scotia, 1973

Physician Profile For 12 months ending Dec. 31/73			Specialty 00 Family Practice / Location 19 Anytown	Name Dr. J.J. Jones	Dr. No. 0000	Peer Group XJ	
Totals				Indices			
Services	Pay-ments	Patients	Fee Group and Item	Services	Pay-ments	Patients	PSI[a]
12,069	55,123	1,977	Total	156	132	98	160
20	255	19	001 Major Consult GP	126	126	120	143
5,970	25,363	1,544	103 Office Visit GP	153	153	100	156
12	51	10	105 Well Baby Care GP	18	18	25	26
698	4,138	331	121 Day Home Visit GP	166	166	138	171
76	638	69	123 Night Home Visit GP	73	72	71	73
72	612	61	125 Emergency Visit GP	243	242	220	305
117	986	115	127 Sunday & Holiday Visit GP	132	131	137	135
114	291	71	129 Extra Patients—Home GP	300	307	251	348
135	574	144	151 Initial Hospital Visit GP	319	319	316	334
4,013	12,615	298	153 Subsequent Hospital Visit GP	215	210	185	221
128	326	46	201 Injections	81	81	55	83
112	285	11	202 Hyposensitization	37	36	24	43
21	89	25	249 All Other List I	177	175	229	229
188	799	186	251 Pap Smear	124	124	136	128
15	191	13	252 Sigmoidoscopic Exam	119	114	105	143
33	140	33	255 Vaccination	131	132	134	148
25	319	14	299 All Other List II	70	78	58	72
26	2,060	26	301 Normal Confinement	73	72	73	81
56	213	25	311 Newborn & Premature Care GP	80	66	69	91
5	213	5	321 Diagnostic D & C	76	77	75	115
1	21	1	324 Abortion, Incomp. or Therapeutic	22	9	23	37
6	638	6	423 Appendectomy	166	166	166	551
1	32	1	429 All Other Dig. Tr. Surg. over $50	58	23	58	158
2	102	2	461 Adult Tonsillectomy	55	54	52	120
4	191	4	472 Fractures over $50	78	54	76	91
1	21	1	479 All Other Orth. Pro. over $50	38	11	38	103
16	82	16	501 Incision & Drainage Abscess	166	131	170	173
14	230	13	506 Biopsies	291	261	282	387
2	27	2	511 Excision Sebaceous Cyst	37	36	37	45
23	247	22	526 Excision of Warts	88	75	88	94
42	357	42	531 Suture Lacerations	84	83	85	86
1	34	1	546 T & A (under 16)	7	7	7	18
17	493	17	551 Fractures ($50 and under)	126	135	126	136
10	94	10	561 Circumcision	90	87	90	110
6	142	6	599 All Other Minor Surgery	23	41	27	25
50	1,741	53	600 Surgical Assistant	105	109	109	110
25	357	24	901 Detention Fee	74	105	123	121
2	47	2	905 Independent Consideration	55	47	57	76
3	51	3	909 Group Immunization	51	47	130	119
7	60	6	951 All Other Services	152	150	133	183

SOURCE: *Nova Scotia Medical Bulletin* (Oct. 1974).

[a]PSI = Patient Service Index.

amount of money paid to him for each by the health insurance program, and the number of different patients seen for each. The columns to the right are indices with the average (mean) for all similar physicians as 100. The Patient Service Index to the extreme right divides the number of services by the number of different patients seen. If a physician's index deviates from the mean by more than a specified amount—perhaps two standard deviations—for certain services, the computer exception program is triggered. A great deal of detail is then printed out on this aspect of the physician's services—perhaps every service by day of the week. Inspectors from the licensing body are authorized to visit his office, make further enquiries, and examine his records if necessary. Enquiries may be made of his patients, although since virtually his whole activities everyday are already in computer memory, this is seldom necessary. If he has not been billing for services not rendered, but only providing excessive and unnecessary ones, he may not be disciplined but may only be reimbursed for the services deemed by his peers to be necessary.

This is similar to the type of program developed by Dikewood in Albuquerque, New Mexico, to control overutilization in the state medicaid program.[24] The approach of some Professional Standards Review Organizations in the United States was also similar, until they were dismantled by the Reagan budget cuts.

Canadian physicians have generally acquiesced in such controls over excessive use and abuse, as the price for retaining a fee-for-service method of reimbursement. It is to the economic advantage of the majority of ethical physicians to prevent the bad actors from taking more than they should from the common pool.

PUBLIC HEALTH

Canada is proud of its past record in public health, but in the 1980s local public health services are in transition and their future structure is uncertain. New patterns of collaboration between private practitioners' services under health insurance and traditional local public health services are evolving. In some areas the traditional public health services are still needed and used; in others, such as Quebec, provincial governments are attempting to establish community health centers where primary-care physicians and the public health staff will work together. There are ideological and economic differences to be overcome before this can become an effective pattern in Canada. One needs to know a little of the past structure of Canada's public health services to understand the nature of the present transition.

At the end of the First World War, the province of New Brunswick was the first to establish a Department of Health headed by a cabinet minister. Other provinces and the federal government followed suit, although at various times the health departments were combined with others, notably welfare. The provinces passed public health laws modelled in principle after the landmark English Public Health Act of 1875. The collection of vital statistics and the establishment of environmental programs to control infectious diseases were the major functions; to these were added provision of hospitals for infectious diseases—notably tuberculosis—and for mental illness.

Some industrial provinces also developed advanced occupational health and safety programs. Many large cities had anticipated the provinces and established their own public health programs. In the 1920s maternal and child health programs were added, and the

Rockefeller Foundation in the 1940s and federal public health grants in the 1950s aided in setting up a network of local public health departments across the county. Local boards of health appointed a public health physician to head such departments.Called the "medical officer of health" in some provinces, his appointment and dismissal requires the authorization of the provincial minister of health.

The typical local public health staff consisted of half a dozen public health nurses, half as many sanitary inspectors, and perhaps a nutritionist or a public health educator, working in a small rural health unit or in a district office of a city health department. Bedside nurses and physical therapists were added by some departments as emphasis turned to geriatrics and chronic illnesses in the second half of the century.

At the national level, the Department of National Health and Welfare, established during the Second World War, has the major responsibility for public health. Immigration medical services and medical care for sick mariners, Indians, and Eskimos are federal responsibilities, although some services may be purchased from private or provincial institutions. Control of environmental hazards—such as food and drugs marketed nationwide or for export—is also a federal activity shared in part with the Department of Agriculture. Grants-in-aid to provinces to develop public health and medical care insurance are the major federal services.

Immunization has long been a key element in Canadian public health activities. Tetanus antitoxin and typhoid vaccine were developed before World War I, produced, with many other biologicals (such as tuberculin, smallpox, rabies, and pneumonia vaccines), at the Connaught Medical Research Laboratories of the University of Toronto, affiliated with the School of Hygiene. When Ramon in the 1920s developed diphtheria toxoid by treating the toxin with formaldehyde, Donald Fraser from the Toronto School and Connaught Laboratories went to France, learned the technique, and obtained rights to produce it at Connaught. The Laboratories also held the Banting and Best patents for insulin, another Canadian discovery. The culture medium used by Jonas Salk to produce enough polio vaccine for the first mass trials was developed by Raymond Parker at Connaught and exported to the United States.

As with the insulin, diphtheria toxoid, and many other products, a major contribution of researchers at Connaught—notably Peter Maloney—was the development of methods for mass production, so the products originally produced only in test tube lots could be available to immunize whole populations. In 1928 and 1930, Hamilton and Toronto were the first cities in the world to exist for a year without a case of diphtheria.

By the 1940s Connaught was producing all the penicillin for the Canadian armed forces, as well as ACTH and other hormones. A triple tetanus, diphtheria, and pertussis (whooping cough) vaccine, developed by Connaught, was made available free of charge by provincial governments to private physicians and local health departments nationwide. When in the 1940s the federal government introduced a comprehensive Food and Drug (later also Cosmetics) Act, the regulations relating to drugs were written with major input from the Connaught Laboratories.

During the three critical decades when the greatest advances were made in the control of communicable diseases in Canada, a Dominion Council of Health, consisting of the federal and provincial ministers of health, met regularly and developed nationwide public health policy. The only nongovernmental member for most of this time was Robert D. Defries, director of the Toronto School of Hygiene and Connaught Medical Research Laboratories, where most of the Canadian public health workers were trained and most of the immunizing agents and antisera were produced. Canada pioneered both in scientific advances in public health and in their communitywide application.

Until about 1960, on a typical weekday in a rural public health unit, the local public health medical director and a public health nurse might drive up to thirty miles over back roads to a small rural school to inspect and immunize all the children. Those children with suspicious symptoms of acute illness or malnutrition were identified for referral to a local physician or for a home visit by the public health nurse or nutritionist. In the afternoon, twenty miles away in another direction, a nutritionist and a local private practitioner, assisted by several nurses, would conduct a combined weekly immunization, well baby, and prenatal clinic. Services were free of charge and patronized by all classes of society. On Saturday mornings a staff meeting was held at the health unit offices, and Board of Health and community health education meetings were scheduled in the evenings.

A public health nurse visited every home shortly after a baby was born—having been alerted by the hospital or the birth certificate—and assisted the mother in providing adequate infant care. In isolated areas of the Maritimes and elsewhere in the 1920s and 1930s, the public health nurse was often also the midwife delivering babies at home. By the late 1940s this was no longer necessary—except in Newfoundland and the far north—because doctors had returned from the war and more specialists in pediatrics and obstetrics were trained. During the 1950s and 1960s, especially in the cities and larger towns, more middle and upper income patients turned to private practitioners for maternal and child health and immunization services, with part of the cost met by health insurance. Health departments concentrated on poorer areas and immigrant populations; they also started to develop home care and other services for patients with chronic illnesses.

As universal medical and hospital insurance programs developed, traditional public health services in most provinces were eclipsed. Public officials often did not understand why maternal and child health clinics, or tuberculosis clinics, or mental hospitals, or public health laboratories needed to operate separately from the general hospital and medical insurance programs.

In some smaller provinces the provincial health department became the administrative structure to which the health insurance programs were attached. In most provinces separate hospital insurance commissions and medical care insurance commissions operated under the minister of health, but independently of the traditional Health Department, and were much more powerful. After a decade or two, most provinces have seen some amalgamation of all these health services into a single department, under one minister and often one deputy minister.

The minister, who is elected, sits in the provincial legislative or lower House of Parliament—the only chamber in most provinces. The deputy minister is a civil servant, and may be a public health specialist in medicine; more often, however, this person is a former hospital administrator or other nonphysician manager, and the public health physician heads a small section of the department concerned with preventive medicine.

As epidemiology has been applied to the data base of Canadian health insurance, a new role of medical policy analysis has been emerging for public health in Canada. The Royal College of Physicians and Surgeons of Canada now approves postgraduate medical specialty training in community medicine as well as in public health. At the local level some provinces—notably Quebec—have defined a new role for the local medical officer of health trained in community medicine.

One large hospital, often a teaching hospital, is identified and a catchment area for its outpatient services is defined. The new specialist in community medicine is given responsibilities both for managing that ambulatory care service and for the traditional public health services in the catchment area. It is too early to say where these innovations will lead.

At the federal level it has been noted that most of the conditions requiring expensive hospital care are to some extent self-inflicted. A former minister of health used such data to promote changes in life styles for Canadians.[25]

CONCLUSION

Equal access for all people to medically necessary health care is the basis of the Canadian system. Although the provinces have instituted stringent cost containment measures and have, in a sense, rationed health care, it has been at a very high level of use—perhaps higher than is healthful. Days of hospital care per thousand population and average physician contacts per person per year are substantially higher than in the United States. Differentials between income classes changed in favor of the poor when universal health insurance was introduced. A classic before-and-after study by Enterline in Montreal showed that free access to physicians' offices provided more care to those who needed it most.[26] Physicians reported seeing fewer patients for frivolous reasons, and more for serious complaints, after free medical care was introduced.

Canada retains a single service for rich and poor alikc—not a two-class system. It has proven to be of good quality, yet inexpensive, free to all, yet not abused.

ACKNOWLEDGEMENTS

Lothar Rehmer of Health and Welfare, Canada, provided essential data and informed interpretations of their significance and limitations. Without his disinterested support this chapter would not have been completed. Likewise, Cyril Nair of Statistics Canada provided essential data and was particularly helpful in this scholarly enterprise. The staff of Provincial Hospital and Medical Care Insurance programs in Canada graciously responded to questionnaires on selected aspects of their programs with courtesy, accuracy, and brevity.

To all of these we are indebted. The opinions expressed in the chapter are, of course, our own, and not those of persons who helped us assemble the basic data.

Notes

1. B.H. Curry, J.E. Hastings, G.H. Hatcher, and M.A. Ross, "Administrative Practice in Relation to the Quality of Medical Care Under the Ontario Workmen's Compensation Board," *American Journal of Public Health* 45, no. 8 (Aug. 1955): 1011–15; G.H. Hatcher, "Administrative Factors in the Rehabilitation of Injured Workmen. Some Observations on the Experience of Ontario and Pennsylvania," *Industrial Medicine and Surgery* 31, no. 7 (July 1962): 319.

2. L. Miller and G.H. Hatcher, "Public Medical Care Programs in Newfoundland," *Canadian Journal of Public Health* 55 (Feb. 1965): 69–73.

3. C.R. Rorem, *The Municipal Doctor System in Rural Saskatchewan,* Committee on the Cost of Medical Care, publication no. 11 (Chicago: Univ. of Chicago Press, 1931).

4. Saskatchewan Hospital Services Plan, *Annual Reports,* 1948 to 1982 (Regina, Saskatchewan, 1949–

1983); Saskatchewan Medical Care Insurance Commission, *Annual Reports,* 1963 to 1982 (Regina, Saskatchewan, 1964–1983).

5. Government of Canada 5–6, Elizabeth II. Chapter 28 (1975), "Hospital Insurance and Diagnostic Services Act," 1957. Statutes of Canada, Chapter H-8. (Ottawa: Queen's Printer).

6. Government of Canada 14–15, Elizabeth II. Statutes of Canada, Chapter 64, "The Medical Care Act," 1966. (Ottawa: Queen's Printer).

7. Government of Canada, "The Federal Provincial Fiscal Arrangements and Established Programs Financing Act" (Ottawa: Queen's Printer, 1977).

8. Hon. Emmett E. Hall, *Canada's National Provincial Health Program for the 1980's—A Commitment for Renewal,* report to ministers of health (Saskatchewan: Universal Bindery Ltd., 1980).

9. Canada, House of Commons, *Fiscal Federalism in Canada. Report of the Parliamentary Task Force on Federal-Provincial Fiscal Arrangements* (Ottawa: Minister of Supply and Services, 1981).

10. G.H. Hatcher, "Health Insurance, Health Care Costs, and Mortality in Selected Industrial Nations" (Paper presented at the Annual Meeting of the American Public Health Association, Montreal, Quebec, 15 November 1982).

11. G.H. Hatcher and S. Constantinou, "Manpower Supply Surgical Rates and Health Care Costs in Selected Canadian Provinces," in *Dimensions in Health Service* (Toronto: Canadian Hospital Association, 1979).

12. National Committee on Physician Manpower, *Report on Manpower Requirements for Physicians in Canada* (Ottawa: Health and Welfare, Canada, 1975).

13. G.H. Hatcher, "Access to Medical Care and the Remuneration of Physicians," *The Lancet,* 23 May 1981, 1143–46.

14. Statistics Canada, *Hospital Statistics,* Vols. I, II, and III (Ottawa: Publications Distribution Unit of Statistics Canada, 1981).

15. G.H. Hatcher, *Universal Free Health Care in Canada. Utilization and Quality Aspects of Cost Controls as Canada's "zero price" National Health Insurance Evolves into a Comprehensive Health Service,* U.S. DHHS, NIH Publication no. 81–2052 (Washington, D.C.: Gov. Printing Office, 1981).

16. Saskatchewan Hospital Services Plan, *Annual Report, 1980–81,* pp. 11–13.

17. McKinsey and Co. Inc., "Setting Hospital Operating Budgets," in *The Implications of Canadian Health Regulatory Experience for U.S. Health Regulatory Policy,* Report on DHEW Contract No. HRA 231–77–0122 (Washington, D.C., 1978), pp. 61–91.

18. Health and Welfare Canada, *Salaries and Wages in Canadian Hospitals 1970-77,* with data for 1979 in Appendix (Ottawa: Policy Planning and Information Branch, 1980).

19. Hon. Emmett E. Hall, *Canada's Health Program,* p. 55.

20. Hon. Monique Begin, "Opening Statements to Conference of Federal and Provincial Ministers of Health, Ottawa, 26 May 1982" (Ottawa: Health and Welfare Canada Office of the Minister).

21. William A. Mennie, "Health Insurance and Long-Term Health Care in Canada" (Paper presented at the Annual Meeting of American Public Health Association, Montreal, Quebec, 15 November 1982).

22. Milton Roemer and Ruth Roemer, "Health Manpower Policies Under Five National Health Care Systems" and "Health Manpower Policy Under National Health Insurance—The Canadian Experience," U.S. DHEW Publications HRA 77–37 and 78–43 (Washington, D.C.: Health Resources Administration, USPHS, 1977 and 1978).

23. M.L. Barer et al., *Controlling Health Care Costs by Direct Charges to Patients* (Toronto: Ontario Economic Council, 1979).

24. R. Brook and K. Williams, "The New Mexico Peer Review Program," *Medical Care* 16, no. 9, suppl. (1978).

25. Hon. Marc Lalonde, *A New Perspective on the Health of Canadians: A Working Document* (Ottawa: Health and Welfare Canada, 1974).

26. P.E. Enterline et al., "The Distribution of Medical Services Before and After Medicare—The Quebec Experience," *New England Journal of Medicine* 289 (1973): 1175–76.

Table 1 Canadian population by age and sex in 1980

Age	Number (thousands)			%		
	Male	Female	Both	Male	Female	Both
All ages	11,887.1	12,049.3	23,936.3	100.0%	100.0%	100.0%
0 to 4	914.9	868.9	1,783.8	7.7	7.2	7.5
5 to 13	1,689.9	1,607.0	3,296.9	14.2	13.3	13.8
14 to 17	929.3	887.2	1,816.6	7.8	7.4	7.6
18 to 24	1,673.1	1,621.9	3,295.0	14.1	13.5	13.8
25 to 34	2,030.7	2,024.7	4,055.5	17.1	16.8	16.9
35 to 44	1,432.0	1,405.1	2,837.0	12.0	11.7	11.9
45 to 54	1,236.0	1,234.7	2,470.7	10.4	10.2	10.3
55 to 64	999.3	1,099.8	2,099.1	8.4	9.1	8.8
65 and over	981.9	1,299.9	2,281.8	8.3	10.8	9.5
Median age	28.4	29.9	29.2	—	—	—

SOURCE: Statistics Canada, Postcensal Estimates of Canadian Population (based on 1971 census).

NOTES: Data are estimates of resident population as of 1 June 1979 and 1 June 1980. Information on race is not collected in Canada. Available data on national origin and language groups is still based on 1971 census; results of 1981 census are not expected until 1983 at earliest. Percentages calculated by Hatcher Research Associates. Due to rounding, age groups do not add exactly to totals.

Table 2 Live births, birth rates, and fertility rates, Canada

	Number of Live Births	Birth Rate	General Fertility Rate
1979	366,046	15.5	58.2
1978	358,852	15.3	58.0

NOTES: Rates on an annual basis. Birth rates per 1,000 population and fertility rates per 1,000 women aged 15 to 49 years.

Table 3 Infant mortality rates by age, selected years, Canada

	Under 1 Year (IMR)	28 Days to 1 Year (Post-Neonatal)	Under 28 Days (Neonatal)
1950	41.5	17.1	24.4
1955	31.3	12.0	19.3
1960	27.3	9.7	17.6
1965	23.6	7.3	16.3
1967	22.0	6.8	15.2
1970	18.8	5.3	13.5
1973	15.5	4.8	10.8
1975	14.3	4.6	9.7
1977	12.4	4.1	8.3
1978	12.0	3.9	8.0
1979	10.9	3.7	7.2

SOURCE: Statistics Canada, *Vital Statistics, Volume III, Deaths, 1977* and *Volume I, Births and Deaths, 1979,* catalogues 84–206 and 84–204.

NOTE: Rates are per 1,000 live births. Data for 1975 is estimated. Data for 1980 was not available.

Table 4 Infant mortality rates by major causes, selected years, Canada

Causes of Death	1960	1965	1970	1975	1976	1977
Total, under one year	2,732.6	2,356.0	1,882.0	1,430.5[a]	1,346.7[b]	1,238.2
Congenital anomalies	433.8	435.0	382.0	298.4	310.3	308.5
Birth injury	264.3	237.9	224.2	136.6	135.0	112.9
Asphyxia and atelectasis	318.0	258.7	155.7	97.9	101.1	93.8
Pneumonia and influenza	415.4	275.2	153.5	65.3	61.3	45.9
Suffocation	94.2	95.6	68.0	31.2	26.4	24.4
Gastrointestinal diseases	119.7	49.0	26.9	21.7	19.4	20.2
Other diseases of early infancy	200.7	156.4	128.7	75.2	62.5	64.0
All other causes	886.2	848.1	740.3	704.1[a]	630.3[b]	569.2

SOURCE: Statistics Canada, *Annual Vital Statistics, Volume III, Deaths, 1977,* catalogue 84–206. (Figures for 1978 to 1980 are not yet available.)

NOTE: Rates for "cause of death" are calculated per 100,000 live births.

[a]Includes 228 deaths "cause not stated."
[b]Includes 116 deaths "cause not stated."

Table 5 Leading causes of death 1979, Canada

Rank[a]	Male	Rate	Female	Rate
1	Ischemic Heart Disease	299.6	Ischemic Heart Disease	97.1
2	Lung Cancer	86.5	Breast Cancer	40.4
3	Cerebrovascular Disease	49.7	Cerebrovascular Disease	36.0
4	M.V.T. Accidents	30.7	Lung Cancer	22.9
5	Bronchitis, Emphysema, Asthma	30.2	Colon and Rectum Cancer	22.0
6	Suicide	28.9	Cancer of Ovary	11.9
7	Cirrhosis of Liver	28.2	M.V.T. Accidents	11.7
8	Colon and Rectum Cancer	27.2	Cirrhosis of Liver	11.7
9	Stomach Cancer	16.6	Diabetes Mellitus	10.3
10	Cancer of Pancreas	14.4	Suicide	10.2
11	Cancer of Prostate	13.9	Bronchitis, Emphysema, Asthma	9.6
12	Diabetes Mellitus	12.3	Cancer of Pancreas	8.3

[a]Ranked by 1979 ASMR (Age 25–74) per 100,000 population.

Table 6 Average length of stay (and rates of separation) for selected operative procedures, 1977, Canada

Operation	ICDA Listing	Male			Female		
		Procedures (in Thousands)	Rates of Separation (Per 100,000 Pop.)	Average Length of Stay (Days)	Procedures (in Thousands)	Rates of Separation (Per 100,000 Pop.)	Average Length of Stay (Days)
Appendectomy	411	20.243	175	6.3	17.601	151	6.1
Biopsy	XVII (A1–A2)	16.231	141	14.3	18.180	156	12.0
Cardiac catheterization	302/303	7.040	61	6.4	3.493	30	7.0
Cardiac revascularization	298	3.640	32	17.6	.686	6	20.4
Cesarean section, all	77				42.947	368	9.2
Cholecystectomy	435	16.475	143	12.9	46.143	396	10.7
Dilation and curettage of uterus	703				63.843	574	2.9
Excision and ligation of varicose veins	244	3.798	33	6.7	9.670	83	6.3
Excision of intervertebral cartilage (prolapse disc)		7.117	62	14.1	4.266	37	16.4
Excision of semilunar cartilage of knee joint	865	14.917	129	5.3	5.185	44	6.5
Extraction of lens, infrascapular	145	10.124	88	7.4	13.740	118	7.7
Hemorrhoidectomy	513	8.798	76	6.8	8.424	72	6.9
Hysterectomy, all	69				62.871	539	10.1
Inguinal hernia repair	382/383	44.796	388	5.7	5.662	49	5.6
Ligation and division of fallopian tubes	685				64.167	550	3.7
Local excision of lesion of skin and subcutaneous tissue	921	9.006	78	9.6	9.927	79	7.6
Operations on muscle, tendon, and facia except of hand	88	10.523	91	5.7	9.926	85	5.6
Operations on ovary	67				12.156	104	8.6
Partial mastectomy	652	.334	3	5.0	12.057	103	4.1

Table 6 *Continued*

Operation	ICDA Listing	Male			Female		
		Procedures (in Thousands)	Rates of Separation (Per 100,000 Pop.)	Average Length of Stay (Days)	Procedures (in Thousands)	Rates of Separation (Per 100,000 Pop.)	Average Length of Stay (Days)
Prostatectomy, transurethral	582	23.580	204	14.2			
Reduction of fracture and fracture dislocation of ankle and wrist	83	7.263	63	6.0	6.530	56	7.0
Reduction of fracture and fracture dislocation of hip	82	2.836	25	30.9	5.590	48	31.4
Reduction of fracture and fracture dislocation of other than hip, ankle, and wrist	84	18.685	162	10.4	10.044	86	13.2
Tonsillectomy	211/212	42.415	368	2.1	49.046	420	2.2

SOURCE: Statistics Canada, *Surgical Procedures and Treatments, 1977,* catalogue 82–208.

Table 7a For Canadian males twenty leading causes of hospitalization, days of hospital care, and average length of stay in 1978

Subgroup Number	Subgroups of Diseases and Conditions ICDA–8 (Description)	Rank	Separations[a] (in Thousands)	Days of Hospital Care	Average Length of Stay[b] (in Days)
410–414	Ischemic heart disease	1	87.660	1,196,680	13.7
780–789	Symptoms referable to systems or organs	2	71.121	419,705	5.9
500–508	Other diseases of upper respiratory tract	3	69.991	178,092	2.5
550–553	Hernia of abdominal cavity	4	55.022	325,713	5.9
600–607	Diseases of male genital organs	5	51.293	435,052	8.5
300–309	Neuroses, personality disorders, and other nonpsychotic mental disorders	6	50.012	664,133	13.3
720–729	Osteomyelitis and other diseases of bone and joint	7	47.981	463,787	9.7
460–466	Acute respiratory infections except influenza	8	44.778	232,808	5.2
490–493	Bronchitis, emphysema, and asthma	9	42.293	367,251	8.7
480–486	Pneumonia	10	37.762	451,618	12.0
590–599	Other diseases of urinary system	11	37.074	327,250	8.8
570–577	Diseases of liver, gallbladder, and pancreas	12	36.452	481,626	13.2
560–569	Other diseases of intestine and peritoneum	13	33.754	324,360	9.6
530–537	Diseases of oesophagus stomach and duodenum	14	33.688	—	—
420–429	Other forms of heart disease	15	32.558	441,681	13.6
430–438	Cerebrovascular diseases	16	30.014	1,141,182	38.0
000–009	Intestinal infectious diseases	17	29.174	164,415	5.6
820–829	Fracture of lower limb	18	28.771	450,901	15.7
450–458	Diseases of veins and lymphatics, and other diseases of circulatory system	19	26.212	269,928	10.3
370–379	Other diseases and conditions of eye	20	25.237	147,438	5.8
(1–20)[c]	Leading 20—total		870.847		
(21–98)[c]	Residual—total		614.526		
(1–98)[c]	All groups—total		1,485.373		

SOURCE: Statistics Canada, *Hospital Morbidity*, 1978, catalogue 82–206; Government of Canada.

[a]Causes of hospitalization ranked by number of separations, not by days of hospital care.
[b]Average length of stay figures calculated by Hatcher Research Associates Corporation and Statistics Canada staff.
[c]These numbers are not subgroups, but refer loosely to the 98 categories of ICDA–8 listings.

Table 7b For Canadian females, twenty leading causes of hospitalization, days of hospital care, and average length of stay in 1978

Subgroup Number	Subgroups of Diseases and Conditions ICDA–8 (Description)	Rank	Separations[a] (in Thousands)	Days of Hospital Care	Average Length of Stay[b] (in days)
650–662	Delivery	1	353.684	2,050,272	5.8
620–629	Diseases of the uterus and other female genital organs	2	113.800	662,173	5.8
780–789	Symptoms referable to systems or organs	3	86.446	568,889	6.6
Y00–Y15	Supplementary classifications	4	82.726	616,840	7.5
630–634	Complications of pregnancy	5	65.823	215,824	3.3
500–508	Other diseases of upper respiratory tract	6	65.181	163,250	2.5
570–577	Diseases of liver, gallbladder, and pancreas	7	62.672	678,661	10.8
640–645	Abortion	8	57.692	129,602	2.3
300–309	Neuroses, personality disorders, and other nonpsychotic mental disorders	9	55.220	822,517	14.9
410–414	Ischemic heart disease	10	51.573	1,019,357	19.8
210–228	Benign neoplasm	11	43.965	313,346	7.1
610–616	Diseases of breast, ovary, fallopian tube, and parametrium	12	40.604	208,274	5.1
590–599	Other diseases of urinary system	13	40.411	323,966	8.0
560–569	Other diseases of intestine and peritoneum	14	40.156	456,308	11.4
720–729	Osteomyelitis and other diseases of bone and joint	15	36.617	495,529	13.5
460–466	Acute respiratory infections except influenza	16	34.617	190,687	5.5
450–458	Diseases of veins and lymphatics, and other diseases of circulatory system	17	33.754	365,899	10.8
490–493	Bronchitis, emphysema, and asthma	18	33.360	272,415	8.2
000–009	Intestinal infectious diseases	19	30.191	180,494	6.0
480–486	Pneumonia	20	29.812	388,103	13.0
(1–20)[c]	Leading 20—Total		1,358.304		
(21–98)[c]	Residual—Total		719.569		
(1–98)[c]	All groups—Total		2,077.873		

SOURCE: Statistics Canada, *Hospital Morbidity*, 1978, catalogue 82–206; Government of Canada.

[a]Causes of hospitalization ranked by number of separations, not by days of hospital care.
[b]Average length of stay figures calculated by Hatcher Research Associates Corporation and Statistics Canada staff.
[c]These numbers are not subgroups, but refer loosely to the 98 categories of ICDA–8 listings.

Table 7c Standardized hospital separation rates, Canada

Reason for Admission	ICDA Listing	Standardized Rates 1976	1977	1978
Total		15,390.8	14,974.1	14,627.9
Infective and parasitic diseases	000–136	457.7	452.8	441.9
Neoplasms	140–239	932.9	934.7	890.0
Endocrine, nutritional, and metabolic diseases	240–279	292.7	300.5	290.3
Diseases of the blood and the blood-forming organs	280–289	107.5	101.1	78.2
Mental disorders	290–315	616.1	609.3	628.5
Diseases of the nervous system and the sense organs	320–389	690.1	684.0	658.6
Diseases of the circulatory system	390–458	1,570.5	1,591.7	1,487.9
Diseases of the respiratory system	460–519	1,960.1	1,910.2	1,834.6
Diseases of the digestive system	520–577	1,676.4	1,618.1	1,548.5
Diseases of the genito-urinary system	580–629	1,413.9	1,245.7	1,193.6
Complications of pregnancy, child-birth, and the puerperium	630–678	1,977.5	1,916.4	1,861.9
Diseases of skin and subcutaneous tissue	680–709	257.0	251.8	242.3
Diseases of the musculoskeletal system and the connective tissue	710–738	693.9	702.8	683.2
Congenital anomalies	740–759	193.9	194.1	189.3
Symptoms and ill-defined conditions	780–796	719.1	664.5	760.0
Accidents, poisonings, and violence	800–999	1,460.6	1,435.0	1,408.8
Supplementary classifications	Y00–Y29	370.9	361.5	409.0

SOURCE: Statistics Canada, *Hospital Morbidity,* 1978, catalogue 82–206.

NOTES: Hospital separation rates are standardized to the 1971 Canada population, using five-year age groupings. Standardized rates are per 100,000 population.

Table 8a Active major health care workers, selected years, Canada

Year	All Health Professions	Physicians		Dentists	Registered Nurses	Optometrists	Pharmacists	Podiatrists	Veterinarians
		MD[a]	MD[b]						
1970	—	31,166	25,656	7,115	104,258	1,497	11,084	123	—
1975	207,118	39,104	32,561	8,738	140,388	1,685	13,872	143	3,188
1978	235,279	42,238	—	10,451	161,125	1,869	15,709	139	3,748
1979	—	43,192	36,444	10,763	—	1,919	16,052	271	3,909

SOURCE: Health and Welfare Canada, *Canada Health Manpower Inventory,* 1980, Ottawa, March 1981.

[a]Includes interns and residents.
[b]Excludes interns and residents.

Table 8b Allied health care workers, selected years, Canada

	1970	1975	1979
Dieticians[a]	1,668	2,443	3,164
Health record administrators[a,b]	1,265	2,274	2,160
Health record technicians[b]	156	160	130
Medical technologists			
Medical laboratory technologists[c]	6,502	11,274	13,655
Medical radiation technologists[a]	4,186	7,211	8,055
Respiratory technologists[a]	346	1,054	1,736
Occupational therapists[c]	—	1,178	1,439[d]
Physical therapists[a]	2,210	2,802	3,208
Speech pathologists and audiologists[c]	—	973	1,324
Dental assistants[a,e]	1,531	1,519	3,381
Dental hygienists[f]	746	1,566	3,506
Nurse graduates of basic baccalaureate programs	413	845	1,440
Nurse graduates of initial diploma programs	8,212	8,933[g]	5,647[g]
Nursing assistants[f]	46,227	69,541[h]	77,439[h]
Full-time and part-time qualified nursing assistants employed in public general and allied special hospitals, tuberculosis sanatoria, and mental institutions	34,098	40,660	—

SOURCE: Health and Welfare Canada, *Canada Health Manpower Inventory,* 1980.

[a]Number of registered members of Canadian associations of specific occupation. These numbers may not always reflect the number of persons working in certain fields because all do not belong to their respective associations, dependent on the year, the province, and changes in provincial laws regarding mandatory membership. (See notes for specifics.)
[b]Certificants of Canadian College of Health Records Administrators (CCHRA), formerly called registered record librarians. Accredited record technicians are now termed "Associates," CCHRA.
[c]Number actively certified.
[d]Figure for 1978.
[e]Association members constitute an estimated 10% of the total number of dental assistants in Canada.
[f]Number licensed.
[g]Figures low due to missing data (schools not reporting).
[h]Estimated figures high due to inclusion of inactive members.

Table 9 Operational medical schools, medical students, and medical school graduates by sex, 1980, Canada

	Number	
Medical Schools	16	
Male Medical Students	4,710	(63.8%)
Female Medical Students	2,677	(36.2%)
Total	7,387	
Male Medical Graduates	1,182	(67.8%)
Female Medical Graduates	561	(32.2%)
Total	1,743	

SOURCE: Association of Canadian Medical Colleges, *Canadian Medical Education Statistics 1980/81,* Source Tables 19, 21, 38, and 39 (Ottawa: 1982).

Table 10 Canadian physicians, population, and physician population ratios

Year	Total Physicians[a]	Total Population (in Thousands)	Population Per Physician
1951	14,325	13,984	976
1961	21,290	18,238	857
1965	25,481	—	779
1970	31,166	21,465	689
1972	34,508	21,942	636
1974	37,297	22,569	605
1975	39,104	22,884	585
1976	40,130	23,175	577
1977	41,398	23,436	565
1978	42,238	23,667	558
1979	43,192	23,932	551

SOURCES: *Canada Health Manpower Inventory,* 1980, from the Health Information Division, Health and Welfare, Canada and the Royal Commission on Health Services, 1964, Vol. 1.

[a]Includes interns and residents.

Table 11a Physicians by place of practice, 1979, Canada

	Total
Office-based practice	29,000
Hospital-based patient care	5,700[a]
Administration and research	1,700
Residents	4,900
Interns	1,800

SOURCE: L.W. Rehmer, Director, Health Information Division Health Resources, Government of Canada.

NOTES: Data are estimated by Director Rehmer from Canadian government health and welfare statistics. Canada does not have data which permits us to distinguish precisely between "office-based" and "hospital-based" patient care.

[a]This number includes 1,500 physicians with appointments in teaching.

Table11b Active civilian physicians by type of appointment, 1979, Canada

	Total
Family physician	18,469
Specialist	17,975
Research (medicine)	256
Teacher (medicine)	1,520
Administration (government)	1,437
Administration (business)	223
Medical director (pharmaceutical industry)	44

SOURCE: Health and Welfare Canada, *Canada Health Manpower Inventory,* 1980.

NOTE: This table does not include physicians with staff appointments in hospitals or physicians with part-time appointments.

Table 11c Physicians by specialty, 31 December 1979, Canada

	Number of Physicians
Total physicians[a]	36,444
General practice family medicine	18,469
Medical specialties	7,551
Allergy	24
Cardiology	201
Dermatology	306
Gastroenterology	127
Internal medicine	2,178
Pediatrics	1,299
Pediatric cardiology	5
Pulmonary disease	6
Psychiatry	2,089
Surgical specialties	6,474
General surgery	2,137
Neurosurgery	156
Obstetrics/gynecology	1,330
Ophthalmology	820
Orthodontic surgery	732
Otolaryngology	501
Plastic surgery	221
Thoracic surgery[b]	148
Urological surgery	429
Other specialties	3,927
Anesthesiology	1,452
Pathology	790
Radiology	1,427

SOURCE: Statistics Canada, *Canada Health Manpower Inventory*, 1979, table 21.15.

[a]Excluding interns and residents.
[b]Includes cardiovascular surgery.

Table 12a Average net professional income of self-employed physicians, by specialty, 1979, Canada

	Average Professional Incomes		
	Net	Gross	
	(in Thousands)	Mean	Median
General practice	45.4	82.1	79.3
All specialties	63.2	95.1	89.2
All physicians	53.5	88.3	84.1
Medical specialties	56.3	86.1	78.8
Paediatrics	51.3	90.7	85.7
Internal medicine	59.8	93.3	84.5
Psychiatry	52.4	61.4	56.1
Dermatology	64.2	114.7	112.5
Neurology	61.6	90.2	80.4
Allergy	52.1	56.7	—
Physical medicine	61.4	56.7	—
Surgical specialties	66.8	108.2	103.5
General surgery	61.3	99.6	96.9
Cardiovascular and thoracic surgery	81.9	148.1	139.5
Orthopaedic surgery	78.1	107.7	103.7
Plastic surgery	80.2	101.9	96.0
Neurosurgery	70.7	93.7	87.0
Obstetrics and gynecology	63.4	109.4	104.3
Urology	65.6	107.2	101.1
Ophthalmology	67.1	113.5	107.2
Otolaryngology	72.3	127.9	120.6
Ophthalmology/otolaryngology	50.4	—	—
Other specialties	68.4	—	—
Radiology[a]	75.6		
Pathology[b]	69.0		
Anesthesiology	61.7	75.1	73.8

SOURCE: Net data compiled by the Health Insurance Division, Health Services and Promotion Branch, on the basis of unpublished statistics received from Revenue Canada Taxation.

NOTES: (1) "Net professional income" generally consists of net fee-for-service incomes only, i.e., excludes professional income received in the form of salaries and wages, as well as all nonprofessional incomes. (2) "Self-employed physicians" generally refers to physicians for whom net fee-for-service receipts were the largest single source of income; may also refer to physicians in part-time practice (limited average number of hours per week, or limited number of weeks per year). (3) In Canada classification as a specialist generally depends upon certification by the Royal College of Physicians and Surgeons or the Professional Corporation of Physicians of Quebec. All noncertified physicians are counted as general practitioners, regardless of the specialty-orientation, if any, of their actual practice. (4) Depending upon the fiscal year adopted by physicians (the fiscal year must end in the taxation year), the earnings reported for 1979 may have been partly earned in 1978. That is, the figures are likely to understate true 1979 incomes.

[a]Some provinces reimburse radiologists from the hospital insurance program payments to hospitals rather than through medical care insurance payments to physicians, so data are not available for gross incomes.

[b]Likewise, some provinces reimburse pathologists from the hospital insurance program payments to hospitals rather than through medical care insurance payments to physicians, so, again, data are not available. One province reported gross payments of over $1 million to a pathologist in a teaching hospital.

Table 12b Payment per phys cian receiving fee-for-service payments, by specialty, fiscal years ending March 31, Canada

	1972	1973	1974	1975	1976	1977	1978	1979
General practice	$33,250	$34,125	$37,742	$41,401	$45,047	$49,061	$53,263	$58,561
All specialties	46,553	48,113	51,478	56,875	59,651	63,968	68,749	74,700
Medical specialties	36,884	38,354	41,967	46,606	49,461	53,612	57,978	63,016
Internal medicine	37,980	39,333	43,291	47,866	51,874	57,080	61,806	68,592
Neurology	40,517	41,100	44,599	49,763	53,793	60,319	65,653	70,637
Physiatry	27,226	28,229	31,535	35,139	36,996	39,124	41,391	43,868
Pediatrics	40,884	42,256	44,086	48,304	52,061	55,728	59,910	64,697
Dermatology	58,178	61,376	67,189	73,044	78,903	83,662	92,088	96,165
Psychiatry	49,013	59,032	70,246	87,546	66,481	76,269	94,679	97,137
Surgical specialties	56,612	58,492	61,866	68,449	71,610	76,555	82,250	89,857
General surgery	50,989	51,981	55,267	60,032	62,443	66,614	72,023	80,038
Thoracic and cardiovascular	65,013	72,757	76,461	83,541	91,417	99,799	105,566	123,052
Urology	58,123	58,020	62,504	68,240	73,252	78,580	85,017	94,101
Orthopedic surgery	56,893	59,398	63,312	73,902	74,522	78,498	83,667	91,507
Plastic surgery	53,788	57,144	57,335	66,276	69,437	74,948	79,003	90,739
Neurosurgery	46,792	49,294	51,395	57,009	60,363	65,018	73,778	78,403
Ophthalmology	58,713	61,258	64,388	72,554	77,423	83,753	88,628	95,665
Otolaryngology	67,761	71,863	74,139	82,057	83,586	91,799	98,533	106,290
Obstetrics and gynecology	61,098	62,638	66,230	71,803	75,770	79,648	85,526	90,272
Technical specialties	41,112	42,710	46,103	50,837	52,725	56,503	60,390	64,860

SOURCE: Net data compiled by the Health Insurance Division, Health Services and Promotion Branch, on the basis of unpublished statistics received from Revenue Canada Taxation.

Table 13a Hospitals, beds, admissions, average daily census, and percentage occupany by type of hospital, Canada

	Hospitals[a]		Beds[a]		Admissions[b]		Average Daily Census[b]		Percentage Occupancy[b,c]	
	1979–80	1980–81	1979–80	1980–81	1979–80	1980–81	1979–80	1980–81	1979–80	1980–81
Total	1,241	1,239	165,440	167,477	3,566,471	3,617,902	128,414	134,153	80.77	81.64
Federal	132	131	4,166	3,329	34,739	26,154	2,014	1,808	68.83	67.96
Public (includes teaching)	1,047	1,049	158,105	160,744	3,514,493	3,568,507	123,405	130,792	80.79	81.75
Public general (includes teaching)	859	856	121,393	122,660	3,338,634	3,380,899	93,337	97,014	78.11	79.39
Public general (nonteaching)	810	802	87,955	86,239	2,498,806	2,442,713	67,528	67,962	77.52	79.07
Without long-term units	525	490	37,110	34,186	1,200,356	1,106,406	26,963	25,014	73.10	73.40
1–24 beds	197	183	3,028	2,793	90,913	82,277	1,751	1,610	58.17	58.16
25–49 beds	142	132	4,882	4,520	151,238	135,784	2,838	2,581	58.78	58.17
50–99 beds	84	78	5,882	5,369	186,980	174,601	3,883	3,554	67.71	66.20
100–199 beds	51	48	6,949	6,418	222,661	211,083	5,074	4,790	73.22	74.64
200–299 beds	26	27	6,009	6,249	203,420	209,410	4,855	5,043	79.82	80.69
300 + beds	25	22	10,330	8,837	345,144	293,251	8,562	7,436	83.11	84.15
With long-term units	285	312	50,845	52,053	1,298,450	1,336,307	40,565	42,948	80.77	82.79
1–49 beds	61	83	1,905	2,473	50,499	64,763	1,235	1,649	66.03	67.83
50–99 beds	65	68	4,607	4,835	118,768	124,378	3,352	3,529	73.76	75.11
100–199 beds	63	67	8,832	9,336	238,111	244,989	6,829	7,519	78.42	80.53
200–299 beds	37	39	9,096	9,832	237,818	264,696	7,643	8,490	84.26	86.36
300 + beds	59	55	26,405	25,577	653,254	637,481	21,506	21,761	82.61	85.08
Proprietary	62	59	3,169	3,404	17,239	23,241	2,995	1,553	97.32	92.75

SOURCE: Data from Statistics Canada, as calculated by the Health Information Division, Health and Welfare Canada.

[a]Figures for all operating hospitals.
[b]Figures for reporting hospitals (preliminary data).
[c]Figures based on approved bed complement.

Table 13b Canadian hospitals for psychiatric disorders: reporting hospitals, beds, admissions, average daily census, and percentage occupancy by type of hospital

	Reporting Hospitals[a]		Rated Bed Capacity		Beds Set Up		Average Daily Census		% Occupancy[b]	
	1978–79	1979–80	1978–79	1979–80	1978–79	1979–80	1978–79	1979–80	1978–79	1979–80
Public										
Mental	28	23	11,757	10,863	10,820	9,984	9,667	8,924	82.8	82.1
Psychiatric	7	7	1,038	1,038	974	928	827	781	79.7	75.2
Other[c]	6	4	1,189	989	1,061	759	901	728	75.8	73.6
Proprietary	3	3	342	342	337	337	319	318	93.4	93.1

SOURCE: Statistics Canada, *Mental Health Statistics, Volume III, Institutional Facilities, Services, and Finances, 1978–79,* catalogue 83–205, annual, July 1981; additional calculations by the Health Information Division, Health and Welfare Canada, from figures provided by the Institutional Statistics Section of the Health Division of Statistics Canada for 1979–80.

[a]All operating hospitals reported in 1978–79 and 1979–80.
[b]Figure based on rated bed capacity.
[c]Includes hospitals for alcoholics and epileptics.

Table 14 General and allied special hospitals and beds by type of ownership, 1981, Canada

Ownership	Hospitals	Beds
Lay Corporation	505	98,801
Municipal	320	22,272
Religious	116	25,976
Health and Welfare Canada (HWC)	101	832
Provincial	89	16,703
Proprietary	57	3,351
Department of National Defence (DND)	28	890
Red Cross	16	176
Industrial	4	63
Department of Veterans Affairs (DVA)	2	1,606
Total	1,238	176,670
Beds per 1,000 population		7.1

SOURCE: Data by province from Health and Welfare Canada, Division of Health Information, adjusted by Hatcher Research Associates Corporation.

Table 15a Special care facilities and maximum beds by selected principal characteristics, Canada

Categories (Principal Characteristics)[a]	1979		1980	
	Number	Beds	Number	Beds
Aged persons	2,048	127,257	2,017	129,546
Physical handicap	206	12,490	190	11,866
Retarded	370	18,704	383	18,735
Mental handicap	868	23,834	842	23,507
Emotionally disturbed children	599	11,730	690	12,668
Alcohol/drug	148	4,190	148	4,119
Total (includes above and other designated and undesignated categories)[b]	4,570	206,174	4,713	210,420

SOURCE: Hon. Emmett M. Hall, Special Commissioner, *Canada's National Provincial Health Program for the 1980s,* "A Commitment for Renewal," Health Services Review, 1979.

NOTES: This table deals exclusively with Residential Special Care Facilities, which maintain four or more beds for residents other than members of staff and which provide care to at least one resident. These facilities are, in general, maintained for residents who are chronically ill or disabled.

[a]Residents are classified into ten categories. Each category is the principal characteristic of the predominant group that comprises the largest number of residents.

[b]Includes "Delinquent," "Unmarried Mother," "Transient," and "Other."

Table 15b Beds in Canadian special care homes

	Beds				Beds Per Thousand Population			
	1962	1972	1976	1978	1962	1972	1976	1978
Nursing homes	18,685	43,100	49,145	53,739	1.0	2.0	2.1	2.3
Homes for the aged	39,189	70,489	85,297	87,642	2.1	3.2	3.7	3.7
Homes for the mentally retarded	14,805	16,939	16,853	—	0.8	0.8	0.7	—
Other special care homes	—	6,719	13,289	30,886	—	0.3	0.6	—
Total	72,679	137,247	164,584	172,267	3.9	6.3	7.1	7.3

SOURCE: Hon. Emmett M. Hall, Special Commissioner, *Canada's National Provincial Health Program for the 1980s,* "A Commitment for Renewal," Health Services Review, 1979.

NOTES: Data are as at 31 December for 1962; 1972 and 1976 at totals as at 31 March of the subsequent year. Figures for 1978 are as at 31 March 1979. Table excludes hostels, homes for child protection, and homes for unwed mothers; excludes hospital beds for acute short-term care, rehabilitation–convalescent, extended care (chronic), psychiatric units in general hospital, and tuberculosis sanatoria. Data compiled by Health Economics and Data Analysis Division, Health Services and Promotion Branch, 28 April 1980.

Table 15c Institutional beds in Canada

	1962	1972	1976	1978	1980
All institutional beds (per thousand population)	13.7	14.9	14.7	14.5	14.8

SOURCE: *Canada's National Provincial Health Program for the 1980s.*

NOTES: Includes all beds in hospitals and homes for special care—*except* hostels, homes for child protection, and homes for unwed mothers. Data for 1980 calculated from table 15a.

Table 16 Operating expenses per patient day in reporting Canadian acute care hospitals and in public general and in specialty hospitals

	Operating Expenses per Patient Day			
Type and Size of Hospital	1978–79	1979–80[a]	1980–81[a]	% Change[b] 1979–80 to 1980–81
General total	167.69	182.18	208.89	14.66
Public general				
Nonteaching total	146.91	160.13	182.23	13.80
Nonteaching with long-term units	141.34	153.93	174.15	13.14
By bed-size category (all public general hospitals)				
1–49 beds	131.60	151.65	157.17	3.64
50–99 beds	140.34	147.13	163.18	10.91
100–199 beds	139.33	153.57	177.67	15.70
200–299 beds	142.42	156.63	177.62	13.40
300+beds	142.34	157.27	174.62	13.19
Specialty total	283.35	301.22	335.42	11.35

SOURCE: Compiled by the Health Information Division, Government of Canada; derived from Statistics Canada publication.

[a]Preliminary data, excludes medical staff salaries and fees in Quebec.
[b]Percentage change calculated by Hatcher Research Associates Corporation. Estimated expenses for outpatients represent about 15% of total operating expenses. Smaller hospitals are mostly in rural areas.

Table 17 National health expenditures: amount and per capita amount by major sources of funds and percentage of Gross National Product, selected years, Canada

	1979	1977	1975	1970	1965	1960
National health expenditures						
(thousands)	$18,836,389[a]	$15,395,216	$12,340,324	$6,255,917	$3,414,974	$2,136,525
As % of GNP	7.20%[a]	7.37%	7.46%	7.30%	6.17%	5.57%
Aggregate amounts by sector[b]						
Private	—	$ 3,683,728	$ 2,906,908	$1,863,906	$1,636,295	$1,232,851
Public	—	11,711,488	9,433,416	4,392,011	1,778,679	903,674
Federal	—	5,241,685	3,971,108	1,816,170	673,112	341,172
Provincial	—	6,265,189	5,298,476	2,477,355	1,035,051	498,877
Local	—	204,614	163,832	98,486	70,517	63,625
Per capita expenditures						
Aggregate amounts by sector	$794.74[a]	$661.30	$542.98	$293.38	$173.54	$119.30
Private	—	158.23	127.91	87.41	83.15	68.84
Public	—	503.06	415.08	205.97	90.39	50.46
Federal	—	225.16	174.73	85.17	34.21	19.05
Provincial	—	269.12	233.14	116.18	52.60	27.86
Local	—	8.79	7.21	4.62	3.58	3.55
GNP and population						
Gross National Product[a]						
(millions of current dollars)	261,961	208,868	165,343	85,685	55,364	38,359
Population (thousands)[c]	23,768.7*	23,286.8*	22,697.1	21,297.0	19,644.0	17,870.0
Annual percentage change (increase)						
Population[d]	0.99%	1.27%	1.48%	8.41%	9.92%	—
GNP[d]	13.72	9.33	12.07	54.76	44.33	—
Per capita health expenditures	10.5	8.0	18.7	12.0	9.6	—
Aggregate national						
health expenditures	11.4[a]	9.3	20.4	13.6	11.6	—
Private[d]	—	12.25	13.07	13.91	32.72	—
Public[d]	—	8.37	22.88	146.92	96.82	—

SOURCE: Data compiled by the Health Information Division of Health and Welfare, Canada, from Statistics Canada figures, Government of Canada.

[a]Provisional figures.
[b]This amount is the Canadian approximation to the U.S. terminology "major source of funds."
[c]Population figures are final intercensal estimates, as of June 1 of the respective years. * indicates which figures are intercensal preliminary estimates.
[d]Percentages calculated by Hatcher Research Associates Corporation.

Table 18a National health expenditures in Canada by type of expenditure and source of funds

	1978						1979[a]
			Public				
Type of Expenditure	Canada	Private	Total[b]	Federal	Provincial	Local	Canada
Total health expenditures	$16,902,517	$4,137,364	$12,765,153	$5,936,529	$6,590,544	$238,080	$18,836,389
Institutional care[c] (all institutions)	9,293,467	1,028,781	8,264,686	4,329,109	3,838,128	107,449	10,259,454
General and allied special care hospitals	6,773,035	548,982	6,224,053	3,585,730	2,579,780	58,543	7,519,852
Mental hospitals	399,761	18,865	380,896	1,786	377,456	1,654	433,366
Homes for special care	2,035,099	460,934	1,574,165	682,527	844,386	47,252	2,211,445
Professional services	3,712,461	1,074,135	2,638,326	1,227,401	1,408,698	2,227	4,159,436
Physician services	2,535,608	114,737	2,420,871	1,203,068	1,217,803	0	2,822,600
Dental services	954,095	856,214	97,881	23,045	73,033	1,803	1,090,352
Other services[d]	222,758	103,184	119,574	1,288	117,862	424	246,484
Drugs and appliances	1,823,174	1,494,068	329,106	44,818	283,149	1,139	2,012,106
Other health expenditures							
Prepayment administration	243,385	71,340	172,045	6,885	165,160	0	273,751
Government public health	562,173	0	562,173	114,921	384,578	62,674	627,724
Capital expenditures	825,761	311,359	514,402	53,748	396,063	64,591	1,000,370
Health research	186,226	37,464	148,762	108,124	40,638	0	212,629
Miscellaneous health costs	255,870	120,217	135,653	51,523	84,130	0	290,919

SOURCE: Health Information Division, Health and Welfare Canada, and Statistics Canada.

[a]Data are provisional; data by sector are not yet available for 1979.
[b]Figures tallied by Hatcher Research Associates Corporation.
[c]"All institutions" figures include federal hospitals and tuberculosis hospitals as well as listed hospitals.
[d]"Other professional services" category includes chiropractors, optometrists, podiatrists, osteopaths, and nurses.

Table 18b National health expenditures in Canada by type of expenditure and source of funds, per capita amounts

	1978						1979
			Public				
Type of Expenditure	Canada	Private	Total	Federal	Provincial	Local	Canada
Total health expenditures	$719.46	$176.11	$543.35	$252.69	$280.53	$10.13	$794.74
Institutional care[a] all institutions	395.58	43.79	351.79	184.27	162.95	4.57	432.86
General and allied special care hospitals	288.30	23.37	264.93	152.63	109.81	2.49	317.27
Mental hospitals	17.02	.80	16.22	.08	16.07	.07	18.28
Homes for special care	86.63	19.62	67.00	29.05	35.94	2.01	93.30
Professional services	158.02	45.72	112.29	52.24	59.96	.09	175.49
Physician services	107.93	4.88	103.05	51.21	51.84	.00	119.09
Dental services	40.61	36.45	4.17	.98	3.11	.08	46.00
Other services[b]	9.48	4.39	5.09	.06	5.01	.02	10.41
Drugs and appliances	77.60	63.60	14.01	1.91	12.05	.05	84.89
Other health expenditures	88.26	23.00	65.26	14.27	45.57	5.42	101.49
Prepayment administration	10.36	3.04	7.32	.29	7.03	.00	11.55
Government public health	23.93	.00	23.93	4.89	16.37	2.67	26.48
Capital expenditures	35.15	13.25	21.90	2.29	16.86	2.75	42.21
Health research	7.93	1.59	6.33	4.60	1.73	.00	8.97
Miscellaneous health costs	10.89	5.12	5.77	2.19	3.58	.00	12.27

SOURCE: Health Information Division, Health and Welfare Canada, and Statistics Canada.

[a] "All institutions" figures include "federal hospitals" and "tuberculosis hospitals" as well as listed hospitals.
[b] "Other professional services" category includes chiropractors, optometrists, podiatrists, osteopaths, and nurses.

Table 19 Information not available; Canada does not tabulate data in terms of payments made by third-party payers.

Table 20 Percentage of Canadian population covered by private health insurance, selected years

Year	% of Population
1950	19.0
1955	37.2
1960	51.1
1965	60.6
1966	59.4
1967	59.5
1968	52.2
1969	9.4
1970	0.7
1971	0.1

SOURCE: Data compiled by the Health Information Division, Government of Canada.

NOTES: Tabulations made in early years were of the percentage of the population covered by insurance for physicians' services. The above data are drawn from these records. The last such tabulations were those made for 1971.

Health Services in the People's Republic of China

Teh-wei Hu

INTRODUCTION

The population of the People's Republic of China (the PRC) was approximately 980 million at the end of 1980.[1] The population distributions are uneven both in terms of geographic location as well as in the urban and rural difference. An estimated 95% of the population lives in a thousand-mile belt along the east coast; furthermore, about 80% of the population live in rural areas.

The Chinese government has emphasized the following four basic principles in delivering health care services to its people: (1) put prevention first, (2) combine Western and traditional medicine, (3) combine health with mass movements, and (4) concentrate on the rural areas. These features make China's health policy unique as compared to those in other developing countries.[2]

By the mid-1960s the Chinese government had already carried out many "patriotic" health campaigns. Involving millions of people, these campaigns aimed at getting rid of the "four pests" (flies, mosquitoes, bed bugs, and rats), improving environment sanitation, preventing parasitic diseases (schistosomiasis), and eliminating venereal disease. However, the government had failed to extend curative services and to provide medical insurance coverage to over 80% of the rural population. In retrospect, Mao Zedong's directive of 26 June 1965, issued on the eve of the Cultural Revolution, marks the turning point toward an emphasis on rural health care. In it Mao said, "In medical and health work, put the stress on the rural areas," and called for the modification of health care delivery and medical education. This directive had a more far-reaching impact on recent health care services than did earlier health policies. This chapter therefore focuses on health care in China since the Cultural Revolution, examining how resources are allocated in the provision of services for the majority of the Chinese people.

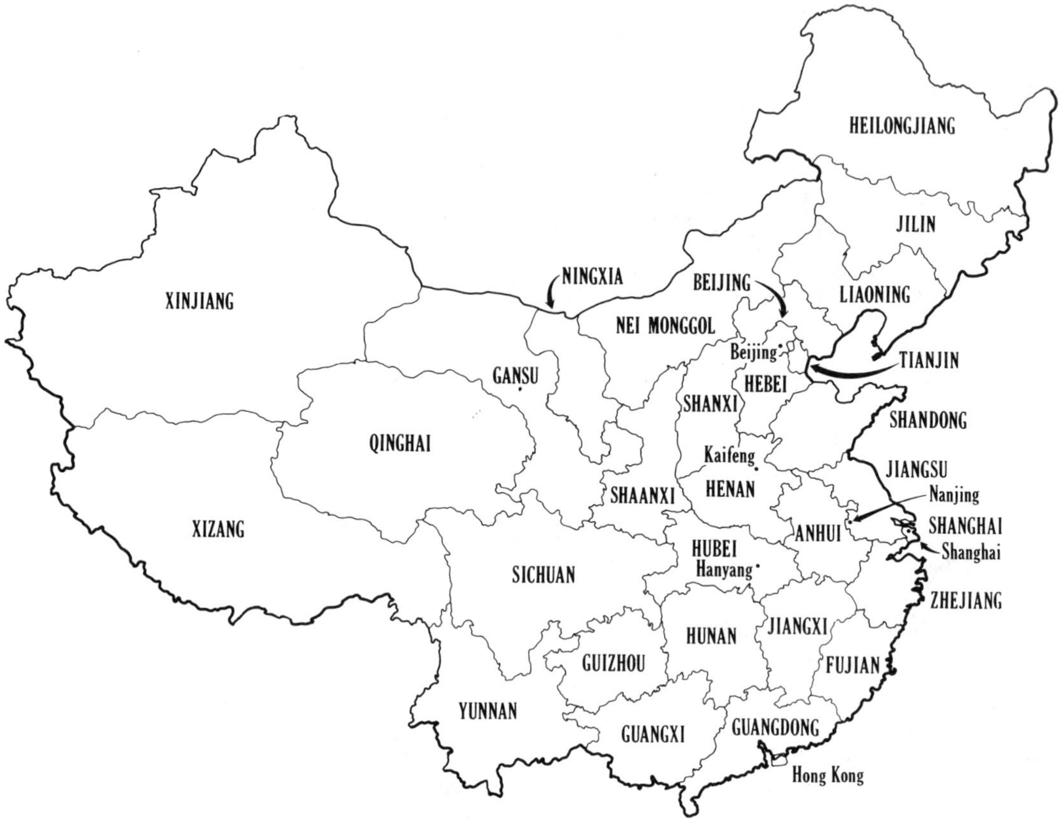

HEALTH CARE ORGANIZATION

It will be useful to first examine the Chinese political structure and the organization of the country's health care services. China is a socialist country, ruled by the Chinese Communist party. Its land mass comprises twenty-one provinces, five autonomous regions, and three centrally administered metropolitan areas, Beijing (Peking), Shanghai, and Tianjin (Tientsin). Within each of these provincial-level administrative units, a health department (or bureau) operates under guidelines from the ministry of health in Beijing, which has primary responsibility for formulating health care policies and supervising health research institutions throughout the PRC. The provincial department is in charge of medical schools in its area, oversees the provincial hospital system, works out annual plans at provincial health conferences, and supervises the activities of lower units; however, it does not directly manage the local hospitals or health activities. The major tasks of financing and delivery of health services are left to the local political units.

The sub-provincial political unit in rural areas is the *hsien,* or county; in urban areas it is the city. The political structure and health care organization within counties is shown in figure 1. The average county has about 300,000 people, although some counties may have populations of close to one million. The organizational levels descend from county to commune to production brigade to production team. The commune is the basic political unit; production brigades and teams are not parts of the governmental hierarchy—they serve mainly as accounting units for purposes of production and management, and their

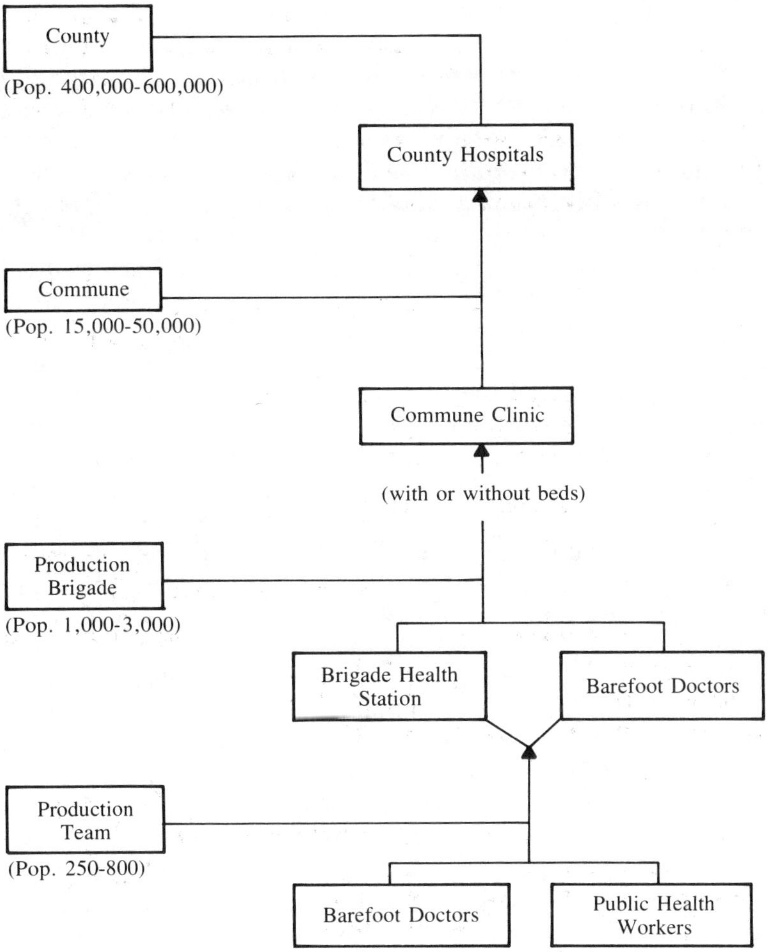

Figure 1 Rural health care and its referral system in China

leaders draw not salaries from the government but work-points, as do other peasants. On the average, a commune has a population of fifteen to fifty thousand persons, although the largest has as many as sixty to seventy thousand. A commune contains ten to twenty-five production brigades, each of which is divided into five to twenty production teams with populations of 250 to 800. A production team (or several teams, depending on the population) shares a barefoot doctor and a number of public health workers. A barefoot doctor is a peasant who receives three to six months of medical training and then returns to the farm to treat his or her fellow members' "light diseases": minor injuries, gastrointestinal illnesses, colds, bronchitis, and the like. He or she also administers immunizations and birth control, and oversees other activities carried out by public health workers who are trained and supervised by the barefoot doctor.

It is reported that each production brigade has a health station within which two or three barefoot doctors provide health care services. The health station also has a referral function, for if a patient's illness is too serious for the barefoot doctor to treat, the health station either requests the services of a mobile medical team or sends the patient to the commune clinic, which usually includes both traditional Chinese and Western-trained doctors, along with nurses who perform minor operations. A more serious illness may be further referred to a county hospital. The arrows in figure 1 show the direction of the referral system in rural China.

From time to time there are two adjuncts added to the implementation of rural health care: one is the mobile medical, or army medical, team, which stays in the rural area for variable periods of time while training barefoot doctors and treating patients; the other is the permanent relocation of doctors or nurses from urban areas.

In the PRC, cities of over 100,000 are divided into districts. Each district is subdivided into neighborhoods, which, in turn, are further subdivided into resident areas, or lanes. In the Chinese urban health care system (shown in figure 2), each lane has a street doctor and some public health workers. These street doctors are not formally trained physicians; their training is similar to that of the rural barefoot doctors. Within each lane is a lane health station, and every neighborhood has a health station with street doctors in charge. The neighborhood station serves as a unit for organizing the neighborhood outpatient clinic or small hospitals. Seriously ill patients are referred by the street doctor to the district hospital, where the staff includes traditional Chinese doctors and Western-trained doctors. The district hospital can refer cases to the municipal hospital or the specialized hospital, both of which belong to the municipality as a whole. The arrows in figure 2 show the direction of the referral system in the urban area.

It should be noted that the street doctors usually take care of the workers' dependents, while the workers, during the working period, are treated by their fellow worker doctors in the factory. Again, the duties and training of worker doctors are similar to those of barefoot or street doctors. Depending upon its size, a factory may have a clinic or hospital from which a seriously ill patient can be transferred to a district or municipal hospital.

The available descriptions of county and municipal health care systems indicate extensive autonomy within each local political unit. From local news reports it is apparent that administrative coordination among the various levels is effected by periodic regional and national conferences which are attended by various health administrators.

Aside from its governmental organization, the PRC has a medical professional association, the Chinese Medical Association (CMA). Although the CMA performs functions similar to those of many medical associations in other countries—such as journal publication, research, and international medical exchange—it has political activities that are influenced by the central government. Medical associations in European countries often try to assert their influence on government medical policy; the Chinese situation is reversed: the CMA follows medical policies set by the government.

MEDICAL PROVIDERS

Most developing countries experience shortages of physicians. The physician-population ratio in East Asia (excluding Japan) was about 1:5,200, as reported in the late 1970s, and 1:1,800 in Latin America.[3] China is no exception: the 1979 official estimate of the physician-population ratio was about 1:2,500.[4] By Western medical care standards this signals an inadequate supply of doctors. The distribution of physicians in rural China was worse before 1966, when 60 to 80% were located in urban areas where only 15 to 20% of the

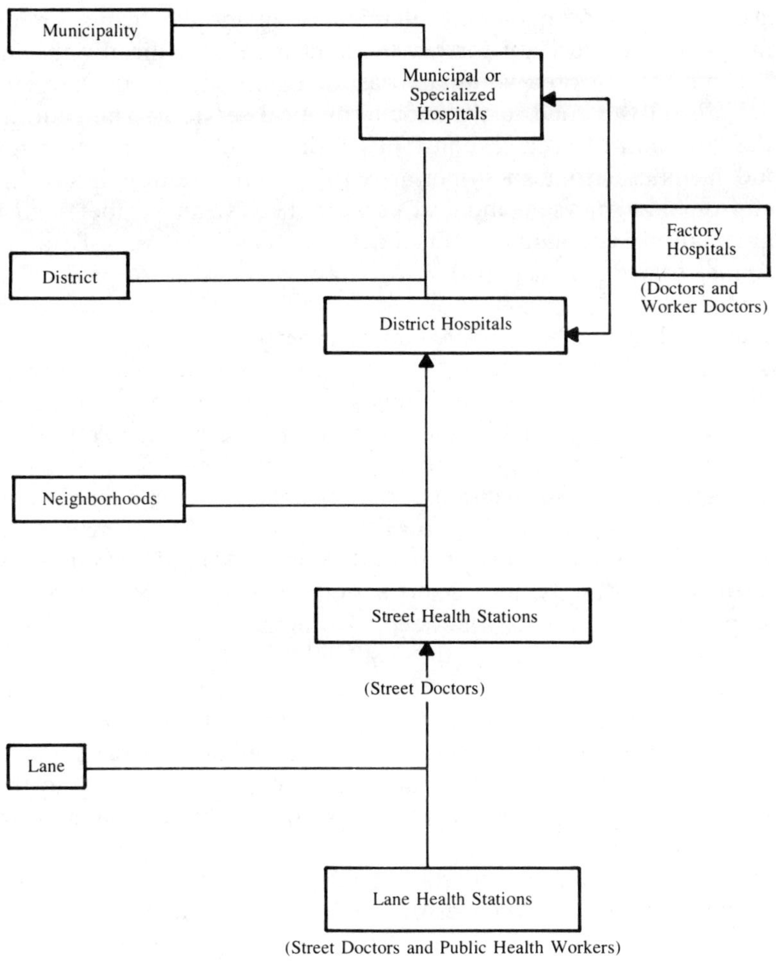

Figure 2 Urban health care and its referral system in China

total population resided. In other words, the estimated physician-population ratio in the rural areas was 1:8,000 to 1:15,400, and 1:680 to 1:890 in the urban areas.[5] This shortage and disproportionate distribution of medical manpower was a major concern of the central government at the time of the Cultural Revolution. To overcome the problem, the country's leaders chose to train barefoot doctors and public health workers rather than to concentrate resources on the training of regular doctors. This strategy can be interpreted as the Chinese way of adopting their particular set of factor endowments: the training of regular doctors requires large numbers of experienced physicians, capital equipment, and extended periods of time. China has a scarcity of capital and highly skilled medical personnel but an abundance of labor and the know-how of traditional medicine. The Chinese strategy, therefore, is to distribute their scarce resources as widely as possible and to substitute less skilled labor for capital and more advanced skills. This strategy has apparently improved the accessibility of primary health care to China's rural majority.

Several approaches to the task of increasing availability of health care services in rural areas have been adopted in the PRC. First, urban medical personnel have been relocated to rural areas, either by permanent settlement or in mobile teams for periods of six months to one year. The decision for resettlement is made either by the urban hospital revolutionary committee or on a voluntary basis. In general, one-third of an urban hospital's personnel are on the road in the mobile medical services. The central government encourages the "division of area responsibility," direct subsidies (or transfers of medical manpower and facilities) from an urban area to a rural or autonomous region. For example, the city of Shanghai sent medical personnel to Xizang (Tibet) and Heilongjiang (Heilungkiang);Tianjin sent medical personnel to Guangxi (Kwangsi); and Beijing sent medical personnel to Gansu (Kangsu).[6,7] All travel expenses are paid by the respective city governments.

By 1973 China had dispatched 800,000 medical personnel to rural areas.[8] This redistribution approach not only increases health care services but also facilitates the training of barefoot doctors in the rural areas. The Chinese Communist party argued that the reallocation of urban medical personnel would improve the doctors' ideological education and induce them to learn about disease problems in rural China and to adopt or modify medical technology so that rural peasants would benefit from their services. However, the redistribution of medical personnel to rural areas has weakened health services in the urban regions. Physicians there have increased their work loads, resulting in more rotation of night shifts in hospitals, less time for outpatient treatment, fewer surgeries, and longer waiting periods for patients who need treatment.[9]

The second approach to increasing the availability of health care in rural areas is to integrate traditional Chinese and Western approaches to medicine. The traditional Chinese physician serves as a complement to Western-trained physicians. The government has built special hospitals and clinics for traditional medicine and has created special wards for it in existing hospitals. Many rural Chinese are accustomed to the practice of traditional physicians, and their openness to this kind of treatment, along with the promotion of it by the government, can increase health services to rural areas in a short period, given the relatively large number of traditional physicians already available. In many cases, despite the availability of Western medicine, the Chinese prefer to avoid surgery and look instead to traditional medicine. Sometimes when Western medicine fails they look to traditional medicine as a last resort. Especially in rural areas, a large majority of patients are treated by traditional medicine.[10]

The third approach is to modify the medical college curriculm from five or six years of training to three so that more graduates will emerge from these colleges. Furthermore, new three-year medical colleges have been created within major hospitals (such as the Shanghai First Hospital or the Beijing Worker-Peasant-Soldier Hospital). This approach can be considered a tradeoff between quantity and quality, given the same resource constraints, but it will obviously affect future medical research advancement in the PRC. (The Chinese have more recently extended medical training to five to eight years.)

The fourth and most important approach to increasing rural health care availability is seen in the expansion of the training of barefoot doctors, who are trained locally by mobile team urban doctors or are sent to urban areas for training. Experienced barefoot doctors, especially those in northwest China, also train new barefoot doctors. Thus, the quality of training received by barefoot doctors varies greatly among regions.

Official Chinese statistics indicate that as of 1979 there were about 1.575 million barefoot doctors, 395,000 senior western physicians, 435,000 middle-level physicians, 258,000 clinic medicine physicians, and 421,000 nurses—this is a drastic increase in medical care manpower since the 1950s (as evidenced by the figures in table B at the back of this chapter). Because of the importance of barefoot doctors in Chinese medical care, the

Chinese government has computed a regional distribution of these workers during 1979 (as seen in table C). The barefoot doctors are not equally distributed among various provinces, the barefoot doctor/population ratio ranging from 1:300 in Beijing (municipality) to about 1:927 in Guizhou. On an average, the ratio is lower in the north region than it is in the east, south, and northeast.

Within the hierarchy of medical services, public health workers are supervised by barefoot doctors. Thirteen provinces or regions have reported their number of public health workers by means of newsprints or radio. Based on these figures, the public health worker/population ratio is estimated to be 1:265. Given this estimated 1970–72 ratio, and assuming a total population of 826.8 million in 1970, the estimated number of public health workers is about 3.1 million. The average ratio between barefoot doctors and public health workers is now about 1:3. There are relatively more public health workers per capita in the east —Guangdong and Guangxi (Kwangtung and Kwangsi)—than in the southwest or northwest regions. This could be explained by the nation's important Schistosomiasis Control Program launched in the past decade, since this program's massive public health campaigns have been concentrated in the schistosomiasis epidemic areas of the east and southeast regions. No figures are available to indicate the numbers of public health workers in the northwest and in parts of the central south regions of China.

The above estimated figures of barefoot doctors and public health workers lend credence to the claim that there is at least one public health worker in each production team, and an average of two or three barefoot doctors in each production brigade in rural China. The great increase in the number of barefoot doctors and public health workers over a period of fifteen years is indeed an impressive achievement, however, questions about the possible trade-off between quantity and quality in the training of medical personnel, the costs and effectiveness of medical services provided by barefoot doctors instead of trained physicians, and the impact of redistribution of medical manpower on health services in urban and rural areas are difficult to answer, especially when political aspects of this type of health care delivery system in the PRC may outweigh the system's economic aspects.

MEDICAL EDUCATION

Formal medical schools were established in China by Western missionaries more than one hundred years ago. With a limited number of medical educational facilities, China did not have sufficient personnel to meet medical care needs. Soon after the 1949 Communist Chinese liberation the central government decided to increase the number of physicians. In that period they adopted the Soviet medical training model, by splitting medical schools into various specialties.[11] Training usually lasted from five to eight years. During the Cultural Revolution, however, the medical schools admitted no new classes. Students already enrolled in medical schools were given accelerated training and then sent to the countryside. As a result the quality of medical education and the quantity of trained medical students were drastically reduced. During the early 1970s medical schools again began to admit students, many of whom were graduated within two to three years. There were no grades and no competition; therefore, there was no attrition for academic reasons. Some of these students were former barefoot doctors or assistant doctors. After

Figure 3 Health care personnel education and role

Position	Education	Typical Role
Senior Western doctor	Varied over time; currently 5 to 8 years postsecondary	Work in county general hospitals
Doctor of Chinese medicine	Currently 5 years postsecondary	Work in county general hospitals
Public health doctor	Same as senior western doctor except less clinical training and more in public health	Staff and manage county and provincial anti-epidemic stations
Junior Western doctor	Varied over time; currently 3 years post-secondary	Work in commune hospitals and comparable urban facilities
Assistant doctor	Senior secondary school specializing in health education	Play assisting roles in city hospitals (principally before the Cultural Revolution)
Barefoot doctor	Highly variable primary education (or more) plus 3- to 6-month special course plan plus continuing education	Serve in brigade health stations

mid-1970, the government recognized the need for rigorous medical training, and has since returned to the five- to eight-year training program. There are also postgraduate residency training programs in clinical specialties in the teaching hospitals.

There are six basic categories of medical personnel: the senior Western doctor, the doctor of Chinese medicine, the public health doctor, the junior Western doctor, the assistant doctor, and the barefoot doctor. The differences in their educations and their typical roles are shown in figure 3. The Chinese medical profession also places great emphasis on continuing education through conferences and workshops. Western medical journals and textbooks are often available in county hospitals.

HOSPITALS AND MEDICINE

Chinese hospitals are always crowded. By western standards the country has a shortage of hospital beds, although compared to its neighbors—India, Indonesia, Thailand, and Korea—China has much less population per bed, about 500 population per bed as of the late 1970s. Between 1952 and 1979, the number of hospital beds in China increased more than ten times, from 180,000 to 1,932,000. Regional distributions of hospital beds show wide variations, from a high 766 population per bed in Gwanzi, to a low 237 population per bed in Shanghai.

Hospital construction is a major capital expenditure. Most of these expenditures are financed by the central and provincial governments. The local government often cannot afford such expenditures. It was estimated in 1979 that the cost of construction of one hospital bed was about 5,000 yuan (about U.S. $3,000). Since 1978 the emphasis on modernization has led many urban hospitals to adopt advanced medical technology and import foreign medical equipment. The trend also seems to favor medical hospitals in urban settings.

There are specialized hospitals for particular diseases or for particular professions (railroad or army, for example), but most major hospital services are provided in county general hospitals. Each county has a hospital, which serves as the general referral hospital for the entire county, receiving and treating referred patients from the commune health centers. The county hospitals are staffed by college-graduated physicians (both western and traditional). In addition to its curative service, the county hospital has the responsibility of training and improving the quality of physicians at the commune level. The county hospital thus plays a primary role in providing hospital care services as it becomes a focal point for patient referrals and for medical knowledge diffusion to rural areas.

Hospitals are also the major medicine distribution center in China. One striking difference between Chinese and Western medical care costs is the overwhelming amount of medicine expenditures in China: about 60% of total health care costs is spent on medicine. In 1979 the General Bureau of Medicine, which is responsible for pharmaceutical production, reported that China used about 5 billion yuan of Western medicine and 1.4 billion yuan of Chinese herbal medicine. The large medicine consumption in China could be explained in several ways. First, the Chinese are more inclined to take tonic medicines than westerners and will even give them as gifts among friends and relatives. Second, there are fewer restrictions on prescribing medicine than in Western countries. So long as the medicines are available at the dispensary, physician prescriptions are not always required to obtain them. Finally, hospitals are administered by the local government but financed by the province, and medicine is a free commodity under the public expenses medical insurance. As a result, in recent years the central government and some official publications have publicly denounced the rapid cost increase in medicine.

HEALTH CARE FINANCING

The major issue of health care financing in China is how to allocate limited resources to provide effective health care for a population of about 980 million. To understand the issues of health care financing in China, a brief discussion of the systems of health care financing is necessary.

It would be misleading to say that health care services in the PRC are free or virtually free to all people.[12] Chinese health care insurance is neither a uniform nor a well-planned system. A delegation of the Canadian Medical Association visiting China in 1973 was most surprised to find that the country's health care system is not a socialized one. The Canadians claimed that the Chinese system is in fact even less socialized than theirs.[13]

There are essentially three types of health care insurance coverage in the PRC: (1) public expenses medical insurance, (2) labor medical insurance, and (3) cooperative medical services. Each will be discussed here in turn. A more detailed discussion of these financing schemes are shown in author's earlier paper.[14]

"Public expenses medical insurance" (*Kung-fei Yi-liau*), introduced in 1951, covers the medical expenses of the state cadres and the students fully, without any contribution by them to the insurance premium. Coverage includes visits to clinics and costs incurred during hospitalization, although hospital meal costs are excluded. It is estimated that about 2% of the population is covered by this insurance plan, excluding family dependents.[15] Family members of state cadres are not covered by the scheme, their insurance being financed by the government.

"Labor medical insurance" (*Loa-poa Yi-liau*) covers the workers or staff members in factories and state-owned firms. Introduced in 1951 and revised in 1953, this insurance is funded by factory employers' contributions—about 2 to 3% of the total factory income before salaries are distributed to workers. The percentage varies among factories and over time. In general, the percentages are mandated by the province through the same process that approves the factory's annual production plan. Factory workers receive medical services at no charge. Thus, the labor medical insurance fund is regarded as a noncoinsurance system since the employer's contributions to the insurance premium are not considered a reduction in workers' salaries or wages.

Beijing health officials have estimated that about 10 to 12% of the country's population are covered by the labor medical insurance fund, including the dependents of the factory workers. These people are located primarily in urban areas. It should be noted, however, that this type of insurance provides 100% coverage for only the workers themselves, not for their dependents, who must pay about 50% of their medical expenses under this system.

The "cooperative medical services" (*Ho-tso Yi-liau*), the third type of medical care insurance, is intended for the inhabitants of the rural agricultural areas. About 80% of China's population lives in rural areas, and to implement its planned expansion of rural health care services to these people, the Chinese central government needed vast financial resources. Although the central government could have reallocated health care expenditures from urban to rural or from rich to poor provinces, the total amount required would still be very difficult to finance. Thus, officials decided that a decentralized approach to health care was the economical way to relieve the central government of its financial burden. As a result, the cooperative medical services concept was actively advocated and promoted at the commune level, commencing in 1966. It is claimed that 70% of China's 50,000 communes have now adopted this self-reliance financing approach.[16]

The main forces for establishing the cooperative medical services are poor and lower-middle-class peasants. Participation is voluntary—in the early years of the service, commune members had the option of joining the system; in recent years, the decision to join is made at the commune level. Once a commune decides to join, everyone in the commune must participate.

The annual membership fee varies both among and within communes over time. The annual fee is calculated from the individual commune's expenditures for treatment and medicine during the previous year. For instance, in 1972 Pujiang (Pu-chiang) Commune in the Province of Zhejiang (Chekiang) had fewer serious illnesses than before, and because the commune used herbal medicine extensively (a major cost-saving factor), the annual membership fee was reduced from 1 yuan in 1972 to .35 yuan in 1973. About fifteen communes across the country have reported their annual membership fees in various news sources, and these ranged from .35 to 3.60 yuan per person in 1973; the average was about 1.50 yuan per person per year.[17–20] The average family have five members; thus, annual expenditures for membership fees are about 7.5 yuan per family. Take-home income varies among communes, ranging from 150 to 350 yuan per worker annually. Assuming both that an average worker makes 250 yuan and that a family has two workers (husband and wife), the family income will be 500 yuan per year. The financial burden of the medical services premium therefore, is about 1.5% of the family's disposable income. It should be noted that there is considerable variation in medical services premiums and incomes among communes. Based on a survey by P. Chen, the ratio of premium to disposable personal income varies from .6 to 3.0% in different parts of the country.[15] Again, these results indicate that 1.5% of the family's disposable income is a reasonable average figure. A lump-sum payment of 7.5 yuan in a given month would take about one-fifth to one-sixth of a family's monthly income. Thus, it seems that 1.5% of the annual disposable income is not an insignificant figure for poor and lower-middle-income peasants, as many visitors to the PRC have claimed. In fact, there are reports that peasants in some areas avoid participation in the cooperative medical services, save the membership fee, and chance staying healthy.

In addition to contributions by commune members, each production team pays a certain amount from its collective welfare fund for each member subscribing to the medical services. The production team's contribution varies from .10 to 1 yuan per member, depending upon that year's agricultural production and the utilization status of its commune members. Each commune has a "public accumulated fund," contributed by the production teams, which comprises reserve and welfare funds. The reserve fund—about 7 to 10% of the gross income—may be used to buy farm equipment or to finance hospital construction, which is supplemented by state funds. Approximately 2 to 3% of the gross income, the welfare fund is used to pay for education costs, cooperative medical services, and social welfare assistance.[21] These percentage figures vary among communes.

Under the self-reliance principle, when high-income communes accumulate larger public welfare funds, they share larger amounts of health costs and can reduce the medical service premiums paid by individual members. On the other hand, low-income communes are without large public welfare funds, so their members have to pay higher premiums.

To the extent that poor rural areas are not financially able to carry out cooperative medical services, the central government's policy is to provide additional health service resources for the relatively poor and rural areas. This policy is implemented in two ways: (1) through direct subsidies from the central government and (2) through subsidies from urban to rural areas.

It is reported that since the Cultural Revolution the central government has allocated about 60% of its health expenditures to rural areas, compared to only 20 to 30% before 1965. Although the redistribution of health funds is initiated by the central government, the actual implementation takes place at the provincial and county levels. The national budget is a unified fiscal plan that includes the expected revenue and expenditures of central, provincial, and local governments. The simultaneous determination of national and provincial financial budgets provides the central government with an important influence on the geographic distribution of health care resources. Once a province receives its revenue, it allocates the resources to various counties and municipalities. In turn, the counties allocate funds to various communes. Therefore, it appears that local communes obtain subsidies directly from the county government, but these funds are in fact transferred from the central government via the provincial government.

It is rather difficult to discuss the shares that various levels of government have in financing local health care services. One important feature of state financing of local health care services is that these funds are used mainly for capital expenditures of local health hospitals or clinics. In many instances the state contributes about 50% of total construction funds; the balance of costs are then paid by brigade health station funds or by cooperative medical services funds. These funds represent surplus revenue from local health services, after maintenance costs of the health station have been paid. Therefore, it can be safely argued that the largest share of health care services expenses is paid at the household, brigade, and commune levels, the higher levels of government—county, province, and central—merely provide portions of funds for capital expenditures. Only during a poor harvest or a depletion of commune welfare funds does the state provide additional support for local health services.

The second approach to financing rural health care services involves subsidies from urban areas to rural or poor regions. The central government encourages these direct subsidies, which take the form of medical manpower or facilities. Upon a relocation of manpower, as discussed previously, the urban area pays all travel expenses as well as the salaries of urban medical personnel while they are stationed in a rural region. Therefore, it is concluded that the central and the provincial governments play important roles in forming the redistribution policy, but that they are of relatively minor importance in financing health services. The job of actual policy implementation is left to the local government, which uses local manpower and financing. This decentralization approach is intended to maximize community participation and investment in health services and to reduce the financial burden on the central government, enabling it to assist wider areas without increasing their budgets.

According to statistics from the 1980 State Statistical Bureau, China expended about 9.6 billion yuan on health care costs in 1979. Per capita costs were about 10 yuan per person (approximately U.S. $6.40). About two-thirds of the expenditures were on Western and traditional medicine, close to 10% on hospital capital expenditures, and the rest on medical manpower. China spent about 2.5% of its national income on health care. This figure is certainly much smaller than corresponding figures for Western countries. However, compared to other developing Asian countries, China actually spends a higher proportion of her income on health care (see table H).

STRATEGIES FOR COST CONTAINMENT

During the past few years China has experienced a rapid increase in health care costs. Alternative strategies have been developed for controlling these increases.

Visit Fee

When a peasant or his family joins the cooperative medical service, they pay a fee of .05 to .10 yuan for each visit to the brigade health station. This payment helps to cover maintenance expenses incurred by the station (excluding the salaries of barefoot doctors and public health workers, which are paid by production team funds). The registration or visit fee also serves to discourage indiscriminate use of available services. Certain communes reported that during the early days of cooperative medical services, when registration fees were not charged, there was overutilization of the services, including unnecessary visits and requests for tonic herbs. As a result, several commune cooperative medical services had to be discontinued due to their large deficits.

Referral System

One mechanism for controlling health costs in the brigade is the use of barefoot doctors for patient referrals to county or city hospitals. Patients seeking care at these hospitals on their own initiative cannot receive reimbursement from brigade health funds. Conversely, if the barefoot doctor refers a patient to one of these hospitals, part of the patient's medical expenses will be reimbursed by the brigade health fund. Certain communes pay 50% of the costs, while others pay fixed amounts of 30 to 40 yuan and the patients pay the rest of the expenses, including the food costs.[22] Again, it must be noted that these payment schemes vary among communes. All of these examples indicate that free medical services or unlimited amounts of medical finances are not feasible, even in a socialized country. A limit must be set so that medical expenses can be minimized.

Herbal Medicine

One important health services campaign for reducing costs and financing local cooperative medical services during the Cultural Revolution has been to promote the use of herbal medicine and acupuncture. Most herbal medicines can be grown and processed locally, so the costs of the medicines can be greatly reduced in comparison to Western-type remedies or herbal medicines imported from other communes. Local surplus herbs are sold to other communes or to the province, with the proceeds going into the local cooperative medical funds. Cost reductions have been seen either in lower state subsidies to the local communes or a reduction in the membership fees of the local cooperative medical service.

Payment System

During the early period of cooperative medical services a system was in operation in which an account established by a commune at the county or city hospital covered the costs of treatment for commune patients at those institutions. This type of credit system resulted in some unnecessary expenses being incurred by the patient's commune. Hospitals now require patients to pay all expenses while they are receiving medical services; no credits are allowed for the commune. The patient must then request a refund from the commune for his or her medical expenses. Each refund request is reviewed by a peer group in the commune. The communes appear to believe that this modification may reduce their medical expenses at county or city hospitals.

Hospital charges vary according to the location of the hospital and the type of illness. The average daily room charge is .6 yuan for Luda (Dalien) Second Hospital, 1 yuan for the Beijing Worker-Peasant-Soldier Hospital, and 1.5 yuan at the Norman Bethune International Peace Hospital. The average charge is about 1 yuan per day, excluding meal expenses. Surgery fees range from 8 to 30 yuan among several hospitals in Beijing and Shanghai. A tonsillectomy costs 8 yuan; chest surgery is about 30 yuan. In these hospitals the average length of stay per admission is about two weeks. Thus, a serious illness may cost a patient more than 45 yuan, which is more than a month's income for a poor or lower-middle-income peasant. Because hospital expenses are not easily affordable to Chinese peasants, some urban hospitals in Beijing, Luda, and Shanghai offer a lower room rate (about 50% less) for poor and lower-middle-income peasants by putting more beds in a ward.

HEALTH STATUS

Major outcomes of the health care inputs—manpower, facilities, and costs—are the health status of a population. Health status can be measured in terms of life expectancy, infant mortality, mortality rate, and causes of death.

Life expectancy is perhaps the best indicator of a country's health status. In China in the mid-1950s it was estimated at about fifty-seven years. In 1979 the life expectancy was about sixty-four, which is well above the average life expectancy among the low-income developing countries and a bit above the middle-income developing countries. The infant mortality rate in China was 56/1,000 during 1979.

Current crude death rates are available for various communes or rural areas; several are 7.3/1,000 for Shajiao (Sha-chiao) Commune, Sunde Xian (Sun-Te Hsien), Guangdong; 5.2/1,000 for Chiyi (Chi-yi) Commune in the Shanghai area; 5/1,000 for Dongting (Tung-ting) Commune, Wu Xian (Wu Hsien), Jiangsu (Kiangsu); 4/1,000 for Nayin (Nan-ying), Shanghai area; and 6/1,000 for the Nanjing (Nanking) area.[23] The national average was 7.8/1,000. A comparison of these rates with those of other developing or developed countries (table I) indicates that China's health status is well above that of many other countries, granted that the crude death rate is only one of many indicators of a nation's health status. For example, India has a crude death rate of 14/1,000; Indonesia has 17/1,000; the United States has 9.4/1,000; Russia has 7.9/1,000; and Japan has 6.6/1,000.[24]

Chinese health officials now claim that the leading causes of death are cancer and cardiovascular, cerebrovascular, and respiratory diseases, instead of infectious diseases and malnutrition, which were the country's leading killers two decades ago. These current causes of death are comparable to those of the United States and other developed countries. These health statistics suggest that the PRC has received substantial benefits from its health care services, particularly from the preventive nature of its health care.

CONCLUSION

Medical services in socialist China are not entirely socialized, or free to all of the population. It is a costly task for a central government to provide health care services to an entire country. Therefore, the government has strongly emphasized preventive medicine and public health work while it encourages self-reliance at the local level. The decentralization approach in health care services has been adopted. A unique feature of the Chinese health care system is its incorporation into the political structure. In other words, the structure of the health care delivery system is a part of the national administrative system, running from the commune to the county, province, and the central government. Thus, the system has become very efficient.

By Western standards, health care manpower, facilities, and expenditures in China are much lower than in developed countries; however, these health inputs are far better than the average for developing countries. The Chinese Cultural Revolution from 1965 to 1975 forced a setback on advanced training of medical manpower. On the other hand, the emphasis on rural health care and the development of barefoot doctors proved very useful for the care of the rural population. With its efficient use of limited resources for health care, China has improved the health status and life expectancy of its people.

Notes

1. State Statistical Bureau, *1980 Communique of the Statistical Bureau* (Beijing: People's Republic of China, 1980).
2. Teh-wei Hu, "The Financing and Economic Efficiency of Rural Health Services in the People's Republic of China," *International Journal of Health Services* (1976).
3. Agency for International Development, *Proposed Foreign Aid Program* (Washington: U.S. Gov. Printing Office, 1967), table 3.
4. State Statistical Bureau, *Renmin Ribao,* May 1980.
5. C.Y. Chen, "Health Manpower: Growth and Distribution," in *Public Health in the People's Republic of China,* ed. Wegman et al. (New York: J. Macy Jr. Foundation, 1973), pp. 139–57.
6. U.S. Department of Commerce, *Foreign Broadcast Information Services Daily Report, People's Republic of China* (Washington, D.C., 11 June 1974).
7. *Renmin Ribao,* Beijing, 27 June 1973.
8. *Peking Review,* February 1975.
9. These negative impacts were revealed by Chinese physicians who recently left China and were interviewed by this author in Hong Kong.
10. Ralph C. Croizier, "Traditional Medicine As a Basis for Chinese Medical Practice," in *Medicine and Public Health in the People's Republic of China,* ed. J. R. Quinn, DHEW Publication no. (NIH) 72–67 (Washington, D.C.: National Institutes of Health, U.S. Dept. of Health, Education, and Welfare, 1972), pp. 3–17.
11. V.W. Sidel and Ruth Sidel, *Serve the People: Observations on Medicine in the People's Republic of China* (New York: Josiah Macy Jr. Foundation, 1973), p. 82.
12. L.G. Reynolds, "China as a Less Developed Economy," *American Economic Review* 63 (1975): 418.
13. *China Report: Health Care in the World's Most Populous Country* (Ottawa: Canadian Medical Association, 1973).
14. Teh-wei Hu, "Health Services and the Economic Development in the People's Republic of China," in *China's Development Experience in Comparative Perspective,* ed. Robert Dernberger (Cambridge, Mass.: Harvard Univ. Press, 1980), pp. 229–60.
15. P. Chen, *Public Health Development and Birth Planning Programs in the PRC* (Washington, D.C.: Smithsonian Institution, 1976).
16. U.S. Dept. of Commerce, *Foreign Broadcast Information Services Daily Report, People's Republic of China* (Washington, D.C., 1969–1974).
17. *Guang Ming Ribao,* Beijing, 1969–1975 (in Chinese).
18. *Renmin Ribao,* Beijing, 1968–1974 (in Chinese).
19. *China Reconstructs,* Beijing, 1968–1974.
20. *Red Flag,* Beijing, 1969–1974 (in Chinese).
21. J.B. Gordon, "The Organization and Financing of Health Services in the PRC," in *China Medicine as We Saw It,* ed. J. Quinn, DHEW Publication no. (NIH) 75–684 (Bethesda, Md.: Fogarty International Center, 1974).
22. Changwei Administrative Region Revolutionary Committee, "Thriving Cooperative Medical Service," *Chinese Medical Journal* 54 (1974): 328.
23. Personal interview in Nanjing.
24. World Bank, *Health: Sector Policy Paper* (Washington, D.C., 1975).

Table A Health manpower in China, 1979

	Number	Population Per Health Personnel
Barefoot doctors	1,575,000	616
Senior Western physicians	395,000	2,458
Middle-level Western physicians	435,000	2,232
Practitioners of traditional medicine	258,000	3,763
Nurses	421,000	2,306
Total	3,084,000	

SOURCE: State Statistical Bureau, *Renmin Ribao,* May 1980.

NOTE: Figures are also cited in Chen, Pi-chao, *Rural Health and Birth Planning in China* (North Carolina: Research Triangle Park, 1981), p. 14.

Table B Personnel changes in China

Year	Physicians	Population Per Physician	Auxiliary Health Personnel (Excl. Barefoot Doctors)	Population Per Auxiliary
1952	52,000	10,417	988,000	548
1957	75,000	8,620	1,833,000	353
1979	395,000	2,458	2,689,000	365

SOURCES: For 1952 and 1957 figures, see D. Perkins and S. Yusuf, *Rural Development in the People's Republic of China;* for 1979 figures, see *1979 Communique of the State Statistical Bureau* (April 1980), p. 48.

Table C Regional distribution of barefoot doctors, 1979, China

	Population Per Barefoot Doctor
Southwest region	
Sichuan	530
Guizhou	927
Yunnan	861
Xizang (autonomous region)	319
Northwest region	
Shaanxi	332
Gansu	429
Qinghai	356
Ningxia (autonomous region)	595
Xinjiang (autonomous region)	684
Central south region	
Henan	438
Hubei	505
Hunan	539
Guangxi (autonomous region)	795
Guangdong	726
East region	
Shanghai (municipality)	471
Jiangsu	650
Zhejiang	479
Anhui	679
Fujian	649
Jiangxi	606
Shandong	371
North region	
Beijing (municipality)	300
Tianjin (municipality)	406
Hebei	387
Shanxi	326
Nei Monggol (autonomous region)	490
Northeast region	
Liaoning	632
Jilin	595
Heilongjiang	633

SOURCE: The ministry of public health, Beijing, 1980.

Table D Distribution of public health workers in China's thirteen provinces, 1970 to 1972

Province or Region	Population[a]	Public Health Workers: Total	Public Health Workers: Population Per Worker
East			
Anhui	41.4	189,000	219
Fujian	18.7	63,000	296
Jiangsu	65.6	290,000	226
Shandong	69.8	200,000	349
South central			
Guangxi	26.9	190,000	141
Guangdong	46.2	200,000	231
Southwest			
Sichuan	89.6	375,000	238
Yunnan	23.5	60,000	392
North			
Hebei	61.8	200,000	309
Northeast			
Heilongjiang	24.3	50,000	486
Jilin	18.4	83,392	220
Liaoning	36.8	13,000	541
Nei Monggol	6.7	13,000	515
Estimated national total (35 provinces)	826.8	3,120,000	

SOURCE: Teh-wei Hu, "Health Services and the Economic Development in the People's Republic of China," in *China's Development Experience in Comparative Perspective,* ed. Robert Dernberger (Cambridge, Mass.: Harvard Univ. Press, 1980), pp. 229–60.

[a]John S. Aird, *Population Estimates for the Provinces of the People's Republic of China,* Series P-95, no. 73 (Washington, D.C.: U.S. Dept. of Commerce, 1974), p. 22, appendix table 1.

Table E Medical personnel and facilities in China and other countries

Country	Population Per: Hospital Bed	Population Per: Physician	Population Per: Nursing Person
China, 1979	503	2,458	365[a]
India	1,620	3,620	5,680
Indonesia	1,560	14,580	2,820
Sri Lanka	330	6,270	2,260
Nepal	6,630	35,120	51,220
Korea	1,510	1,960	510
Thailand	800	8,170	3,540
Low-income developing countries	—	9,900	8,790
Middle-income developing countries	—	4,130	1,860

SOURCES: World Bank, *World Development Report 1980,* pp. 152–253, and World Bank, *Health Sector Policy Paper,* February 1980, pp. 79–82.

[a]Includes barefoot doctors and all health auxiliaries.

Table F Regional distribution of hospitals, 1979, China

	Population Per Hospital Bed
Southwest region	
Sichuan	557
Guizhou	683
Yunnan	536
Xizang (autonomous region)	444
Northwest region	
Shaanxi	527
Gansu	565
Qinghai	349
Ningxia (autonomous region)	512
Xinjiang (autonomous region)	297
Central south region	
Henan	676
Hubei	426
Hunan	452
Guangxi (autonomous region)	766
Guangdong	547
East region	
Shanghai (municipality)	237
Jiangsu	517
Zhejiang	633
Anhui	660
Fujian	543
Jiangxi	479
Shandong	626
North region	
Beijing (municipality)	325
Tianjin (municipality)	413
Hebei	587
Shanxi	368
Nei Monggol (autonomous region)	398
Northeast region	
Liaoning	320
Jilin	366
Heilongjiang	345

SOURCE: The ministry of public health, Beijing, 1980.

Table G Costs of health care in China, 1979

	Annual Cost (Million Yuan)	Annual Cost (Y Per Capita)	% of Total Cost
Barefoot doctors	661.5	0.68	6.9
Senior Western physicians	568.8	0.59	6.0
Other health personnel	1,074.4	1.11	11.1
Hospital beds	881.5	0.91	9.2
Western medicine	5,040.0	5.19	52.4
Chinese (traditional) medicine	1,400.0	1.44	14.5
Total	9,626.2	9.91	100.0

NOTE: The *1979 Communique of the State Statistical Bureau* (April 1980, p. 33) indicates that 41,700 tons of chemical pharmaceuticals were produced in 1979, a 2.5% increase over 1978. The 1980 figure decreased by 3.8% to 40,100 tons *(1980 Communique of the State Statistical Bureau).*

Table H Public expenditures on health care in China and other countries

	Per Capita Public Expenditure	
	In $	% of Per Capita Income
China, 1979	6.4	2.5
India, 1976	2	1.2
Indonesia, 1976	1	0.7
Sri Lanka, 1975	4	1.9
Nepal, 1976	1	0.8
Korea, 1977	1	0.2
Thailand, 1976	2	0.7

SOURCE: Figures for countries other than China from the World Bank, *Health Sector Policy Paper,* February 1980, pp. 75–78.

NOTE: Figures for China at the rate of 1.54 yuan/dollar and a per capita income of $260 assumed.

Table I Mortality and life expectancy in China and other countries

	Crude Death Rate (Per Thousand Population)	Infant Mortality Rate (Per Thousand Live Births)	Life Expectancy (Years)
China, 1979	7.8	56	64
India, 1978	14.0	—	51
Cuba, 1977	6.0	25	72
Korea, Dem. Rep., 1977	8.0	—	63
Indonesia, 1978	17.0	—	47
Sri Lanka, 1978	6.0	—	69
Nepal, 1978	21.0	—	43
Thailand, 1978	8.0	68	61
Low-income developing countries, 1978	15.0	—	50
Middle-income developing countries, 1978	11.0	—	61

SOURCE: World Bank, *World Development Report 1980,* pp. 144–45 and 152–53.

Health Services in Denmark

Willy Søndergaard and
*Allan Krasnik**

SUMMARY

The Danish health services operate on three main levels.

The *primary health services* are centred upon the general practitioner, who though working independently in private practice, earns the greater part of his income from the public health insurance scheme. The general practitioner is primarily performing a curative function, but at the same time has a predominant role in the process of referring patients to practising specialists, to hospitals, or to institutions or welfare arrangements in the nursing homes and social sectors.

The primary health sector includes also dental services, retail chemists, home nursing services, and industrial health services, etc.

The *secondary health services* are synonymous with the hospital services, which almost without exception are operated by public authorities, namely, the fourteen county councils in Denmark, plus the city councils of Copenhagen and Frederiksberg.

The *tertiary health services* include the nursing homes and social welfare sectors.

Financing and Expenditure

The Danish health services are free of charge for all residents in the country, with the exception of certain services provided by the nursing homes and social welfare sector, which must be paid for according to income. The counties and the municipalities have the main economic responsibility, but their expenditure is partly reimbursed by the state in

*The account of health services in Denmark was authored by Dr Søndergaard while a member of the Danish Hospital Institute, and is reprinted with permission from the institute. Minor editing was undertaken to bring the text into conformity with the other chapters. The discussion section ("The Best Health Services in the World?") was recently authored by Dr. Krasnik, who also provided the account of medical education in Denmark and most of the tables which appear at the end of the chapter. The other tables and the charts were part of Dr. Søndergaard's account.—Ed.

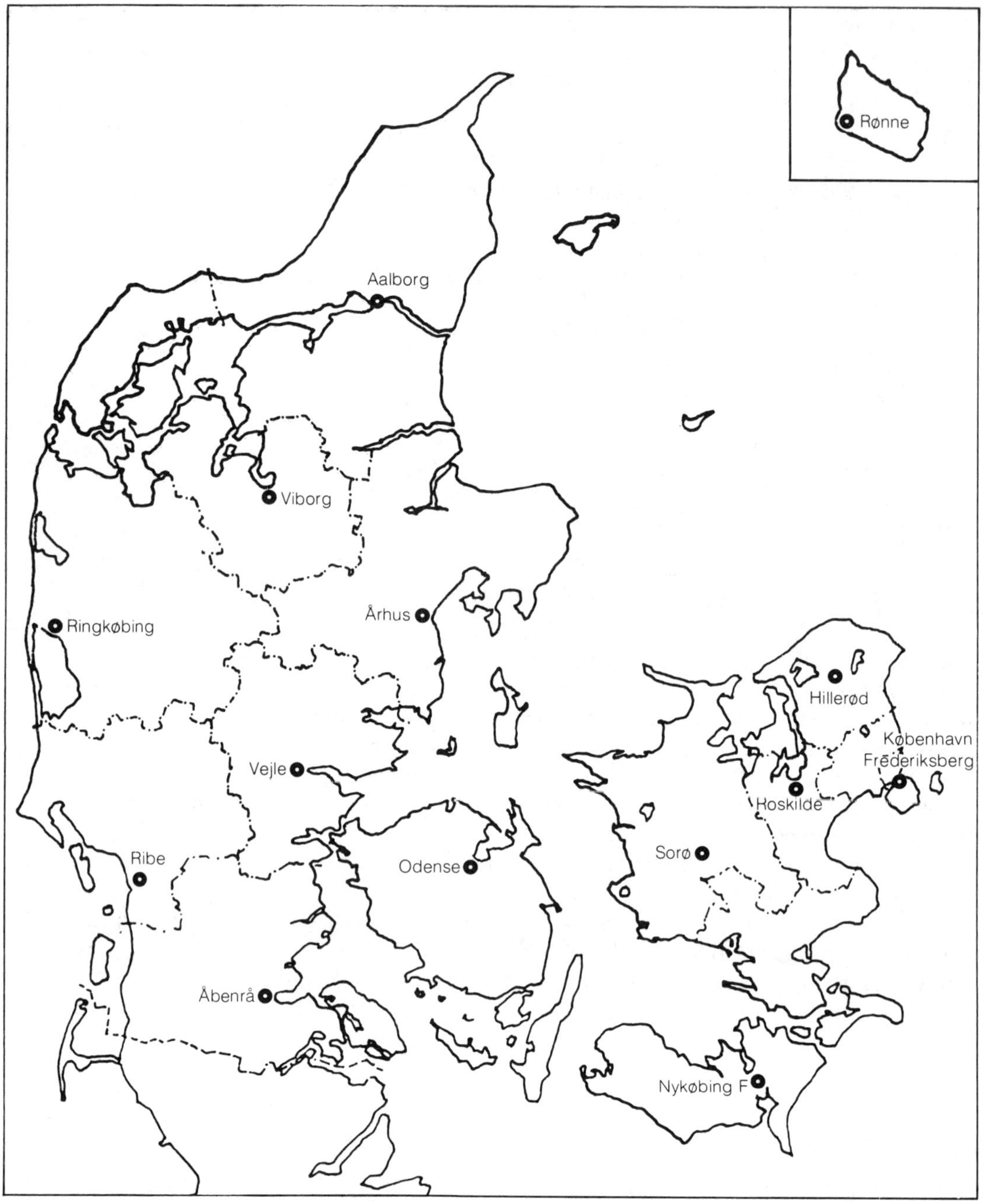

the form of lump sum subsidies. The Danish health services are in this way financed essentially out of rates and taxes.

The total public expenditure for health services for the financial year of 1979 was estimated at 25.5 milliard Danish crowns, which corresponds to 8.8% of the estimated gross national income for that year (289 milliard Danish crowns).

DENMARK'S GEOGRAPHY AND POPULATION

The kingdom of Denmark consists of approximately 500 islands, together with the peninsula of Jutland. The largest islands are Zealand, with the capital Copenhagen, Funen, Lolland, Falster, and Bornholm. The Danish state also includes two self-governing dependencies, the Faroe Islands and Greenland.

Distances are relatively short and the transport systems are well developed. However, the "Storebælt" straits, between Zealand and Funen, create a barrier to rapid surface traffic between the eastern and western parts of the country.

The country has a total area of 43,000 square kilometres, and a population which reached 5 millions in 1975, 2 million living in the area of Greater Copenhagen. Over 14% of the total population are over 65 years of age. (For the population distribution according to age, see figure 1.)

The Faroe Islands have had self-government within the Danish state since 1948. The Faroes determine their own foreign policies, and are responsible for the defence, religious, police, and legal systems. Health services are also under the jurisdiction of the home government, but the Danish state provides subsidies for both capital and current expenditure.

The total area of the Faroe Islands is 1,400 square kilometres, and the population approximately 40,000.

Greenland has had self-government within the Danish state since 1979. However, health services have not yet been taken over by the home government, and are still fully controlled and financed by the ministry for Greenland in Denmark.

DENMARK'S ADMINISTRATIVE ORGANISATION

With the exception of the capital city, Denmark is divided into 14 county authorities of very varying size. A typical county has approximately 250,000 inhabitants, whilst the smallest has nearly 50,000 and the largest over 600,000. Each county is divided into a number of municipalities which also vary in size of population from small county municipalities with about 5,000 inhabitants, to large city municipalities with about 200,000 inhabitants.

The cities of Copenhagen and Frederiksberg are outside the county divisions and have functions and responsibilities of both the counties and the municipalities.

The 14 county authorities are administered by a politically elected county council, the city of Frederiksberg by a city council, and the city of Copenhagen is administered by a council of representatives with a central administration. The 14 county councils are amalgamated as members of the Danish County Councils Association, which supports and promotes the county councils' affairs by carrying out planning and development activities of common interest, and undertaking wages and conditions negotiations. The association represents the counties' interests in relation to the executive political and administrative authorities. In 1973 the Metropolitan Council was established, comprising the city councils of Copenhagen and Frederiksberg, together with the county councils of Copenhagen, Frederiksberg, and Roskilde. The Metropolitan Council is elected by and consists of

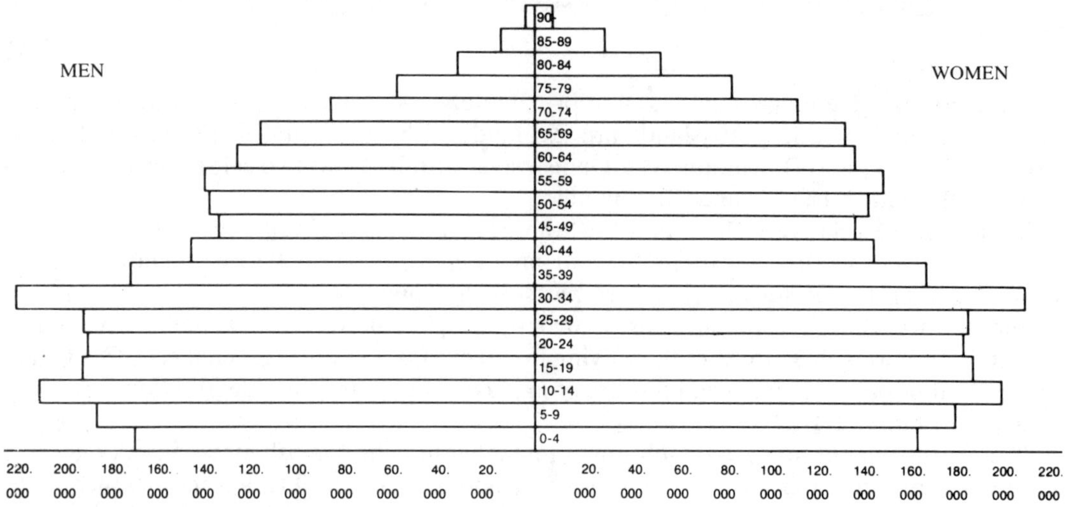

Figure 1 Population according to age and sex: 1 January 1979

politicians sitting on the various county and municipal councils within the area. The council's main objectives are in a variety of areas such as regional planning, transport, protection of the environment, water supply, and the future planning of hospital services within the metropolitan area of Copenhagen.

With regards to health services, the Metropolitan Council is responsible for the preparation of a unified plan for the development of hospital services for the area within the jurisdiction of the five authorities. This plan will include proposals for collaboration and distribution of activities between the hospital authorities and between hospitals in the area. The Metropolitan Council must be informed by the ministry of the interior (in the case of Rigshospital, the ministry of education) of any proposals for significantly revising the function or capacity of the hospital services of the various authorities within the area, before these proposals can be finally approved.

THE ADMINISTRATIVE ORGANISATION OF HEALTH SERVICES IN DENMARK

Introduction

The administrative organisation of health services in Denmark is the product of a very long development process both within national and regional administration. For instance, there is no ministry of health, with the sole executive authority for health services, and there are no clear demarcation lines between those health services for which the state is responsible and those which are the responsibility of the county or municipal authorities. In principle, the state lays down the legislation and bylaws under which the various

Figure 2 The three levels of health services in Denmark

Level	Definition	Services Provided
Primary health services	General practise, individual preventive care, etc.	General practitioners, practising specialists, dentists, visiting nurses, retail pharmacists, physiotherapists, occupational therapists, chiropractors, child health care services, school health services, industrial health services
Secondary health services	Hospital services	Somatic hospitals, Psychiatric hospitals
Tertiary health services	Nursing home and social welfare services	Nursing homes, psychiatrical nursing homes, protected residences, home health services, meals delivery services, day centres

activities of the health services are carried on and developed, and undertakes supervision and control. The county councils, with responsibility for hospital services, and the National Health Insurance Scheme, are responsible for the *curative* health services and their associated activities, whilst the municipalities' main areas of authority are within nursing and care of the aged and disabled, the greatest part of preventive activities, and matters concerning public health and hygiene. With all three levels there are, however, essential exceptions to these main principles.

Ministry Level

The national government's interests within the health services are taken care of by different ministries, i.e. several social and health activities are placed in different ministerial departments. The chief responsibility for conventional health services is undertaken by the ministry of the interior and the responsibility for the greatest part of primary health services by the ministry of social affairs.

Ministry of the Interior

The ministry of the interior is divided into two departments, one dealing with the municipalities, and the other with health. The Department of Health takes care of the health service activities which are the responsibility of the ministry. This involves legislation regarding hospitals, and concerns, for example, the future planning of hospital services, approval of hospital projects, and other matters concerning hospital services, legislation regarding pharmaceutical services, and general questions regarding health services, such as coordination at ministry level of the planning and development of preventive and prophylactic measures together with other ministries and administrations. To this should be added the basic and further education of nonacademic staff, together with the post-graduate education of doctors and dentists, etc. To advise the ministries there are at present three permanent committees.

The National Hospital Council advises the minister on questions regarding the future planning and administration of the hospital services. The council is composed of representatives from county hospital authorities. The Hospital Services Educational Tribunal, which is made up of representatives from the county hospital authorities, and the trade unions, etc., advises on questions referring to the education and training of nonacademic health staff. The Central Committee for the Further Education of Doctors, which includes representatives from the county hospital authorities, the National Health Insurance Scheme, different ministries, and the Doctors' Association, advises the minister with regards to the training of specialists and the conditions in which it is undertaken.

The National Board of Health falls under the ministry of the interior, but, in terms of the Parliamentary Act for the Central Administration of Health Services, is vested with the supreme authority in the field of public health and is the chief advisor to the state on all medical and pharmaceutical matters. In this capacity, the National Board of Health must be consulted by the central administration's different departments in all cases which require medical or pharmaceutical expertise; likewise, the service is able to deal with and pronounce on any case which it deems to be of interest for the health services. The National Board of Health is in the charge of the medical director, who is a doctor and who, besides the above-mentioned primary responsibilities, undertakes various administrative and managerial tasks.

The district medical officers services are under the ministry of the interior, and operate in close collaboration with the National Board of Health, especially with regard to the district medical officer's responsibilities as local supervising authority in matters concerning medical staff and health care.

The State Serum Institute is the country's central laboratory for human bacteriology, virology, serology, etc., and comes under the ministry of the interior. It undertakes a series of highly specialised diagnostic, preventative, and consultative tasks within the health services; at the same time the institution carries out an extensive research activity.

As the only hospital in the country which is an independent institution, the Finsen Institute comes under the ministry of the interior in that the institute's activities are financed solely by the state.

Ministry of Social Affairs

Within the ministry of social affairs, the National Social Security Office and the National Board of Social Welfare both carry out a number of central administrative tasks within health services. The Insurance Department is responsible for various matters dealing with disability pensions, accident insurance, and national health insurance.

Wage and conditions agreements with doctors, dentists, etc. within the national health system are negotiated by the Insurance Negotiation Committee, made up of representatives from the Association of County Councils, the city councils of Copenhagen and Frederiksberg, and the state. The Social Department is responsible for various matters within health services, for example, child welfare, home nursing, and the school medical services.

Ministry of Education

The ministry of education, through the universities and colleges of higher education, is responsible for the training of academic staff within the health services. Further, the School of Midwifery, with departments at the Rigshospital in Copenhagen and in Ålborg, is under this ministry.

The Rigshospital in Copenhagen, as the only state teaching hospital, comes under the ministry of education. The Rigshospital carries out to an exceptional degree highly specialised treatment functions, and collaborates in teaching and research activities between the university's main disciplines within the medical sciences, and various country and city hospitals.

Ministry for Greenland

Health services in Greenland are the responsibility of the ministry for Greenland. It has still not been decided when these will be handed over to the home government. The medical staff in Greenland are under the National Board of Health's jurisdiction, and the medical officer for Greenland is appointed in the same way as district medical officers in general, by the ministry of the interior and the National Board of Health. The national medical officer for Greenland further pariticipates in the day-to-day administration of the health services.

Ministry of Labour

The Industrial Safety Act delegates responsibility for the establishment of the Industrial Health Service, and the Industrial Inspection Scheme to the ministry of labour. These activities, which make up part of the total health services, are under the leadership of a senior physician, and the various factory inspection districts have permanently seconded factory physicians.

Other Ministries

Public health and environmental hygiene, certain aspects of food inspection, etc. are under the responsibility of the ministry of the environment. The ministry of justice has set up a permanent medical-legal committee; the ministry of defense is in charge of the military medical services; and the ministry of agriculture has some influence on the health services through its interests in foodstuffs.

County Council Level

Whilst the tasks of the above-named ministries within health services are essentially to initiate, coordinate, and supervise, the responsibility for setting up and running the health services on a day-to-day basis is decentralised. In accordance with the Hospitals Act, each county council is required to provide hospital services, which meets the requirements of the society, and similarly establish those areas of health services, which come under the National Insurance Scheme, in accordance with the Health Insurance Act. To undertake the political leadership of these activities, the county councils appoint permanent committees, the Hospital Committee, and the Committee for Health and Social Welfare.

In addition to the activities mentioned above, the county councils are responsible for the welfare of various groups of handicapped, such as the mentally handicapped, the blind, and the deaf. These activities are delegated to either the Hospital Committee or the Committee for Health and Social Welfare, depending on their character.

Over 50% of a county council's total expenditure goes to the day-to-day running of health services. The state allocates the individual county councils a block grant, which serves as a subsidy to finance partially the councils' expenditure. The remainder—the larger part—of the expenditure is raised by the county councils by means of taxes on incomes and property.

The individual county councils are delegated the responsibility to provide free transport by ambulance, special vehicles, or taxis as required—both in connection with the admittance of patients to hospitals and for the transport of outpatients. With the exception of the municipal councils of Copenhagen, Frederiksberg, Gentofte, and Roskilde, where ambulance and transport services for the sick are provided by the municipal fire authority, the remainder of the country is provided with this type of transport on a contract basis by a private contractor (*Falcks redningskorps*).

The Municipal Level

The municipalities also undertake several activities which are part of health services, mainly those areas affected by the Social Security Act, and preventive medical measures. The provision of nursing home facilities is usually the responsibility of the municipalities, as are also the various home nursing and home help services. The municipality further has responsibility for preventive medical activities such as child health services, school medical and dental services, etc.

The Danish Hospital Institute

With the main purpose of collecting, analysing, and disseminating information in the hospital and health services field and undertaking research and development into aspects of planning, rationalisation, and management—with the aim of providing a better basis for solving the problems faced by the planning and governing authorities within the health services—the Danish government, in association with the Association of County Councils and the city municipalities of Copenhagen and Frederiksberg, in 1975 founded an independent organisation, the Danish Hospital Institute. The institute is governed by a board of directors in consultation with an advisory council. The day-to-day management of the institute is under the responsibility of the institute's director, and the institute's staff is multidisciplinal, including doctors, nurses, economists, sociologists, technologists, etc.

Figure 3 The various institutions within the three administrative levels of the health services

Level	Institutions
Ministerial	Ministry of the Interior
	Ministry of Social Affairs
	Other ministries
	Ministry of Labour
	Ministry of Defense
	Ministry of Justice
	Ministry of Agriculture
	Ministry of the Environment
	Ministry of Education
Supervising and advisory	The National Board of Health
	The National Hospital Council
	The National Social Security Office
	The National Board of Social Welfare
	The Metropolitan Council
Management	County Councils/Metropolitan Council
	City of Copenhagen
	City of Frederiksberg
	Municipalities
	Ministry of Education

MEDICAL EDUCATION IN DENMARK

Of the five universities in Denmark, three are providing medical training: the University of Copenhagen, the University of Åarhus, and the University of Odense. The training programmes differ slightly, but graduates from all three universities have equal rights and receive a general authorisation as medical doctors from the National Board of Health.

Until the early 1970s, entry to a medical education was open to all high school graduates and was free of charge. As overproduction of medical graduates became imminent, access to the training programmes was restricted, and admission has now become dependent on high school grades. Higher educations in Denmark in general, are still free of charge. The figures for overall admission and graduation have now stabilised (see table 9). The late 1970s were characterised by a growing unemployment among younger medical doctors, but a reduction of working time for younger hospital doctors in 1981 to a 40-hour week, and the following increase in numbers of physicians employed in the hospital sector, has resulted in a situation of full employment today. The present level of graduates, combined with an age curve displaced towards the younger group of medical doctors in the country, will probably again lead to a growing unemployment in a short time. As there is some political reluctance to further reduce educational possibilities for the Danish youth, this trend will probably not change for some years unless new employment possibilities are introduced for doctors in Denmark or abroad.

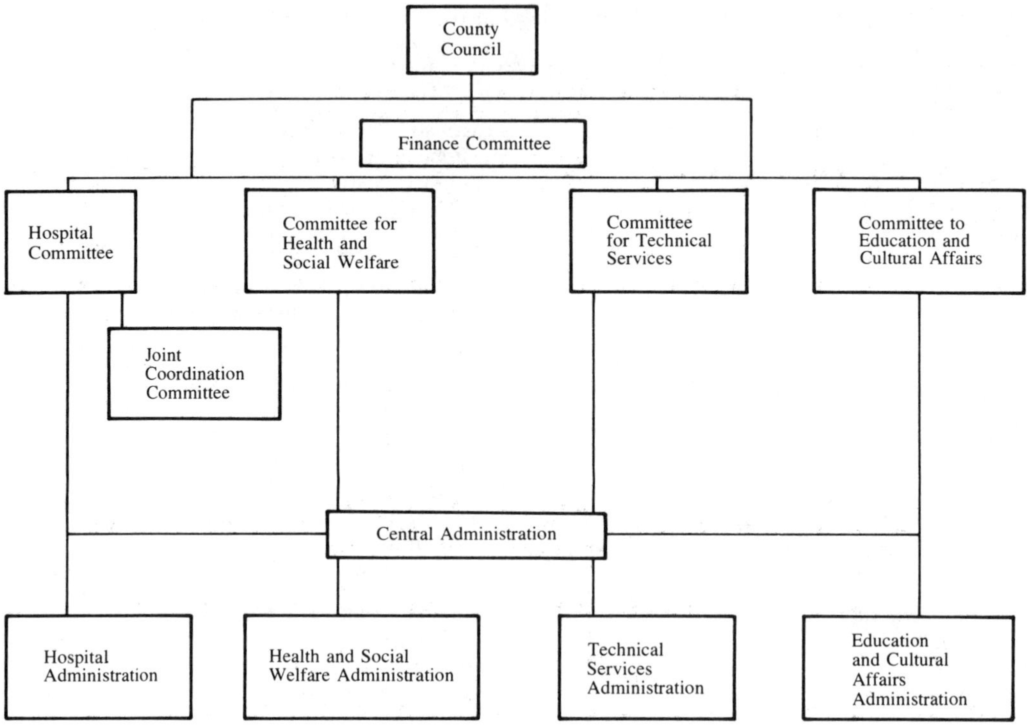

Figure 4 Organisation of a county

THE ORGANISATION AND FUNCTION OF PRIMARY HEALTH SERVICES

General Practitioners

In Denmark primary health services are built up around the general practitioners' services, which are based on the family doctor principles—that is, the individual family or person chooses themselves which doctor they will use. Some families often keep the same doctor for a considerable number of years, which enables the establishment of a valuable relationship of trust between the doctor and his patients, and at the same time ensures the practitioner a comprehensive insight into the families' social and medical conditions.

The general practitioner operates in principle in private practice, and carries on his business independently of the hospital services. In practice, however, his income derives from the services he carries out for the public health insurance, calculated according to the scale of fees agreed to by his own professional organisation and the Public Health Insurance Board.

General practitioners often carry on their practices in collaboration with other doctors, either in partnership, with common facilities and a single list of registered patients, or in group practices, where the individual doctors carry on their own practices but in premises shared with others. As a rule the general practitioner owns the clinic and the facilities and is also responsible for the employment and salaries of assistants such as secretaries, nurses, etc. It is normal for a doctor to establish himself as a general practitioner by taking over an existing "vacant" practice, for which he will usually pay a lump sum for "goodwill." This is approximately the equivalent of 1 to 1½ year's gross income. Another method is for the doctor to be taken into partnership in an existing practice, where he will as a rule be expected to invest capital as required by the other partners in the practice. The freedom to set up a new practice is today restricted, in that the establishment of general practitioners is controlled and regulated according to an agreement with the public health insurance, and each new practice requires approval by the parties to that agreement. In the same way, a doctor who takes over an existing practice must first receive endorsement from the same organisations.

According to existing agreements, a general practitioner is required to hold open consultation sessions four times a week in the mornings and once a week late in the afternoon. He is under obligation to give consultation to all those patients who report during consultation hours; further, without any extra remuneration, he must undertake home visits, so long as he is notified between the hours of 8 and 9 in the morning.

On the average, between 30 and 40 patients attend the private practitioner every day, and he visits 3 to 4 patients at their homes. The visits and consultations cover everything from the more complicated clinical examinations of new ailments, to the renewal of prescriptions and other minor tasks.

In the case of the majority of patients, the general practitioner will be able to undertake the necessary examination and treatment himself, with the facilities available to him in his consulting rooms. A small proportion of the patients will be referred for further examination and/or treatment to either practising specialists or the hospital.

The general practitioner has a considerable degree of contact with the municipal or county social welfare services. It is often the general practitioner, in his capacity as family doctor, who is aware of social problems which the family will be unable to solve without the help of the Department of Social Affairs. Further, he is responsible for issuing medical certificates in connection with sickness benefits, and the provision of visiting nursing services, etc., and he has similarly an important function with respect to recommending patients for nursing homes and applying on the patients' behalf for disability or other pensions.

Certain preventive activities within health services are also undertaken by the general practitioner.

Practising Specialists

The primary health service also includes the practising specialists who are connected to the National Health Insurance Scheme.

The largest group of specialists working within primary health services are the ear-nose-throat specialists and ophthalmologists. Both these disciplines have entered into special agreements with the National Health Insurance Scheme, which in the case of the Copenhagen and Frederiksberg City councils, differs from the rest of the country. The largest proportion of the total outpatient acitivity for ENT and ophthalmology is undertaken by practising specialists.

A large number of other disciplines also have agreements with the National Health Insurance Scheme, and general practitioners are able to refer their patients for examination and, if necessary, treatment to practising specialists in psychiatry, internal medicine, surgery, gynaecology-obstetrics, dermatology, physiology, etc. In the cities of Copenhagen and Frederiksberg there exist a large number of private clinics in diagnostic radiology, whilst the outpatient facilities for this discipline throughout the rest of the country are to be found in the hospitals.

In all, about 1,900 specialists have agreements with the National Health Insurance Scheme and are therefore permitted to treat the patients who are referred to them by general practitioners. Only approximately one-third of these specialists rely on their private practices as their sole source of income—these are mainly the ENT specialists and the ophthalmologists. Most of the others have other positions, usually in hospital services, and carry on their private practices on a part-time basis. In many parts of the country the catchment population is not sufficient to provide the basis for full-time private practice in the case of most disciplines.

Dental Services

Child Dental Health Care

The Act on Child Dental Health Care, which was passed in 1972, guarantees all children of school-going age the right to free dental care, including both preventive and curative treatment. The children's dental services are provided by the municipalities, who as a rule provide the dental clinics and employ the staff who work in them. In smaller municipalities the services are provided by dentists in private practice, in agreement with the local authorities. From 1981 the free dentistry concession will be gradually extended, so that by 1987 all children aged 0 to 16 years will be encompassed by the service. To this must be added that the municipalities have the possibility to extend the dentistry service to include adolescents up to 20 years of age.

Adult Dentistry

The National Health Insurance Scheme gives subsidies of various forms for dental examinations and treatment carried out by dentists in private practice. The subsidies are paid for cleaning, fillings, and extractions, but not for cosmetic treatment or artificial dentures. The subsidy covers two-thirds of the dentist's bill, whilst the patient pays the rest.

Visiting Nursing Service

The municipal visiting nursing service is considered as a supplement and sometimes an alternative to the nursing facilities available at a hospital or nursing home. The visiting nurse carries out treatment, as directed by the doctors, and other nursing activities in the patient's own home, making it possible for the patient to stay at home throughout the period of his illness, where he otherwise would have to be admitted to hospital or a nursing home.

The visiting nurse collaborates closely with the Home Help Service, which ensures that the practical problems in the home can be solved, even during prolonged illness.

Medical products are dispensed to the consumers by retail chemists and, in some cases, by their branches and depots.

The manufacture, import, export, storing, distribution, and packaging of drugs can only be carried out in Denmark with the permission of the National Board of Health, which is further able to lay down rules and regulations for the technical management, in-house expertise, the establishment, and the operation of concerns which are given that permission.

The retail chemists in Denmark operate as private enterprises carried out on the basis of concessions granted by the public authorities. Each retail chemist is obliged either to stock or be in a position to obtain, without delay, all the medical products which are certified as suitable for prescribing by the general practitioner and which can legally be retailed in the country. The chemists' hours of opening are stipulated by agreement with the public authorities, encompassing also the necessary duty service, which ensures that every district in the country has at least one retail chemist operating a 24-hour service.

The retail chemists service is further the subject of economic redistribution by the public authorities, in that their profits are regulated in such a way that there is effected a form of income distribution from the large retailing concerns with a considerable turnover, to smaller concerns in lowly populated areas. In this way it is possible to maintain services in keeping with the standards set down, even though the necessary population to attain liquidity is not available.

Other Forms of Treatment Available

There are several other groups of health practitioners who have agreements with the National Health Insurance Scheme for the reimbursement in part or in total of fees paid by their patients. This includes first and foremost physiotherapists who, outside of Copenhagen and Frederiksberg, are permitted to establish private clinics and receive patients for treatment after being referred by their general practitioners. Occupational therapists are also permitted to practise in terms of the same agreement. In the city councils of Copenhagen and Frederiksberg, physiotherapy clinics are run by the Health and Social Welfare Administration.

Chiropractors can receive patients for treatment, whereby the patient qualifies for subsidies. Patients are permitted to seek treatment from chiropractors without being referred by their general practitioners.

Preventive Activities

There are several areas of health services where preventive activities are carried on; some are under the supervision of the general practitioner, while others are the result of special arrangements, such as the school medical services.

Maternity Care

All pregnant women have the right to three medical examinations before giving birth and two after. Advice is also given on how to avoid future, unwanted pregnancies. As a rule, these examinations are carried out by general practitioners, but in close collaboration with the hospital services' departments of obstetrics, where the patients can go for control in those cases where it is considered necessary. There is further provision for at least five examinations by a midwife.

Maternity care and delivery services are organised by the county councils according to a plan, which they are required by law to draw up. The National Health Services have set out directives for the organisation of maternity care services, to ensure that women in all parts of the country are provided with facilities of a comparable standard.

Health Care Services for Children

All births are notified by the midwife to the health services authorities in the municipality where the mother lives. They, in turn, offer health care facilities to the mother in the form of home visits by a health worker. On the average, each child is visited on between seven and nine occasions during its first year, but this can vary considerably, depending on the needs of the individual child or family.

The main aim of the health workers' visits is to give basic and individual health guidance to the parents, and, in cases where there are deviations from the progress expected, to arrange for the family doctor or social welfare expertise to be brought in.

The health worker shall, in cooperation with medical and social welfare workers, strive to prevent the occurence of illness and to recognise potential development and growing problems in the children at the earliest possible stage.

Child Examination and Vaccinations

All children are able to take advantage of a programme which provides ten health examinations before reaching school age and vaccinations against whooping cough (pertussis), diphtheria, tetanus, and poliomyelitis. These examinations and vaccinations are carried out by the private practitioners, often in close collaboration with health workers. The great majority of families in Denmark take advantage of these facilities.

School Medical Services

The municipalities are required by law to employ school medical officers and school health workers with the task of undertaking preventive medical examinations of all children of school and nursery school age. All nursery children and children in the first, second, and fifth school years undergo medical examinations. Children in the ninth school year also undergo medical examinations, at which time the school medical officer offers guidance as to the child's suitability for employment in different fields.

The school medical service does not undertake any treatment, but can, where it is shown to be necessary, refer the child to his family doctor, who will perform the necessary treatment or possibly refer the child further to a practising specialist or to a hospital.

The school medical services also include school dental services.

Occupational Health Services

Legislation has been passed to give all industrial concerns the opportunity to establish occupational health services. In factories with special safety problems, these services are mandatory. Occupational health services are still in the development stage but are intended to encompass medical, economical, and technical expertise, which will be offered in close collaboration with the concern's Industrial Safety Organisation.

Occupational health services get support in the form of advice and supervision partly from the industrial inspection services and partly from the industrial medical clinics and outpatient departments, which are gradually being established within hospitals in all the hospital authorities.

THE NATIONAL HEALTH INSURANCE SCHEME

The Act on National Insurance stipulates that all residents in Denmark are guaranteed the right to free medical treatment by a medical practitioner or a practising consultant. This right is independent of the person's income, the costs of the service being paid through rates and taxes by the 14 county hospital authorities and the city councils of Copenhagen and Frederiksberg.

At present, the health insurance regulations permit patients to choose to be insured in one of two insurance groups: group 1 and group 2. Patients insured in group 1 are covered for all medical expenses but have to choose one particular private practitioner, who they should use in order to get their expenses fully covered. Normally, these patients are allowed to change their doctors once a year. They may not themselves go directly to a practising specialist but must be referred by their private practitioners. Those patients who choose group 2 must pay part of the consultation expenses themselves, usually in the order of 25% of the full amount. However, the patient is not obliged to be registered with one particular doctor and is not dependent on the doctor's referral to attend a practising specialist. Everyone in the country is free to choose which of the two insurance groups he wishes to belong to. At present (October 1979) about 93% belong to group 1.

General practitioners in Copenhagen and Frederiksberg are remunerated by the National Health Insurance Scheme annually with a sum which relates to the number of patients who are registered with them. This sum is in no way affected by the number of times the patient visits the doctor or by which services the doctor renders the patients.

General practitioners throughout the rest of the country are remunerated by the National Health Insurance Scheme, partly according to the numbers of patients on their lists and partly according to the services which they render to the patient, for example, consultations, home visits, etc. The fees are fixed so that about one-half is determined by the number of patients and one-half by the services provided.

Practising specialists usually receive their fees from the Insurance Scheme in the form of payment for services rendered, for example, per consultation, examination, operation, etc. Certain practising specialists in Copenhagen and Frederiksberg are paid a lump sum per year for each outpatient registered with them.

In accordance with the regulations drawn up by the ministry of social affairs, the

The national health insurance budget and expenditures for 1979

	Million Crowns
Fees, etc. to private practitioners	1,361.8
Fees, etc. to practising consultants	498.1
Fees, etc. to dentists	651.1
Pharmaceuticals	864.0
Other services[a]	167.0
Total	3,542.0

[a]Other services includes mainly physiotherapy treatment.

National Health Insurance Scheme covers part of the expenses paid by the patient for drugs and medicine. The subsidies are given according to a list drawn up by the ministry, where some preparations receive a 50% subsidy and others 75%. In the case of certain preparations, their use for specific ailments must first be authorized before the insurance scheme can pay the agreed subsidy.

EXPENDITURE AND MANPOWER RESOURCES

General Practitioners and Practising Consultants

At the end of 1979 there were 2,700 general practitioners and 1,900 practising specialists in Denmark. Only about one-third of the specialists practised on a full-time basis; the remaining group carried on their practice part time, at the same time being employed in hospital services.

Dentists

In 1978 there were about 5,200 dentists actively employed in Denmark, of whom over one-half were self-employed and the rest were employed in private or public clinics.

Retail Chemists

At the end of 1979 there were 320 private retail chemists in Denmark. Their owners had in 1978 a gross turnover of over 1.9 milliard crowns and had dealt with over 36 million prescriptions.

In special cases subsidies may be paid for preparations not included in the list after consultation with the national health service.

SECONDARY HEALTH SERVICES (HOSPITAL SERVICES)

Introduction

Hospital services in Denmark are in almost all respects financed from public funds. The majority of hospitals are publicly owned, and the few private hospitals that are to be found are almost 100% subsidized by the local authorities and are subject to the same legislation and standards as the public hospital. The county council through its Hospital Committee is responsible for the day-to-day administration of the hospitals.

As in other European countries, the first hospital services in Denmark were provided during the Middle Ages, usually by the monasteries. The first public hospital in modern terms was King Frederik's Hospital, established in Copenhagen in 1757 and still in existence today as the Rigshospitalet. Most Danish towns during the second half of the 19th century established public hospitals at the same time that private hospitals were set up in various places, usually by religious organisations. The first local hospitals were either basic general hospitals, providing medical and surgical care, or isolation hospitals. They were established and run by the councils in the provincial towns or the counties, or by the towns and counties in collaboration.

The local government reforms carried out in 1970, and the consolidation of the counties into 14 county councils, transferred all publicly owned hospitals to these political-administrative units, which thereby were given the responsibility for the administration of hospital services as well as the planning work to meet future needs. The city councils of Copenhagen and Frederiksberg are on a par with the counties in this respect; there are, therefore, in all 16 political-administrative authorities with responsibility for hospital services.

The Structure of Hospital Services

The structure of hospital services in Denmark is in principle determined partly by the terms set out in the Hospitals' Act and partly by the authority granted by the act to the guidelines drawn up by the ministry of the interior for the planning of future services within the general somatic services (Guidelines for the planning of the future development of hospital services—1971) and the psychiatric services (Guidelines for the planning of psychiatric services—1977). On the basis of these ministerial recommendations, every hospital authority is required to prepare future plans for their hospital services. These plans must be revised/updated and sent to the ministry of the interior for approval every four years.

The above recommendations set out that each hospital authority should establish within its area one main hospital, which shall be the centre for the authority's specialised hospital services. The county's (or city council's) remaining hospital services, covering the more general hospital functions, can beyond this be provided for by smaller hospitals, though with at least four basic specialities: surgery, internal medicine, anaesthesiology, and radiology. The local hospitals, with only surgical and medical specialities, play an increasingly minor role in the hospital system.

This structure of the hospital services varies somewhat from one hospital authority to another. There are some counties where the main specialised functions are undertaken by two hospitals, usually of similar size, which divide the different specialities between them; in some cases the high density of population around the larger cities means that the hospital services are built up around several large specialised hospitals. Some of these hospitals are at the same time university teaching hospitals and undertake several highly specialised functions, as well as their teaching functions.

The different types of hospitals found in Denmark and their number are shown in figure 5.

National and Regional Hospitals

The large hospital units found in the larger cities, as described above, undertake by means of their highly specialised facilities, several regional tasks, which require a larger population basis than the smaller counties usually have. These duties are divided into national and regional functions.

By national functions are understood the diagnosis and/or treatment of:

a. Ailments that occur so seldom that it is reasonable that the facilities and expertise required to treat them are placed in only one or two hospitals in the country.
b. Ailments that require access to diagnostical or therapeutical facilities that are either so new or expensive that they are only to be found at one or two hospitals in the country.
c. Ailments that are complicated by the presence of other ailments, requiring collaboration between different specialists of a nature that can only be found at one or two hospitals in the country.
d. Outpatient consultation, or admission of the patient to control, before or after treatment of any of the categories or ailments mentioned above.

By regional functions are understood the diagnosis and/or treatment of ailments that in the case of some hospital authorities necessitate the transfer of the patient to another hospital authority, but cannot be classified as either national function or normal county hospital function.

Regional functions are carried out by 5 to 7 hospitals in Denmark. National and regional hospital functions are a present located in Ålborg, Århus, Odense, the county of Copenhagen, the city of Copenhagen, and the Rigshospitalet.

An example of a regional function is neurosurgery, which is to be found at all the places mentioned above. Examples of national functions are the burns unit at the city of Copenhagen hospital at Hvidovre and the department of paediatric surgery at the Rigshospital. These are the only special departments for these respective disciplines, and as such receive patients from the whole of Denmark.

Specialising Somatic Hospitals

Over and above these types of hospitals there is further to be found a limited number of specialising hospitals. This category includes, on the one hand, hospitals established to accommodate the treatment of a particular category of patients, as, for example, at the

Figure 5 Categories and numbers of hospitals in Denmark with complements of staff and number of beds

	General and Specialised Hospitals	Smaller General Hospitals	Nonspecialised Hospitals	Other Hospitals	Somatic Hospitals in All	Psychiatric Hospitals and Psychiatric Nursing Homes	Hospitals in All
Number of institutions	42	30	24	20	116	16	132
Number of beds	25,091	4,402	1,665	2,355	33,513	9,442	42,955
Staff (calculated in full-time posts)	60,486	8,146	2,670	3,616	74,919	10,805	85,723

rheumatism hospitals, and on the other hand, general hospitals that during reorganisation are used for special services such as rehabilitation or geriatric care.

Psychiatric Hospital Services

From the middle of the nineteenth century until 1976, the care and treatment of psychiatric patients has predominantly been undertaken by the state, which through the state hospital service was responsible for a network of large special psychiatric hospitals called state hospitals. These psychiatric hospitals were by law handed over to the county hospital services in 1976 and are now a part of the various hospital authorities' hospital services, together with the departments of psychiatry which had already been established within the hospital system. At the present (1979) moment psychiatric hospital services are undergoing an extensive reorganisation.

Hospital Services Statistics

The total hospital services administrates approximately 43,000 beds, of which about 9,500 (or 22%) are psychiatric beds. Over and above these are approximately 6,500 beds in institutions for the mentally deficient, the majority of which will from 1 January 1980 be transferred to the hospital authorities' social services, whilst only a small proportion were incorporated into the hospital services.

In 1978 the hospital services had the following capacity and usage:

Somatic beds	
Number of beds	33,513
Total admissions	920,000
Number of bed days	9,534,000
Average bed occupation	79%
Total number of outpatient visits	3,177,000
Psychiatric beds	
Number of beds	9,442
Total of admissions	25,000
Number of bed days	3,183,000
Average bed occupation	90%
Total number of outpatient visits	68,000

The use of hospital facilities is increasing. Most hospitals cater for acute outpatient functions in the form of an accident and emergency department, which deal with patients involved in all types of accident, together with some categories of sudden illness. Further to this, the outpatient departments deal with examination of patients before and after they are admitted to hospital for treatment. Finally, many departments carry on outpatient functions in day wards, where the patients are admitted for a limited number of hours for examination or treatment. Typical examples are psychiatric patients and patients with chronic kidney failure who require dialysis treatment.

Hospital Staff

The various county councils' hospital services are under the administration of a central hospital administration department with local management departments in the different hospitals. The allocation of responsibilities and the form of organisation used in the different county councils is dependent on the extent of the hospital services provided and the size of the different hospitals. The central hospital administration also serves as a secretariat to the hospital board.

Administration

The day-to-day management of the individual hospital is carried on under the auspices of a hospital administrator, who is responsible for forward planning, budgeting, staff administration, the daily running of the hospital, and maintenance.

Clinical Staff

Of the almost 10,000 doctors in Denmark, about 6,000 were employed within hospital services in January 1979. There are approximately 2,000 heads of departments who are permanently established as "public servants"; the remainder are called "junior doctors" and are employed according to various agreements.

Registrars are employed for one year at a time, the maximum time that they may stay in any one position being 3 years. Senior registrars are appointed for periods of 5 years. In addition, there is a smaller group of doctors who are appointed on other conditions.

Every hospital department has a head of department, who is responsible for the examination and treatment of the patients in that department. The remaining medical staff in a larger clinical department will consist of assisting heads of departments, senior consultants, registrars, and possibly clinical assistants. The hospital as a whole or a county hospital service does not have a superintending chief doctor or a medical director. The head of a department does not appoint staff in his own department (though he may recommend junior doctors for appointment); neither is he himself allowed to directly place orders for larger apparatus or equipment, which can only be done with approval of the hospital administration.

Doctors who work in Danish hospitals are employed on a full-time basis and are paid a salary according to national wage agreements. They are not allowed to demand fees from the patients who are treated at the hospital. However, specialists employed by the hospital are allowed to carry on private practice outside normal working hours, either on premises of their own or at the hospital. In case of the latter, there are rules for the time, the extent, and the payments to be paid by the doctor to the hospital for the use of rooms, instruments, and staff for the treatment of private outpatients.

The medical staff's interest are looked after on both local and county levels by medical councils who also act as advisors to the political and administrating hospital authorities. The medical council is elected by and among the doctors employed in the area that it represents, and normally the majority of its members are heads of departments.

Nursing Staff

The senior leader of nursing at a hospital is the chief nursing officer, who is the professional and administrative leader of the nursing staff, which is made up of nurses and

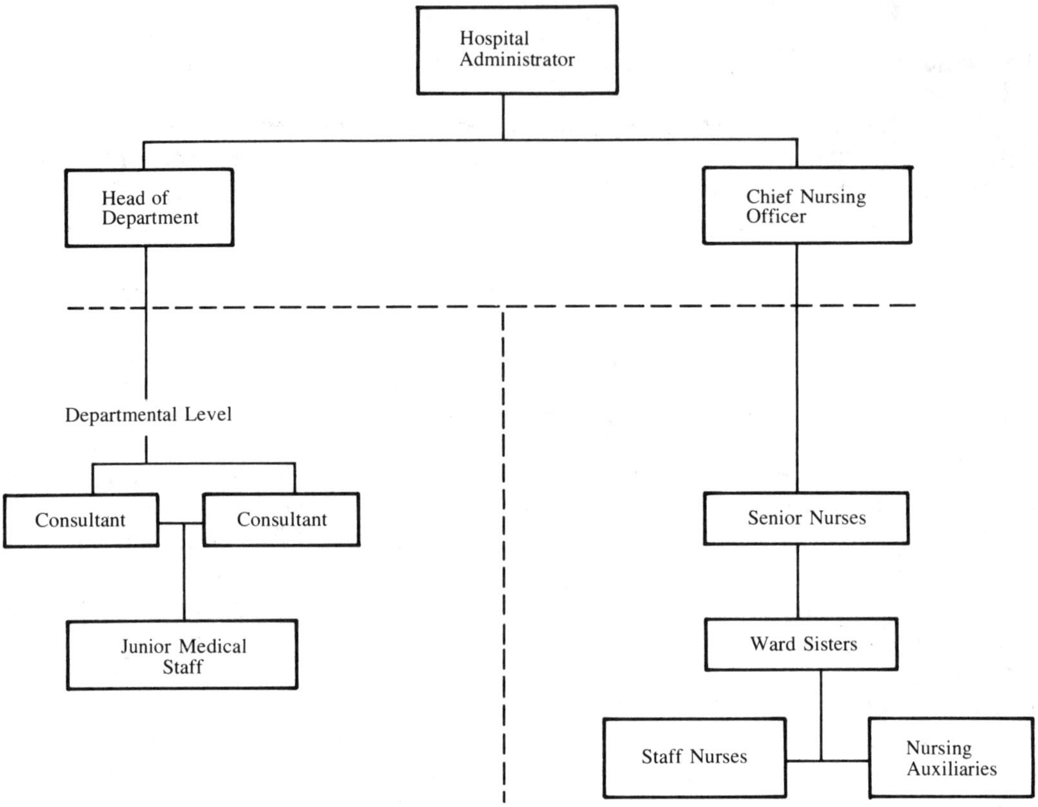

Figure 6 Example of the organisation of staff at a larger hospital, executive level

nursing utilities. Nurses are appointed as nursing assistant, nurse, ward sister, and senior nurse.

There are over 22,000 nurses and over 19,000 nursing *utilities* employed in the Danish hospital services.

Other Hospital Staff

Apart from the administrative, medical, and nursing staff are to be found the following categories of personnel.

Other professional health staff. Examples here are pharmacists, dentists, physio- and occupational therapists, laboratory technicians, and radiologists.

Clerical staff. The clinical departments employ both doctors' secretaries and secretaries to relieve the nurses in the ward of clerical work.

Supply services. Internal transport and supply services are undertaken by hospital porters. In more modern hospital building complexes, there is an increasing tendency towards mechanising some of the transport functions, such as the transport of pharmaceutical supplies, instruments, and food.

Kitchen, laundry, and cleaning staff. In recent years there has been an increasing tendency to contract out laundry and cleaning duties to private firms on a tender basis.

Figure 7 Staff categories working in Danish hospital services, January 1979

	Full Time	Part Time
Doctors	6,139	95
Other graduates	510	236
Nurses	12,381	10,249
Staff with other nursing training	10,800	12,355
Staff with other health training	7,254	6,932
Other staff without health training	530	612
Student nurses	7,425	
Administration	2,455	1,470
Staff in service departments (kitchen, cleaning, laundry, supply and works departments, pharmacy, etc.)	16,859	11,797
Total	64,353	43,764
Total calculated in terms of full-time posts	86,226	

Hospital works. This function includes staff who are employed to control the hospitals' heating and electrical systems, and to carry out the technical maintenances of diverse apparatus and installations.

The Total Manpower and Expenditure in the Hospital Services

The total number of employed (in terms of full-time posts) within the hospital services was in 1979 approximately 86,000, which is equal to about 2 full-time posts per bed.

The distribution of staff into different categories is shown in figure 7. In 1979 the budget for total expenditure for hospital services in Denmark was approximately 15 milliard crowns.

TERTIARY HEALTH SERVICES (NURSING HOMES AND CARE FOR THE INFIRM AND AGED)

Introduction

The tertiary health services—which includes the provision of nursing homes and care for the infirm and the aged—are closely allied to social services, with no clear lines of demarcation between the two. The following describes some of the social welfare arrangements which, when applied as an extension of the care of an illness, relate to hospital services, but which are also available to all residents in the country (even when they are not sick) as part of the function of the social services.

Institutions

Nursing homes receive patients who are not in need of hospital treatment but who require intensive nursing and certain assistance to an extent that they are not able to manage in their own homes. Psychiatric nursing homes receive patients whose psychiatrical disabilities are of a character that the need for nursing and supervision make it impossible for them to stay at home.

The nursing homes have permanently seconded doctors, who are usually general practitioners.

Social Welfare Arrangements

Protected residences can be placed at the disposal of patients who require limited nursing or assistance. The home help service gives temporary or varying assistance with domestic chores to people or patients who are so disabled that they would otherwise not be able to manage to stay at home.

Meal services in several municipalities are delivered to pensioners, who in this way are able to manage in their own homes even if their infirmities make it impossible for them to manage to buy or prepare their meals themselves.

Day centres are found in various parts of the country. Here nursing and welfare facilities are provided during the day, whilst the rest of the time is spent at home.

Financial Status and Remuneration

Certain psychiatrical nursing homes are part of the hospital services, and are financed as such by the county councils. The majority of the nursing homes, both general and psychiatrical, are run either by the municipalities or by private institutions under contract to and supervision by the municipalities.

Those who live in a nursing home and who receive disability or old age pension have to pay that pension plus a certain part of any other income to the authorities. They receive, however, "pocket money" to pay for various daily expenses. Those who use the day centres pay a fixed sum per day, which also covers the meals that are provided there. Those living in protected residences pay rent which is equal to 25% of their (combined) income.

The payment for home help is dependent on the income of the recipients, the low income groups getting the services free of charge. Meals delivered by the home meal service are paid for at a constant price per portion.

Capacity, Staff, and Expenditure

In January 1979 there were 1,354 nursing homes in Denmark, providing over 49,000 places, which is equal to approximately 700 places per 10,000 population aged 65 or over. There were the equivalent of 39,000 full-time employees in the nursing home sector, which is equal to 0.8 members of staff per nursing home place. The total public expenditure for the nursing home and social care sector for 1980 is budgeted at approximately 6.9 milliard crowns.

COLLABORATION BETWEEN THE THREE LEVELS OF HEALTH SERVICES

Between the Primary and Secondary Health Services

A report published by the ministry of interior states: "Every patient, regardless of where they live, should have access to the best possible treatment at the nearest hospital that fulfills the requirements hereto." This principle is the basis for the referral process, the main aim of which is to ensure that the hospital services' technical and manpower resources are utilized to the greatest possible effect.

In the referral process from the primary sector to the secondary sector, general practitioners play the dominating role in that, on the basis of clinical, social, and geographical criteria, they make the final decisions on whether the patient should be referred to hospital and whether admission to the hospital should be classified urgent or normal. The hospital concerned, however, also plays a part in the referral question in that it decides whether the patient should be treated as an inpatient or outpatient and whether the necessary facilities are available.

The general practitioner has, in principle, no influence on the examination, treatment, and nursing methods used in the hospital. However, some hospital authorities have started collaboration schemes with general practitioners, using a standardised routine when patients are referred to the hospital.

The different hospital authorities have drawn up regulations for referral procedures both in their own areas and between their own and other areas. The Hospital Act stipulates that the costs incurred when treating patients in the hospital of a county outside of that in which they live, shall be borne by their home county; this implies that the latter consents to the treatment which is being given. This consent is given either after the recommendation of one of the county's own chief physicians, or by the general practitioner's formal application either to the county's central hospital administration or to the relevant hospital department.

Certain county councils have, however, introduced directives which require the general practitioner to refer the patient to one of the county's own hospitals in all cases where the decision for further referral will be made.

The continuity of the patient's treatment is safeguarded in that the hospital sends a "discharge certificate," in which the necessary information concerning the results of the examination and treatment is given to the patient's general practitioner, together with proposals for control or further treatment of the patient.

Between the Primary and Secondary Levels of Health Services, and the Tertiary Level

Referral to the tertiary health services can be made from both the primary and secondary levels. Both hospital departments and general practitioners can recommend patients for admission to a nursing home or prescribe home help and/or home nursing. Often the patient is evaluated by a hospital geriatric department, which in that way participates in the referral to the tertiary health services.

The county councils and the city councils of Frederiksberg and Copenhagen are required to set up a procedure ensuring that both social and clinical expertise is brought in in every case where an assessment is being made for referral to a nursing home or protected residence. All the above-named authorities have therefore established "referral committees," with representatives from the social hospitals and the public medical services.

Bibliography

References have not been given in the text. The following publications have been used as a basis for this report.

Amtskommunernes organisation og funktion. Amtsrådsforeningen i Danmark, 1972.

Bekendtgørelse af lov om offentlig sygesikring, nr. 94 af 9. marts 1976. Socialministeriet.

"Betænkning om befolkningens tandsundhedsstatus og tandlægevæsenet." *Betænkning nr. 756,* 1976. Indenrigsministeriet.

Bistandsloven. Juristforbundets forlag, 1976.

"Delbetænkning vedrørende lands- og landsdelsfunktioner." *Betænkning nr. 791,* 1977. Indenrigsministeriet.

Grannik, D., E. Holst, & M. Wagner. *The National Health System in Denmark.* Washington: U.S. Department of Health, Education, and Welfare, Public Health Service, National Institutes of Health, 1976.

Health Services in Denmark. Amtsrådsforeningen i Danmark, 1976.

Lov om sygehusvæsenet, nr. 324 af 19. juni 1974. Indenrigsministeriet.

"Lægestillinger og sengepladser på institutioner maj 1979." *Medicinalstatistiske meddelelser 1979: 6.* Sundhedsstyrelsen.

"Personale- og økonomistatistik for sygehusvæsenet, 1979." *Medicinalstatistiske meddelelser 1979: 7.* Sundhedsstyrelsen.

"Prioritering i sundhedsvæsenet," *Betænkning nr. 809.* Indenrigsministeriet, 1977.

Redegørelse vedrørende planlægning og administration af den offentlige sygesikring. Amtsrådsforeningen i Danmark, 1972.

Speciallægeuddannelse i samfundsmedicin, Betænkning afgivet af en arbejdsgruppe, nedsat af speciallægekommissionen, København, 1977.

Undersøgelser over apotekernes driftsforhold. Apotekerfonden, 1979.

"Vejledende retningslinier for planlægning af psykiatrisk sygehusvæsen." *Cirkulære af 4. april 1977.* Indenrigsministeriet.

"Vejledende retningslinier for planlægningen af sygehusvæsenets fremtidige udbygning." *Cirkulære af 8. juni 1971.* Indenrigsministeriet.

"Ydelsesstatistik for sygehusvæsenet 1977." *Medicinalstatistiske meddelelser 1978:7.* Sundhedsstyrelsen.

The Best Health Service in the World?

THE DANISH CASE

For several decades now, most Danes have had a strong belief that the Danish health services are among the best in the world—if not the best of all. Free of charge with equal access for everybody to an evenly distributed primary care system and from there, whenever needed, immediate referral to the advanced technology of the hospital. Well-trained physicians in all corners of the country, and hospital centres never more than one hour's drive away. The best possible treatment was expected to be available for everybody regardless of cost—and the Danes seemed to be willing to pay these costs, mainly through taxation—without questioning the use of resources or the outcome.

This sublime picture of what foreigners sometimes call "the Danish Case of Successful Socialised Medicine" is now beginning to wither away. Although the basic organisational picture has not been changed since the early 1970s, we have in recent years been facing a radical shift in attitude and health policies by politicians and health administrators.

In the mid-1970s it became clear that health expenditure was rising faster than the Gross National Product, and forecasts anticipated that by the year 2000, all the Gross National Product would be used by health services if the trends continued. The Committee on Priorities within the Health Services was appointed in 1974 by the Danish ministry of the interior, consisting of members of Parliament, municipal and county politicians, administrators, representatives from the trade organisations, etc., and supplemented by experts from the public authorities, university institutes, hospitals, and so on. A unique opportunity was provided to establish the basis for setting general priorities for treatment and prevention of illness with the aim of exploiting the limited resources available in the best possible way.

The report by this committee was presented in 1977 and has since served as a general reference when discussing health policy in Denmark. A number of basic issues were raised in the report, implying problems and needs in the following areas: (1) the role of primary health care and ambulatory services; (2) emphasis on prevention and health promotion; (3) coordination of the functions of health services and the planning systems for the entire health sector; and (4) development of relevant and useful information systems. In the following section the present situation of the health services in Denmark will be discussed in relation to these basic issues which seem to have obtained a broad consensus in the Danish population. These will be seen in the light of, on the one hand, the growing economical constraints in a country with a long tradition of public welfare services and, on the other hand, recent ambitions to decentralise the political and administrative power in all sectors.

PRIMARY HEALTH CARE AND AMBULATORY CARE

Thanks to the development of cheap nationwide health insurance schemes on a cooperative basis in the late 19th century, Denmark has been favoured by a well-developed primary health care system with the general practitioner as the key person. The principle of the free choice of family doctor has gone hand-in-hand with the principles of equality and free service for everybody. These services are still based on the "free enterprise system," financed through agreements with health insurance schemes, originally cooperative organisations receiving support from the public authorities. The schemes were eventually nationalised in 1973, the structure and operation of the health services remaining unchanged.

With the general practitioner supported by a network of dentists and physiotherapists organised on a similar basis, as well as municipal health agencies of public health nurses, home visitors, school physicians, and so on, primary health care in Denmark can be said to have a very solid basis for strengthening the role of local health care as a community-oriented service. The fact that general practitioners see more than 60% of the population at least once a year and perform the role of gatekeepers to the much more expensive hospital services through the referral systems, should provide an excellent opportunity to control the balance between primary health care and secondary care.

How has the development actually been in the country? In spite of the general consensus on the need for more and better primary health care to improve the quality of care and to reduce the pressure on hospital services, we face a situation today where primary health care is stagnating and hospitals are using still more and more resources. The number of general practitioners is now under the joint control of council authorities and local medical associations, who have seen it as their main task to guard against a potential increase in either the use of the services or in the services available for use. The result has been that the level of income has been ensured for existing general practitioners and rises in costs for the health insurance scheme have been prevented.

At the same time, we have seen a steady increase in hospital costs due to ambitious regional hospital building activities, uncontrolled development of medical technology, and agreements between counties and the Medical Association that have guaranteed more medical positions at hospital departments in order to achieve a 40-hour working week for all medical staff. Where locally an increase in the number of professionals in primary health care has been possible, the result has not been a reduction in the consumption of secondary services but rather an increasing demand for specialist care. The conclusion here might well be: Medical care creates more medical care—at least when the actual content of services is unchanged.

As a rather unique feature, the Danish health insurance scheme offers free specialist service outside hospitals to patients referred by general practitioners, as an alternative to hospital ambulatory care. This type of service has grown significantly where sanctioned by the county authorities (through permission to establish new specialist practices), but, again, a parallel growth in ambulatory care activities in hospitals has occurred with a total lack of systematic coordination. Although ambulatory care is encouraged as an alternative to inpatient treatment, it is today an open question whether these services should be integrated in hospital departments or be placed in the community as part of health insurance schemes. Which gives a better quality of care? What is preferred by the patient? And what is more cost-effective? Although these basic questions today can be heard in the discussion, the actual setting of priorities is based on the prevailing political views on private practice as an alternative to nationalised services, rather than on scientific facts produced by data.

In discussing the problems of primary health care as an alternative to secondary care, one can perhaps refer to the Mattheus formula: "To those who have, shall be given." The growth of primary health care is strongly inhibited by the ever-expanding hospital system. At the same time, another challenge seems to have emerged.

Research data indicates that alternative forms of medicine—for example, faith healers, acupuncturers, zonal therapists—have in the last decade become a real, growing enterprise as a substitute for authorised medicine. Physicians seem to have lost their authority in the eyes of the population and their patients, who, frustrated by the incapability of medicine to cure chronic diseases and cancer, turn to alternative care based on simplified disease models or mysticism. This phenomenon was thus manifested in a population having the offer of free medical care, and indicates a growing uncertainty as to the actual benefits of modern medicine.

PREVENTION AND HEALTH PROMOTION

The growing emphasis on prevention has been described as another reaction to the difficulties of modern medicine in demonstrating a reasonable output of the immense public investments in health. Prevention is seen as the way to reduce the need for curative care that is expensive and inefficient. Health care services should engage much more in screening, case finding, and health education, as well as community work and activities, to ensure a more healthy environment. Again, the Danish situation should be very favourable, with a widespread primary health care service already responsible for successful preventive activities regarding maternity and child health as an integrated part of curative services.

Unfortunately, the effect of preventive work is very hard to demonstrate, and conclusive results can be expected only over a rather long period of time. Contrary to curative work, no identified patients can complain when services are removed. Thus, whenever politicians are looking for savings, the preventive services are in danger—even if their actual costs are relatively small compared to huge budgets of curative care. What has actually been seen, therefore, is a continuous cutting down of expenditure on public preventive services. First, the consultative physicians at day care institutions for children were abolished. Next, one of the preventive examinations for preschool children by the general practitioner was cut out. And recently, the functions of the school physician were reduced drastically to save municipal expenditure on health, leaving the public dental services as the major preventive effort still in operation among school children.

During the last few years, occupational health services have been established in many branches of industry as a result of legislation on industrial safety. This new service is financed and administered by both parties in the labour market, and is completely separate from the general health care systems. The problems created by this have been intensified by the fact that very few physicians have been employed in occupational health services due to very high wage claims by the medical profession and a general uncertainty about the capability of doctors in this field. The result has been that occupational health services today are run mainly by technicians and physiotherapists, and physicians seem to have lost an opportunity to achieve an important new role.

The concept of prevention has recently obtained yet another dimension through the still-increasing problems concerning the elderly in our society. Institutionalisation has become an easy but still more expensive solution to the health problems of the growing number of elderly as a consequence of family disintegration and demographic changes. Hospital beds are to a large extent occupied by elderly in no need of acute treatment but without the ability to care for themselves at home; these people are often only waiting for a spare bed in a nursing home. At the same time others are waiting to get hospital treatment: waiting lists have become an important practical and political issue.

Prevention of institutionalisation of the elderly has become a popular solution to waiting lists and rising hospital costs. All over the country, municipal health authorities are building up systems of day- and night-home care by visiting nurses and general practitioners, based on various referral systems and technology for continuous surveillance and alarm in the homes of the elderly.

The establishment of those new services is rather costly, and the interesting question today is whether an effect can in fact be shown on waiting lists and hospital costs—a problem which is just now subject to a huge research effort by Danish researchers in the field.

To stimulate preventive activities, the Committee on Health Priorities proposed the establishment of a central prevention council. Although its establishment was delayed for several years and given a very small budget, the council is actually now in existence as a result of legislation. This is today a multidisciplinary central body linked to the ministry of the interior but free to propose preventive measures in all sectors. Until now, the prevention council has been dealing with subjects such as basic health education, smoking, accident prevention, back pain diseases, and infant nutrition, mainly in the form of seminars and reports. Whether the council is just another way of demonstrating public interest without real interference with actual practice, or whether new preventive measures will actually be established, is yet to be seen.

PLANNING AND COORDINATION

As was pointed out by the Committee on Health Priorities, the political-administrative system in Denmark is characterised by segmentation, both vertically and horizontally. The reform to reorganise political-administrative power in the country in 1970 gave a very high level of autonomy to both municipal and county authorities. Responsibility for health services is now partly in the hands of county authorities (hospital services and health insurance schemes, including general practitioners, dentists, and physiotherapists) and partly of municipal authorities (the rest of primary health services), and there are no effective systems of coordination and joint planning between these levels. The central national authorities in practice have very little more than advisory functions and the responsibility for determining various minimum standards. As a result, each county today can plan and build their hospitals disregarding advice from the ministry and the National Board of Health. The main tool the state authorities have for influencing levels of service activities is mainly the setting of levels of the general financial support from the state to the counties.

As a number of administrative activities cannot be adequately run by each local authority independently (such as negotiating employment contracts with the professional associations), the country has witnessed the building up of new centralised authorities parallel to the former political-administrative system, the Association of County Councils and the Association of Municipal Councils, which have become a powerful force in the formal and informal planning and steering of health services in Denmark. Thus, efforts to decentralise have to some extent led to a new type of centralisation based on a rather weak democratic structure and only partly integrated into the formal political-administrative system.

The problems created by vertical segmentation are mainly of the political-administrative type, whereas horizontal segmentation adds serious functional problems to the actual carrying out of services. At the state, county, and municipal levels, the administration and running of health services are separated into various departments and institutions. Planning systems have been developed separately for hospital services, health insurance schemes, and primary health services under public administration, and useful devices for the coordination of these are lacking.

Seen from the point of view of health professionals, cooperation and coordination of actual services involve interaction with various professional groups working under a number of different administrative and financing systems, varying from completely free enterprise through publicly financed service systems to civil servants administrating a fixed budget. The population and patient basis is very different for the various professionals, in some cases involving geographical limitations, in others patient criteria, such as age, occupation, or even the free choice on the part of the patient. Thus, one public health nurse might have to cooperate with ten to twenty general practitioners to discuss her children population, and the social welfare office often needs to communicate with dozens of general practitioners.

Seen from the patients' point of view, the system offers a family physician as the key contact to obtain the individual preventive and curative services. Where further treatment is needed, the patients are sent off to specialist services, losing contact with their general practitioner for awhile. In school, a separate preventive service will take care of them, unless treatment is needed (since no curative activities are allowed for in-school health services); the same is true in occupational health. Finally, the nursing home offers another doctor to take care of their basic medical needs. Although Denmark certainly has a better starting point than most countries, the ideal of the family physician following the patient from cradle to grave is hard to preserve in a society where the concept of comprehensive local communities is losing its real content.

In primary health care, the reaction to these kinds of problems is—centralisation. The general practitioners move away from their villages and suburbs, and gather in health centres in the urban areas. Two, three, four, or more general practitioners often cooperate by serving a joint population basis and are in some cases offering facilities to visiting nurses, midwives, physiotherapists, etc. to establish the basis for some kind of teamwork. The loss of the neighbourhood doctor will have to be weighed against the potentials of a multidisciplinary team, which, in spite of different employment systems, might work out a community-oriented approach of a new type.

In relation to hospital services, another type of reaction is seen as a result of shortcomings in health planning and coordination. This is manifest in the growing frustration of patients who are on waiting lists (average waiting time in December 1982: varicose veins—5 months, hip arthrosis—8 months, gall stones—4 months, inguinal hernia—5 months) and in the closing down of hospitals, along with the uncoordinated, impersonal service offered by the big, new, centralised hospital institutions fragmented into the many subspecialist departments; it is also manifest in medical profession frustration, resulting from savings and administrative cost-containment exercises. Together, these frustrations have created a basis for building up private alternatives to the public hospital system. An attempt by the former social democratic government to stop such a development, through legislation against private hospitals, fell in Parliament.

Various groups are now working on the establishment of such a new private hospital sector in Denmark based on patient payment partly through private insurance systems (as, for example, has been seen in the United Kingdom), and a number of new perspectives have been outlined for hospital care in the country as the result of such developments:

Overall planning and coordination, of course, will be still more difficult when a private hospital sector will have to be taken into account and local coordination of care will have to involve another dimension; the overall control of national resource allocation to health will suffer, and efforts to change and control balance between primary and secondary care will be weakened. Even more radical is the consequence for the previously ruling general principle of equality in access to medical care in Denmark. Introducing a private, patient-financed hospital service means that waiting lists to public hospitals can be overhauled by individual payment, and in time, you might be able to buy advanced types of care not offered by public hospitals.

Although this might not seem very radical in countries that have had major private hospital enterprises, it is certainly a new outlook in the Danish welfare system with its tradition of a public delivery of services to everybody in need, regardless of the economic potential of the individual.

POTENTIALS FOR PROGRESS

A number of problems in the Danish health service system have been outlined, demonstrating the lack of consistence between generally accepted health policy statements and principles, and real life. How do we from here transform ideals to reality? How do we change and improve health services in times of scarce resources, when savings are all the time high up on the agenda? Among many specific answers, at least four general issues are prevalent in Denmark: information systems, consumer participation, health personnel educations, and local experimental developments.

As a rather small country with a well-established public sector, Denmark has developed a number of information systems on the various public activities, including health services. Both in primary and secondary health care, these information systems are primarily directed towards the daily accounting and administrative activities, rather than towards planning and evaluation purposes. As was already outlined by the Committee on Health Priorities, the data normally illustrate the measurable demand as indicated by number of contacts or bed days broken down by age and sex (only lately supplemented with the actual diagnoses as far as hospital statistics are concerned). This means that there is very little information on the actual content of services and no data on effects. Thus, evaluation of services today is based on general impressions and statements by the medical profession rather than on real knowledge. For setting priorities and for planning, it is necessary to go even further, including data on actual needs, realising that, even in a welfare society, health services consumption is not necessarily reflecting the actual needs of the population.

The growing understanding of the necessity of developing and coordinating comprehensive information systems on health needs and demands on the one side, and services performance and effect on the other, is counteracted by an increasing opposition in the population towards registration. Legislation has made exchange of information between registrars very difficult because of the greater social concern to maintain confidentiality. In a computerised welfare society, this seems reasonable from the individual's point of view, but the establishment of continuous health surveillance systems—including social demographic data and health indicators, as well as information on health services consumption—has now met a significant hurdle that will have to be taken into consideration.

Besides these kinds of general problems, the medical profession in Denmark, as in many other countries, to some extent opposes the development of detailed "quality control" systems in fear of administrative take-over of power and the building up of regulation systems which might narrow their traditional clinical freedom. But it seems that the present demand from the political-administrative system for a rational resource allocation based on valid information is slowly overriding the various obstacles. The challenge now is to develop information systems that will give continuous and valid quantitative and qualitative data on health and health services in the country to help local, regional, and national authorities.

Thus, the medical profession is presently feeling strong pressure from the political-administrative system while, at the same time, another interest group is making demands for a share of power: the consumers. Consumer participation has also become a real issue in Denmark as a new impetus for change. Although the Danish health system as a publicly financed service has certain political involvement at all levels, the role of consumers is now under debate. There is a growing demand for more consumer influence on many levels of the health services: the individual doctor-patient relationship, the general service rendered by health centres and hospital wards, and the overall planning of the organisation of services at the municipal and county levels.

Consumer groups are successfully opposing the closing down of small hospitals. Maternity wards have changed radically through pressure from nationwide "parent-infant" organisations which are demanding better service and new rights for mothers in delivery. Patient participation groups are beginning to influence general practitioners on their policy towards both individual patients and the community. Although health services are far behind in regard to consumer participation in Denmark compared to other public sectors (for example, educational services, social services, environmental protection and planning), the present development seems to favour the role of consumers (both actual and potential patients) in the health sector, probably involving strong potential for change.

Besides the organisational and financing systems, probably one of the most important influences on professional behavior is the actual educational background. Presently, health personnel educations do not in general seem to support development of health services towards a greater emphasis on either primary health care and prevention or planning and cost containment. The learning experiences give health professionals a profound basis for providing advanced hospital technology to individual patients, whereas community medicine, epidemiology, preventive medicine, and health economy barely exist as elements in the curricula. Although general practice has been an important element of the Danish health services for more than a century, departments of general practice have only been established at Danish universities a few years ago—and they are so small that students hardly realise their existence. When the universities have to economize every year, the establishment of new chairs is only possible by cutting down others—and power structures at universities in Denmark have not allowed for that. Only now, because of strong pressure from the ministry of education, things have begun to move, probably resulting in more up-to-date curricula in the years to come.

Although this gives some hope for the future, it is often forgotten that health services will only benefit from these changes in the early 1990s. Producing the physician is a long-term investment. Therefore, how can we expect a health service frozen by reduced budgets and out-of-date educations to change in the coming years? Will the health services be able at all to react positively to pressure from politicians and consumers? Fortunately, there seem to be some bright spots on the map of Danish health services. Local innovators have established here and there a number of exciting local experimental models, involving radical changes in organisation and functions. Often through unorthodox teamwork and local political support, groups of health workers have become engaged in trials for new approaches. As examples of these one could mention surgical hospital wards that are establishing short-stay units to shorten waiting lists; health centres that are organising group therapy for diabetics to facilitate self-care; home visitors who are arranging for terminal cancer patients to get sufficient medical and social support to die in their homes rather than in hospital wards; school physicians who are participating in parent education programmes aimed at, for example, preventing juvenile delinquency.

Central authorities and professional associations are sometimes reluctant and have to be pushed for some time to allow for such deviations. However, at present there seems to be a growing understanding of the value of local experiments for improvement of the general system, even if extra costs must be provided locally for awhile. Unfortunately, tools for evaluation of such trials are not well developed. Multidisciplinary health services research is often necessary to describe and analyse content and consequences of such local changes before the general value can be judged. As research activities in Denmark are slowly moving in this direction, the need for international cooperation and exchange of experiences and ideas is becoming more important.

CONCLUSION

The image of "the best health service system in the world" has probably faded away forever. The growing consciousness of the limits of any health service will probably prevent such an ideal from becoming manifest once again; instead a new ideal is spreading in the country: a flexible health service that is sensitive to changes in health problems, expectations, and resource allocations.

This review probably gives the reader an impression of a health system that, like an oil tanker, is only very slowly shifting its direction. It has also been illustrated, however, that new winds are blowing in the country, and with significant national and international support, there can be no doubt that the coming years will be a period of fruitful change.

Guide to sources for the following statistical tables on Denmark, Finland, Iceland, Norway, and Sweden

Denmark	Danmark
Central Statistical Office	Danmarks Statistik
Statistical Reports	*Statistiske Meddelelser*
Vital Statistics	*Befolkningens Bevægelser*
Statistical Yearbook	*Statistisk Årbog*
National Board of Health	Sundhedsstyrelsen
Vital Statistics	*Vitalstatistik*
Hospital Statistics	*Sygehusstatistik*
Primary Care	*Statistik om den primære helsetjeneste*
Statistical Surveys	*Statistiske oversigter*
Finland	Finland
Central Statistical Office	Statistikcentralen
Statistical Yearbook	*Statistisk Årsbok*
Series OSF (Official Statistics of Finland):	Serien FOS (Finlands offisiele statistikk):
Vital Statistics	*Befolkningsrörelsen*
Life Tables	*Dödlighets- och livslängdstabeller*
Causes of Death in Finland	*Dödsorsaker*
National Board of Health	Medicinalstyrelsen
Health Services	*Hälsovård*
Iceland	Island
Statistical Bureau of Iceland	Hagstofa Islands
Statistical Reports	*Hagskyrslur Islands*
State Social Security Institution	Tryggingastofnun Rikisins
Social Security Matters	*Félagsmál*
Director General of Public Health	Skriftstofa Landlæknis
Public Health of Iceland	*Heilbrigdisskyrslur*
Norway	Norge
Central Bureau of Statistics	Statistisk Sentralbyrå
Series NOS (Norway's Official Statistics):	Serien NOS (Norges offisielle statistikk):
Statistical Yearbook	*Statistisk Årbok*
Population by Age	*Folkemengden etter alder*
Vital Statistics	*Folkemendgens Bevegelse*
Health Statistics	*Helsestatistikk*
Causes of Death	*Dødsårsaker*
Health Institutions	*Helseinstitusjoner*
Health Personnel	*Helsepersonell*
Sweden	Sverige
National Central Bureau of Statistics	Statistiska Centralbyrån
Series SOS (Official Statistics of Sweden):	Serie SOS (Sveriges officiella statistik):
Statistical Abstract of Sweden	*Statistisk Årsbok*
Population Changes	*Befolkningsförändringar*
Causes of Death	*Dödsorsaker*
National Board of Health and Welfare	Socialstyrelsen
Public Health in Sweden	*Allmän hälso- och sjukvård*
The Federation of Swedish County Councils	Landstingsförbundet
Statistical Yearbook	*Statistisk Årsbok*

Table 1 Mean population (in thousands), 1980

Age (Years)	Denmark	Finland	Iceland	Norway	Sweden
Males					
0–4	160.6	163.8	10.6	133.7	249.7
5–9	186.0	153.3	10.8	159.4	285.0
10–14	200.0	178.9	10.7	170.9	299.6
15–19	202.3	194.9	11.5	161.1	291.2
20–24	190.2	196.8	11.1	158.3	284.0
25–29	191.4	208.7	9.7	155.8	298.5
30–34	211.8	227.8	8.5	163.4	342.1
35–39	190.5	162.5	6.6	130.2	311.7
40–44	150.8	144.9	5.3	102.8	241.8
45–49	135.6	134.7	5.6	98.8	218.8
50–54	134.6	135.9	5.5	107.6	227.6
55–59	138.7	114.9	4.9	118.9	250.8
60–64	124.5	87.2	4.1	107.6	228.6
65–69	113.2	83.1	3.4	93.2	210.7
70–74	88.9	63.5	2.7	71.3	170.8
75–79	58.1	36.3	2.0	48.2	112.6
80–84	32.5	16.7	1.2	27.8	61.2
85 and over	18.9	6.9	0.8	15.7	32.8
Total	2,528.6	2,310.8	115.0	2,024.7	4,117.7
0–14 years	546.6	496.0	32.1	464.0	834.3
15–64	1,670.4	1,608.2	72.8	1,304.4	2,695.2
65 and over	311.6	206.5	10.1	256.3	588.2
Females					
0–4	153.3	156.5	10.2	127.3	237.8
5–9	178.1	146.3	10.2	152.5	271.8
10–14	190.1	171.8	10.2	161.9	284.4
15–19	193.3	186.9	11.0	152.8	277.8
20–24	181.5	187.3	10.4	151.3	272.0
25–29	182.4	197.9	9.0	147.8	284.9
30–34	201.5	214.0	7.8	152.7	325.5
35–39	182.2	155.3	6.5	123.1	292.1
40–44	147.8	142.3	5.3	100.3	232.0
45–49	136.8	134.9	5.5	97.2	217.5
50–54	138.7	144.2	5.4	107.3	231.6
55–59	147.1	143.2	4.9	122.8	258.6
60–64	135.2	122.1	4.2	117.2	241.2
65–69	131.1	124.6	3.8	106.9	234.0
70–74	115.0	107.9	3.1	91.8	208.4
75–79	87.4	72.8	2.5	72.0	158.4
80–84	56.3	40.7	1.8	46.5	99.2
85 and over	36.6	19.9	1.3	29.5	65.6
Total	2,594.4	2,468.7	113.1	2,060.9	4,192.8
0–14 years	521.5	474.6	30.6	441.6	794.0
15–64	1,646.5	1,628.1	70.0	1,272.6	2,633.2
65 and over	426.4	365.9	12.5	346.7	765.6
Total male and female	5,123.0	4,779.5	228.1	4,085.6	8,310.5

SOURCE: D: DS, *Befolkningens Bevægelser*
F: FOS, *Befolkningsrörelsen*
I: HI, *Statistical Reports*
N: NOS, *Folkemengdens Bevægelse*
S: SOS, *Befolkningsförändrangar.*

Table 2 Live births and birth rates, selected years

	Denmark	Finland	Iceland	Norway	Sweden
Live births					
1970	70,802	64,559	4,023	64,551	110,150
1975	72,071	66,662	4,392	56,345	103,632
1979	59,464	63,428	4,475	51,580	96,255
1980	57,293	63,064	4,528	51,039	97,064
		Per 1,000 Inhabitants			
Live births					
1970	14.4	14.0	19.7	16.7	13.7
1975	14.2	14.1	20.1	14.1	12.6
1979	11.6	13.3	19.8	12.7	11.6
1980	11.2	13.2	19.8	12.5	11.7

SOURCE: *Nordisk Statistisk Årsbok*
D: DS, *Befolkningens Bevægelser*
F: FOS, *Befolkningsrörelsen*
I: HI, *Statistical Reports*
N: NOS, *Folkemengdens Bevegelse*
S: SOS, *Befolkningsförändringar.*

Table 3 Late fetal deaths and infant mortality, selected years

	Late Fetal Deaths	Infant Deaths	Fetal Death Rate	Deaths Per 1,000 Live Births			
				−24 Hours	−1 Week	−4 Weeks	Total Under 1 Year
Denmark							
1971–75	529	855	7.2	4.1	7.8	9.1	11.7
1978	364	545	5.8	3.2	5.1	5.9	8.8
1979	309	522	5.2	2.4	4.8	5.7	8.8
1980	253	484	4.4	2.9	4.6	5.6	8.4
Finland							
1971–75	450	681	7.3	3.2	7.7	8.9	11.2
1978	314	484	4.9	1.9	4.4	5.5	7.6
1979	269	486	4.2	2.5	5.2	6.0	7.7
1980	266	481	4.2	1.9	4.2	5.1	7.6
Iceland							
1971–75	40	51	8.8	3.6	8.4	9.2	11.6
1978	30	47	7.2	1.9	6.0	6.2	11.3
1979	17	24	3.8	2.9	4.2	4.6	5.4
1980	21	35	4.6	2.9	4.2	6.0	7.7
Norway							
1971–75	560	714	9.1	4.5	7.4	8.4	11.6
1978	346	446	6.6	2.6	4.5	5.5	8.6
1979	382	447	7.4	2.2	4.5	5.4	8.8
1980	363	411	7.1	2.3	4.0	5.1	8.1
Sweden							
1971–75	758	1,102	6.8	3.2	6.9	7.9	10.0
1978	455	727	4.9	1.9	4.7	5.5	7.8
1979	445	721	4.6	2.0	4.5	5.4	7.5
1980	436	671	4.5	1.8	4.2	4.9	6.9

SOURCE: D: DS, *Befolkningens Bevægelser*
F: FOS, *Befolkningsrörelsen*
I: Skriftstofa Landlæknis, *Heilbrigdisskyrslur*
N: NOS, *Helsestatistikk*
S: SOS, *Befolkningsförändringar.*

Table 4 Information not available.

Table 5 Causes of deaths, 1980

B List (ICD. 8th Rev.)		Denmark	Finland[a]	Iceland	Norway	Sweden
	Number of deaths	55,939	43,818	1,538	41,340	91,795
	Per 100,000 population	1,091.9	922.0	674.1	1,011.8	1,104.6
B 19	Malignant neoplasms	13,832	8,796	333	8,627	20,108
B 21	Diabetes	578	627	4	414	1,670
B 26	Chronic rheumatic heart disease	254	320	9	598	832
B 28	Ischemic heart disease	17,235	13,014	482	10,711	33,316
B 29	Other heart disease	1,472	2,529	37	1,900	2,422
B 30	Cerebro-vascular disease	5,139	5,309	147	5,284	9,177
B 32	Pneumonia	1,907	1,571	131	2,471	2,859
B 33	Bronchitis, emphysema, and asthma	1,837	1,081	18	866	1,824
B 34	Stomach and duodenal ulcer	360	164	5	214	640
B 37	Cirrhosis of liver	586	268	2	248	813
B 42	Congenital anomalies	265	301	24	184	426
B 47	Motor vehicle accidents	710	633	24	379	872
B 48	All other accidents	1,210	1,553	87	1,705	2,440
B 49	Suicide and self-inflicted injuries	1,618	1,200	24	507	1,610

SOURCE: *Nordiske Statistisk Årsbok,*
D: Sundhedsstyrelsen, *Dødsårsagerne i Danmark*
F: FOS, *Dödsårsaker*
I: Hagstofa Islands
N: NOS, *Dødsårsaker*
S: SOS, *Dödsorsaker.*

[a] 1978.

Tables 6 and 7 Occupancy and average stay in hospitals, 1980

	Denmark[a]	Finland	Iceland	Norway	Sweden
Discharges (1,000) total	934	980	38	619	1,440
Internal medicine	282	343	—	219	524
Surgery	557	445	—	258	742
Psychiatry	41	36	—	19	121
Patient days (1,000) total	12,247	19,388	891[b]	8,680	18,604
Internal medicine	3,740	4,558	—	2,605	5,503
Surgery	4,228	3,082	—	2,889	5,700
Psychiatry	3,457	6,229	—	2,326	6,869
% Occupancy total	81	85	—	81	77
Internal medicine	81	79	—	83	80
Surgery	82	73	—	77	73
Psychiatry	89	90	—	84	86
Average stay (days)[c] total	9	14	—	11	9
Internal medicine	13	13	—	12	11
Surgery	8	7	—	8	8

SOURCE: D: Sundhedsstyrelsen, *Aktiviteten i sygehusvæsenet*
F: Medicinalstyrelsen, *Hälsovård*
I: Skriftstofa Landlæknis, *Heilbrigdisskyrslur*
N: NOS, *Helseinstitusjonsstatistikk 1980*
S: Landstingsförbundet, Socialstyrelsen *LKELP 81.*

[a]Figures are for 1979.
[b]Figure for 1978.
[c]Somatic hospitals.

Table 8 Active health personnel, 1980

	Denmark	Finland	Iceland	Norway[a]	Sweden
Physicians	11,143	7,641[b]	510	7,813	16,650[a]
Dentists	4,800	3,938[c]	173	4,084[c]	8,263
Professional nurses and midwives	35,900	28,432	1,304	26,796	58,790
Qualified auxiliary nurses	19,882	21,023	—	18,387	23,096
Physiotherapists	2,822	2,146	75	4,246	4,599
Inhabitants per active					
Physician	460	531	449	522	499
Dentist	1,067	1,216	1,326	996	1,005
Professional nurse and midwife	142	168	175	152	141
Qualified auxiliary nurse	257	226	—	221	360
Physiotherapist	1,814	2,231	3,060	960	1,809

SOURCE: D: Sundhedsstyrelsen
F: Medicinalstyrelsen
I: Skriftstofa Landlæknis
N: NOS, *Helsepersonellstatistikk*
S: Socialstyrelsen, *Läkares arbetstider och tjänster 1979*
SCB: *Statistiska meddelanden Serie HS 1982,* Riksförsäkringsverket.

[a]Figures refer to 1979.
[b]Excluding part-time work, etc.
[c]Including economically inactive.

Table 9 Medical school admissions and graduates in Denmark

	Admissions				
	University of Copenhagen	University of Åarhus	University of Odense	Total	Graduates
1979	470	250	130	850	660
1980	470	250	130	850	650
1981	340	250	130	720	695
1982	340	250	130	720	710

SOURCE: The National Board of Health, Denmark.

Tables 10 and 11 Active physicians by occupational group, 1980

	Denmark	Finland	Iceland	Norway[a]	Sweden[a]
Physicians total	11,143	7,641[b]	510	7,813	16,650
Of which in					
Hospital health service	6,581	4,097	365	4,178	12,010
Nonhospital health service	3,559	—	135	2,761	3,880
General practitioners	2,876	1,881[c]	—	1,971[d]	1,480
Practising specialists	683	—	—	485	806
Administrative medicine	73	63	10	316	95
Medical research, education, etc.	499	420	60[e]	355	265[f]
Other medical work	431	44	—	203	400

SOURCE: D: Sundhedsstyrelsen
F: Medicinalstyrelsen
I: Skriftstofa Landlæknis
N: NOS, *Helsepersonellstatistikk*
S: Socialstyrelsen, *Läkares arbetstider och tjänster 1979.*

[a]Figures refer to 1979.
[b]Excluding part-time work, etc.
[c]Physicians in health centers.
[d]Including district health officers and general practitioners.
[e]Including physicians working in hospitals.
[f]Physicians working only in research and education, mainly in theoretical institutions.

Table 12 Information not available.

Table 13 Beds in hospitals by speciality, 1980

	Denmark[a]	Finland	Iceland[b]	Norway[c]	Sweden
Total	41,842	62,733	2,505	29,370	66,232
Internal medicine	12,841	15,796	494	8,636	18,782
Of which					
Neurology	1,430	887	23	524	524
Dermato-venereology	263	389	14	222	579
Pediatrics	1,444	2,378	112	839	2,348
Tuberculosis and lung diseases	385	2,323	37	489	1,444
Rheumatology	1,271	330	—	708	1,227
Surgery	14,398	11,551	520	10,340	21,431
Of which					
Thoracic surgery	277	135	—	—	274
Orthopedics	2,150	698	33	715	2,920
Plastic surgery	215	28	—	158	360
Urology	441	—	—	—	640
Obstetrics and gynecology	3,011	3,725	149	2,556	5,427
Oto-rhino-laryngology	919	717	14	643	1,357
Ophthalmology	363	585	12	503	971
Psychiatry	10,849	20,140	393	7,649	21,829
Of which					
Adult psychiatry	10,684	19,884	379	—	21,183
Child psychiatry	165	256	14	—	646
Radiotherapy	469	479	—	439	848
Rehabilitation	1,089	952	408	648	519
Mixed med.-surg.	1,072	—	502	1,040	392
Other	1,124	13,815	188	618	2,431
Beds per 100,000 population, total	817	1,311	1,117	718	796
Internal medicine	251	330	220	211	226
Surgery	281	241	232	253	258
Psychiatry	212	421	175	187	262
Radiotherapy	9	10	—	11	10
Rehabilitation	21	20	182	16	6
Mixed med.-surgery	21	—	224	25	5
Other	22	289	84	15	29

SOURCE: D: Sundhedsstyrelsen, *Aktiviteten i sygehusvæsenet*
F: Medicinalstyrelsen, *Hälsovård,*
I: Skriftstofa Landlæknis, *Heilbrigdisskyrslur*
N: NOS, *Helseinstitusjonsstatistikk 1980*
S: Landstingsförbundet, Socialstyrelsen *LKELP 81.*

[a]Figures for 1979.
[b]Figures for 1978.
[c]Excluding beds out of use.

Table 14 Information not available.

Table 15a Beds in nursing homes and old-age homes, 1980

	Denmark	Finland[a]	Iceland[b]	Norway	Sweden
Beds, total[c]	49,915	32,953	665	46,329	115,946
Of which in					
Somatic nursing homes	—	1,008	—	17,019	48,141
Mental nursing homes	1,482	744	—	4,685	8,422
Nursing homes for other special diseases	789	—	—	893	—
Combined institutions	47,644[c]	31,201	—	15,581	1,284
Nursing ward	—	7,647	—	9,690	350
Old-age ward	—	—	—	5,891	934
Old-age homes	—	—	—	8,151	58,099
Beds per 100,000 population	975	693	293	1,133	1,394
Of which in					
Somatic nursing homes	—	21	—	418	579
Mental nursing homes	29	16	—	114	101
Nursing homes for other special diseases	16	—	—	22	—
Combined institutions	930	656	—	381	15
Nursing ward	—	161	—	237	4
Old-age ward	—	—	—	144	11
Old-age homes	—	—	—	199	698

SOURCE: D: DS, *Statistiske Efterretninger*
F: Medicinalstyrelsen
I: Skriftstofa Landlæknis
N: NOS, *Helseinstitusjoner og Sosialstatistikk*
S: Landstingsförbundet, Socialstyrelsen, *LKELP 81 og SCD Statistiska Meddelanden,* Serie S Ålderdomshemmen.

[a]Figures for 1978.
[b]Figures for 1979.
[c]Including combined old-age and nursing homes and old-age homes.

Table 15b Care of mentally retarded in 1980

	Denmark[a]	Finland	Iceland[a]	Norway	Sweden
Beds, total	9,251	5,771	349	5,936	11,222[a]
Of which in					
Central institutions	5,172	5,297	—	3,676	963[a]
Other treatment homes	4,033	474	—	2,260	10,259[a]
Convalescent homes	46	—	—	—	—
Beds per 100,000 population	181	121	154	145	135[a]
Patients in private/family care	10,875[b]	489	—	838	20,448[b,c]
Patients in day nurseries/day care services	6,295[d]	4,693	—	2,477	14,861[c]

SOURCE: *Nordisk Statistisk Årsbok*
D: Socialstyrelsen
N: NOS, *Helseinstitusjoner*
S: Socialstyrelsen, *Antal utveclingsstörda den 1. november 1980,* og upublisert materiale.

[a]Figures refer to 1 October 1979.
[b]Including own home, parents' homes, and other private homes.
[c]Figures refer to 1 November 1980.
[d]Including 3,231 patients from treatment homes.

Table 16 Information not available.

Tables 17, 18, and 19 Public health expenditure in 1979

	Millions of National Currency Unit				
Item of Expenditure	Denmark	Finland	Iceland	Norway[a]	Sweden
Health, total	27,065	9,455	67,212	19,450	52,326
Cash allowances	7,105	1,852	14,237	4,845	20,471
Public health insurance	3,605	395	1,092	2,475	20,471
Other cash allowances	3,500	1,457	13,145	2,370	—
Public health and hospital services	17,111	7,235	47,741	13,639	27,031
Hospital expenses	13,569	4,058	35,538	8,226	—
Consultations, etc. outside of hospital	2,933	2,961	3,282	1,914	—
Other expenses	609	216	8,921	3,499	—
Care of mentally retarded	1,525	368	2,887	537	2,090
Dental care	1,324	—[b]	2,347	429	2,734
	Private Consumption: Medical Expenditures (Current Prices)				
Year					
1976	2,497	1,699	—	2,878	3,732
1977	2,805	1,844	—	4,400	4,115
1978	2,961	2,068	—	4,900	4,444
1979	3,214	2,197	—	5,228	4,930
1980	3,466	2,490	—	6,380	5,628

SOURCE: *Nordisk Statistisk Årsbok 1981.*

[a]Figures refer to 1978.
[b]Included in "Consultations, etc. outside of hospital."

Table 20 Information not available.

Health Services in England

David Allen

INTRODUCTION

There are several important characteristics that distinguish the organisation of health care in England from the organisation of health care in most other countries.* Health care in England is overwhelmingly financed and organised by the central government. Health care outside of the government National Health Service represents only 2 or 3% of the total expenditure on health care in England, so this chapter mainly describes the National Health Service. The finance and control of health care in England differs from that in other countries, such as the United States, as does the organisation of medical practice. In England there is a division between primary and secondary health care. Primary medical care is provided largely by general medical practitioners, and almost everyone in England is "registered" with a "GP," whom they normally visit first when they have a medical problem. The GP can, if he thinks it necessary, refer his or her patient to a specialist. This secondary care is based in the government hospitals. This, then, is the basis of health care in England: the government-financed and government-controlled National Health Service, based on the primary care system, provided partly by general medical practitioners in the community who may refer their patients to doctors working in hospitals.

Vital Statistics

The population of England, counted at 46.5 million in 1980, has been growing slowly during the last twenty years; this slow increase is expected to continue. England covers an area of 130,400 square kilometers and is a very urbanised country, with a population

*For the sake of clarity and simplicity, this chapter deals with England. The other three countries of the United Kingdom—Scotland, Wales, and Northern Ireland—have different constitutional positions, so legislation is specific to each country. However, the National Health Service in the four countries differs only in detail, and the general principals are the same in all four countries.

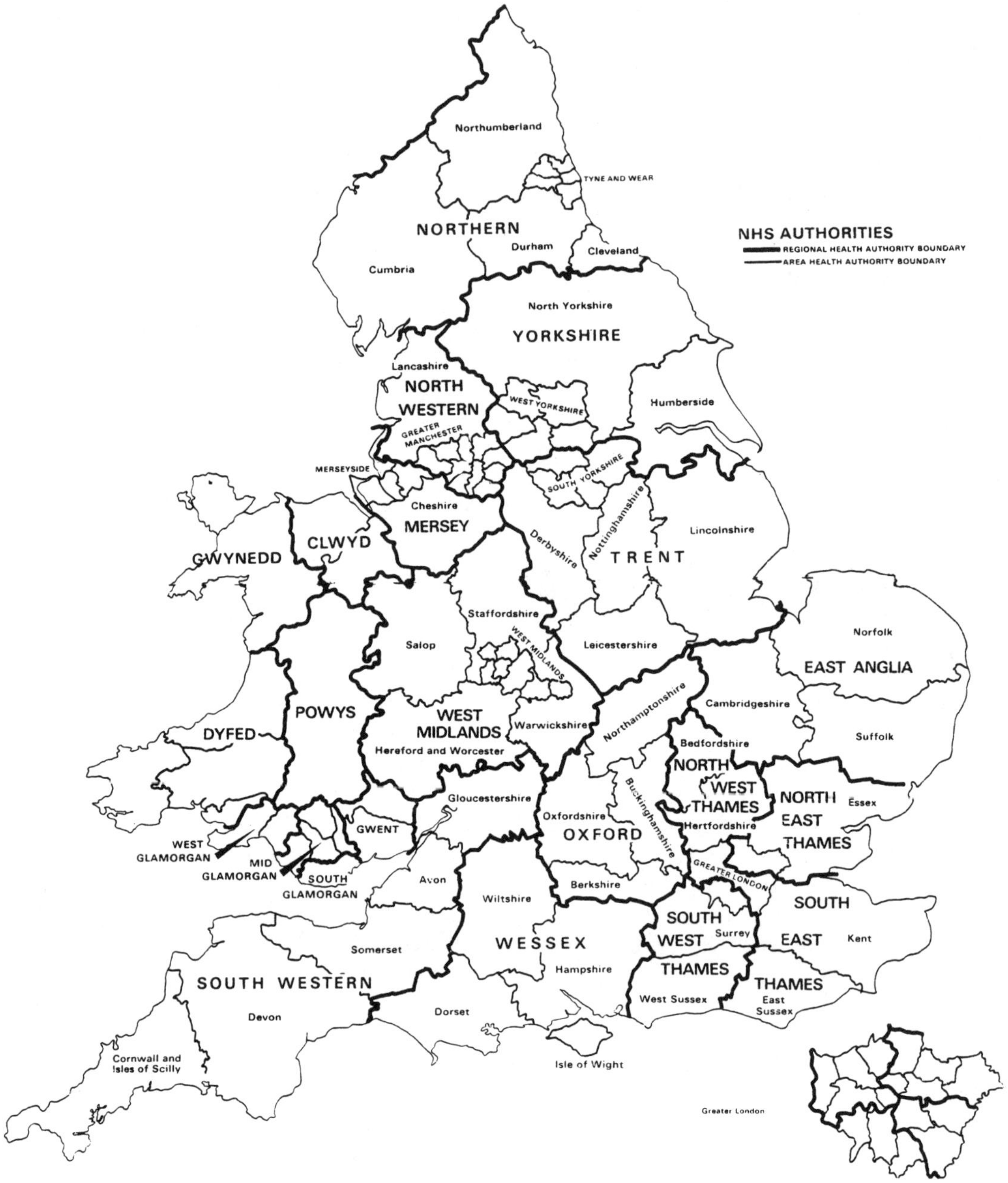

density of 365 persons per square kilometer. (Of the industrialised countries only the Netherlands, with a population of less than a third of England's, has a greater density.) Over one-third of the inhabitants live in seven large urban conurbations; however, the least densely populated regions have the fastest growing populations. England's populace is largely homogenous, with only about 6% of the people born outside of the United Kingdom. Those born abroad appear to be concentrated in the urban areas.

In common with other industrialised countries, England has experienced a decline in birth and age-specific death rates, particularly infant mortality rates, during the last 100 years or so. In 1980 the birth rate was 13.3 per 1,000 population (having started to rise since 1978, reversing the trend of the early 1970s, it is now falling again), the crude death rate was 11.7 per 1,000, and the infant mortality was 12 per 1,000 live births. Life expectancy at birth has risen from 48 years for men and 52 years for women in 1901 to 70 years and 76 years, respectively, in 1977.

About one-sixth of the population is over the retirement age (60 for women and 65 for men), and this proportion is growing slowly. However, the number of those persons over 75 will increase by about one-fifth before the end of the century. There are more than twice as many women as men aged 75 and over. The elderly tend to form a higher proportion of the population in inner urban areas and in the coastal belts.

The principal causes of death in 1980 were ischaemic heart disease (26%) and cerebro vascular disease (12%). The second biggest group of causes, accounting for over one-fifth of the deaths, were malignant neoplasms, the most important sites being the trachea, lungs, and bronchus (6%). Respiratory conditions are responsible for about one in seven of all deaths, the main element being deaths attributed to pneumonia (9%). A most striking change in the last thirty years has been the great reduction in deaths due to communicable diseases. Among children and young adults, accidents and violence now account for a much higher proportion of death. Lethal congenital malformation of children and infants of very low birth weight contribute disproportionately to the total of perinatal deaths.

The number of abortions almost doubled between 1970 and 1980, and was 130,000 in 1980 in England and Wales. The number of spontaneous abortions is not known, but about one-sixth of the other pregnancies were terminated.

Political Organisation

The United Kingdom has no written constitution like that of the United States. The law is based on Acts of Parliament and case law, and can be changed at the will of Parliament. The queen is the constitutional monarch. In law she is head of the executive, an integral part of the legislature, and head of the judiciary. In practice her role is purely formal: "she reigns, but she does not rule." In all important respects she acts only on the advice of her ministers.

Parliament consists of the queen, the House of Lords, and the House of Commons. Over the centuries the balance between the three parts has changed so that the queen's role is now only formal and the House of Commons is paramount. The United Kingdom is divided into 635 constituencies, each returning one member of Parliament to the House of Commons. Since the seventeenth century, two political parties have usually been predominant. While the Tories (Conservatives) have remained, the Whigs, and to a certain extent the Liberals, have disappeared to be replaced by the Socialists (Labour) and recently by the Social Democrats. Whichever party obtains the majority of seats in the House of Commons has the right to have its leader form the government and become the prime minister. The prime minister appoints members of either the Commons or the Lords to be ministers. A minister is responsible for a government department. Leading ministers form the cabinet and, because of the party system, the initiative in government lies not in Parliament, but in the cabinet.

Ministers, the heads of government departments, are answerable to Parliament. Their departments are staffed by civil servants who are permanent officials and administer the policy of the government. These employees are nonpolitical in that they serve whichever political party forms the government. As a minister often has no previous experience of the details of the field to which he is appointed and his tenure of office may be short-lived, great responsibility falls on the shoulders of the civil servants.

Local government in England is the creation of Parliament, its structure being laid down by that body. The ancient tradition, established by the Norman Kings of England persists in the combination of local autonomy and central control that characterises the provision of public services. Local authorities are not instruments of central government: they receive substantial financial help from that parent, but they can raise further revenue locally; some of their actions require ministerial approval, but they are authorities in their own right. Local councillors are elected to local authorities, whose functions include responsibility for education (except in the universities), most personal welfare services, housing, environmental hygiene, and transport, in each case subject to some control by the central government.

HISTORICAL DEVELOPMENT OF THE HEALTH CARE SYSTEM

Health care in England can only be understood as a product of evolution, its roots reaching back into history. The first general hospital recorded in Britain was St Peter's, York, founded by the Saxon King Athelstan in the tenth century. The oldest hospital still functioning is St Bartholomew's, Rochester, which began in 1078 as a leper hospital. It was followed by St Bartholomew's, London, founded in 1124 by Rahere, the monk.

In the Middle Ages hospices for the sick were developed from guest houses provided by the monasteries, or from lazar houses in which lepers were housed. In the seventeenth century philanthropy replaced religion as the motivating force in ministering to the sick. The following century saw some private ventures running a sort of doctors' club among the well-to-do in return for an annual retention fee. In 1800 there were only 3,000 patients in hospital. Illnesses of any kind were normally endured at home.

The present-day medical profession evolved from the nineteenth century. Early in that period there were three long-established professions with different functions and social standings: apothecaries, who charged for the medicines they made, gave advice, and later became the general practitioners; surgeons, who were descended from barbers (who took care of fractures and rudimentary surgery); and an elite of university-educated physicians, who charged for advice, gave medicines, and later became the hospital specialists. These were outnumbered, however, by persons practising medicine without qualification. The Medical Act of 1858 established what is now the General Medical Council, formed primarily of doctors not chosen by the government, with the duty of registering the medical practitioners it considered suitably qualified.

By the nineteenth century hospital treatment was provided by either hospitals, voluntary or public-supported, or the Poor Law Infirmary. Voluntary hospitals provided free treatment for the poor, often through the patronage of subscribers, in part to correct some of the worst consequences of increased urbanisation caused by the industrial revolution. England became covered with small hospitals: "The pattern of provision depended upon the donations of the living and the legacies of the dead." In the early voluntary hospitals local physicians gave their services just as local benefactors gave their money. This made little demand of their time, most of the work being done by their apprentices and the apothecaries. In the nineteenth century hospitals became central to the doctors' interests, for they provided access to patients both for teaching (which earned fees) and for research; in addition, hospital appointments, while honorary, endowed the physicians with the reputation and contacts necessary for a flourishing private practice. These "honorary" hospital doctors were not under contract; consequently, the managers of many hospitals did not control the medical staff.

Despite the formal unification of the medical profession, it was divided into those elite holding hospital posts and the general practitioners. (In places where there was not enough private practice to support a full-time specialist, some general practitioners served as part-time specialists in the local hospitals). Later in the nineteenth century there were conflicts between the GPs and the hospital doctors, particularly over the retention of patients referred for consultation and the free treatment in outpatient departments of patients who could have afforded a GP. The dispute was eventually resolved by a convention that a consultant saw patients only by referral from a GP, while the consultants retained the hospital beds apart from those in small cottage hospitals outside the main urban centers. This division has had a lasting effect on health care in England.

Until the last years of the nineteenth century the state had neither the finance nor the administrative machinery to provide health care for the population in general, and there was no expectation that it should do so. Yet, despite the general assumption that health care was the individual's own responsibility, and despite a general distrust of state action and a reluctance to increase public expenditure, the state undertook both hospital provision through the Poor Law and provisions relating to lunacy and infectious diseases, which together provided more beds than the voluntary sector. The state's motive was not so much charity to the needy as the protection of society. State provision did not mean provision by the central government. Hospitals were financed and administered by existing local authorities, so government control was limited and conditions varied greatly from place to place. (The wish for greater equality became a principal motive for a National Health Service and remains a concern today).

After 1870 compulsory education made visible the health of the country's children and after 1907 there was the administrative machinery through which a school health service could be provided. In 1888 a comprehensive elected system of local government for the whole country was established for the first time. This new local government machinery began the development of what are now called the community health services.

At the turn of the century, because of, among other circumstances, unexpected difficulties of the Boer War and the realisation that the industrial lead was being taken by the United States and Germany, England was much concerned about national efficiency, physical degeneration, and the problems of poverty. Several reports published by social investigators showed the desperate "condition of the people." The Liberal government followed Germany's example and passed the National (Health) Insurance Act of 1911—originally "the National (Sickness) Insurance bill"—which covered manual workers and other workers up to a certain income but did not insure their dependents. Financed by contributions from employees, employers, and the state, it provided free care by general practitioners, free drugs for insured persons, and a maternity benefit for the wives of insured persons.

The National Insurance Act, like other arrangements for health care before and since, had to build on existing arrangements. The friendly societies and industrial insurance companies were already powerful interests and were incorporated in the arrangements as "approved societies." Each insured person had to belong to such a society, which paid the financial benefits at centrally determined standard rates. Physicians were remunerated by capitation fees for patients registered with them and could not charge fees.

The administrative and financial arrangements for general practice—established in 1911 and combined with the convention about the relationship between generalists and hospital specialists—have served to preserve general practice in England while it has declined in most other countries. The demands made by the returning casualties of World War I exposed the deficiencies of the hospital service. The case for an integrated approach to the nation's health became widely accepted, and in 1919 the ministry of health was established.

The same act that gave birth to the ministry of health had provided for the Council on Medical and Allied Services, which, under the chairmanship of Lord Dawson, produced in 1920 a report outlining a scheme of primary and secondary health centres. This report largely ignored the entire history of the development of medical care and started from first principles. It had no immediate influence, but its comprehensive thinking influenced all future discussions of the health services.

The interwar years was a period of uneven development of health care. The national insurance system came under increasing pressure, since it satisfied neither user nor provider. General practitioners in the scheme were poorly paid and users were poorly served. A Royal Commission in 1926 criticised the scheme because it did not cover enough people and included wide variations in the provision of additional benefits between societies, having, therefore, no national uniformity of service. Also, societies could reject members, so that those in most need received least protection. By 1939 health insurance covered only one-half of the population. Health care on the eve of World War II was inadequately financed, lacked coordination to provide a rational geographic distribution of facilities that were inadequate and decaying anyway, and was plagued by costly competition between voluntary and municipal hospitals. Because the war and the possible saturation bombing were expected to make heavy demands on the country's hospital services, the government created the Emergency Medical Service. The EMS took over the coordination of the hospitals, but not their management, and paid for the treatment of patients for whom the government had responsibility—broadly, civilian and military casualties and evacuees from the bombed cities. It established a national blood transfusion service and actively developed hospital laboratories. A National Public Health Laboratory Service was set up separately to help combat epidemic diseases.

The EMS brought specialists from the leading hospitals into contact with hospitals outside of the main centres, and the bad impression they gained was confirmed by official surveys carried out between 1942 and 1945. It was apparent that hospitals could not be allowed to revert to their former state of incoordinate duplication and waste after the war. In 1941 the coalition government announced its decision to create a national hospital service after the war, and in February 1943 the government made known its acceptance of the assumptions of the Beveridge Report, which included a comprehensive medical service. A white paper outlining the proposals for a health service was published in February 1944. The basic objectives stated were to ensure that everybody in the country should have "equal opportunity to benefit from the best and most up-to-date medical and allied services available, to provide—for all who wanted it—a comprehensive service covering every branch of medical and allied activity, and to divorce the care of health from questions of personal means." The services would be free to all, the costs being met by both local and central public funds.

With the advent of the Labour government in 1945 the task of building the National Health Service fell to one man, Aneurin Bevan. There was little effective opposition with one major exception: the medical profession, led by the British Medical Association, opposed details rather than the principle.* Agreement was reached, partly because the profession was itself divided and partly because Bevan made some concessions—including that general practitioners were to be independent contractors and that doctors were allowed private practice. As he said, "He stuffed their mouths with gold." Such concessions have also had a lasting effect on the NHS's finances and industrial relations.

The United States emerged from the war as the richest nation in the world, with an affluent middle class which believed in the capacity of science to alter man's destiny, including his chances of survival, and consequently encouraged the growth of specialist medical practice. By contrast, Britain emerged impoverished from the war. Not affluent, the middle class opted for a form of access to general medical practice, which had served the manual worker before the war. Their wartime experience had emphasised not so much the value of highly instrumental scientific activities as that of national unity and egalitarianism. The nation generally supported and wanted the National Health Service, which came into being in July 1948.

The NHS was an initiative supported in principle by all political parties. Proposals for it had been announced by a Conservative minister; the 1944 White Paper on a National Health Service Act was published by the coalition government. Labour Minister Bevan inherited the initiative when he became a minister in 1945. The NHS was a product of a long socio-economic process; it has been said that the structure of "the service owed more to the opinions of doctors than to political and public opinion."

Like all previous and subsequent reforms, the NHS built onto existing services. It did, however, make three important innovations: (1) that the comprehensive medical service should be available to everybody; (2) that the service was, for the most part, to be financed from general taxation with little or no charge to the user at the point of delivery; (3) that all voluntary hospitals (with certain exceptions) and all local authority hospitals were vested in the minister—that is, he "nationalised" the hospitals. (The medical profession in particular was against local authority control.) Services were to be provided in three ways: the basic primary services, the community services, and the hospital service—hence, a tripartite structure. The basic primary services were to be provided by independent contractors. The arrangements for the general medical and pharmaceutical services were in many ways a continuation of those established in 1911. The insurance committees, which had managed national health insurance locally, were replaced by executive councils with similar functions. Two services which had been only partly available were now made general: the general dental and the ophthalmic. For these two services, unlike for general practice, members of the public did not have to register with a certain practitioner but could attend any practitioner they wished. Payment was accordingly by item of service, not per caput as for the general medical service. Fees were agreed upon by the various professions, the amount depending on the numbers of patients presenting themselves and the treatments prescribed.

Community services were to be provided by local government, including the provision of maternity and child welfare services, health visitors and home nursing, vaccination and immunisation, health centres, home domestic help, chiropody, and ambulance services.

*The BMA was founded in 1832 to promote "the medical and allied sciences and to maintain the honour and interests of the medical profession." With a membership of approximately 64,000 in the United Kingdom and overseas, the association deals with all matters of a socio-political or medico-social nature and is recognised as the representative organisation of the medical profession in matters concerning their material interests.

The support services for community care were thus available to general practitioners but were not controlled by them.

The National Assistance Act of 1948 placed various welfare responsibilities on local authorities, including residential care for the elderly, the infirm, and the handicapped, and provision of meals for old people in their homes. Local authority health services were not financed from general taxation but rather in the same way as other local authority services: by rates (taxes paid by local residents) supplemented by the central government rate support grant.

The plan to reorganise the hospital and specialist services was the most far-reaching feature of the NHS. An entirely new structure was introduced for these services, which were among the most expensive parts of the NHS. The 1946 NHS Act set up regional hospital boards and required them to appoint hospital management committees to administer the hospitals on behalf of the minister. This relation of agent and principle—with the centre issuing guidance in broad policy and priorities, and health authorities carrying out the work—has remained the theme.

The "tripartite structure" of the NHS was subsequently much criticised, and, in fact, the main purpose of a later reorganisation was to unify it. The arrangements were, however, far simpler and more rational than anything that had existed before. They probably represented as much change as was acceptable at the time and, in any case, were not unreasonable, given the very different types of service provided by the three parts.

The NHS so quickly established itself as an accepted part of the country's life that it is easy to overlook what a new departure it was. Whereas in other countries (such as the United States) it is believed that the government should not undertake the production of goods and services that can be viably produced for profit, that belief in private enterprise ideology had long been breached in Britain. That was not the innovation. The innovation was that for the first time the central government took direct responsibility for a type of service which had previously been administered by local authorities or by ad hoc bodies. The extent of the new departure was disguised by the fact that the new hospital service was not administered directly by the civil service but by committees of voluntary members in the usual British fashion. Hospital authorities, however, unlike local authorities, were agents of the ministers and were without power to raise their own revenue.

The establishment of a national service had a number of consequences, particularly from the hospital service, which continue to this day. First, because of government financing, the government had to decide what should be spent on the service. Second, the new service became one of the largest employers in the country. National financing brought national salary scales, and the obvious model for negotiation was the existing civil service system of Whitley councils. As with finance, the deeper consequences of being a very large employer were appreciated only gradually. All staff groups have their interests and influences, and there may be a touch of truth in the cynical view that the service existed for the sake of the staff. Third, the central department for its part had little experience in the type of work it now had to undertake. Existing civil service practices, such as the use of circulars, were available but were not enough. For advice on difficult or contentious matters, ministers looked to committees with some or most members drawn from the service. For day-to-day advice, the department assembled professional staffs, their members drawn from most of the professions working in the service. The other approach was, finally, regular meetings between ministers, civil servants, chairmen, and senior officers of hospital authorities.

In 1948 the administration of the English hospital service was divided into fourteen regions, which were responsible to the minister of health for planning and policy. Hospitals within each region were grouped and administered by hospital management committees (about 330 in all), most of which found themselves in charge of a number of hospitals that had previously been managed independently or as parts of local government systems. It was only gradually that they came to think of and organise their services as a group rather than as individual units. With this change came (1) an increase in the number of group rather than individual hospital management posts, (2) the development of functional management, and (3) fundamental change in nursing organisation. Following the recommendations of a report in 1966, nursing services, hitherto the responsibility of the matron of each hospital, were organised on a group basis under a chief nursing officer.

During the 1960s there was much criticism of the tripartite structure. In many spheres the functions of the district organisations were interdependent, if not actually overlapping. For example, the maternity services—the hospital authorities, the local health authority, and the family doctor service—all had responsibilities for the care of mothers and their babies, and yet the three services were each concerned with different local populations; they were separately financed, separately planned, and developed according to different assessments of priorities. Many locales had informal arrangements, but there was no single authority responsible for providing the population of a given area with the right combination of comprehensive health services. There was a lack of continuity of care. The difficulties were felt particularly in the care of psychiatric and geriatric patients (where several scandals were uncovered), as value was increasingly put on short inpatient care and the return of the patient to the community wherever possible. The solution, it was argued, was a unified rather than a tripartite service.

After a preliminary discussion paper issued in 1968, a new secretary of state for social services, who was responsible for the Department of Health and Social Security (formed in 1968 by the merger of the ministry of health and the ministry of social security), issued proposals in 1970 for a unified administrative structure, taking into account the government's intention to reorganise local government. Functions were reallocated between health and local government authorities, so that all social workers would be employed by local government and all medical and nursing staff by health authorities. Local government also retained responsibility for other personal social services, such as home domestic help and home meal deliveries. The secretary of state proposed ninety area health authorities to match the new local government units to improve collaboration. Each area was responsible for every aspect of planning and administration of a comprehensive health service for its population. The number of areas was too great to relate to the central Department of Health, so the need for a regional tier remained to coordinate and plan. Areas too large to manage were divided into districts (about 200) In view of the complexity of the NHS and the diversity of its staff, each level was to be managed by a multi-disciplinary management team. The emphasis was on effective management and on the attempt to make the NHS more responsive to public policy, with "maximum delegation downwards matched by accountability upwards."

Community health councils were established to represent the public and separate the management of the health service from representation of its users. Because of the way in which the NHS is financed, those who spend money within the service have no responsibility for raising it. Some have suggested that the greater emphasis on managerial qualities in the final plan has rendered the Treasury more willing to allow the NHS greater financial flexibility after 1974.

The reorganised National Health Service came into operation on 1 April 1974. The reorganisation exposed inequalities, an imbalance between services, and opportunities for change and redeployment of resources that were obscured by the old structure, from which later initiatives on resource allocation and planning sprang; the timing, however, could not have been worse, for the economy and, in turn, public expenditures were being battered by the oil crisis. Some of the problems which occurred, however, were intrinsic to reorganisation. The upheaval involved was considerable and every health service was affected; therefore, disenchantment was not long delayed. Until 1973 the service had had very little experience with strikes and other industrial action; from then on these actions became fairly common and sometimes serious. While the somewhat more distant, larger-scale management might have increased the problems of personnel relations, this new development was mainly due to discontentment over pay and conditions of service and also to action against the treatment of private patients in NHS hospitals. Spokesmen for the medical profession called for the appointment of a Royal Commission on the NHS, which, they thought, would support both their criticisms of the reorganised structure and their belief that the service was seriously underfinanced. In 1976 a Royal Commission was indeed appointed, "to consider in the interests both of the patients and of those who work in the national health service the best use and management of the financial and manpower resources of the national health service."

Reporting in 1979, the Royal Commission proposed no great changes and concluded that, although it had shortcomings, there was little shameful in the NHS and much to be proud of. Soon after publication of the commission's report, the new Conservative government responded by rejecting many of the Commission's proposals, such as direct accountability of the regional health authority to Parliament and abolition of the family practitioner committees. However, the government did accept the Commission's criticisms of the NHS regarding excessive bureaucracy and failure to take quick decisions and agreed upon its proposals to simplify the structure by removal of area tier and substitution of multi-district areas by single districts, each accountable to their own authorities. The government also proposed to strengthen local management by creating several "units" within a district, each responsible for services to a client group (say, psychiatry) or for a major hospital. The separate units would be managed by an administrator and a nurse with help from a medical representative. Staff in the "support functions" (catering, cleaning, etc.) would report to the unit administrator, not as before to a district functional manager. These reorganisations reflect the problem faced by any organisation, but particularly by such a diffuse and complicated one as the NHS, of how to use the managerial talent available. The rationale of the 1974 reorganisation was to create units to provide comprehensive care that required experienced NHS managers to be moved away from hospital-based patient care duties and become planners and coordinators. There was a reaction to this after 1974 because the administrators at the hospital level were too junior and inexperienced to cope. The 1982 reorganisation was an attempt to reverse the balance somewhat and provide greater administrative talent at the hospital level. Therefore, the NHS is now managed through 14 regional and 192 district health authorities (figure 1 shows its structure).

THE NHS: ORGANISATION AND STRUCTURE

Patterns of health care provision in England today differ considerably between different localities, according to their resources, the facilities they have inherited, and the needs of

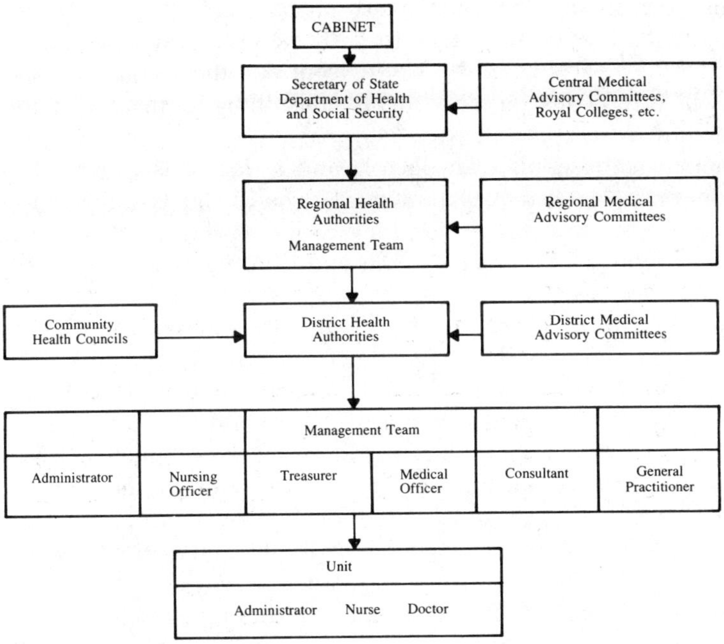

Figure 1 Structure of the NHS

the population as they see them. However, the basic types of service provided by the National Health Service are the same.

Primary Care Services

The aims of the primary care services are (1) to promote good health, both physical and mental, and improve health through education and early detection; (2) to provide treatment or advice; (3) to refer to the specialist services for examination, diagnosis, and treatment those patients who need it and to continue care after advice is obtained from specialists in outpatient departments; (4) to provide treatment and support to patients after their discharge from the hospital.

Primary care services consist of the general medical service, the primary health care teams, the general dental service, and the pharmaceutical, ophthalmic, and chiropody services.

The General Medical Service

The general practitioner as family doctor distinguishes the NHS from health care organisations in most other countries. Few other health care systems (with the possible exception of Denmark's) have a GP service as closely integrated with community support services, as extensive, and as crucial as that of the NHS. The GP is an independent practitioner under contract with the family practitioner committee (FPC) to provide services, practising sometimes alone but mostly in partnership or in group practice; he is normally the patient's first point of contact with the NHS. He acts as a gateway between the patient and other parts of the NHS (except for the dental, optical, and accident services). He will attend his patients in his consulting room and in their homes, and sometimes in a clinic or a hospital.

Each person may choose his own doctor, and a doctor is free to decide whether to accept a person onto his list as a patient. However, he is obliged to give necessary treatment to any person applying to him for treatment who is not on another doctor's list or who needs emergency treatment. Of the entire population, 97% is registered on the NHS lists of family doctors.

It is estimated that three out of four people who feel ill deal with it themselves, but of those who seek help from the NHS, GPs care for about 90% unaided. They deal with all illnesses, both physical and mental. It is only recently that the Royal College of General Practitioners has explicitly defined a comprehensive approach to the physical, psychological, and social aspects of patients' illnesses. Many people expect such service from their GP, but this is not always reflected in his attitude, nor in the way in which general practice is run. Sympathetic personal attention is time consuming, and some patients complain that their GPs do not give them enough time and explanation, and also that it is sometimes difficult to see their GP when they want to. Patients may find it hard to have a genuine dialogue with their GP. The average consultation lasts six minutes, and four out of five patients receive a prescription, of which one in five is not presented for dispensing. On the other hand, a minority of patients do overuse the service, attending for minor ailments that should be coped with privately.

Family doctors are remunerated through a combination of allowances, capitation fees, and fees for item of service. The GP can render maternity services, and will receive an additional fee for them, either independently or in cooperation with a hospital obstetric department; he also can offer to patients free family planning guidance and supplies. An additional fee is payable for certain family planning services. If a second opinion is required from a specialist in a particular field, the GP may refer his patient to the specialist, who is usually at a hospital though the GP can ask a specialist to visit the patient at home. Some X-rays and pathological tests are in some places directly available to the family doctor.

GPs are not employees of the NHS; they contract with family practitioner committees to provide all necessary and appropriate services within the scope of general practice to patients registered with them. There are variations within this contract; for example, not all GPs provide maternity services. They have considerable freedom to choose their own premises, methods of work, and availability. They may practise privately or may hold part-time hospital or other appointments within the NHS, such as working in industry or for an insurance company. It is also open to a GP to arrange for a locum tenens, or deputy, to stand in for him when he is sick or on holiday or when he chooses not to be available; however, the responsibility for his patients remains with him, except where a deputy is on the same FPC list.

Most GPs contract to provide a 24-hour service, although such availability would be rare. They cover for each other and may be on call only one or two nights during the week. Moreover, the use of commercially organised deputising services has grown rapidly over the last ten years: about one-third of all GPs now employ them at least occasionally. In large cities the proportion is much higher. Public concern over the use and quality of such deputising services has recently grown.

The use of appointment systems in general practice has increased substantially over the last fifteen years. One study suggests that the GPs of three-fourths of all patients surveyed used them, yet, in spite of this, surgery waiting times have not declined substantially. Continuity of care is a key concept for general practice, but may simply not exist in many large cities. A study on access to primary health care suggests that in one year 15% of the people had occasion to use (or to take their children to) the accident and emergency departments of large hospitals rather than consult their GP.

There has been an increase in the number of GPs in the last ten years; the average list size has been falling (2,250 in 1980), as have the number of home visits. Because GPs are free to select and reject patients, they can, for the most part, adjust the size of their lists to suit themselves and there is considerable variation in list size.

Although there have been great improvements in the last ten years following the "GPs Charter" in 1966 (which gave the GPs better conditions of service) and although the new generation of GPs have a higher level of motivation, the quality of care provided by a minority of GPs is poor. There are three main reasons for this: (1) GP training is not always adequate, but is slowly improving; (2) there is no mechanism for setting national standards in the selection of principals in general practice; (3), GPs are often isolated and they lack the close contact with professional colleagues available to those who work in hospitals. In some places, forms of audit of GP services have already been introduced or are under consideration. Better record keeping, systematic self-criticism, and inspection of training practices should lead to improvements in standards.

In 1977–78 the total cost of drugs, dressings, and appliances prescribed by GPs in the United Kingdom was £539.5m, which was more than the salary cost of the general practitioners. The cost of all other prescriptions was about £127m, most of which was incurred in hospitals. The bulk of the £539.5m went for drugs. The GPs are subjected to massive pressure from the drug companies. There is one drug company salesman for every five GPs, and one-tenth of the NHS drug bill is spent by the drug companies on promotions. From time to time, health ministers have exhorted the public not to request medicines for which a prescription is unnecessary, but most of the effort in keeping the GP drug bill down is directed at the GPs themselves. GP's prescribing is monitored, but subsequent comment reaches the individual GP very slowly.

Primary Health Care Teams

The role in the primary health care service played by health visitors, district nurses, and midwives is helped by the integration of these health authority-employed staff into primary health care teams, where they work in partnership with general practitioners. In a few places the multi-disciplinary team extends to include dentists, chiropodists, and local authority-employed social workers. The first step towards the formation of primary health care teams is the attachment of district nurses and midwives to general practice, which means that they work with the patients on the list of that practice. About 25% of general practitioners now practice from health centres designed to accommodate the full primary care team, and many others work from premises adapted or purposely built for team working. The concept of the integrated team remains an objective rather than a fully developed aspect of the National Health Service, for many health visitors are not yet fully integrated into general practice.

There has been a rapid expansion of the health centre programme in recent years, from 212 in 1972 to 950 health centres in 1981 with more than 200 planned for the future. However, there is evidence that health centres are by no means universally popular with the GPs or their patients. The increase in the number of health centres has been less rapid in the conurbations, where they are most often needed, and is slowing down in places where there are already high concentrations of centres.

The General Dental Service (GDS)

Like family doctors, general dental practitioners are contracted independently to provide, or to arrange provision, for their patients all the treatment needed to ensure a reasonable standard of dental efficiency and oral health. General dental practitioners are remunerated by the FPC mainly by fees for item of service and not per capita as for medical services. Since the mid-1960s the amount of treatment provided by the GDS has increased by 3% per year. Within this increasing volume there has been a shift away from extracting teeth and providing dentures and towards tooth conservation and periodental treatment. However, emergency dental services are not readily available in many areas.

The Pharmaceutical Services

Everyone using the services of a family doctor under the NHS is entitled to the supply of medicines and certain appliances prescribed by his doctor. Almost all chemists dispense medicines and appliances under the NHS. These chemists and appliance suppliers, who enter into arrangements with their FPC to provide pharmaceutical services, are independent contractors and cannot be compelled to provide dispensing facilities in any particular place. In 1982 patients were charged £1.30 per item supplied, with the exceptions of certain surgical appliances for which the charge was higher and of items for conditions requiring continuous treatment, for which there was no charge. There are exemptions from charges for certain groups such as the elderly, the young, the poor, and pregnant women. In 1980, 67% of prescriptions were dispensed free.

Ophthalmic Services

Eye problems may be dealt with under the NHS by hospitals or in the general ophthalmic services (GOS). The GOS provides sight testing and replacement and repair of spectacles. Opticians, like pharmacists, derive part of their income from NHS work, but perhaps three-fourths of their profits come from other activities, including private practice.

Chiropody (Podiatry) Services

Like pharmacists and opticians, chiropodists engage partly in NHS work, partly in private practice. Access to a chiropodist is normally by referral of a GP; however, while the NHS aims to provide pharmaceutical and ophthalmic services to all who need them, chiropody service is restricted to priority groups, like the elderly.

Hospital Services

Hospital services are responsible for around 10% of patient contacts but account for about 70% of total NHS expenditures. Hospitals provide the specialist elements of health care that are beyond the scope of primary care services. Hospital services include the main specialities, internal medicine and surgery, and their various branches: obstetrics and gynaecology, paediatrics, psychiatry, geriatric medicine, mental handicap, accident and emergency services, and the clinical support services (radiology, pathology, etc.). Services may be provided on an inpatient (both long and short stay), outpatient, or day-patient basis, according to the severity of the illness concerned. Hospital clinical services are supported by the "hotel" services (e.g. catering, domestic, and laundry services).

Except in an emergency, access to the specialist services is normally obtained through the patient's family doctor or dentist. Clinics for sexually transmitted diseases, "special clinics," do not require a GP referral. Compulsory hospital admission is sometimes, though rarely, necessary, perhaps under the Mental Health acts, or the Public Health Act for notifiably infectious diseases, or the National Assistance Act, for chronic incapacity to manage at home. Admission to mental handicap hospitals is often in consultation with the social services department of the local authority; otherwise, patients are referred to hospitals by their family doctors. The hospital consultant will normally see the patient in the outpatient clinic before admitting him to hospital. Only 20% of outpatients become inpatients.

In 1948 the NHS inherited a heterogeneous collection of some 2,400 local authority and voluntary hospitals with about 428,000 beds. Approximately 45% of the buildings were erected before 1891 and 21% before 1861. In the early years of the NHS there was little money available for hospital building, and, despite a substantial capital programme since around 1962, a large proportion of floor space is still in accommodation built before 1919. The aim has been to achieve a more rational system, in addition to correcting the worst local deficiencies and adjusting to changes in medical knowledge and practice and development of supporting skills.

The policy that has evolved since 1948 is to build up a network of district general hospitals providing for the entire district population both a full range of specialised treatment for acute specialties and the necessary diagnostic and supporting facilities. Some specialties (such as cardiac and neurosurgery) are concentrated at one or two hospitals and serve the population of a region. The objective has been to create a network of about 250 district general hospitals with associated community hospitals where appropriate and annexes for long-stay care. A reduction in the capital programme since 1973–74 has contributed towards a shift in policy away from "whole hospital" schemes involving the comprehensive development of district general hospitals on single sites and towards better integration of existing facilities.

In 1980 there were about 2,000 hospitals, ranging from the large psychiatric hospital with over 1,000 beds and about 800 staff, drawing its patients from a wide area, to the cottage or general practitioner hospital with under 50 beds and a handful of full-time staff providing local service to a small community. The total number of hospital beds is about 360,000, of which 80% are occupied on any one day. Outpatient and accident and emergency departments serve some 130,000 patients daily.

Waiting lists in general, and the size of waiting lists in particular, attract a good deal of attention in Parliament and in the press. However, the number of people recorded as waiting for hospital admission is not by itself a useful figure because it does not by itself indicate how long people must wait for hospital treatment, especially treatment which they require urgently. In addition, interest tends to focus on inpatient admissions, while the waiting period for an outpatient appointment may be just as or even more significant. Also, waiting lists are one mechanism for controlling access to services free at the time of use. The patient who becomes acutely ill is well cared for by the NHS. Generally, the acute hospital services provide excellent and rapid treatment of urgent cases. Problems are greatest for nonurgent cases where the longest waiting lists and waiting times are, in the main, for inpatient surgery; and within surgery, for orthopaedics and for some of the commonest operations, for example, tonsillectomy, hernia repair, and cataract removal.

Waiting times are affected by strikes, longer holidays, and shorter working hours for staff. Shortages of theatre staff, particularly anaesthetists and trained nurses, and theatre facilities are among the causes of long waits. A survey found that 45% of all inpatient admissions took place within one month of the patient's enter onto the waiting list, but 6% had to wait more than one year. The Royal Commission on the Health Service questioned patients about their attitude toward the NHS but did not hear a great deal about waiting lists; their survey found that most patients were not greatly distressed by waiting for their admissions. The distress caused by waiting lists has been exaggerated, partly for political reasons, but may be real enough for some patients, like those needing hip replacement or removal of cataracts. The scope for increasing the amount of day surgery is, however, considerable.

The number of new outpatients has remained relatively stable in recent times, but there has been a considerable growth in the number of day patients, normally for minor surgery or investigation, who do not stay in hospital overnight.

Most patients are satisfied with the treatment they receive in NHS hospitals, as they are with other parts of the service, but two complaints have been both frequent and long-standing. (1) Patients are not given enough information about their treatment, and (2) despite continuous protests, they sometimes still feel ignored when doctors discuss their problems with colleagues. Also, some hospital staff persist in waking patients very early.

While the replacement of old hospital buildings has been disappointing, expansion of hospital activity—despite a decline in the total number of beds—has been dramatic. There have been big increases in staff, although the increases have not been proportionate among all staff groups, and the intensity of labor has allowed a much greater throughput of patients: the number of inpatients has risen from 2.8 million in 1949–50 to 5.5 million in 1980.

Special Boards and Committees

There are a number of other advisory and executive agencies that perform specific specialised functions.

The Public Health Laboratory Service Board

Originally established to provide surveillance and control of infective diseases, the Public Health Laboratory Service is principally concerned with the monitoring of microbial disease. It performs specialist diagnostic services for hospitals, general practitioners, and environmental health officers from its fifty-four laboratories; provides specialist diagnostic facilities in its hospital laboratories; and produces the weekly communicable disease report. Other functions of the PHLS include the provision of a quality-control service for microbiology, and research and development in both epidemiology and technology.

The Medical Practices Committee

The Medical Practices Committee is responsible for the distribution of GP practices; it attempts to achieve a more equitable arrangement by stopping NHS doctors from practising in districts that are already well served.

The Prescription Pricing Authority

The Prescription Pricing Authority prices prescriptions and calculates the amounts due to chemists and dispensing doctors.

The Dental Estimates Board

The Dental Estimates Board considers dental estimate forms for prior approval of treatment or for approval of payment.

The Health Advisory Service

The Health Advisory Service (originally the Hospital Advisory Service) was established in 1969 after the public showed concern over conditions in a number of long-stay hospitals. The remit of the Hospital Advisory Service was originally confined to long-stay hospitals (which in Britain undertake many of the functions of nursing homes), but in 1976 the HAS was renamed the Health Advisory Service and its remit was extended to cover related community services, including those provided in collaboration with local authorities. The services consist of a director, who reports directly to the secretary of state, together with teams of doctors, nurses, administrators, and other staff who are seconded to work with the service from the NHS and who visit and evaluate mental illness, geriatric, and mental handicap services. The HAS is, in a sense, an inspectorate for long-term care services, although in its style of operations it stresses advisory rather than inspectorial functions.

The Development Team for the Mentally Handicapped

In 1975 the secretary of state for social services set up the National Development Group for the Mentally Handicapped, which subsequently prepared a series of reports covering a wide range of health and personal social services for mentally handicapped people. At the end of 1979 it was announced that the group would be withdrawn, but the Development Team for the Mentally Handicapped, which had been associated with the group, would continue.

The team consists of a director and three associate directors assisted by a panel of specialists in psychiatry, paediatrics, administration, nursing, psychology, social services, etc. It offers advice and assistance to individual health and social services authorities on the planning and operation of services in their locality. It visits authorities either by their invitation or by decision of the secretary of state.

The Medical Research Council

The Medical Research Council is outside the NHS but collaborates with it and has far-reaching influence on its activities. Incorporated under royal charter in 1920, the council is responsible to the secretary of state for education and science. Its objective is to promote research into all aspects of health and disease. The MRC conducts research in its own establishments and supports researchers in universities and elsewhere by long-term and short-term grants for specific programmes or projects.

Management of Health Care at the National Level

The NHS is the responsibility of a government minister, the secretary of state for social services, who is a member of the cabinet and is responsible for health and personal social services and for social security. He is supported by ministers of state and parliamentary under-secretaries whose number, titles, and responsibilities vary with governments; his duty is "to promote a comprehensive health service designed to secure improvement (a) in the physical and mental health of the people and (b) in the prevention, diagnosis, and treatment of illness, and for that purpose to provide or secure the effective provision of services." He or she has specific duties to provide some services, duties qualified by the phrase "to such extent as he considers necessary to meet all reasonable requirements."

The secretary of state's responsibilities are for providing services and facilities, not for providing diagnosis and treatment. This reflects the view taken from the outset that it was for the patients' doctors (or other professionals with clinical responsibility) and not the minister to decide what treatment was appropriate. The principal function of the Department of Health and Social Security in relation to the NHS, is to assist ministers in providing central leadership in the health and social services, to advise them on choices about the nature and scale of the NHS, and to take decisions on the development of national policies, objectives, and priorities. Much of the work of the central department, particularly that performed by the most senior staff ("the top of the office") is concerned with supporting and advising ministers in relation to government policy on health matters and on health service development. A major preoccupation is supporting the minister in his relations with Parliament and, in particular, handling parliamentary questions and enquiries from members of Parliament. Although ministers have a permanent civil service to advise them, they sometimes appoint for special subjects further political advisers drawn from outside civil service.

The main division of the DHSS's functions into groups indicates the activities that it undertakes: regional activities, services development, NHS personnel activities, and finance and support services. These divisions work with three large professional sectors: medical, nursing, and works.

The National Health Service is funded by "votes" approved by Parliament. For each parliamentary vote, one specified individual is personally responsible, and that responsibility cannot be delegated. For the health and personal social services "votes," the senior civil servant, the first permanent secretary of the DHSS, is the accounting officer personally accountable to Parliament and can personally be surcharged for the misapplication of funds. The effect of the accountability principle on the NHS and the central department is considerable. The parliamentary watchdog over this principle is the Committee of Public Accounts and its agent, the comptroller and auditor-general. Accounting officers have to appear personally before this committee to account for their vote and for any irregularities—any apparent misuse of funds or any waste recorded in the report of the comptroller and auditor-general. Consequently, much detailed work is undertaken to brief the permanent secretary for his appearances before the Committee of Public Accounts. In 1979 the House of Commons established the Select Committee on Social Services to monitor these services.

The health and personal social services (HPSS) side of the DHSS is responsible for government functions relating to the National Health Service, general health matters, and personal social services. The total staff engaged on these functions is approximately 9,300, about 3,000 of which are involved in the direct provision of services in the special hospitals and artificial limb and appliance centres, the remainder in central administration.

These staff are civil servants, including doctors and nurses employed directly by the Crown. Occasionaly, staff are seconded from the NHS to the central departments, or from the central departments to the NHS, but the administrative workers of the central department are essentially part of the central civil service machinery and are liable to be transferred to other departments of state.

Personal social services (PSS) are administered by 108 local authorities who are answerable to their electorates. They must, however, under statute, act according to the "general guidance" of the secretary of state. These services are paid for partly by rates (locally raised taxes) but mostly by money from the central government through the rate support grant. The rate support grant does not provide the Department with direct financial control.

In broad terms, the major tasks of the DHSS are to formulate policies in relation to the general health and welfare of the nation: to assess needs, balance needs with resources, and determine priorities. In translating these central tasks in terms of the NHS, the Department not only issues general guidance based on the policies determined by the secretary of state and the government, but it also allocates funds, monitors the use of those funds, and is accountable for them in Parliament.

Ministers have ultimate power to direct health authorities but are loathe to use this power; they can remove authority members but have only done so when confronted with outright refusal to accept a direction. Much work of the Department is in the form of policy statements, or guidance, to authorities. It would be a mistake to assume that the policy or guidance was always translated into action, for there have been matters on which ministers have found it difficult to persuade authorities and their staffs to follow the spirit or even the letter of national policies (such as the central government's wish to establish "secure units" for dangerous mental patients, which has been frustrated).

There has been considerable criticism about the extent to which the central department has involved itself in matters concerning the management of the hospital service. The involvement was not unnatural given the national character of the service, the wide powers placed on ministers, the pressure on the departments by all bodies interested in changing the service or in preserving pieces of it, and, not least, the fact that the service is centrally financed, so that governments had a strong incentive to direct and control the activities of hospital authorities. Nevertheless, ministers and the central departments, no less than the members of staff of hospital authorities, deplored the tendency for decision making to move upwards, and various schemes have been proposed to stress the importance of keeping as much decision making as possible at the local level.

NHS Management: Regional and District Levels

Apart from a relatively small range of centrally provided services, the secretary of state's responsibilities are delegated to the National Health Service, composed in England of 14 regional and 192 district health authorities. Regional populations vary between 1.8 million and 5.1 million; district populations are from less than 100,000 to more than 800,000. This highlights one of the problems of the NHS: can any structure be designed which is generally applicable to such large variations in population and need?

Regional health authorities (RHAs) are responsible for strategic planning and resource allocation for their regions, while the district health authorities (DHAs) have operational responsibility. The RHAs also provide certain specialised services that can be more rationally or economically organised on a regional basis. Health authorities, corporate bodies with appointed members, appoint a management team, known as the regional, or district, team of officers. This team comprises an administrator, a medical officer, a nursing officer, a treasurer, and, for the region, a works officer. While the work of most members of the team is self-evident, that of the medical officer may not be clear. He is a community physician who "tries to measure and predict the health care needs of the population, and plan and administer services to meet those needs." At the district level the team is supplemented by a consultant and a general practitioner elected by their colleagues (see figure 1 above). The team is jointly accountable to its authority for advising the authority and carrying out on its behalf its directions. This joint accountability means that members of the team must arrive at decisions by consensus—that "no decision can be taken by the team which overrides the opposition of a member." Decisions not agreed upon by the team are referred to the health authority for resolution. In practice the power of veto is rarely exercised and the consensus approach amounts to "having one's say and not one's nay." Each appointed member of the team is individually accountable to the authority for the management of staff and for the performance of specific functions in his or her own professional field. The consultant and GP members are answerable to their electorates.

The structure of the NHS has certain key features: (1) It is population based; regions and districts have defined geographical boundaries, although these boundaries are not rigid barriers to the movement of patients for treatment. (2) It is a national and nationally financed service, organised hierarchically with ultimate accountability to the central government. (3) Local management is the responsibility of appointed corporate bodies (health authorities), separate from the elected local government authorities. (4) Day-to-day running of both regional and district levels is in the hands of management teams. (5) Public representation is separated from responsibility for management of the service and is the responsibility of district-based community health councils (CHCs), specially established for the purpose. The NHS is structured to enable comprehensive health services to be planned, organised, and operated in a manner consistent with both the secretary of state's accountability to Parliament and the need for the local management of the services. The secretary of state directs regional and district health authorities to perform his functions; nevertheless, the secretary of state retains some important powers and places some restrictions upon the freedom of health authorities in the exercise of their delegated functions. Therefore, each health authority is free to decide whom it will employ, but no authority may pay more or less than the rates of pay agreed upon by national negotiating machinery.

Regional health authorities are also empowered to issue directions to district health authorities. Health authorities are required to ensure that their annual expenditure does not exceed the amounts allotted to them. The principle functions of an RHA are—in consultation with DHAs—formulation within national guidelines of regional strategic plans, allocation of resources to DHAs, and monitor of the performance of DHAs in achieving agreed upon plans. The planning of some medical services is done on a regional basis because individual districts are not large enough to be self-sufficient for all services. In addition, RHAs have some direct executive functions which are better exercised on a scale larger than that of the average health authority. The most important of these are the design and construction of major new building works, the operation of the blood transfusion service, and in the case of six regions, the management of an ambulance service for the metropolitan counties within their region.

The secretary of state appoints chairmen and members of regional authorities and chairmen of district health authorities. The RHA appoints DHA members except for the chairmen and members who are appointed directly by the local authority. Individual RHAs are responsible for establishing community health councils within their regions and appoint one-sixth of their membership, the remaining five-sixths being appointed by the local authorities and voluntary organisations.

Public Participation in the NHS

There has been some means for public participation and control of the National Health Service since its inception in 1948. At the broadest level it is provided by the statutory powers and duties of the secretary of state, who is accountable to Parliament and ultimately to the electorate. Lay participation in the day-to-day management of the service is provided by the membership of health authorities and public participation more directly through the community health councils.

Community health councils (CHCs) were introduced in each district as part of the 1974 NHS reorganisation to represent the interests in the Health Service of the people in the districts. CHCs do not have executive functions, but they do have statutory rights—to acquire information, to visit health premises, and to be consulted on substantial changes in the local health services. The DHA must meet the CHC at least once a year. DHAs are required to comment on the annual reports of the CHCs, and both the CHC report and the DHAs comments on it must be published. CHCs also have a special role in relation to closures or changes of use of health buildings. If the council accepts a proposed closure or change of use, the health authority no longer needs to seek the secretary of state's approval.

Many other volunteers make a variety of contributions to the NHS that are complementary to the services of the paid staff. They provide the additional comforts, the amenities, the companionship, and the contact with the outside world which the paid staff may not have time to provide, such as hospital libraries, shops, canteens, and visits. They are particularly valuable in long-stay hospitals where the need for voluntary effort is especially great; however, larger efforts are needed to attract volunteers.

Complaints Procedures

There about 200 million contacts between GPs and their patients each year and a similar number of contacts between patients and dental, pharmaceutical, and ophthalmic services. In 1978, 1,253 complaints filed about these services got as far as a hearing. (All GPs and hospital doctors are required by their contracts to belong to a protection organisation, which provides doctors with indemnification for compensation claims involved in negligence cases. The typical doctor's fee for these organisations is about £135 per annum in 1983.) A complaint is made in writing to the FPC. Where it cannot be resolved informally, it is referred to the appropriate FPC committee. A breach of contract has been found in just under one-third of the cases brought.

In 1982 there were about 15,000 written complaints resulting from hospital treatment (less than .1% of inpatient admissions). No statutory procedure is laid down for complaints about hospital services, but the DHSS has published guidance for health authorities on handling complaints. Generally, oral complaints by members of the public which cannot be dealt with on the spot to the complainant's satisfaction are recorded and a senior member of the staff takes action. If a complainant remains dissatisfied, he must be advised of his right to go to the commissioner of the Health Service Commission.

The Parliamentary Commission for Administration (PCA) can investigate any action taken by or on behalf of the health departments in the exercise of their administrative functions if a complaint by a member of the public is referred to the commissioner by a member of Parliament and the complainant claims to have sustained injustice in consequence of maladministration. However, the PCA has no power to investigate actions taken by health authorities; this is the function of the Health Service Commission (HSC), which can investigate a complaint by a member of the public if the complainant claims to have suffered injustice or hardship because of a failure in a service, or a failure to provide a service, or maladministration.

The commissioner cannot investigate the actions of family practitioners or actions taken solely in the exercise of clinical judgement. The commissioner must make an annual report to the secretary of state and may make other reports as well. The secretary of state is required to lay each report before the House of Parliament. The Select Committee on the Parliamentary Commission for Administration examines the commissioner's reports. The commissioner of the HSC received some 700 complaints in 1982, although only about 100 were within his terms of reference, and upheld just over one-third of these. There is now provision, outside of legal proceedings, for the independent review of complaints about the exercise of clinical judgment. A complaint that involves the exercise of clinical judgement by a hospital doctor and that does not seem likely to lead to litigation may be reviewed by two independent doctors. This is an important innovation, because doctors have now accepted responsibility for assessing the clinical actions of their colleagues.

The secretary of state has statutory powers to set up an inquiry into any matter arising under the NHS acts. These powers are normally used only when serious incidents or shortcomings in the NHS give rise to national concern. The NHS is not, of course, the exclusive provider of personal health services; care is also provided by a variety of other agencies, public and private. In addition to the possibilities already mentioned, patients may have recourse to use one of the practitioners of "fringe medicine." Someone feeling ill has a range of alternatives to the NHS, extending from taking patent medicines to admission to a private hospital.

PRIVATE MEDICINE

Private medical practice in England is small but arouses considerable controversy. It is estimated that expenditure on hospital-based private health care in 1980 was between £300 and £350 million and that the private sector treats about 300,000 inpatients annually, or 6.5% of the total. Private health care is divided between health care provided in private beds in NHS hospitals and health care provided in the independent sector in private hospitals and nursing homes. The independent sector exists in competition, or at least in parallel with the NHS, though the image is misleading: the independent sector is as much intertwined with as alongside the NHS. There are private beds in NHS hospitals, while many of the small voluntary hospitals treat NHS patients—mainly the elderly and the mentally handicapped (but also special groups with epilepsy, drug, or alcohol problems) under contractual arrangements with health authorities.

Private Practice Within the NHS

The NHS Act of 1946 empowered the minister of health to set aside NHS hospital accommodation for private patients and to allow the medical staff of NHS hospitals to treat private patients and charge for their professional services (university teaching staff generally surrender their fees to the medical school, which uses the proceeds for medical research and development). Any person admitted as a private patient is required to pay the full cost of accommodation and services provided by the hospital authority. The doctor's fees are a private matter between doctor and patient.

In 1949 the number of authorised pay beds in NHS hospitals in England was about 6,400 out of a total 428,000 beds in NHS hospitals. By 1979 the number had declined to 2,400 and represented less than 1% of all beds. Despite these changes, the number of private inpatients increased steadily from 78,000 in 1950 to 113,000 in 1974; in 1979 there was a drop to 91,000. The average length of stay of private patients decreased from 14.5 days in 1953 to 6 days in 1979. While NHS patients may not have comparable domestic circumstances, it is noteworthy that patients who pay for their treatment seem to spend less time in hospitals than do comparable NHS patients.

In 1971–72 the House of Commons Expenditure Committee investigated the National Health Service's facilities for private patients. The Committee's report was not unanimous, though the majority favoured the continuation of private practice within the NHS. Although the Conservative government of the day accepted the majority report, the Labour government of 1974 started to phase out the pay beds and to separate private medical practice from NHS hospitals. The Conservative government elected in 1979 stopped the phasing out and now wishes to "facilitate the use of private medical care."

Private Practice Outside the NHS

In 1948 the independent sector comprised the old, established institutions left out of the NHS. Since then a number of developments have been seen, possibly the most important of which has been the appearance and growth of provident schemes (BUPA, the Private Patient Plan, and the Western Provident Association). Their expansion has enabled an increasing number of people to pay for private medical care, mainly through employment groups.

Some expansion of private hospital beds took place in the 1970s, mainly but not exclusively in London. For a long time that city has had a number of hospitals, not all operating for profit, where private patients are treated. More recently a number of new hospitals have been established, operated by limited companies for profit and catering mainly to patients from overseas, particularly the Middle East. (A quite different development has been the provision of hospices for the terminally ill. While hospices are not a new idea, the need for more attention to the care of the dying has been appreciated in recent years.) The Abortion Act of 1967 placed a new demand on the independent sector. Nearly one-half of the 130,000 abortions performed on women residents in England—as well as practically all on nonresident women—are performed in private clinics and nursing homes.

Determining the scale, and nature, of private practice is far from easy. There are no routinely collected statistics. In 1977 there were 1,110 registered nursing homes with 30,400 beds, mainly for long-term care. The majority of the beds in registered private nursing homes are used for nonacute treatment, for example, care of chronically sick or elderly patients, convalescence, or rehabilitation. Health authorities can make contractual arrangements for NHS patients to be treated in these beds, and about 4,000 beds are occupied by NHS patients (mainly nonacute). The number of beds used or suitable for acute treatment—surgery, maternity, acute general medicine—is thought to be about 3,000 in England. In 1977 over 60% of these beds were situated in London and the counties around London. Elsewhere distribution is very uneven.

Although very little is known about the size of the market for the private sector, there are probably three main constituent groups: (1) members of the provident association and other United Kingdom residents who use the private sector for routine acute treatment; (2) people who receive mainly nursing care and nonacute treatment in charitable or religious nursing homes, many of whom are residents; and (3) wealthy foreigners who visit the country to use the most expensive private hospitals for acute treatment, some of it sophisticated. People turn to the private sector for a number of reasons: they may want the privacy of a single room, or they may desire the guarantee of seeing a particular consultant; the convenience of being able to book an admission date to suit business or personal commitments is important to many, while others may seek private treatment to reduce the time they spend waiting for an outpatient appointment or for an inpatient treatment, particularly where elective surgery is involved. It has been said that "NHS patients wait to avoid payment, while private patients pay to avoid waiting."

About 50% of private patients treated in NHS pay beds or receiving acute treatment in private hospitals are covered by private, nonprofit-making insurance schemes. Altogether there were some 1.3 million subscribers to these schemes in the United Kingdom in 1979. As subscriptions often cover more than one person, a total of 2.75 million people were covered in 1979, or 6% of the national population. This does not mean that almost three million people have opted out of the NHS. First, three-fourths of members belong because of their employment, not because of personal choice, though employers would not arrange group schemes if they did not think them attractive to staff. Second, it is likely that the majority use the NHS for most purposes (family practitioner services, maternity care, emergency admissions, etc.) and use their membership for "cold" surgery. Contributory schemes are used to pay for treatment both in the independent sector and in NHS pay beds.

Except for a dip in the mid-1970s, private medical care is an expanding market: the number of subscribers doubled between 1962 and 1978, rose very fast in 1979 and 1980, and is now said to be levelling off. The subscription income of the three main provident associations came to over £154 million in 1980 and the average subscription was £94. Group schemes now represent 80% of the income. The number of employer-paid subscriptions has expanded the fastest, and health insurance, no longer a "perk" for only top managers, is now more widely used, with an estimated quarter of a million trade unionists eligible. A popular explanation for the growth of company-paid schemes is the restriction of wage and salary increases imposed by successive government incomes policies. During the 1970s companies were generally allowed to offer increases in incomes in kind in the form of health insurance without breaking the pay code. Insurance coverage of illness is normally not total, with typically 75 to 85% being refunded. One-half of the cost is taken by accommodation; another quarter is paid to surgeons.

The arrangements for medical staff are somewhat similar to arrangements in voluntary hospitals before 1948, when honorary consultants treated private patients either in the private wing of the hospital or in nursing homes. The extent to which NHS consultants undertake private practice is not exactly known, but an indication can be found in the number who hold part-time rather than full-time NHS appointments. Following an agreement with the profession in 1948, health authorities may not insist on full-time contracts for medical staff. The new consultants' contract introduced in 1980, which permits "full-time" medical staff to undertake limited private practice, has been seen as an encouragement by the Conservative government to take on private practice, but, as the Royal Commission has pointed out, an increase depends not only on its attractiveness to doctors but also on the demand from patients.

In 1978, 94% of geriatricians and 85.3% of pathologists were full time, but only 14.4% of general surgeons and 15.5% of ENT surgeons. "Cold" surgery is the type of health care most likely to attract the private patients. Specialty is not the only factor determining the choice between full-time and part-time contracts; the uneven distribution of facilities for private care is also relevant. General practitioners are free to undertake any other work they wish, provided it does not interfere with their obligations under their NHS contracts. It is probable that nearly all undertake some work—such as examination for insurance purposes—for which they charge fees; however, while a few live entirely by private practice, the great majority have few or no private patients. In 1971–72 (the latest available figure) about 6% of general practitioners' income was from private practice. General dental practitioners are equally free to take private patients, and more of them do so. In 1977 some 11% of their time was spent on work other than that in the general dental service, probably concentrated on private practice. Some patients receive both NHS and private treatment from the same dentists. Some members of the various health care professions work in independent hospitals, and some, such as nurses, physiotherapists, and chiropodists, live by private practice outside of hospitals. Also in private practice are members of professions not employed in the NHS, such as osteopaths and chiropractors.

Nursing Homes Act

The 1975 Nursing Homes Act defines a nursing home as "any premises used, or intended to be used, for the reception of, and the providing of nursing for, persons suffering from any sickness, injury or infirmity"; this includes maternity homes and any other premises used for surgical procedures, the termination of pregnancy, endoscopy, haemodialysis, or peritoneal dialysis. All nursing homes must obtain registration, which is granted by the secretary of state, but application is made to the relevant DHA. Registration can be refused, or cancelled, on various grounds (including unsuitability of applicant or premises and the failure to have in charge a qualified doctor or nurse or midwife). Regulations require nursing homes to maintain registers of patients and various records; medical officers or authorised persons have power to inspect these.

Conclusion

Although the private sector is too small to have an impact on the NHS except locally and temporarily, the Royal Commission concluded that it "responds much more directly to patients' demands for services than the NHS and that it provided a useful pointer to areas where the NHS is deficient." The arguments for and against private health care reflect different political views, and the size of the private sector is likely to change with changes in government; it is likely, however, to remain small compared with the NHS, which will probably continue to provide health care for the majority of the population.

FINANCING THE NATIONAL HEALTH SERVICE

The basic underlying financial concept of the National Health Service is to provide a mechanism for people to pay for health services when they are well and working so that they can use them virtually free of charge when they are ill and not working. The NHS cost about £11.1 billion in 1981–82, or about £250 per person. (Personal social services provided by local authorities but financed by the central government to the extent implied by the Rate Support Grant cost a further £2.1 billion in 1981–82. The health and personal social services programme is the second largest government programme, much smaller than social security and just larger than defence and education.) Rapid inflation, however, makes money figures practically meaningless; more significant is the proportion of the Gross Domestic Product spent on the NHS, and that is about 6%.

Despite the financial problems of British governments, the amount of money spent on the health services has increased in practically every year since the services started in 1948. The cost has risen from £314 million in 1949 to £11.1 billion in 1981–82; if one allows for inflation, the total real expenditure has more than doubled. Similarly, the percentage of the Gross Domestic Product spent on the NHS has risen in almost every year—from just under 4% in 1949 to about 6% now. Although total expenditure has never been cut significantly, what has suffered is capital money spent on buildings and major equipment, Governments have seen it politically expedient to cut money not spent on direct patient treatment and not having immediate effects on employment in the NHS.

Why Have Costs Increased?

There has been a major alteration in the structure of the population of England and, thus, a consequent change in demand on the NHS is seen. Although the English population has risen from 41 million in 1951 to over 46 million in 1980, more significant for the NHS is the growing number of old people, particularly the very old. The number of people over 74 has gone from 1.5 million in 1951 to almost 2.7 million in 1980, not because those who survive to old age are living much longer but because more children born in this century have survived the first years of life. This trend will continue and increase, so that by 1986 there will be approximately 24% more people aged 75 and over than now. At the same time the number of women in the 45 to 60 age group, who provide the main source of support for old people in the community, will fall. The average cost of care and treatment of a person over 75 is seven times that of a person of working age. Although only about 2½% of old people are in the hospital at any one time, they occupy more than one-half of the beds, those over 75 taking up nearly one-third. The rise of the birth rate from 1978 to 1981 acted to increase costs. It is estimated that the NHS needs an extra .7% of resources per year just to cope with demographic changes.

The level of service provided by the NHS has increased from about 2.8 million inpatients in 1949–50 to over 5.5 million in 1980. The number of outpatient and accident and emergency attendances rose from about 25 million in 1949–50 to over 48 million in 1980.

Rapid advances in medical science in the last thirty years have meant that "high technology" medicine can achieve much more. Although some technological advances reduce costs, benefits of recent advances have been mainly to increase the diagnostic powers and the range of treatment. Many of these advances are costly; indeed, to pay for this process of innovation costs rise by a least ½% per year.

Consequently, the public's expectations have grown. Combined with greater affluence, these expectations render people less willing to suffer minor ailments and more expectant of the NHS support; therefore, a larger number of less severe cases are coming forward for treatment. To care for this growing volume of patients the NHS staff has more than doubled in size since 1948, rising from 324,000 in 1948 to 792,000 in 1980 (whole time equivalents). At the same time, however, as the NHS is employing more labour, the real cost of that labour, as for other government departments, is rising and the hours spent working is decreasing, so that unit costs have been climbing even more.

Another factor that compounded the increasing costs of the health service was equality legislation. The NHS employs nearly 600,000 women. Legislation to equalise male and female wages has increased costs.

Sources of Finance

The NHS derives its income almost entirely from public funds: about 89% comes from government taxation; revenue from NHS Insurance contributions (a leftover from the Social Insurance System of 1911–48) paid by employers and employees represents about 9%; and about 2 or 3% comes from charges for certain services including prescriptions, dental and optical treatment, and private beds in NHS hospitals.

When the NHS was established, some believed that the cost of providing free service would not increase, but eventually diminish; people who were then sick and were made better would be able to return to work, thus increasing the total contributions to the National Health Service Insurance Fund and reducing the drawings from it. We now realise that health is a relative term and that the more health care becomes available, the more will be demanded. Also, the longer we live, the more health care we will need and use.

In the early years of the NHS the actual costs turned out to be much higher than forecast. In an attempt to control costs and to pay for rearmament for the Korean War, the Labour government introduced charges for prescription, dental, and ophthalmic services in 1950. Charges have occasionally been raised, and the current Conservative government has indicated its intention to increase the proportion of the NHS cost covered by charges to 5% and has already boosted prescription charges by 500%. It will now be cheaper to buy some drugs without prescriptions.

Charges are made for prescriptions, appliances, dental and ophthalmic services, treatment of road accident victims, welfare foods and milk, private patients in NHS hospitals, and amenity beds (NHS beds which provide some privacy). Government cash benefits (such as sickness and retirement benefits) are reduced when the beneficiaries are in the hospital. In addition, beginning in 1982 foreign residents whose governments have no reciprocal arrangements with the NHS were charged for medical services. It is estimated that the gross revenue will be about 6 million pounds per annum. Various groups—particularly children, the aged, the poor, and expectant mothers—are exempt from some of these charges. In addition, contraceptive prescriptions are free of charge. About two-fifths of the population were exempt from prescription charges in 1980 and over two-thirds of all prescriptions were dispensed free.

Besides the official funding arrangements, there are trust funds (mostly small) that are administered by health authorities and are entirely at the discretion of those authorities. These originate in gifts and bequests to hospitals, many made before 1948. The older teaching hospitals tend to have fairly substantial trust funds, but even the most wealthy of these would not be able to increase their total income by more than about 1% through this means. Groups of people can raise money for equipment, alterations, or new hospital departments either by appeals to the public or by a lottery. They need the agreement, if not the active encouragement, of the health authority, because the authority has to decide whether or not to accept a gift. In recent years authorities have occasionally agreed to accept a gift of expensive equipment (such as a whole body scanner) only if the campaigners also raised the money to meet the running costs. For the first time in 1980 health authorities were themselves allowed to raise money by appeals, collections, and other such methods.

Method of Allocation

Between 1948 and 1965 the amount of money spent on the NHS was the same each year, allowing for inflation plus a small increase of up to 3% for development. Budgets were prepared by each hospital management committee (HMC) and submitted to the regional boards; there were some negotiations between these two bodies, and once the budgets were agreed upon, the boards produced their regional budgets and sent them to the ministry of health. Again, negotiations ensued, and then the ministry submitted its bid to the Treasury. If the total amount of money the government wanted to spend was less than that requested by the ministries—which it normally was—the budget for the NHS was cut, the ministry of health clipped the regional budgets, and the regions trimmed the HMC budgets. This "bottom-up" budgeting was wasteful and caused much disappointment and ill will.

In 1961 a government committee proposed to reverse the procedure, and now government budgeting is done under the Public Expenditure Survey Committee System (PESC). The purpose was to simplify government budgeting but also to allow decisions about one area of government expenditure to be taken in relation to the levels of government expenditure in other areas and also in light of future expenditures. Now each year total public expenditure is determined by the cabinet with the help of estimates made several years ahead. The cabinet divides the available money between government departments. The Department of Health then allocates the money to the regions, and so on.

This system had one major weakness: it did not take inflation into account. PESC was based on an allocation of real resources—that is, each claim was allocated a given volume of goods and services. This was a workable approach when the value of money was fairly stable, but with high inflation the method proved somewhat defective, and "cash limits" were introduced in 1976. This means that the government's decision about the NHS volume allocation is expressed in cash terms at the present value of money; this amount is then increased by what the government expects inflation to be, and the "cash limit" figure which the NHS is allowed to spend up to is thus determined. If inflation is less than the expected rate, the NHS has a bonus; if it is more, the NHS suffers a cut. Most public expenditure is now planned and announced in terms of cash—the so-called cash planning.

The effect of cash limits showed in a reduction of £160 million worth of services in 1979–80. It is now clear that the cash limit formula is more important in determining how much money a government department receives than the expenditure forecasts that the government gives. Therefore, spending can be cut and the government can evade responsibility for unpopular decisions by setting the cash limit figures so that spending authorities have to determine how to cope with the effects of unexpected price increases. What cuts should be made are thus decided by administrators, not politicians.

The latest public expenditure survey shows that hospital and community services and family practitioner services were planned to grow by 4% between 1978–79 and 1981–82, personal social services by about 7.6%. Because of cash limits, future growth is hard to estimate, but it is unlikely to be as large as it has been.

International comparisons show that England spends relatively little on health services. Whether it should spend more is difficult to say. It should be pointed out that while it spends relatively little, the country's mortality and life expectancy rates are comparatively good. So, on that basis, the NHS is good value for money. The financial strengths of the NHS are several. First, the primary care system, through general practice and outpatient clinics, treats patients in the community rather than in the hospital. Second, being practically the only buyer for doctors' and nurses' services and for many kinds of drugs and equipment, the NHS has been able to use its monopoly position to contain costs better than have other health care systems. Third, its centralised financial control system has kept costs from going out of control: the NHS controls not only the cost of treatment but also the number of doctors employed and the amount of treatment provided.

The Search for Greater Efficiency

Attempts have been made through administrative measures—such as cost accountancy and examination of the number of beds needed for a population and the length of stay for the patients—to achieve greater financial efficiency. There is now some interest within both the Health Service and the government in something approaching "Quality Assurance." The government's motive is almost certainly defensive, having been stung by Parliament's critical statements about its failure to relate in any way policies, expenditures, and results.

A number of mechanisms—for example, medical audit and clinical budgeting—are being increasingly discussed and put into practice. There have been a number of innovations in financial control and accountability introduced recently. Mrs. Thatcher invited a private businessman to scrutinise the management practices of the National Health Service and other government departments to see whether there is any scope for greater efficiency. A management advisory service is being used in several regions to try to improve the quality and efficiency of service provision. Performance indicators are being developed by the Department of Health and Social Security as a way of assessing and comparing the efficiency of health authorities. Finally, regional reviews are being instituted; these will involve meetings of ministers, civil servants, regional chairmen, and officers, who will discuss regional plans for service development and past performances. This procedure will be matched by similar reviews between the regions and districts. Therefore, the greater delegation achieved by the 1981 reorganisation will be matched by this system of accountability.

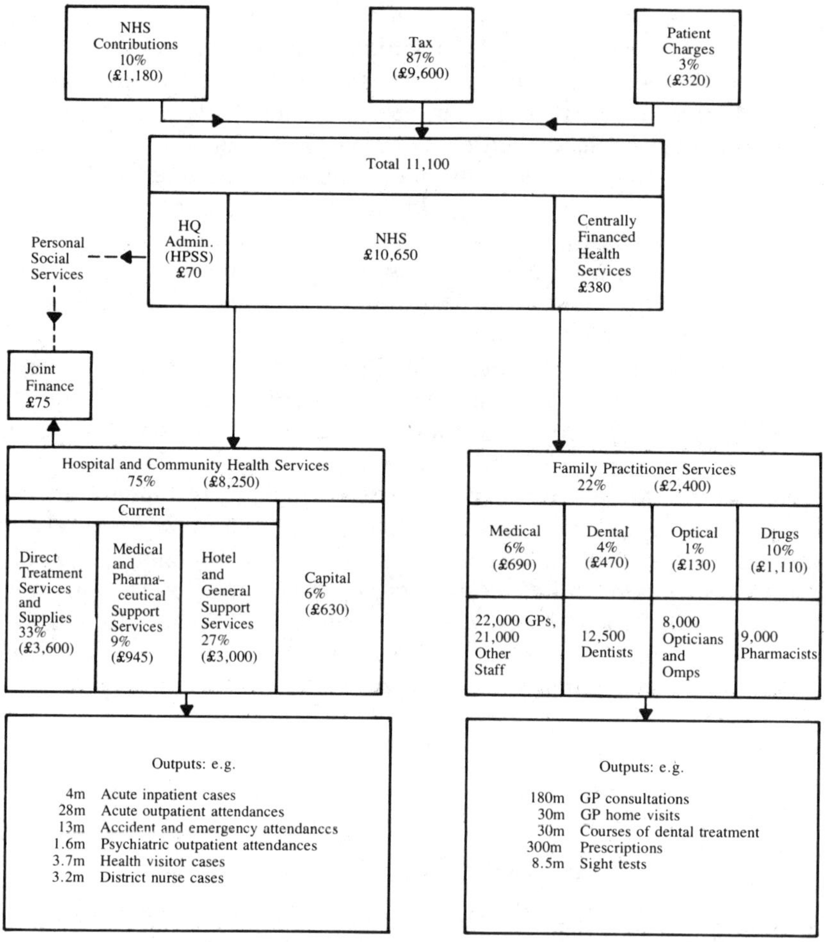

Figure 2 National Health Service in England: source of money (in millions), expenditures, outputs, 1981–82

How the Money Is Spent

About three-fourths of the NHS budget is spent on salaries, a further tenth goes for drugs, and about 6% is spent on buildings and major equipment (see figure 2). Over half the cost of the NHS is spent on running the hospitals, and this has been taking an increasing proportion. The share for general medical services, covering general practice, has been falling and is now about 6%; the share for dental services has fallen to 4%.

Considerable attempts have been made to control administrative expenses, which are closely monitored by the DHSS. This overall cost was reduced to 5% of the total cost in 1980, and there is hope it can be lessened to 4.5% by 1984–85. The price of medicines for the GP services are negotiated centrally with the manufacturers under the Voluntary Price Regulation Scheme, which is so designed as to enable the department to satisfy itself that profits are fair and reasonable. The manufacturers supply the department with audited financial returns of their business with the NHS, from which the necessary assessments can be made and adjustments negotiated.

Geographic Distribution of Expenditure

Some parts of England receive more money for health services than others. The richest region, North West Thames, received £122 per head in 1976–77, while the poorest region, West Midlands, received £91 per head. These differences in figures did not reflect variances in need, in fact almost the reverse—what has been called the "inverse care law." The region with the lowest revenue allocation had among the highest standardised mortality ratios (regional mortality rates standardised for differences in age and sex distributions). These differences were due to the historic way in which the NHS had been funded. In 1948 the ministry of health took over the existing health services and expenses, and with each year added a little more to them. The regions around London and others started in 1948 were better provided with health services, and so they continued. Attempts were made to redistribute the available resources on a more equitable basis and some success was met, particularly in the redistribution of consultant manpower and, to a lesser extent, in general practice.

However, although the gap was closed, we have seen that even in 1976–77 there were still considerable differences which were certainly not justified on the grounds of differences in need. Thus, in the mid-1970s the government set up the Resource Allocation Working Party (RAWP), which proposed that resources be allocated on the basis of need (the RAWP formula). Need was measured in terms of population and adjusted for age and sex variations; for some services this was further adjusted by standardised mortality and fertility rates. Revenue was allocated to regions on this basis, with adjustments for patient flows between regions and consideration of the high cost of providing services in London and the expense of training medical students. The RAWP formula provided the target allocations. It takes time, however, to recruit and re-train staff, so money could not simply be transferred from one region to another; therefore, it was decided that the gap should be closed over a period of six years, which was later increased to ten. Capital allocation has also been adjusted to equalise the regions' capital stocks, but this has even further to go. No region was supposed to suffer a cut, even the best supplied being allowed a minimum growth, but other factors, particularly inflation, caused cuts. On the other hand, some regions, in applying the formula to their authorities, have enforced quite drastic cuts in some areas in order to accelerate development in their worst-funded areas.

RAWP has helped a great deal in the deprived districts within poor regions. However, the rich regions, which are not gaining much under RAWP, are not enthusiastically applying RAWP to redistribute their money within the region. The main achievement of RAWP has been to reduce the variation in regions' revenue resources from a gap of 36% between rich and poor regions in 1977–78 to 18% in 1982–83 in terms of the formula used.

These measures towards equalising revenue expenditure do not affect the family practitioner services, where expenditure depends on the number of practitioners practising in an area and the demands made on their services. Thus, a "deprived" district that is building up its hospital and community services has no means of doing the same with the family practitioner services.

If and when equality is achieved, it will be financial equality, not necessarily equality of service. As would be expected, such redistributions have caused considerable controversy, particularly among those areas which have lost relative to others. Criticisms of the basis of the reallocation are inevitable, and it remains a source of considerable debate. It does, however, represent an attempt to reduce inequalities in health care—which was one of the original objectives of founding the NHS.

SOCIAL EQUALITY IN THE NHS

Equality of distribution between social groups was another early objective of the Health Service. There are still great differences in mortality and morbidity between social classes, with little sign of these health inequalities diminishing. The risk of death before retirement is two and one-half times greater for unskilled workers and their wives than for professionals, and the gap has increased since the 1950s. The gap in infant mortality rates has also increased. However, while the health of the poorest social classes *relative* to the professional classes has not improved, and in some cases has worsened, the *absolute* level of health of all classes has improved—except for mortality among women in the poorest social classes, which has risen since 1960. Whether these disparities can be corrected by changes in the NHS is, of course, questionable.

Setting Priorities

In 1976–77 about 40% of NHS and personal social services expenditure was allocated for general and acute hospital and maternity services, about 20% on primary care; 12% was spent on services specifically for the elderly and physically handicapped (in addition to services designed specifically to meet their needs—the elderly make considerable demands on the acute services), 7% on services for the mentally ill, 6% on services for children, and 4% on services for the mentally handicapped.

There is no conceptual basis on which to allocate resources between patient groups. The absence of objective criteria for settling health priorities means that decisions are mostly a matter of judgement. Ministers and MPs are vulnerable to lobbying from various quarters and may be subject to the influences of the many pressure groups. The health professions, particularly doctors, play an active role in this process. Ultimately it is Parliament that decides, but health ministers—especially the secretary of state for social services—probably have more influence than any other individuals on determining priorities in the NHS.

Since about 1975 the DHSS has set priorities and attempted to persuade health authorities to redistribute resources in line with these. A number of factors influence the department's decisions on priorities. Diseases which require the most care nowadays are different from the main diseases of forty or fifty years ago (such as tuberculosis), so some types of treatment that were provided are now less frequently required.

There has also been much attention paid to the conditions of treatments of long-stay geriatric and psychiatric patients. The average cost per patient bed day in an acute hospital has been between two and three times the cost of that in long-stay, geriatric, and psychiatric hospitals. This has led the government to attempt to shift resources away from the expensive "high technology" acute medicine to services for the elderly, the handicapped, the mentally ill, children, and the "Cinderella services." Maternity and neonatal care have recently become priority services.

The main mechanism for implementing the government's priorities in the NHS is the planning system. A systematic planning process was introduced in the DHSS in 1974, and the NHS planning system and a system of social services planning were initiated in 1976. The planning process in the NHS starts each year with the issue of "Guidelines" from the secretary of state to the regional health authorities on policies and priorities and on the resource assumptions within which planning should proceed. The planning system enables a check on the consistency of health authorities' plans with national policies and an assessment of the development of services. Divergence from the national pattern may be justified in particular circumstances, but reasons for it "may merit exploration," and that may lead to a review of the national guidance itself. In February 1982 a new secretary of state announced a new series of meetings with regional chairmen and officers to examine whether national guidelines were being complied with.

Perhaps the most difficult part of the planning and budgeting system is the monitoring aspect. NHS treasurers have difficulty in relating their budgeting system to planning guidelines because the accounting information in the NHS is in terms of individual hospitals and community services, not of client groups. In conjunction with the planning system, the DHSS has developed a programme budget approach as a means of costing policies for services development across the board. Expenditure can be allocated to broad patient and client groups and can show the trends in spending on the groups. However, this initiative is yet to be followed by the NHS.

A more direct method of implementing national priorities is to earmark part of the funds allocated to authorities for use in particular services. In the period of 1971 to 1976 additional capital allocations totalling more than £44 million were made to health authorities to be spent on mental handicap, mental illness, and geriatric services; these allocations, however, had little noticeable effect on the overall proportion of capital expenditure devoted to services for those three groups. Health authorities have received funds specifically allocated for the development of regional secure units, but the monies have sometimes been diverted to other purposes. A variation is to make additional funds available outside of the normal allocation for use on specific projects, such as capital funds for the development of health centres. These funds are separately administered and cannot be diverted to other uses, but may not be fully taken up.

The problems of the NHS are worst in the deprived urban areas of the inner cities. Large numbers of old people and single-parent and poor families make large demands on the health service, but in many inner cities the provision of services, particularly those for chronic patients, is at its weakest. In these areas more patients commit suicide or die from pneumonia or bronchitis, and there are more accidents than elsewhere in the country. Here patients are often served by elderly general practitioners in poorly equipped surgeries with little nursing help.

To encourage the provision of services across administrative boundaries, some NHS funds have been specifically designated since 1976–77 for use in projects planned and funded jointly with local authorities. Money for jointly financed projects totalled about £80 million in 1981.

One further area of great current debate is the increased importance of prevention.

Many of today's health problems are self-inflicted and can be prevented, and we are now more aware that psychological and social problems influence our health. There has been a shift of emphasis away from the hospitals and towards areas where the problems are rooted—in the home and at work—and towards prevention and care as much as cure. Through laws and exhortations the government has tried to promote personal behaviour that will improve health. These measures have yet to show any great effect. Preventive health catches few votes and is even politically unpopular. Prevention works best when the desire of the government and the Health Service to act in a situation coincides with the public's wish to be controlled. The problem of how to adapt the NHS to cope adequately with this need has not yet been solved.

NHS PERSONNEL

In 1980 just under one million people were employed by the NHS in England. Many of these are part-timers; it is estimated that this is equivalent to 792,000 full-timers (up from 760,000 in 1978), and the service is continuing to expand by about 10,000 employees per year. This total represents about 4% of the national workforce and includes a great variety of skills and knowledge, ranging from highly trained medical staff to the semi-skilled or unskilled manual workers in some ancillary grades. Staff costs account for over 70% of the total NHS budget. Nursing and midwifery staff account for almost one-half of the workforce, and about half are professionally qualified. Ancillary grades come next at about 22%, while doctors and dentists amount to about 7% of the total.

Some features of the workforce are worth mentioning. (1) There is a high proportion of female staff—over 70%. (2) Use of part-time staff has increased considerably in recent years. (3) Over 60% of the NHS workforce—unqualified nursing staff, "hotel" staff, maintenance workers, and certain administrative and clerical staff—are recruited in competition with other employers from the local labour market. For most of the more highly skilled personnel—medical and dental, qualified nursing, professional, and technical staff—the NHS is virtually a monopoly employer (although these staffs have limited opportunity for employment overseas, in industry, research, the universities, and the armed forces). (4) The NHS relies heavily on team working; therefore, any changes in duties, skills, working hours, or deployment in one group affects others. (5) The total staff has grown steadily since 1949. This growth has not been uniform between the different occupations. The 1980 numbers of hospital medical, nursing, and administrative staff were each more than double the 1949 figures, while professional and technical staff had more than trebled. The numbers of GPs and community nurses have not increased as much. Among hospital staff only ancillaries showed a substantially lower growth. In the 1960s medical and dental manpower increased more slowly than did the population, while in the 1970s the increase has been much greater, with an almost zero growth in population. A vital factor affecting growth rates has been the economic climate. When unemployment is high, the increase in staff numbers is significantly above those forecast. (6) The management structure established in April 1974 provided a number of new functions within the NHS.

Doctors

Among the group considered as doctors are hospital medical staff; general medical practitioners; specialists in community medicine; child health specialists, including school health service medical officers; and other NHS medical staff. All doctors in the United Kingdom are required to spend a year in preregistration house officer posts in hospitals in order to become fully registered medical practitioners.

Almost all doctors spend at least a few years in hospital grades. Typically, the graduate trained in the United Kingdom will take his first post, as house officer, when he is about twenty-four years old. Those who intend to make a career in the hospital service will work for about five years in the house officer, senior house officer, and registrar grades, and another three or more years in the senior registrar grade before being appointed as a consultant. However, for a number of reasons, the median age for the first consultant appointment is about thirty-six. In the future doctors who go into general practice will be required to have had three years of training, including at least twelve months as a trainee general practitioner, two periods of at least six months each in hospital specialties, and the remainder in approved posts in hospital or community medicine.

A hospital doctor may go on working past the normal retirement age of sixty-five. Nationally applied terms and conditions of service mean that there is likely to be little incentive for a consultant to move once he is appointed, and he may stay in his first post for thirty or more years. Often appointed when in their twenties, GPs may spend even longer in the same place. They can go on working past retirement age.

In 1980 hospital medical staff were composed of 12,134 consultants, 2,855 senior registrars, 5,552 registrars, 9,197 senior house officers, and 2,726 house officers. There were 22,300 fully qualified general practitioners and 1,561 trainees.

General medical practitioners are remunerated through a combination of allowances, capitation fees, and fees for items of service. Hospital doctors are salaried employees of the health authorities; those in the career grades (mainly consultants) may be full-time or part-time, the latter group being paid the appropriate proportion of the full-time salary. Those in the junior, or training, grades are predominantly full-time employees. There are also a number of part-time grades in the hospital service, mainly filled by general practitioners. Doctors in community medicine and the community health service are salaried employees, though some do clinic work remunerated on the basis of sessional fees.

The geographic distribution of doctors is uneven both in general practice, where there is a system of restraints and incentives to steer doctors towards the underdoctored areas—the designated areas, and in the hospital service, where systematic consultant targets and a general policy of preference for the understaffed regions has not removed staffing disparities. The best provided-for region in 1980 was North West Thames with 57 general practitioners per 100,000 population; the poorest region was the Trent area with 48 per 100,000. Similarly, North West Thames had 83 hospital doctors per 100,000 population, while Trent had 58 per 100,000. Broadly speaking, London and the South East of England are better staffed than the North and Midlands, but there are significant variations within the regions.

Within the hospital service, some specialties appear to be unattractive and recruitment for them is difficult. These include psychiatry and geriatrics, where policies of the DHSS require considerable growth, and anaesthetics and radiology. In recent years there have been larger than average increases in several of the shortage specialties; however, these may be made up in part by recruits who have taken the jobs because career prospects are good, and such recruits may bring little enthusiasm to their work. In 1977 consultant geriatricians on first appointment spent only four years in the specialty; the average for all specialties was seven years. There are various reasons for shortages. Some shortage specialties, like radiology and anaesthetics, have been created by a rapid increase in demand combined with attractive opportunities abroad; some, like the laboratory specialties, lack opportunities for private practice; while others, like the psychiatric specialties, may appeal to relatively few doctors. On the other hand, the surgical specialties have the smallest growth rate, and competition for senior registrar and consultant posts is fierce. In 1979 there were an average of 4.4 candidates for each consultant post and 9.3 for each senior registrar position. There is also strong competition in most medical specialties, with the notable exception of geriatric medicine. The demand for psychiatrists, however, continues to grow and career prospects are generally good, as are prospects in anaesthetics and radiology.

The creation of new consultant and senior registrar posts is controlled by the Central Manpower Committee. A number of factors, such as availability and recognition of posts for training purposes, will influence this decision, but probably the most important will be the number of vacancies in the existing establishment and the funds available.

A clinical specialty is one recognised as such by the Royal Colleges and their faculties (which are concerned with standards of medical practice and education and grant qualifying and postgraduate diplomas. The oldest Royal College is the Royal College of Physicians in London, founded in 1518). There are currently forty-nine hospital clinical specialties, thirteen of them introduced in the last fourteen years and some having only tiny numbers of consultant posts so far.

Staffing structure agreements with the medical profession regulate the career progression of hospital doctors. Broadly, they provide that consultant is the normal career grade in the hospital service. There are increasing conflicts between training, service, and career demands, which the present structure does not satisfactorily resolve. The existing medical career structure is, in fact, criticised on a number of grounds. It is claimed that there are too many doctors in the training grades below senior registrar for the number of consultant posts available. Indeed, there has been an increase in the number of unemployed doctors, but medical unemployment remains small (about 1,500 in 1982). The central manpower machinery controls the number of senior registrar posts, so doctors appointed to that grade can be reasonably sure of being appointed as a consultant in due course. But below senior registrar there is no such certainty. Because a consultant may spend over thirty years in the grade, there should be many more consultants than juniors to achieve equilibrium. In fact, registrars and senior house officers together outnumber consultants, and the overall ratio of junior to senior staff is about one and a half to one. Calculations are complicated by the existence of doctors from overseas, who comprise over one-half of the senior house officers and registrars, and who are often not intending to make careers in the United Kingdom.

One-third of hospital doctors and almost one-fifth of general practitioners are from overseas. Their contributions have been greatest in the areas of the country and in the certain specialties in which recruitment is difficult. There are twenty-two overseas universities whose medical qualifications are recognized by the General Medical Council (GMC) for both full and provisional registration. These universities annually provide information on changes in their undergraduate medical curriculum, student numbers, facilities, staff, and resources. In 1980, 2,990 overseas doctors (mostly from Australia or South Africa) were granted full registration. The GMC may grant full registration to doctors from overseas who have practised in the United Kingdom under limited registration, if they are suitable. In 1980, 657 doctors were granted full registration via this route. The GMC may grant limited registration to overseas qualified doctors, only for employment supervised by a fully registered doctor in an approved hospital. Before limited registration is granted, a doctor must have passed or been exempted from a test of competence in English. In 1980, 1,684 doctors were granted limited registration and 5,308 doctors were so registered. Most of these doctors came from India, Sri Lanka, Egypt, and Pakistan.

Another criticism of the medical career structure is that patients are not always treated by fully trained staff. Much of the service is provided by junior staff, who are appointed to be trained. Junior doctor training is unsatisfactory in some places because there are too few consultants to supervise their work properly, and juniors are used simply as pairs of medical hands.

The present policy of the health department is to double the number of consultant posts and hold steady the number of senior house officers, so that, in time, the two will be brought into equilibrium; this will also reverse the current ratio to result in almost twice as many consultants as juniors in the mid-1990s. However, the plan is unpopular with many existing consultants and senior registrars. It will mean that in the future consultants will lose part of their retinue of juniors, while some in the major centres may have to work in "unsocial hours" as their less fortunate colleagues in peripheral hospitals often do now. Many consultants appointed in their thirties have then no higher grading to look forward to, and their only financial incentive to excellence is the possibility of a distinction award. All consultants are eligible for distinction awards, which are made by the health ministers on the advice of the Advisory Committee on Distinction Awards. This is a predominantly professional body, traditionally headed by a distinguished and respected doctor. Members and the chairman are appointed by the health ministers on nomination from the Royal Colleges and the MRC. The total value of awards is about 10% of total consultant remuneration. The highest level of individual awards can almost double a consultant's salary, although these are very rare. Once allocated, awards are held until the consultant leaves the NHS. These increase his retirement pension.

Nurses, Midwives, and Health Visitors

The group of nurses, midwives, and health visitors is the largest staff group in the NHS and commands the largest salary bill, accounting for over one-fourth of the total current expenditure. At present the NHS employs the equivalent of over 370,000 "whole-time" nurses, midwives, and health visitors, almost one-half of all NHS workers. About 50% of these are in training or are auxilliaries.

Nurse training aims to produce different levels of skill. There are courses that last up to two years and lead to state enrollment (SEN) and—for those who desire more technical qualification—ones that last three years and lead to state registration (SRN), with the General Nursing Council. (Like the General Medical Council, the General Nursing Council controls the register of nurses by setting the standards of entry and the qualification to the nursing profession. These responsibilities are being taken over in 1983 by a Central Council and National Board for Nursing, Midwifery, and Health Visiting.) The SRN course has the greater theoretical content. About one-fourth of all nurses are registered nurses working in hospitals, about 15% are enrolled, and a further 15% are student nurses working in hospitals.

There are also a small number of courses that combine SRN training with an undergraduate degree programme. The nursing registers are divided into general, mental, and mental subnormality parts. Early specialisation is encouraged by this arrangement, but flexibility in deploying nursing staff is reduced.

Hospital nurses work in acute, long-stay, children's, psychiatric, maternity, and other specialised units. Outside of the hospital, health visitors, home nurses, midwives, and nurses work in clinics and in general practice as part of the primary health care team. Nurses serve in administration in the NHS and health departments, in education and in research. Extended roles for nurses are developing as a result of specialisation, for example, in renal dialysis, care of spinal injuries, and special care baby units. This has brought into question the professional relationship between doctors and nurses. *Who* initiates *what* is a matter of increasing controversy.

There is increasing recognition that nursing care is the major health need of groups such as the chronic, the long-term sick, and the elderly. While there has been a growth of clinical nursing specialties, there has also been a parallel and sometimes conflicting growth in the increased responsibility of the nurse as a manager in the NHS. Complaints are frequently heard about shortages of nurses despite considerable national increases in their numbers over the years. The increases have been partly offset by a lessening of availability of staff. Factors contributing to a reduction in nurses' availability include a shorter working week, longer vacations, additional national holidays, and revised training schemes that have been expanded to include community and psychiatric aspects. The sense of a nursing shortage may be produced by the greater throughput of patients in hospitals, more people being cared for in the community, and the nurses' increasingly specialised and technical roles. Finally, the increase in the number of doctors has resulted in a greater demand for other services, including nursing.

The NHS has long been dependent on unqualified staff. About 50% of the nursing workforce is unqualified, this group fairly equally divided between nurse learners, nursing auxiliaries, and assistants, some of whom receive only a short basic in-service training. Student and pupil nurses are employees of the NHS and form some 25% of the total nursing staff employed in the hospital service.

Definitely going through a difficult period, the profession has suffered major structural modifications and was considerably influenced by the management changes introduced at the 1974 reorganisation.

Other Staff

The eight professions covered by the Professions Supplementary to Medicine Act, 1960 (the PSM Act) employed in 1980 about 2,000 chiropodists, 715 dieticians, 13,600 medical laboratory scientific officers, 2,800 occupational therapists, 400 orthoptists, 6,800 physiotherapists, 6,000 radiographers, and 350 remedial gymnasts. Speech therapists, numbering 1,600, are usually included in this group though they are not covered by the PSM Act. The professions fall into two broad groups: the remedial group, consisting of occupational therapists, orthoptists, physiotherapists, remedial gymnasts, and speech therapists; and the scientific group, consisting of dieticians, medical laboratory scientific officers, and radiographers.

For each of the eight professions the PSM Act established registration boards in order to promote high standards of professional education and conduct. Concerned with all areas of the United Kingdom, the boards are responsible for maintaining registers and approving the training institutions, the courses of training, and the qualifications of graduates. The PSM Act does not prevent unregistered members of the professions from practising, but it limits the use of the titles "state registered," "registered," and "state," and it prevents the employment of unregistered members in the NHS, though not outside of it. The registration machinery gave control of standards and qualifications to the professions themselves.

There is widespread concern about shortages in these professions, although the shortfall has been taken up to some extent by the appointment of helpers, particularly in the occupational therapy and physiotherapy departments. The growing number of elderly and pressure on the rehabilitation services will increase demand for most of the PSM Act professions.

Scientific and Technical Staff

There are over twenty separate staff groups in the scientific and technical services of the NHS. They range in size from the whole-time equivalent of eight medical artists to nearly 13,000 medical laboratory scientific officers, and include university-trained biochemists, physicists, and psychologists, and grades for which there are no specific educational requirements. Numbers of these groups have grown rapidly, and new groups have emerged.

Administrative and Clerical Staff

The 105,000 administrative and clerical staff are employed in all branches of the health service and are still broadly generalist, though functional specialisation exists and is increasing. The main specialties at present are finance, supply, personnel, and management services, including computer staff and medical records management. A large number within the group have clerical and secretarial functions.

Ambulance Staff

Control of the ambulance service was transferred from local authorities to the NHS at the time of the 1974 NHS reorganisation. Before that, there was considerable local variation in the quality of services provided. Most services were administered by local authorities through their medical officer of health and his ambulance officer, a few were under the aegis of the Fire Service, while others relied upon agency methods for their provision.

The 1974 reorganisation reduced the number of separate services from 142 to 53. In 1980 there were 18,000 members of the ambulance staff. Their work falls into two distinct parts. First, they provide transport for emergency and urgent cases. Second, they provide a nonemergency service, which accounts for about 90% of their work: they take to and from the hospitals outpatients and day patients who are unable to get there by other means. The emergency service accounts for only 10% of the demand, but half the cost. The ambulance service includes the hospital car service, which is usually manned by volunteers and deals with some 14% of the nonemergency work.

Ancillary Staff

The NHS employs the equivalent of over 172,000 (whole-time equivalents) ancillary staff; only the nurses form a larger group. Nearly one-half of them work as domestics or ward orderlies, but there are many catering workers and porters. Other ancillary workers include laundry workers, telephonists, vehicle drivers, stokers, storekeepers, and workers in central sterile supply departments and gardens. Over 70% of ancillary workers are women, and over half work part-time.

The traditionally low status of this staff group, as the "forgotten" members of the Health Service, has resulted in an increasingly agressive attitude. Having been taken for granted for so long, they have realised that their contribution is an essential one and have "flexed their muscles" on many recent occasions.

Works and Maintenance Staff

This group of staff includes architects, surveyors and engineers employed mainly at regional, area and district level; and craftsmen employed on building and engineering maintenance mainly at unit level. There are about 6,000 in the first group about 21,000 in the second. Between them, these staff plan and maintain the stock of NHS property.

Pay and conditions of service for NHS staff (with the exception of doctors, dentists, and maintenance craftsmen) are normally negotiated nationally in the Whitley councils. A General Whitley Council deals with conditions of service (normally excluding pay) common to all grades and eight functional Whitley councils deal with pay and conditions of particular groups. The management sides of the Whitley councils consist of representatives from health authorities immediately responsible for the administration of the NHS, and from the Department of Health and Social Security; the staff sides are made of professional associations and trade unions that represent the staff concerned. There are over forty-six of these bodies, who themselves determine the size and composition of each staff side.

Some associations and unions representing staff employed in the Health Service do not wish to negotiate their terms and conditions of services through the Whitley Council machinery. Doctors and dentists, for example, negotiate directly with the health departments on matters concerning terms and conditions of service. The level of pay is based on the recommendations of the review body on doctors' and dentists' remuneration.

Enforcement of negotiated agreements is ensured by statutory regulations, the principle effect of which is that health authorities must pay neither more nor less than the remuneration approved by the secretaries of state after considering the agreements reached by negotiating bodies. The secretary of state has a veto over agreements reached by the councils. This ensures nationally uniform rates of pay and conditions of service, although the secretaries of state can authorise a health authority to vary the remuneration or other conditions of service from those laid down in the Whitley agreements in the case of an individual officer.

Personnel management, as a specialist service provided by personnel departments, is a comparatively recent addition to the National Health Service. The changing industrial relations climate of the 1970s, however, illuminated the need for professional personnel management in the NHS, and reorganisation gave the opportunity to establish it within the new management structures.

Unfortunately, the NHS has lacked a systematic approach to dealing with industrial relations problems arising at the local level. There are defects on the trade union side as well, interunion rivalries over recruitment and areas of influence occur, and in a few places there are problems with participating in local industrial relations machinery. However, the Whitley councils are too remote to deal with local problems and there is a perennial difficulty of leaving sufficient flexibility in national agreements to enable local problems to be overcome.

The professional ethic is dominant in the NHS and quite naturally invites nonprofessional staff to desire this status. Specialist training has developed in a wide range of fields—theatre attendants and porters, for example, as well as many other groups in the scientific field. While the NHS has benefited from these increased skills, it has meant that the total manpower available is more difficult to redeploy without retraining.

MEDICAL EDUCATION

History

Medical science in nineteenth-century England followed the precepts of Sydenham. Based on careful observation of the patient's symptoms rather than on experiment, this approach to medicine was to have an enduring impact on medical practice and education. Hospital beds were vehicles for teaching apprentices. From 1800 onwards, medical schools grew up concentrated on hospitals rather than universities. Before the founding of teaching hospitals, medical training had been conducted by theoretical instruction and some casual apprenticeship.

Present-day medical education is essentially a partnership. The university medical schools are responsible for providing undergraduate medical education, but they can do this only with the collaboration of teaching hospitals provided by the NHS. In their postgraduate years doctors in training form an essential part of hospital staffing.

The System of Medical Education

Academic qualifications in medicine necessary for the practice of medicine in England are awarded currently by thirty-one medical schools—the medical faculties of British universities. There are presently some 20,000 students in these faculties (18,000 undergraduates for the first academic medical degree and 2,000 postgraduates for higher degrees and diplomas in medicine). The teaching staff consists of nearly 6,000 full-time members. The government, in consultation with the University Grants Committee, determines the overall total of the annual intake of students. As a result of the recommendations by the Royal Commission on Medical Education in 1968, this figure has been speedily increased over the last fifteen years and was due to reach a total of 4,100 new entrants by 1980. (In addition to increasing the numbers of students in existing schools, three new medical schools have been opened in the last few years.) In 1977 about 13,000 students competed for 4,000 places, It is, therefore, not surprising that the intellectual quality of the students accepted for medical study has been very high and the failure rate in undergraduate medical education is correspondingly low: more than 90% of all students entering medical schools are expected to qualify.

Medical education is free to all who are granted admission—with the exception of students from families with very high incomes. Universities receive block grants from the Department of Education and Science. These grants currently provide 75% of the total university income of about £700 million, and the remaining 25% is received as fees for every student enrolled. Although paid by individual students, these, again, are financed by the government, although they are channeled through those local authorities where families of the students are resident.

The curriculum for the undergraduate study of medicine can be developed by each university but must be approved in principle by the General Medical Council. Universities in Britain are constitutionally not part of the state system but are individual organisations under a charter given by the Crown. Medical studies, lasting in total five years, consist of two parts: two years of preclinical studies (the basic sciences) and three of clinical studies. Students normally enter medical school direct from secondary school, at eighteen years of age, and they can, therefore, expect to obtain the basic academic medical qualification at twenty-three years. Since 1953 it has, however, become compulsory for each medical student to complete a preregistration year in an approved hospital, rotating usually in six-month periods from internal medicine to surgery. Only after the university has issued a Certificate of Satisfactory Completion will the new graduate obtain full registration by the General Medical Council.

A student cannot obtain all the necessary knowledge to practice medicine effectively during the six years before full registration. These years of study are only designed to provide the scientific basis and the fundamental skills on which the young doctor's specialised vocational training can be built. The complete study of medicine is conceived to be a continuum consisting of these six years of basic medical education, followed by a further period of vocational or postgraduate studies. Two paths of postgraduate studies can be followed. First, to become a principal in NHS general practice—an independent practitioner with clinical responsibilities for patients—the young doctor will, from 1982 onwards, be required to complete a three-year training programme after full registration. Two years will be spent in hospital on rotating assignments, and one year will be served as a trainee with a qualified general practitioner. Unlike that for any other specialty, this vocational training programme is a statutory requirement for doctors wishing to enter NHS general practice as a principal. The typical age for entering general practice indepently is, therefore, about twenty-seven years. Second, the young graduate who would like to become a specialist in a branch of hospital medicine must undergo postgraduate training in two stages: (1) the graduate will enter into general professional training for three years as a junior member on the staff of a clinical consultant (chief doctor) and will normally be expected to pass, either during or at the end of that period, an examination by one of the specialist Royal Colleges; (2) next the graduate undergoes a higher professional training as a senior registrar, normally lasting four years, when he can apply for a "Certificate of Specialised Training" and his name will be entered by the General Medical Council onto an appropriate list established in Britain, conforming to the directives issued by the European Economic Commission.

Only when both postgraduate stages have been completed can the graduate apply for a post as consultant—as an independent specialist in a clinical department in a National Health Service hospital. The minimum age for this post is thirty years, but most achieve it much later.

The organisation of postgraduate studies has been considerably formalised and strengthened during the last ten years. The Central Council for Post Graduate Medical Education, established in 1972, works through regional committees that are linked with the local universities through a postgraduate medical dean. The latter in turn now appoints consultants working in major hospitals in the region as post graduate medical tutors who can carry out their educational functions in the post graduate medical centres, which are found in all district general hospitals. About 300 of these centres have been built through private donations and public funds. This expansion has also brought a new interest in continuing education for fully-trained practising doctors, allowing them to retain their competence to practice.

A number of experiments are taking place all over the country, including also training programmes about the structure, administration, and finance of the National Health Service.

Financial Integration

The average cost of training an undergraduate medical student from university entrance to MB graduation was estimated at £95,000 in 1980–81. The broad principle has been accepted that the universities will pay for the academic training of the medical students, whereas the National Health Service is responsible for their professional postgraduate training. The students' teachers are a mixture of full-time academics and NHS consultants who devote some of their time to lecturing and to ward rounds.

University financing entails cover of (1) current expenses: The universities completely finance the salaries of full-time academic staffs of their medical faculties; it is assumed that work performed by the university-paid academic staff for the National Health Service will be broadly compensated for by the part-time teaching role performed by NHS-appointed clinical staff; and (2) capital expenditure: Funds for medical school buildings, which are usually physically distinct from the hospital, are entirely furnished by the universities. On the other hand, National Health Service financing provides for the following. (1) Undergraduate teaching: Finance of the costs arising from the provision of educational facilities has long aroused considerable controversy. As recommended by the RAWP committee, a service increment for teaching (SIFT) has been introduced since 1975 for those hospitals that accept clinical undergraduate students, because the cost of treating patients in teaching hospitals is higher than the cost of similar treatment in the rest of the NHS. In 1977 this cost amounted to a global sum of £100 million, accumulated on the basis of about £10,000 per student. (2) Postgraduate training: The NHS pays the salaries of junior medical staff under training, including those who undergo the so-called preregistration training between the completion of the undergraduate studies and the start of their vocational training. (3) Capital expenditure: All expenditures for building and maintenance of hospitals, as well as the necessary equipment used by the NHS, are paid by the Department of Health and Social Security.

Key Issues

How Many Doctors Should Be Trained?

Since the 1940s a number of committees have tried to advise on the number of doctors to be trained. All came to very different conclusions. In particular, the Willink Committee recommended in the mid-1950s a substantial reduction in the intake of medical schools, as at that time many medical organisations expressed a fear of possible unemployment among doctors. The Todd Committee in 1968 reversed this recommendation, advising the government to train a larger number of doctors; as a result, the government decided to increase the number of medical students rapidly in the late 1960s. The figure was based on the capacity of the existing medical schools and the three new ones, which began to admit students in the 1970s.

Curriculum Content

There has been some criticism of the medical curriculum as being inappropriate for the needs of the NHS. Following experiments begun in the United States, British medical schools have also attempted to modernise their curricula. Two attempts are especially noteworthy: (1) by reducing the compulsory part of the curriculum, it is now possible to offer students opportunities for special studies in greater depth; and (2) interdisciplinary teaching, or, as it is often called, "topic teaching," has been introduced.

Issues in Vocational Training

A Balance Between Education and Training

The General Medical Council has warned about excessively burdening the doctor in training with routine activities—making him a pair of hands—to the neglect of his further education. The GMC demanded, therefore, that all training posts, particularly at the preregistration level, " . . . should be regularly supervised, and the holders of the posts should also receive regular supervision of an *educational* nature. . . . The educational nature of the post should be fully understood and accepted by all concerned, and the student should be allowed at least six hours weekly for educational purposes, apart from his free time." This prescription, however, "is more honoured in the breach than in the observance."

The Competing Claims of Training and Service

Young doctors have traditionally been attracted during their training years to the famous teaching hospitals. In recent years this situation has changed because of an increase in the number of medical students under training. Medical schools have been forced to send their students further out into the field by making use of the normal district general hospital. At the postgraduate level this eventually led to the introduction of "rotating residences," where the young doctor in training serves his traineeship alternately in teaching hospitals and district general hospitals, thus having an opportunity to see both the academic practise of medicine in the teaching hospital and the essentially service-oriented practice—which has been termed the pathological reality—in the nonteaching hospital.

Continued Competence to Practice Questioned

The need for continuing education to acquaint the doctor with new knowledge and technology has become more and more compelling. However, the issue of relicensing at predetermined intervals is not yet practical politics. On the other hand, the need for recurrent (continuing) education is more and more acknowledged, and various institutions have already been created to cope with the issues involved.

CONCLUSIONS

It has been mentioned that the underlying concept of the National Health Service is to provide a mechanism for people to pay for health services when they are well and working, so that they can use them virtually free of charge when they are ill and not working. The structure of the NHS is based on regions for planning and resource allocation, with the provision of the service based on districts. This structure was used to distribute resources, particularly medical specialties, and produce an integrated health service that would cover the full range of health services. The resulting organisation is one of the biggest nonmilitary organisations in the world, working in general practices and the community and in 2,000 hospitals of all sizes and ages, some of which were built over a hundred years ago and are spread unevenly throughout the country. The NHS is required by statute to consult the different interests working in the service and is democratically controlled by lay members appointed to authorities, who supervise the workings of the service.

An underlying principle of the original act which set up the NHS was equality of distribution, both geographic and between social classes, but this, though much better now than in 1948, is still far from being achieved. There are great differences in the impact of the NHS on different social groups in society; some argue that the middle classes have gained most from the NHS because they have learnt to use the service better. Attempts have been made to spend more on certain groups of patients—the "cinderella services," for example—but those attempts have met resistance and have not been very successful. All these factors combine in the inner cities to make the problems of providing medical care there, particularly primary care, one of the most pressing for the NHS.

Difficulties also arise in the transfer of money from one area, one group, one type of treatment, and one type of service to another. Employees cannot just be sacked or retrained; it takes time, money, and persuasion to change. What the central department can achieve is limited. What seems to outsiders like one big monolithic system, with the DHSS at the top directing what happens, is in fact a very decentralised system with power spread among many. The government's main means of control is over money, and this is a very imprecise means of direction. However, the DHSS and the NHS are responding to the challenge with new methods of financial control and evaluation.

Current Pressures on the Health Service

In a time of increasing financial stringency, the NHS is facing greater demand from an ageing population, particularly from the very old, where demands on health services are particularly great. Medical technology continues to develop and make the provision of new types of treatment possible, but the expense is always greater. Moreover, people are now less prepared to suffer minor ailments. Affluence and medicine's success early in the century have increased people's expectations.

Since 1948 the number of patients treated has consistently increased and there has been a small improvement in life expectancy, but the greatest impact of the NHS has probably been on the morbidity of the population. International comparisons show that although England spends relatively little and has fewer doctors, nurses, and hospital beds compared to other industrial countries, and although there is much room for improvement, the health of the English people measured by its life expectancy and infant mortality is far from the bottom of the league.

The NHS is nowhere near perfect. Although the occasional polls tell that the vast majority of the public support the NHS (much more so than other government institutions) and patients are generally satisfied with the treatment they receive, there is increasing public concern about the NHS, particularly about waiting list and admission policies for certain conditions, the manner of some doctors, the daily regime of some hospitals, and, for a few patients, the treatment provided. However, even the fallibility of individual doctors or of hospitals does not seem to undermine the public's faith in the NHS as an institution. This faith is revealed in the relatively small number of people who choose to take out private insurance to cover even limited additional medical costs and the generally high public appreciation of the professions of medicine and nursing.

There is often low morale in the service, particularly among the medical staff (who are among the service's most ardent critics) focussing on the quality of care they provide and its poor financing and their modest pay. Certainly by some international standards, doctors in England are poorly paid. Whether this is true after allowing for the low cost of medical education in England and the value of the doctors' NHS pensions is not clear, but high salaries abroad are associated with the extravagant financing of health services in other countries; by English standards, doctors are among the best paid.

Industrial relations have become more difficult in the last ten years. Now many more employees belong to unions and there are many more industrial disputes. One has only to realise that there are forty-six unions looking after the interests of NHS employees, and that the NHS cannot close down a hospital and move elsewhere, to see the problem. Money is short and hospital buildings are neglected, yet, as in every organisation, money is wasted. Unfortunately, the concept of district self-sufficiency is taken to such an extent, particularly in the large urban conurbations, that unnecessary duplication and waste result. The main waste occurs in the areas of clinical decision making in the acute hospitals on such matters as length of stay and consensus on clinical policies. The basic reasons for this are inadequate information and inadequate research and the lack of an effective medical executive in many hospitals. Regular review of outcome is the exception rather than the rule. There is a desparate need for greater effectiveness and efficiency of clinician's decision making.

If, as seems probable, the major investment in the health service has been relatively ineffective in raising health standards, the investment might have been directed at the wrong section of the population and the wrong technology might have been used in the wrong places. While the NHS may not have succeeded in achieving an equitable distribution, it is at least in a position to seek for effectiveness and equality, which other health care systems cannot do.

At a more fundamental level, as Iván Illich reminds us, the NHS has mistaken medical treatment for health care. The NHS concerns itself primarily with disease that is susceptible to medical diagnosis and will be conquered, or at least controlled, by medical intervention. When the curable has been cured and the preventable has been prevented, there is still a good deal left. And what is needed is care. The NHS needs to change to cope with this and should develop prevention and care more effectively.

Attempts made to adapt the NHS have not been greatly successful. Such proposed changes strike at the professional structure of the service and meet deep resistance. The greatest single weakness of the NHS is its largely passive primary care service. Much modern disease is of a type that it is too late when the patient enters the surgery. However, such problems are common to all countries, and at least the NHS is an organisation within which it is possible to tackle such problems—many other countries lack such an organisation. The NHS has many strengths; the quality of the medical and nursing professions is high and the primary care system—while it could be more pro-active, together with the outpatient clinics—provides an effective service for those who seek it. Its financial control system and "monopolist" position does control costs much more effectively than such devices in other systems. The administrative costs of the NHS are low. Its cash limits system provides an incentive for staff to seek efficiency savings. There is a general avoidance of extravagance and duplication of facilities, and the use of medical manpower is probably more efficient than in other countries. The salaried position of hospital doctors removes any financial involvement for them and so they have no incentive to "over provide" services. A salary and consultant status allows hospital doctors in the NHS a great deal of freedom to do their work as they wish.

There have been a number of significant improvements in services to patients: continuity of care between hospital and community services has strengthened since 1974; services for the elderly, the mentally ill, and the mentally handicapped have been improved and expanded, as has been primary health care; activity in acute hospitals has more than kept pace with increased demands; resources are now more evenly distributed; the average cost of acute care has fallen, as has perinatal mortality. But probably the greatest achievement of the Health Service remains the removal for the population of the financial fears of illness.

The Health Service has managed to retain its simple principle: everyone who is ill has the right, irrespective of his means, to whatever treatment is available. Although this treatment may not be the best and the latest, there is no evidence to suggest that anyone is ever denied medical care because of financial circumstances. Perhaps after more than thirty years we are beginning to take the achievements of the NHS for granted; many now do not remember what went before.

The goal is to design a financial system and an organisation which will achieve social equity while it benefits from competition and guards against the dangers of a monopoly organisation and the power of monopoly labour. Given the nature of the need for health services, the general belief that no group in society should be at a great disadvantage in receiving health care, and the realities of the distribution of wealth and income, it has proved difficult to find a better system than the NHS for providing health care.

The remarkable changes that have occurred over the past thirty years make predictions about the next thirty difficult. It is probably prudent, however, not to expect major changes in the next ten years. Private practice will remain; it may increase if more people become eligible for private care—but even if it doubled it would remain small in comparison to the NHS, and although it may affect the NHS in detail, it will leave the service largely undisturbed. There will be no radical changes in financing the service, and if it is financed by taxation, there has to be political accountability—therefore, that role of the government will remain. The NHS is now committed to planning and to making decisions about priorities. Planning thus far has given priority to prevention, development of services for disadvantaged groups, and community services; since resources are likely to allow at best only modest expansion of NHS for some years, giving priority to these services implies that others, particularly acute hospital care, will have less chance for expansion or may have to achieve any developments through economies elsewhere within their own sector. Medical audit and clinical reviews will become more widespread, as will clinical budgets, in an attempt to reduce costs and distribute the limited resources. For a few years at least the NHS must concentrate on getting better value from the money it now spends, rather than on planning to absorb a greater proportion of the nation's resources.

There may be attempts made to improve aspects of prevention by associating acceptable health behavior with government-financed reward. Questions in ethics of treatment will be more numerous with financial stringency. Problems with the medical career structure will increase. The doctors' working relationships with other staff, particularly nurses, will change, and more doctors will work as a member of a team.

There are many imperfections in the NHS, but it is a vast, complicated, highly decentralised organisation, working with advanced technologies, limited in its actions by the legal requirements of consultation and democracy, employing professions that abide by ancient traditions and practises, and further limited by finance and political accountability. It is a marvel it works as well as it does, and it is very good value for money. Despite its shortcomings, the NHS seems to be a permanent, popular part of the welfare state. Despite some murmurings, no government would or could abolish it, and many would agree with the architect of the NHS who called the service "the most civilised achievement of modern government."

Further Reading

Allen, D.E., and D.S. Grimes, eds. *Management for Clinicians.* London: Pitmans Ltd, 1982.

Chaplin, M.W., ed. *Health Care in the United Kingdom.* London: Klumar Medical Ltd., 1982.

Report of the Royal Commission on the National Health Service, Commd 7615, London, HMSO 1979.

Table 1 Population of England by age and sex, 1980

Age	Number (in Thousands) Male	Female
All ages	22,638	23,828
Under 1	309	295
1 to 4	1,124	1,066
5 to 14	3,552	3,364
15 to 44	9,819	9,535
45 to 64	5,087	5,320
65 to 74	1,894	2,452
75 and over	853	1,799

SOURCE: *Health and Personal Social Services Statistics for England, 1982,* HMSO, 1982.

NOTE: Data are estimates of home population.

Table 2 Live births and birth rates in England

	Live Births	Birth Rate[a]
1976	550,383	11.9
1977	536,953	11.6
1978	562,598	12.1
1979	601,316	13.0
1980	618,371	13.3

SOURCE: *Health and Personal Social Services Statistics for England, 1982,* HMSO, 1982.

NOTE: Rates on an annual basis.

[a]Per 1,000 population.

Table 3 Infant mortality rates by age, England

Year	Under 1 Year	28 Days to 11 Months	Under 28 Days
1971	17.5	5.9	11.6
1972	17.2	5.6	11.6
1973	16.9	5.8	11.1
1974	16.3	5.3	11.0
1975	15.7	5.0	10.7
1976	14.2	4.5	9.7
1977	13.7	4.5	9.2
1978	13.1	4.4	8.7
1979	12.8	4.6	8.2
1980	12.0	4.4	7.6

SOURCE: *Health and Personal Social Services Statistics for England, 1982,* HMSO, 1982.

Table 4 Deaths by cause and sex under 1 year, England

Mortality List Number[a]	Cause of Death		1979	1980
F01–F56	All causes (001–999)	M	4,721	4,458
		F	3,440	3,425
F01–F07	Infectious and parasitic diseases (001–139)	M	92	60
		F	63	64
F08–F17	Neoplasms (140–239)	M	18	17
		F	17	26
F08–F14	Malignant neoplasm (140–208)	M	14	
		F	11	
F15–F17	Benign, in situ, other, and unspecified neoplasm (210–239)	M	4	6
		F	6	11
F18–F19	Endocrine, metabolic, nutritional diseases and immunity disorders (240–279)	M	30	37
		F	20	34
F20	Diseases of blood and blood-forming organs (280–289)	M	19	11
		F	10	7
F21	Mental disorders (290–319)	M	1	—
		F	—	—
F22–F24	Diseases of nervous system and sense organs (320–389)	M	99	89
		F	75	63
F25–F30	Diseases of circulatory system (390–459)	M	40	40
		F	38	33
F31–F32	Diseases of the respiratory system (460–519)	M	540	451
		F	384	350
F33–F34	Diseases of the digestive system (520–579)	M	48	66
		F	24	39
F35–F37	Diseases of the genito-urinary system (580–629)	M	19	14
		F	8	13
F42	Diseases of the skin and subcutaneous tissue (680–709)	M	1	1
		F	—	—
F43	Diseases of the musculo-skeletal system and connective tissue (710–739)	M	1	1
		F	1	—
F44	Congenital anomalies (740–759)	M	1,101	1,100
		F	984	1,012
F45	Conditions originating in the perinatal period (760–779)	M	2,061	1,860
		F	1,353	1,283
F46	Signs, symptoms, and ill-defined conditions (780–799)	M	520	626
		F	363	406
F47–F56	Injury and poisoning (800–999)	M	141	97
		F	100	95

SOURCE: Mortality Statistics–OPCS, Series DH3–OPCS, 1980+81.

[a]Mortality list numbers are those set out on pages 757–58 of the *International Classification of Diseases, Injuries, and Causes of Death, 1975.* The "F" prefix and the further breakdown of selected numbers have been added by the Office of Population Censuses and Surveys; the corresponding numbers in the full ICD list are shown in brackets after the description of the cause.

Table 5a Death rates for males per 100,000 population for England and Wales

Cause of Death	ICD	1961 Rate	1977 Rank	1977 Rate	1978 Rank	1978 Rate	%
All causes		1,260		1,210		1,240	100
Ischaemic heart disease	410–414	297	1	374	1	386	31
Cerebro vascular disease	430–438	—	2	116	2	117	9
Lung cancer	162	87	3	112	3	112	9
Pneumonia	480–486	63	4	91	4	91	7
Bronchitis	490–493	101	5	71	5	72	6
Stomach cancer	151	—	6	28	6	28	2
Motor vehicle accident	E810–829	22	8	17	7	20	2
Intestinal cancer	152–153	17	7	19	8	19	2
Hypertensive disease	401–405	32	9	14	9	13	1
Suicide	E950–959	13	10	10	10	10	1
Congenital abnormality	740–759	12	11	7	11	8	1
Accidental fall	E880–888	8	12	6	12	7	1
Undetermined accident	E980–989	—	13	3	13	3	0
Influenza	487	15	14	2	14	2	0
All other causes		—		340		352	30

SOURCE: Office of Population, Censuses, and Surveys, *Population Trends 19,* Spring 1980.

NOTE: Causes from the 9th revision of the *International Classification of Diseases,* 1975.

Table 5b Death rates for females per 100,000 population for England and Wales

Cause of Death	ICD	1961 Rate	1977 Rank	1977 Rate	1978 Rank	1978 Rate	%
All causes		1,140		1,140		1,150	100
Ischaemic heart disease	410–414	210	1	264	1	270	23
Cerebro vascular disease	430–438	—	2	181	2	180	15
Pneumonia	480–486	64	3	118	3	122	11
Breast cancer	174–175	39	4	47	4	47	4
Lung cancer	162	14	5	29	5	30	3
Bronchitis	490–493	36	6	25	6	26	2
Intestinal cancer	152–153	23	7	24	7	24	2
Stomach cancer	151	—	8	19	8	19	2
Hypertensive disease	401–405	41	9	16	9	15	1
Accidental fall	E880–888	14	10	13	10	12	1
Motor vehicle accident	E810–829	8	11	7	11	8	1
Congenital abnormality	740–759	11	11	7	12	7	1
Suicide	E950–959	9	13	6	13	6	1
Influenza	487	15	14	3	14	3	0
Undetermined accident	E980–989	—	14	3	14	3	0
All other causes						378	33

SOURCE: Office of Population, Censuses, and Surveys, *Population Trends 19,* Spring 1980.

NOTE: Causes from the 9th revision of the *International Classification of Diseases,* 1975.

Table 6 Operations per 100,000 population and mean duration of stay for selected operative procedures, 1978, England

	Estimated Operations	Mean Duration of Stay (Days)
All operations and procedures	4,063.3	9.0
Operation on lens	76.1	9.7
Incision of ear drum	49.8	2.7
Tonsils and adenoids	172.9	3.8
Operations on heart and intrathoracic vessels	48.1	12.3
Mastotomy and mastectomy	87.1	6.7
Operations on abdominal wall, peritoneum, and mesentery	109.9	12.7
Inguinal hernia operations	123.4	6.7
Operations on appendix	141.9	7.0
Operations on gall bladder	76.2	14.4
Cystoscopy (with destruction of lesion)	162.2	6.8
Prostatectomy	56.5	16.1
Hysterectomy	116.2	12.8
Diletation, curettage, biopsy, and excision of lesion of cervix	258.6	3.4
Postnatal or post-abortion operations	110.2	2.7
Treatment of fracture by operations	166.4	21.0
Anthroplasty	74.4	26.3
Operation on veins	58.6	5.5

SOURCE: *Hospital Inpatient Enquiry, 1978,* HMSO, 1981.

NOTE: Enquiry based on a one-in-ten sample of inpatient records for National Health Service hospitals of discharges and deaths (not individual patients). This is a condensed list.

Table 7 Discharges and mean duration of stay of sample cases of most frequent medical (nonsurgical) reasons for admission to hospital, 1978, England

		Estimated Per 100,000 Discharges	Mean Duration of Stay (Days)
All causes		4,092	13.6
A1–44	Infective and parasitic diseases	74	11.8
A45–58	Malignant neoplasms	294	15.4
A59–60	Neoplasms of lymphatic and haematopoietic tissues	34	12.5
A61	Benign neoplasms and neoplasms of unspecified nature	96	6.9
A62–66	Endocrine, nutritional, and metabolic disease	85	8.7
A67–68	Disease of blood and blood-forming organs	33	13.1
A69–71	Mental disorders	30	45.8
A72–74, 79 pt	Diseases of nervous system	88	39.4
A75–77, 79 pt	Diseases of eye	92	7.6
A78, 79 pt	Disease of ear and mastoid process	56	4.2
A80–84	Rheumatic fever, hypertensive disease and heart disease	256	19.2
A85–88	Diseases of peripheral circulatory system	215	39.4
A89–96	Diseases of respiratory system	345	10.6
A97–104	Diseases of digestive system	422	6.4
A105–108, 111 pt	Diseases of urinary system	67	10.6
A109, 111 pt	Male genital disorders	73	7.8
A110, 111 pt	Diseases of breast and female genital system	212	5.3
A112–118,[a] Y60–61	Condition of pregnancy, childbirth, and puerperium	131	3.3
A119–120	Diseases of skin and subcutaneous tissue	65	12.8
A121–125	Disease of musculoskeletal system and connective tissue	178	19.9
A126–130	Congenital anomaly	66	9.0
A131–135	Certain causes of perinatal morbidity	62	9.6
A136–137	Symptoms and ill-defined conditions	517	11.9
AN143–150	Other injury and reaction	329	4.9
AY43, Y40–52 rem, Y62–79	Persons undergoing preventive measures and those without current complaint or sickness	75	6.9

SOURCE: *Hospital Inpatient Enquiry, 1978,* HMSO, 1981.

NOTE: Enquiry based on a one-in-ten sample of inpatient records for National Health Service hospitals of discharges and deaths (not individual patients).

[a]There were no cases in the sample of A118 Delivery without mention of complication.

Table 8 Health care workers (work time equivalents), 1980, England

Occupation	W.t.e.
General medical practitioners	23,674
Hospital medical staff	31,421
Community health medical staff	2,821
General dental practitioners	12,415
Hospital nursing staff	308,815
Community nursing staff	33,800
Midwifery staff	20,260
Ophthalmic medical practitioners and opticians	7,636
Dieticians	715
Medical laboratory technicians	13,627
Occupational therapists	2,718
Physiotherapists	6,832
Speech therapists	1,548
Dental surgery assistants	2,976
Dental hygienists	98
Dental technicians	638
Occupational therapists	2,718
Chiropodists	2,068
Diagnostic radiographers	6,023
Biochemists	1,118
Pharmacists	2,614

SOURCE: *Health and Personal Social Service Statistics for England, 1980,* HMSO, 1982; and *Doctors, Nurses, and Midwives in the NHS,* Office of Health Economics, 1981.

Table 9 Operational medical schools, medical student intake and output by sex, and medical school graduates by sex, England

	1978–79	1979–80
Medical schools	26	26
Total medical students		
Intake	2,973	2,986
Output	2,609	2,676
Women medical students		
Intake	—	1,170 (39%)
Output	—	920 (34%)

SOURCE: *On the State of the Public Health, 1980,* DHSS, 1982.

Table 10 Ratios of medical doctors per population, England

	Total Medical Staff	Total Population (Millions)	Medical Staff Per 100,000 Population	Population Per Medical Staff
1972	47,084	46.3	102	983
1973	48,712	46.4	105	952
1974	49,496	46.4	107	937
1975	51,081	46.4	110	909
1976	52,382	46.4	113	885
1977	53,458	46.4	115	867
1980	57,916	46.4	125	801

SOURCE: *Health and Personal Social Service Statistics for England,* HMSO, 1980 and 1982.

Table 11 English hospital medical staff by specialty, 1981

Specialty	Number	W.t.e.
Total all specialties	34,218	32.141.7
General medicine	4,049	3,827.1
Clinical physiology	40	28.5
Nuclear medicine	38	33.7
Rheumatology and rehabilitation	435	394.9
Infectious diseases	81	76.4
Diseases of chest	438	404.1
Dermatology	354	312.2
Cardiology	319	281.6
Genito-urinary medicine	210	195.0
Nephrology	165	150.7
Geriatric medicine	1,453	1,422.4
Ophthalmology	986	890.1
Clinical pharmacology and therapeutics	80	42.1
Neurology	368	337.3
Clinical neurological physiology	64	54.3
Paediatrics	1,815	1,679.0
Paediatric neurology	14	11.6
Endocrinology	56	43.6
Gastroenterology	101	86.2
Medical oncology	71	61.0
Audiological medicine	14	12.0
Clinical genetics	31	22.8
Paediatric surgery	107	100.2
General surgery	3,378.3	3,410.1
Ear, nose, and throat	866	837.2
Traumatic and orthopaedic surgery	1,845	1,796.2
Accident and emergency	1,381	1,372.5
Urology	324	308.6
Plastic surgery	200	193.0
Cardio-thoracic surgery	318	308.0
Neurosurgery	234	226.4
Anaesthetics	3,747	3,597.3
Radiotherapy	406	383.1
Radiology	1,253	1,205.1
Obstetrics and gynaecology	2,475	2,358.5
General pathology	222	205.2
Chemical pathology	306	259.2
Haematology	605	538.6
Histopathology	766	663.5
Medical microbiology	407	321.8
Blood transfusion	78	67.1
Immuno-pathology	56	39.4
Neuropathology	50	36.8
Mental handicap	257	243.4
Mental illness	2,972	2,787.7
Child and adolescent psychiatry	407	361.2
Forensic psychiatry	31	25.6
Psychotherapy	115	84.1
Other	76	45.7

SOURCE: *Health and Personal Social Services Statistics, 1982,* HMSO, 1982.

Table 12a GPs' allowances, England

Revised rates of fees and allowances for general medical practitioners will mean average net remuneration at £18,990 for 1982–83 and reimbursement at average practice expenses at £9,260 per unrestricted principal. The actual remuneration of a doctor involves a combination of fees and allowances. Amounts payable from 1 April 1982 are

Basic Practice Allowance equals sum of the following:	
Full rate	£5.755 p.a. (per annum)
First 100 patients	£1,156 p.a.
Each patient above 100 up to 999	£5.11 p.a.
Leave payment	£1,151 p.a.
Additions (full rate) to the basic practice allowance in respect of	
Practice in a Designated Area	
Type 1	£1,795 p.a.
Type 2	£2,735 p.a.
Practice as a member of a group	£1,005 p.a.
Seniority[a]	
First payment	£1,385 p.a.
Second payment: a total of	£2,360 p.a.
Third payment: a total of	£3,740 p.a.
Vocational training[b]	£1,385 p.a.
Employment of an assistant (full time)	£2,695 p.a.
or	
Where the principal (or in a partnership all principals) receive(s) payment under Practice in a Designated Area	£3,770 p.a.

[a]First payment is made thirteen years after registration and five years of providing unrestricted general medical service. The second payment is made after an additional seven years of general medical service, and the third payment after an additional ten years.
[b]Vocational training is an extra payment for GPs who train GPs.

Table 12b Salary scales of hospital medical staff as of January 1982, England

Training grades	
House officer:	£6,180 per annum for the posts held during the first year; £6,580 per annum for posts held during the second year; £6,980 per annum for posts held during the third year and subsequent years to full registration.
Senior house officer:	£7,700 + £520 (1)[a] – £8,220 + £530 (1) £8,750
Registrar:	£8,730 + £440 (3) – £10,050 + £520 (1) £10,570
Senior registrar:	£10,050 + £530 (1) – £10,570 + £530 (1) – £11,100 + £520 (1) – £11,620 + £530 (1) – £12,150 + £520 (1) – £12,670
Consultant:	£17,370 + £1,220 (1) – £18,590 + £1,230 (2) – £21,050 + £1,220 (1) – £22,270

[a]Base salary plus annual increment. The number in parentheses shows the number of annual increments. Thus, for senior house officers, the base salary is £7,700. There are two annual increments, one at £520 and one at £530, yielding a maximum salary of £8,750.

Table 13 Hospitals, beds, admissions, average daily census, and occupancy rate by type of hospital, England

	Hospitals			Beds (Thousands)			Discharges and Deaths (Thousands)			Average Daily Census (Thousands)			Occupancy (%)		
Type of Hospital	1970	1977	1980	1970	1977	1980	1970	1977	1980	1970	1977	1980	1970	1977	1980
NHS total [a]	2,248	2,125	1,984	433	383	363	5,012	5,345	5,670	351	306	289	82	81	81
NHS psychiatric	334	404	424	172	134	124	191	197	208	161	129	119	84	88	87
NHS nonpsychiatric	1,914	1,721	1,560	260	248	238	4,820	5,148	5,461	190	177	170	78	77	74
Under 50 beds	777	793	727	21	20	18	—	—	—	—	—	—	—	—	—
50–249 beds	1,000	864	802	113	97	90	—	—	—	—	—	—	—	—	—
250–499 beds	251	244	239	89	87	87	—	—	—	—	—	—	—	—	—
500–999 beds	151	175	180	104	116	123	—	—	—	—	—	—	—	—	—
1000–1999 beds	63	49	36	91	61	43	—	—	—	—	—	—	—	—	—
2000 and over	5	0	0	13	0	0	—	—	—	—	—	—	—	—	—
Registered private [b]															
Hospitals and nursing homes	—	1,110	—	—	30	—	—	—	—	—	—	—	—	—	—
Acute hospitals	—	—	—	—	3	—	—	—	—	—	—	—	—	—	—

[a]Figures from *Personal Social Services Statistics for England, 1978* and *1982,* HMSO, 1980 and 1982.
[b]Figures from Royal Commission on the National Health Services, HMSO, 1979.

Table 14 Types of hospitals, England

Besides NHS hospitals, there are 10 military hospitals with about 2,300 beds paid for by the ministry of defence, some of which accept National Health Service patients. There are also 4 special hospitals, which accept psychiatric patients requiring special security, with about 2,300 beds. In 1977 there were 1,110 registered private hospitals and nursing homes with about 30,400 beds. About 73% of these beds were used for medical patients, 15% for surgical, 11% for mental health, and 2% for maternity; however, these classifications are not exclusive and some beds were used for more than one purpose.

SOURCE: *Hospital and Health Services Yearbook, 1980,* and Royal Commission on the National Health Services, HMSO, 1979.

Table 15 Information not available.

Table 16 NHS hospital inpatient and outpatient unit costs, 1980–81, England

	Cost in £s
Cost per inpatient week	
Teaching hospitals (acute)	
London	637.34
Outside of London	532.92
Nonteaching hospitals	
Acute	433.45
Mainly acute	401.32
Chronic sick	200.13
Maternity	462.00
Mental illness	176.52
Mental handicap	152.79
Cost per inpatient case[a]	
Teaching hospitals (acute)	
London	885.73
Outside of London	636.48
Nonteaching hospitals	
Acute	531.71
Mainly acute	601.05
Maternity	372.38
Cost per outpatient attendance	
Teaching hospitals (acute)	
London	27.01
Outside of London	19.42
Nonteaching hospitals	
Acute (with more than 100 beds)	17.13
Mainly acute	17.57
Cost per outpatient case	
Teaching hospitals (acute)	
London	136.55
Outside of London	89.00
Nonteaching hospitals	
Acute (with more than 100 beds)	72.63
Mainly acute	77.36

SOURCE: *Health and Personal Social Services Statistics, 1982,* HMSO, 1982.

[a]Computed only for types of hospitals that have a relatively short average length of stay per inpatient case.

Table 17a National health and personal social services: sources of finance for 1980–81, England

Source	£s (Millions)	%
All services	11,897	100.0
Central government services	10,004	84.1
Consolidated fund	8,871	74.6
NHS contributions	853	7.2
Charges to recipients[a]	250	2.1
Miscellaneous	30	0.2
Personal social services	1,893	15.9
Rates and consolidated fund grants	1,616	13.6
Charges to recipients[a]	277	2.3

SOURCE: *Health and Personal Social Services Statistics, 1982,* HMSO, 1982.

[a]See Table 17b.

Table 17b National health and personal social services charges to persons using the services in 1980–81, England

Services	£s (Millions)
All services	527
Health services	250
Hospital	54
Pharmaceutical	71
General dental	96
General ophthalmic	29
Welfare foods	0
Personal social services	277

SOURCE: *Health and Personal Social Services Statistics,* HMSO, 1982.

Table 18a National health expenditure, year ending 31 March, England

	1975–76		1980–1981	
	£ (Millions)	%	£ (Millions)	%
All services	5,406	100.0	11,897	100.0
Per capita	£116		£256	
Central government services[a]	4,537	83.9	10,000	84.1
Per capita	£98		£216	
Central administration	34	0.6	60	0.5
Health authorities[b,c]				
current	3,129	57.9	6,924	58.2
capital	332	6.1	556	4.7
General medical	280	5.2	619	5.2
Per capita	£6		£13	
Pharmaceutical	390	7.2	975	8.2
Per capita	£8		£21	
General dental	201	3.7	422	3.5
Per capita	£4		£9	
General ophthalmic	62	1.2	104	0.9
Per capita	£1		£2	
Welfare foods	13	0.2	28	0.2
Other[d]	96	1.8	316	2.7
Local authority services[b]				
Personal social services	869	16.1	1,893	15.9
Per capita	£19		£41	

SOURCE: *Health and Personal Social Services Statistics, 1982,* HMSO, 1982.

NOTE: Expenditure includes charges to persons using the services.

[a]The costs of the services provided by the central government contain varying factors (e.g., retrospective pay awards) that prevent them from being strictly comparable from one year to another.
[b]Excluding capital expenditure financed by loans.
[c]Includes (a) administration of family practitioner committee (formerly executive councils), (b) local authority health services, and (c) hospitals.
[d] Including hospitals directly administered by the Department of Health and Social Security, and supply and repair of artificial limbs and appliances.

Table 18b Regional health authorities: current (revenue) and capital expenditure year ending 31 March 1981, England

Units	All Expend-iture	All Revenue Expend-iture	Head-quarters Admini-stration	Hospital Services: Diagnosis and Treat-ment	Hospital Services: Support Services	Community Health Services: Diagnosis and Treat-ment	Community Health Services: Support Services	General Medical Services	Pharma-ceutical Services	General Dental Services	General Ophthal-mic Services	Other Services (Revenue)	Capital Expend-iture
£Millions	9,427	8,864	358	3,564	1,039	472	125	624	942	335	77	325	563
Percentage	100.0	94.0	3.8	37.8	21.6	5.0	1.3	6.6	10.0	3.5	1.0	3.4	6.0

SOURCE: *Health and Personal Social Services Statistics, 1982,* HMSO, 1982.

Table 19 Information not available.

Table 20 Subscribers to private medical provident schemes in the United Kingdom

	1966	1979
Subscribers	700,000	1,300,000
% of population	1.3	2.3
Persons covered (millions)	1.5	2.75
% of population	2.5	6
Subscribers in group schemes	400,000	1,000,000
Individual subscribers	300,000	300,000
Subscription income at 1975 prices	£22m	£75m
Benefits paid at 1975 prices	£20m	£30m

SOURCE: *Social Trends II,* HMSO, 1981.

Health Services in France

Jean-François Lacronique

INTRODUCTION

With an area of 550,000 square kilometers (212,700 square miles) shaped roughly like a hexagon, France is the largest state in Western Europe. Its geographic situation makes it a crossing area between Northern and Southern Europe, and an open gate to the new world: it is bounded by Belgium, Germany, Luxembourg, Switzerland, Italy, and Spain.

The country is surrounded by three seas, the Nord, the Atlantic, and the Mediterranean. Its traditions and culture come from the Latin as well as from the Nordic, the Anglo-Saxon, and even the Arabic invasions, making France one of the most variable countries of the world. Fantastic contrasts can be observed within short distances, between agricultural and industrial regions, between plains and mountains, between rich and poor areas.

Despite the fact that less than 10% of the population lives from agriculture, the classic village stays the nucleus of the social organization—75% of the French live in urban areas, Paris being by far the largest one, with more than ten million people. The vast majority of the population are white and Catholic. France hosts about 4 million foreign workers, mostly from the Arab countries.

The Socio-Political Context

France has a tradition of instability in politics. After centuries of feudalism and despotism, it has been the cradle of democracy. However, after the bloody revolution of 1789, which gave rise to the First Republic, it adopted a new form of authoritarianism and a highly centralized system of government under the rule of Emperor Napoleon the First. This system is still prevalent, surviving many changes that brought, successively, kings, another emperor (Napoleon III), one brief communistic experience in Paris (the Commune of Paris in 1871), and many presidents of four republics.

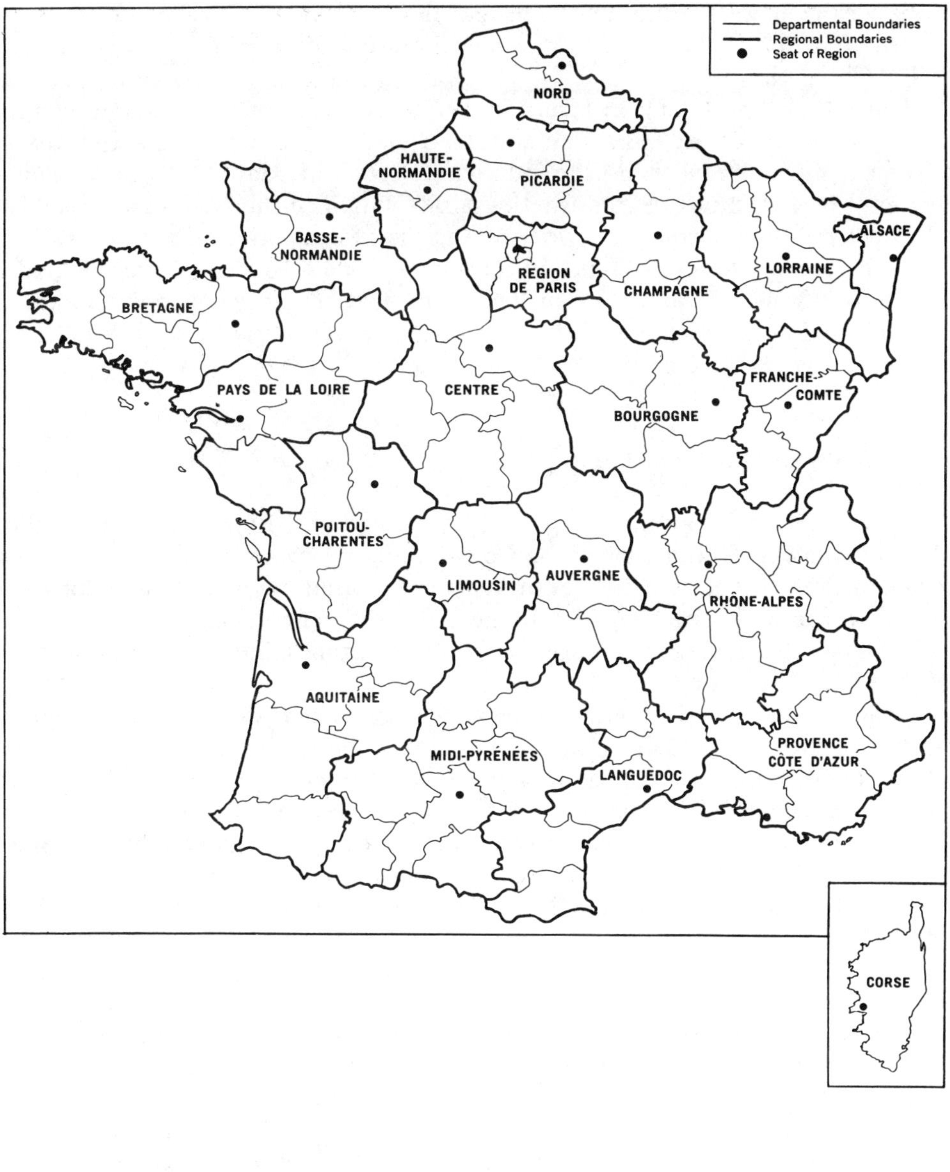

France has recently suffered dramatic wars that have destroyed many cities, taken many lives, and disorganized the economic life. The last war in which France was involved was the Algerian liberation war, which lasted until 1962 and ended a two-century period of imperialistic domination of overseas territories. France still has land in the Caribbean (the Antilles), the Pacific (Nouvelle Calédonie and Polynesia), the Asian Sea (La Réunion), and even in North America (Saint-Pierre et Miquelon). These territories are considered as French "Departements," which means that all the inhabitants hold a full French citizenship.

The political system has been a presidential democracy since the 1958 Constitution ended the Fourth Republic and started the "Gaullist" era: Gaullism meant a system based on the strong authority of the president, elected from full participation election and using referenda for the major political issues, instead of consulting the Parliament. It also meant nationalism (illustrated by the withdrawal of France from NATO), independence, and leadership within Europe.

President Charles de Gaulle resigned in 1970; his successor was Georges Pompidou, who died in 1974. Giscard d'Estaing was then elected president for seven years. His Socialist challenger, François Mitterand, was elected in May 1981, thus ending the Gaullist era. This election was followed by a dissolution of the National Assembly. The new chamber holds an absolute majority of Socialists for a period of five years.

Hence, the scene was set in France in the summer of 1981 for an unprecedented set of fundamental reforms, including one in the health field. The newly appointed minister of health, Jack Ralite, is a member of the French Communist party.

The Role of Central, Regional and Local Governments

Despite a long-lasting opposition to the system set by President de Gaulle, the new Socialist government did not change the Constitution, which gives the executive power to the president, who is elected for seven years. The prime minister is appointed by the president and can be changed by him at once. The cabinet comprises between thirty and forty ministers and secretaries of state, the most important ministers being called "ministers of state" (industry, interior, planning, justice).

The French Parliament has legislative power. It consists of two chambers: the National Assembly and the Senate. The National Assembly, where "deputies" meet, is the more important chamber in terms of political influence. The 491 deputies are elected directly by their constituencies for a period of five years. The Senate is smaller, with 298 senators serving terms of nine years. The senators are elected indirectly by representatives of the local bodies. This system explains why the majority at the Senate is still conservative after the 1981 election, in contrast with a Socialist majority at the National Assembly.

The prime minister proposes new laws to Parliament and can engage public expenditures. Parliament has a censuring power over the government's budget and development plans. However, a special article in the Constitution allows the prime minister to overrule a possible censure, thus guaranteeing a high level of stability to the government.

The administration is highly centralized in Paris. France is divided into ninety-five departments, each of which is administered by a "Commissaire of the Republic" (formerly called a prefect) appointed by the minister of the interior. The commissaire represents all the ministries and must also execute the policies established by the General Council of the department, an assembly elected in each department. A new law aimed at fostering decentralization was passed in 1982, giving this assembly extended powers, particularly over the local budget. The same law also gives new powers to the region, a congregation of several departments, usually associated by cultural or economic similarities. There are twenty-two regions in France, administered by a regional prefect and a regional council that have mostly planning powers.

The basic element of power is exerted by the municipalities, which are administered by an elected mayor and a council, voted in every six years. This council selects the mayor, who is the primary official executive responsible for the public health at the local level as well as for general local policy issues.

The Role of Public and Private Sectors

The French economy is a free enterprise system. As in most of the advanced countries, public funding plays a major role through financial aids, subsidiaries, and loans, and through a social protection system that covers the entire population.

Economic growth was rapid from after World War II until 1976, when it started to flat down and reached about 2% in 1981. The inflation rate has been high in the past five years, climbing to 15% in 1975. Unemployment rose to above 2 million people in 1981. This remains the major political problem facing the Socialist government, which was elected on a platform that gave full priority to a new rise of the national economy.

During the first year of Socialist government, emphasis was essentially placed on a reorientation of economic policy, giving priority to the fight against unemployment. To achieve this objective, the government placed its major thrust into stimulating the general market by elevating the purchasing power of consumers. An illustration of this policy has been the distribution of money to low-income families and the creation of 150,000 new civil servants' jobs, thus expanding the public sector. This policy was in marked contrast with the former government's orientation, which was committed to reducing the role of the administration and imposing a measure of "austerity" in economic life.

The expected outcome of the new policy was a general growth in consumption, which would allow the private sector to invest and thus create jobs. However, after one year of various incentives aimed at convincing private investors that the future was promising, the government realised, in May 1982, that the inflation rate was becoming a major problem and decided to take drastic measures to fight it.

In June 1982 the government decided to devalue the franc and decreed a three-month wage and price freeze. Despite the fact that it meant going back on agreed policies, both Socialists and Communists approved these measures. However, the general climate of confidence in the Socialist government that has prevailed since May 1981 has not been markedly affected. One reason for the lasting popularity lies in the fact that the Socialist government can still blame its predecessor for its "heritage" of the previous situation.

MEDICAL PRACTICE AND MEDICAL EDUCATION

The French health care system is characterised by its ambition to conciliate two major ideological orientations that are classically considered as contradictory. The first is egalitarianism as it is expressed in the preamble of the French Constitution: "The nation guarantees to all protection of health." According to this principle, any person can use any kind of health services under the same conditions. The second is liberalism, since the vast majority of the physicians still work in private practice—that is, they are paid directly on a fee-for-service basis by the patients, who are later reimbursed by the Social Security Administration.

Ambulatory Care and the Role of Medical Practitioners

The vast majority of ambulatory care in France is provided by private practitioners, generalists, and specialists. There is no limitation on access to any of these physicians, nor is there any limit to the prescription of care to the patient. The total freedoms of choosing one's physician, of prescription by the physician, and of setting up practice are three of the four basic principles upon which French liberal medicine is grounded. The fourth principle, freedom to negotiate fees, was abandoned in 1960 (following a decree of May 1960) when the de Gaulle government proposed to the medical profession a system of individual annual contracts (convention) with a fee schedule negotiated annually on a national basis.

In 1982 this system still prevailed, with 92% practitioner participation. Within this group of Medecins conventionné, 28% of the specialists and 5% of the generalists enjoy the privilege of being allowed to exceed the fee schedule because they are considered prestigious by a college of peers. There remains a small number of practioners (2%) who do not accept the "convention." Their patients are thus reimbursed at a very low rate (*tarif d'autorité*) intended to act as a deterrent.

The government in 1979 proposed an intermediate system that would extend the privilege of exceeding the fee schedule to anyone who asked for it, at the expense of a fiscal and social disadvantage. This provision was intended to satisfy those physicians who were penalised by the uniform fee system of payment because they must take more time in their practice (psychiatrists and acupuncturists, for example). There is little doubt that the new system was also intended to open up the possibility of shifting the burden of the rising costs of physicians' fees to the consumer, although it was never presented that way. Only 6% of physicians choose this "free fee sector" where the patient is reimbursed at a fixed rate that is the same as for conventionné physicians. The leading physicians' association, the Confederation des Syndicats Medecins Français (CSMF), fought bitterly against this system and found allies in the most leftist trade unions. Ultimately, during a demonstration in May 1980, police action illustrated the bitterness of the relationship between the Giscard d'Estaing government and the medical profession. Thus, it could have been expected that this "dual sector" would have been abandoned by the socialist government on the grounds that it paved the way to "medicine for the rich and another medicine for the poor." Surprisingly, there have been no attempts to question this system by either the present government or the physicians' associations.

As of January 1982 there were about 120,000 practicing physicians in France. (The number of practicing physicians varies according to the source of information, since there is no official census or registration.) About one-third of them have an exclusively liberal (private) practice; another third have a mixed practice, comprising a salaried part-time position and a liberal practice; the final group is made up of purely salaried doctors, either in hospitals or in other types of institutions. Among the institutions lastly mentioned are the *dispensaires,* or municipality health centres. There are 915 such centres (540 medical, 375 dental care), which are operated by local associations, trade unions, the Red Cross, the mutual aid societies, or municipalities. The originality in the management of these health centres lies in the fact that doctors are salaried, but the centre must be reimbursed by social security on a fee-for-service basis at a lower rate than for private practice (between 7 and 20% reduction) in order to have a fair competition with the private sector. Private practitioners have always been hostile to any expansion of these centres. The preamble of the 1976 Convention states clearly that the Social Security Administration will not create its own health centres; this point led to several months of negotiation.

Today, the discussion over the future of health centres has been reopened, since the Socialist government has declared that it favours the development of "integrated health centres," leaving the initiative of their creation to the local level.

Regulating the Manpower Supply

As has been noted, two-thirds of the registered physicians in France practice private medicine. This supply of physicians is generated by the medical faculties of universities and by teaching hospitals, which are under the oversight of both the education and health ministries. This supply is regulated principally in order to render the supply adequate to and not excessive of the population's need.

Even before 1960 there was concern over the number of doctors serving the French population. At that time young doctors were setting up fees at "bargain prices" to attract clients, creating wasteful competition to established doctors. This competition was severely criticised, particularly by the Associations des medecins, and it was suggested, for the first time, that there might be a surplus of physicians. It was not until twelve or thirteen years afterwards that the question of a surplus was brought up again; in the meantime efforts were even made to increase the supply of physicians.

After the implementation of the *politique conventionelle,* which guaranteed to patients high reimbursement percentages, the demand for health services grew faster than the supply. Despite the increase in annual capacity of medical schools from 4,000 new doctors to 6,000 in 1968, and although an act passed in 1971 embodied a selection procedure for admission to medical training, the general feeling at this time was that there was a shortage of physicians. New medical faculties of universities were thus opened, and the number of doctors per year rose between 1975 and 1980 to over 10,000.

Distributional Issues

While the number of new doctors per year was increasing, concern was expressed by many that such an increase would eventually lead to a surplus, particularly in the southern regions of France and in large cities. At first this concern was considered "conservative" and did not have much impact. In 1975, however, the minister of health proposed a rigorous policy for entrance into the second year of medical school. Despite bitter opposition from medical students, this policy was implemented, and each succeeding year the number of students entering the second year was reduced by 5%. The objective was to stabilize the growth rate of the medical population to aim for an upper limit of 170,000 (one physician per 400 inhabitants) by 1980. Implementation of this policy was not well received, especially since the accompanying reduction in the capacity of medical schools was adversely affecting the budget of these institutions. The leftist opposition was particularly adamant about the selection policy, claiming that it was tailored to the formation of an "elite" while there was a need for more doctors prepared to accept work in underserved areas.

Primarily because the government has always expressed its commitment to the four fundamental principles of the French health care system, the distribution of reduced manpower has not been well regulated: there are more doctors practicing in the south than in the north; there is a higher concentration in urban areas than in rural areas.

Although many solutions to correct this uneven distribution have been suggested during the past ten years, the only effort that has been made was the creation of an information centre intended to inspire doctors to choose an underserved area to set up practice. This centre provides information about underserved areas and about what a physician could expect when setting up practice in a given area.

An experimental centre was first installed in Aquitaine. Then, because students were satisfied with the service (although not so much because it was having a positive effect on the ill distribution of physicians), the government decided to make the information service nationwide. Apart from this effort, measures have not been taken to even out the distribution of physicians. The continued respect for the private practioner's right to establish practice when and where desired has been the main factor in the uneven distribution of physicians.

The new Socialist government has not yet taken measures to correct the distribution problem. Nor has the new government shown any intention of increasing the quota for admission to medical training, although before being elected to office, the Socialists and Communists were against a rationing policy. In 1981 Minister of Health Jack Ralite decided to leave the quota at 6,400 per year and make a thorough study of the population's needs for doctors' services. In June 1982 he decided to follow the line of his predecessors, and set the quota for medical schools at the level of 5,900 per year in 1983.

Medical Schools and Research

The medical schools are under the responsibility of the ministry of national education. There are thirty-seven medical schools in France, nine in the area of Paris alone. All are publicly owned schools and belong to the university system, but the medical schools, as well as the pharmacy school and the dental school, enjoy a privilege by being separate from the main system. According to this privilege, professors receive a second salary from the hospitals and are entitled to less teaching time than the other university professors. They are supposed to take care of patients in the hospitals and do research. One private medical school still remains, in Lille, owned by a private Catholic university, and there are two military schools of medicine. The students admitted to these schools must pass the same university exams as the other public school students.

There were 6,409 new students entering the medical schools in 1981; there were about 10,000 in 1975. This difference shows a concern for regulating the supply of medical doctors in France. A complete change in the curriculum of medical teaching is currently taking place. This change will meet the European requirements set up by the EEC in giving to all students a chance to intern in a hospital. A four-year period of postgraduate training, composed of hospital residency and university teaching, will be implemented. The current system is based on a separation between the hospital practice and the university courses, which sets the scene for heterogeneity in the quality of training of the young doctors.

Generalists and Specialists

There were about 109,000 physicians working in 1980: 48,000 general practitioners in private practice and 51,000 specialists, the majority of whom work jointly in a hospital and in a private office (table 11).

Access to specialists is not limited in France: a patient can consult directly any type of physician without referral. However, the specialists' fees are substantially higher than the GPs', and a sizeable number of the specialists have a policy of not accepting a new patient directly.

There has recently been a trend among medical students to undertake specialist training of three more years rather than start into practice right after the seven-year program of medical school. The consequence has been a decline in the prestige of general practice, enhanced by a half-price fee policy for the services provided in general practice. The government has set up a policy to reverse this trend by way of a proportionally higher increase in the fees of generalists compared to those of specialists. But the most important step in the upgrading of the GP's condition is the forthcoming "Reform of Medical Studies," which will give the future general practitioner a mandatory hospital internship of two years, in accordance with the EEC requirements.

France and Foreign Medical Graduates

Since 1979 an agreement has been signed by the ten EEC countries that allows all practitioners qualified in one country to set their practice in any other EEC country. So far, only a very limited number of foreign graduates from EEC countries have taken advantage of this opportunity.

France has traditionally been a country for refugees from all over the world. Recently, the number of physicians and medical researchers from Chile, Viet Nam, Iran, and from the Arab countries has dramatically increased, forcing the government to set the quota on FMGs at about 150 per year.

Group Practice in France

Although one can expect an oversupply of doctors to stir the need for practicing in groups, this form of practice is not currently developing in France. About 70% of the private practitioners work in solo practice. Among the remaining 30%, one-half only share their premises with another physician.

"Group practice"—consisting of not only sharing the equipment but working in a multidisciplinary spirit with secretaries, nurses, and other health practitioners—is limited to about 3 to 5% of the total. The financial crisis in the health field does not encourage this form of practice, since it increases the fixed cost of management of the group without compensation.

The Physician's Income

There is a growing nervosity among health professionals about the decline of their purchasing power, which has been publicly recognized. An average French GP had a net income of about 200,000 F (francs) per annum (the equivalent of 30,000 US$) in 1980; a specialist made 300,000 (46,000 US$). However, as one could expect, large variations are observed among practitioners in the same type of practice and between specialties. Ranging from 13% to 15% between 1978 and 1981, the rate of inflation has dramatically altered the income of physicians, whose fees were practically frozen during this period. According to the ministry of health, the combined effect of inflation and the evolution of activity has caused a net decline of 14% in the purchase power of the average physician within the past three years.

The Medical Associations

In 1978 the fiftieth anniversary of the creation of the first medical professional association was celebrated in a gloomy mood, in the midst of one of the most important crises that the organized profession ever crossed. Until 1960 the physicians in private practice had been free to set their own fees. The government tried to bargain with the unique "Confederation des Syndicats des Medecins Français" (CSMF) to accept a fee schedule that would guarantee a fixed percentage for the reimbursement of the price paid by patients to doctors. In May 1960 the government, then led by de Gaulle, forced the medical profession into accepting on a personal basis a national bargaining system for contracts of fixed fees. This system was adopted by a majority of practitioners, thus destroying the unity of the medical association; the CSMF became the government's partner in the negotiations, but a minority of opponents founded a rival association, the Federation des Medecins de France (FMF), that refused to negotiate. The division still remains, but the FMF now participates in the setting of the fee schedule, making it only a "matter of principle" that it is attached to the freedom of fee setting. As could be expected, the FMF strongly favored the "dual sector" policy installed in 1980 by the Giscard government.

The change in France's political life had an adverse effect on the activity of the professional trade unions: instead of stimulating the bargaining power with the associations, it placed them in a position of partnership with the new government as a reaction against the preceding government. However, the lasting freeze in the physician's fees forced the associations to show their distances from the Socialist policy. A large and strong demonstration took place in November 1981 to express the discontentment of the majority of health professionals.

There is little doubt that the strength of the professional associations has declined in the past three years, giving rise to the formation of many radical or ultraconservative groups.

HEALTH COSTS AND HEALTH INSURANCE

In order to achieve what may appear as an impossible compromise between commitments to public interest and to private initiative, the financing of health expenditures is assured through a mandatory health insurance scheme, which now covers in principle the whole of the French population. It was stated in 1945, when this system was created, that the social security in France would not merely work as an insurance for health-related risks, but also as a redistribution-of-income mechanism aimed at serving solidarity principles. This last objective was to be achieved by the fusion of the various regimes applicable to the different professional categories into a large and comprehensive insurance plan for every citizen. But this unification was not even attempted, thus leaving a very complex situation where traditional structures survive, mixed together with more modern concepts of health care organisation. However, 80% of the population belong to the "Regime General" of health insurance, which represents the model and the leader in the organization of the whole social security.

Economics

In 1975 the national health expenditure per person was 1,844 F, but by 1981 this figure had increased to 4,506 F. During the same period, the amount of the Gross National Product spent on health care increased from 6.7 to 7.8%. This rise signifies an average annual increase in health care expenditure of 16.8%. Understandably, such a sharp increase has caused considerable concern in the government and has stimulated efforts to identify its causes and control its rate of growth.

One of the most apparent reasons for the rise is the growth in the volume of activity in the health sector. Over the past few years, the volume of activity has been increasing at 7.2% per year. Contributing to this trend has been an increase in the availability of resources. During the past ten years, at least 20,000 new hospital beds were constructed in the public and private sectors, and the number of health professionals rose from 600,000 to 1.2 million. Growth of the general population (0.6% per year) and change in the structure of the population towards a greater percentage of elderly people also account for changes.

Perhaps the most important factor contributing to the growth in the volume of health care activity in France has been a increase in insurance coverage, especially within the last five years. Interestingly, this trend has been the result of a conscious governmental decision. Despite the obvious consequences to the growth rate of expenditure, the government has made efforts to step up coverage. First, a greater number of French citizens are covered by the health insurance scheme, and second, more services are now reimbursed by the insurance scheme. With the intent of assuring equal health protection to all, the national health insurance plan has progressed in recent years to cover the majority of the French population, including migrant workers. Similarly, the tendency has been for an increase in the kinds of services to be reimbursed by the insurance scheme. Although in some cases service coverage has actually decreased, a large number of services have received a greater percentage of coverage. This increased coverage has been a major factor in the rising volume of activity, primarily because it has motivated a greater demand for health care.

The other factors contributing to the rise in the growth rate of expenditure are related to prices. The average price increase per year during the past ten years has been close to 11%. This high percentage is, of course, partly due to inflation, though perhaps more important has been the arrival of modern technology. Facilities and equipment that are expensive to make and to use have resulted both directly and indirectly in price increases. Advanced technology has contributed to rising prices both because it has failed to provide substitutions of care and because it has resulted in a larger group of highly qualified personnel. In recent years nurses and other medical professionals have demanded higher wages, claiming that the level of their technical expertise merits higher pay. Supporting this claim is the tendency in most curricula to add more time for training doctors, nurses, and dentists.

Conversely, governmental efforts to control the escalating rate of expenditure have stepped up considerably in the last five or six years, with the dual policy of supplementing revenue and cutting back spending. Although there were indications even in the late 1960s that health costs and expenditure would pose a problem, the government did not take the issue seriously until five or six years ago. Indeed, it was only in the seventh five-year economic plan (the last to be drafted) that the health expenditure issues were even discussed. One method the government has adopted to cope with rising expenditure is to increase the working force's financial contributions, which is a viable solution in France because the health budget is entirely separate from the other social budgets. This means that when there is an increase in the demand for contributions to the health programs, people are aware that their increased contributions are going to the health budget and not to public budgets that they might not want to support. Hence, the government has been successful in demanding greater contributions based on salaries. It has also demanded that a differential rate be applicable to high-income and low-income workers. Until recently there was a relatively low ceiling in the health taxation system, which meant that high-income workers were paying similar amounts as those workers with lower incomes. Over the past few years, efforts have been made to raise this ceiling to make contributions more a function of direct income levels.

The other principal method by which the government has attempted to stem the tide of increasing costs in the health care system is by restricting spending. Most of the measures that could achieve this objective are still experimental. Although the trend has shown increased coverage, as was mentioned above, insurance for some services has been cut back. The distinction between vital and nonvital medicine, for example, has formed the basis for the policy of allocating insurance reimbursements. The change in reimbursement for the cost of drugs over the past five years is a case in point. Five years ago all medication was covered equally. Since then, laws have been passed that reduce the rate of reimbursement for drugs deemed "comfort drugs" and increase the rate for drugs considered "vital."

In fact, although the government feared that such a cutback could be interpreted as a first attempt to decrease the coverage, there has been very little controversy over this measure, which was extended a year later to a number of nonessential medications.

The government also took action by setting up a *Tableau statistique d'activité des practiciens,* which measured the volume of prescriptions to make physicians aware of how their dispensing compared to that of other physicians of similar status. It was originally proposed that there should be more direct control of prescription dispensing, but this was considered to be a transgression of the privacy rights of physicians.

HOSPITALS

Public and private hospitals are equally open to patients. In both cases, the patient participates by a moderate out-of-pocket payment; 30% co-payment is the limit for the first thirty days of hospitalization. This co-payment is, in most cases, reimbursed by an extra mutual-aid fund or is covered by a public sick fund reserved for low-income persons.

Thus, the most important part of the hospital expenses is covered by the social security, which reimburses the hospitals and the clinics directly. There is no limit to the utilization of the hospitals, and the control exerted by the social security can be considered as quite limited. There is, moreover, no financial incentive for the patient to choose one sector or the other. The main reasons for selecting the public or the private sector are cultural and technical: the public hospitals assure all the emergency care, and thus accommodate current cases as well as the most serious ones; the private clinics are organized to accommodate scheduled surgery and maternity, and cases of middle-ranking gravity.

Although the representatives of the two sectors would deny it, that the low-income families would go more to the public hospitals and the high-income families to the other hospitals has been proven. However, for the most serious cases, or for highly specialized care, the quality of medical care provided in the public sector is quite high and can be compared with the most advanced countries.

Types of Acute Hospitals

There is a large variety of types of hospitals in France. Schematically, most of the hospital care is carried out by government-owned institutions, but there is still an important proprietary sector, which is in competition with the public sector. The voluntary institutions represent only a minority sector, mostly specialized in the care of malignant diseases or run by charity institutions.

The ministry of health classifies the public hospitals into five types:

Regional university hospitals. These large institutions, Centres Hospitaliers Universitaires, or CHU, are located in cities where there are medical schools. There are twenty-eight such institutions in France. Some are composed of several large hospitals: in Paris alone, the CHU represent almost 40,000 beds, divided into forty-six hospitals, ranging from 600 to 1,600 beds.

These hospitals have highly specialized facilities and provide the tertiary level of care for each region. Although Paris is still a place where about 30% of the patients come from outside of the region, each regional centre can claim to have modern, sophisticated equipment that can accommodate any type of medical care.

Hospital centres. Located in the capital city of the department, these hospitals are not supposed to provide specialized care, but many of them do have tertiary care departments. Some are affiliated with a medical school and have interns and residents. There are about 100 of these hospital centres in France; 50% of them are brand new, constructed on a modular basis that allowed an industrial process to be utilized (*composants hospitaliers* type). These hospitals must have an emergency service that is on duty on a permanent basis, with a senior physician on the premises.

Local hospitals. These institutions are usually limited to basic care, provided by part-time physicians. Most are poorly equipped and accommodate elderly people and minor problems; some have maternity services. There are about 400 local hospitals in France.

Specialized hospitals. These institutions provide care for a special category of disease—tuberculosis, mental disorders, physical impairment, and so on. The large majority are psychiatric hospitals, of which some are gigantic in size, reaching 3,000 beds.

Rehabilitation hospitals. These centres aim at providing continuity in the care of patients who have undergone acute treatment. They can accommodate patients for rehabilitation after surgery or during addiction severage, alcoholism treatment, and mental problems.

Number and Capacity of Hospitals

In 1980 there were about 3,483 hospitals for acute care in France: 1,038 public institutions; 1,622 proprietary private institutions; and 823 nonprofit, voluntary private institutions. In terms of capacity, the public sector is prominent—a little more than 400,000 hospital beds in the public sector compared to 175,000 in the private sector; this is because the size of the institutions is very different from one sector to another, since 88% of the private clinics have less than 100 beds, as compared with 80% of the public hospitals having more than 200 beds (8% of the general hospitals in France have a capacity of over 1,000 beds). The relative importance of a strong private sector is thus an original characteristic of the French system. In the past ten years there has been fierce competition between the three sectors—proprietary, nonprofit, and public—with each sector trying to prove that its management provides better care for less money.

As a matter of fact, the evolution in the three sectors was very different during the 1970 to 1980 period; the capacity of the public hospitals increased by only 5,000 beds (up .4% per annum), whereas the private sector constructed 15,000 new beds but closed down about 250 small institutions (maternity mostly). The expenditures in the two sectors show also two different trends, with a 17.6% annual increase in the private sector as compared to a 21% growth in the public sector.

The volume of work performed in each sector, however, is quite different: the private clinics, with 28% of the total bed capacity, are responsible for about 39% of the number of acute hospital days, especially in surgery; the private sector has about 53% of the total surgical activity with 47% of the surgical bed capacity.

These facts have obviously led to some value judgements as regards the productivity of the two sectors; that kind of discussion, however, does underestimate the influence of the case mix, which is very different from one sector to another. Several studies have shown that the private proprietary hospitals perform more "medium range" operations, whereas the public hospitals have a commitment to accept minor operations (that are not well reimbursed) and to perform heavy and costly procedures (open heart surgery, intensive care, etc.). There is also an obvious differentiation among social and professional categories with regards to the selection of private versus public institutions, with a marked preference among high-resource families for private services. An additional factor makes comparisons between public and private sectors very hazardous: the pricing mechanism in each is fundamentally different. In the public hospitals the "hospital day price" is a comprehensive tariff that is calculated on the basis of an anticipated activity and adjusted for an economic hypothesis about the change in the prices of goods and services. It is different from one institution to another. The doctors are usually salaried, and their incomes are totally independent from their activities; with few exceptions, they display a total indifference concerning the price of the different services by the hospitals. The hospital day price in the private clinics is the same in all the institutions in a given regional area; it takes into account only the ancillary services of the clinic. The doctors are paid separately on a fee-for-service basis. Thus, the rules of the economic game are very much different, and any crude comparison is only speculative.

Still, it would not be fair to ignore the rate of growth of the public hospital expenditures, which is indisputably higher than that in the private sector. Moreover, it does not prevent the rise of general dissatisfaction among the health professionals who suffer from excessive workload, which expresses itself in high absenteeism (an average 12%) and occasional strikes and demonstrations.

Hospital Policies and Regulations

The French health administration is highly centralized, and the recent law enacted to decentralize the authority of the government does not include the health services.

It is thought that the solidarity principles that lead the spirit of the social security provides that all French citizens are entitled to the same duties and privileges regarding the funding of the system. Thus, the administration of the health services relies on a hierarchical system led by the ministry of health for its managerial component, and by the ministry of social affairs and national solidarity for its financial component. As can be expected, numerous coordination problems are caused by this double-headed authority.

Each department has a Departmental Directorate of Health and Social Services (DDASS), which serves as a branch of the two ministers, thus bringing about local coordination of the two national agencies. A DDASS can be composed of 200 to 600 civil servants, among which are several medical officers. It holds an authority over public as well as private hospitals, approves the budget, and sets the hospital-day rates.

Health facilities planning, coordination, and technical supervision are conducted at the regional level. Responsibility for decision making in each region rests with the regional prefect, who is advised by the regional director of health and social services (DRASS) and a regional hospital commission. The DRASS performs management advisory functions for the DDASS. It is also responsible for enforcing social security regulations.

The French health care system is still evolving as the regulatory efforts of the government gradually extend to the problem areas of the system. Each wave of governmental intervention and the accompanying legislation has been motivated by a different social condition or concern, with a general goal of offering better, more cost-effective care. Hence, the objectives of the French health care regulation are best presented chronologically, following the course of events since 1965.

The first major reform, the *Loi Debré,* was enacted in 1965 in an attempt to improve the quality of the professional staffs of public hospitals. It called for the affiliation of major hospitals and medical schools, and offered full-time positions at public hospitals to those physicians who would accept the triple function of teaching, practicing, and researching. One of the aims of this law was to upgrade the quality of hospital care by attracting the best possible practitioners to the public sector.

In keeping with this plan, full-time physicians were offered relatively high salaries, the possibility of receiving private patients in public hospitals, and attractive retirement plans. Between 1965 and 1980 more than 15,000 full-time positions were created, altering dramatically the character of French public hospitals. Hence, this law played a significant role in the transformation of public hospitals from the poorly-equipped charity institutions of the mid-1950s to the ultra-modern *centre hospitalier* of today.

The 1970 reform, the *Loi Hospitalière,* was intended to be the institutional equivalent of the *Loi Debré,* reorganising the administration and improving the facilities themselves. It had a fourfold objective: (1) to establish a means of assessing the needs of the population in order to organise a more equitable and sufficient distribution of health services; (2) to make each hospital more responsible for its management by giving directors wider administrative powers; (3) to set up norms for the construction and rehabilitation of facilities and equipment; and (4) to achieve a balance between the private and public sectors in order to avoid wasteful competition between them.

More precisely, the instruments created by the 1970 law were the following:

The planning of facilities. The creation or modification of any hospital bed (public or private) or of any costly equipment should be submitted for authorization by the ministry of health. This authorization would be delivered according to certain criteria, including national norms and local environment data (*carte sanitaire*). For example; "indices" of bed equipment were provisionally set up at 1.7 to 2.3 beds for 1,000 inhabitants for surgery and medicine, and from .4 to .6 beds for obstetrics and gynaecology. Within this range of concentration, each region would have established a regional map of the existing institutions and a plan for expected development in the area. A regional committee for the health equipment (Committee Regionale de l'Equipement-Sanitaire), composed of administrators of both public and private institutions and of representatives of the medical associations, has to advise on the planned equipment. Then, a succession of administrative steps involves the central administration (Direction des Hospitaux) and a national committee for health equipment (Commission Nationale de l'Equipement Sanitaire) and, finally, an approval from the minister of health.

The major objective of this part of the *Loi Hospitalière* has been to avoid costly duplication of equipment to correct the uneven distribution of health facilities. Thus, it has gained the reputation of a "negative" regulation since it has been used much more often to refuse an authorization rather than to facilitate the development of health equipment. However, the objective of the *carte sanitaire* has not been achieved and does not cover long-term care facilities and rehabilitation centres. These institutions are regulated by budgetary measures, set up by the social security administrators.

Costly equipment—such as telegamma therapy, linear accelerators, renal dialysis machines, nuclear medicine cameras, and scanners—are also regulated through the *carte sanitaire* mechanism. For each type of equipment a standard has been set in order to limit the natural tendency to overequip. For example, the diffusion of scanners has been largely limited in France since the standard was set at the level of one machine per million inhabitants. This level was reached in October 1980; at that time it was considered too low, and so was changed immediately to one machine per 600,000 inhabitants to meet the physicians' recommendations. This change in the planned distribution of scanners, however, had no immediate effect, and in 1981 only three new machines were installed, despite the legal authorization of thirty. A cutback in the budget explains this delay.

The management of hospitals. The *Loi Hospitalière* defines the rules for the internal management of the hospitals and establishes the respective responsibilities of the director (an administrator in most of the public hospitals and a physician in most of the nonprofit institutions, such as the oncology centres) and of the board of trustees (Conseil d'Administration), which is composed of representatives of local communities, local social security administrators, and staff members. It also creates a special medical advisory council (Commission médicale consultative, or CMC), which advises the director on the budget of the hospital and the functioning of the medical services.

In summary, this part of the law was intended to give much more initiative to the director and the hospital staff. It is indisputable that it works quite well, and the staff often shows a great deal of interest in the management of the hospital. However, the lasting complexity of the budget setting to a great extent limits this involvement to the sole power of criticism.

Hospital utilization regulations. The law provided that there would be a possibility of closing down hospital facilities if an institution (or a private clinic) failed to meet the criteria that were used to give the initial authorization for opening; for public institutions, the agreement of the board of trustees would be necessary. Thus, this provision of the law was never really applied, except in the case of severe incidents or accidents that could threaten the life of the patients. (Several hundred small maternity and some abortion clinics were closed down through this regulation.) In 1979 it became more and more apparent that the rate of growth of hospital expenditures was not compatible with the corresponding rate of growth of the social security financing. The newly appointed minister of health and social security announced on 25 July 1979 an "emergency plan" to alleviate the deficit of the social security budget. In summary, this plan was intended to fix "global objectives for growth" that would concern hospital care as well as ambulatory care; the objective was to set the rate of growth of expenditures very close to the rate of the GNP, since that rate was a good reflection of the resources available.

In order to complete this plan, a series of amendments to the *Loi Hospitalière* were voted. For example, a law passed on 31 December 1979 gave the minister a discretionary power to close down hospital beds considered as unnecessary (according to a mean rate of occupation inferior to 40%) without asking the approval of the institution's board of trustees. An estimated 7,000 hospital beds were thus scheduled to be suppressed. This new provision of the law was not well received and triggered a fury of criticisms from both the majority party and the opposition, since the mayors of the cities were the presidents of the boards of trustees. Thus, this measure was never really applied.

The search for an equilibrium between the public and the private sector. This last provision of the 1970 law was interpreted by several economists as creating a "legal chimera" by creating a "hospital public service" in which the private sector could be included. According to the law, conventions and contracts could be passed to involve the private clinics in taking care of emergency services or in the provision of specialized care.

In some instances, where the financial situation of the clinic was particularly unstable, the public sector has taken over the management of the private institution. However, despite an initial high interest in this provision of the law (447 private institutions obtained a right to participate in the "public service"), the general mood has been uncertainty rather than satisfaction, and it would be hard to find anyone who believes that the respective role of the public and the private sectors are well defined in the French health care system.

The recent change in the political orientation of the country did not modify the stand-still competition between the two sectors. Communist Minister Jack Ralite made it clear that he would not consider the private sector as "competitive," but rather as "complementary." When the question of the distribution of new scanners was aired, he stated that priority was given to the public sector because the needs of a machine could better be justified in large institutions. Thus, the first thirty-one new authorizations granted in 1981 were all intended for public hospitals. In March 1982, however, he made a reassuring gesture by giving four more authorizations to private clinics. Among those four, one concerns a large clinic in Le Havre, a municipality led by a Communist mayor who obviously would have preferred the machine to be allocated to the public hospital of his town.

Although of minor importance, this decision shows that the new Socialist government has no intention of questioning the existence of a private sector in the delivery of health services. In the *Charte de la Santé,* issued in mid-1982, a paragraph states clearly that "private institutions are an intimate part of the French system. . . ." The two associations of private hospitals reacted to the publication of the *Charte* not because of the content of the paragraph, but because it was considered too short as compared to the place devoted to the public sector. However, there has been an important change in the structure of public hospitals. According to the 1958 law creating "full-time staff positions" for physicians in public hospitals, there was a possibility of keeping a limited private practice within the public institutions. During the past ten years a series of abuses and scandals were reported; some physicians were deriving sizeable amounts of money from such private practice or were not declaring it to the Inland Revenue. There have been some past attempts to "regulate" these abuses, but the question of maintaining such a privilege was often raised on the political scene. During his campaign as a presidential candidate, François Mitterand committed himself to suppress the "private sector in the public hospitals."

Bitter negotiations took place during the fall of 1981, leading to the creation of an association of physicians called "Solidarité Medicale," (which is reminiscent of the Polish union against the Communist government). In June 1982, however, the final decision was made to withdraw the privilege of caring for private patients in public hospitals. This decision will be fully implemented in January 1986. To compensate for such a drawback, salaried physicians in public hospitals will receive better social insurance coverage and a more generous retirement plan.

Hospital Accreditation and Quality of Care

The French hospital system is controlled by professional inspectors who visit the premises on a regular basis and write reports to the minister of health. These inspectors advise the minister as to giving accreditation for the opening of an institution. There are a number of standards concerning the equipment and the personnel that can be used for such inspections. However, the conclusions are usually based much more on personal judgement than on rational and stringent considerations. There is a logical reason for this: more than one-half of the French hospitals are very old, historical constructions, and would not easily pass the criteria for modern equipment. There have been various experiments for control of the quality of medical care in France; but it has been decided that such measures will take place only on a voluntary basis, not systematically. In 1982 one could not say that any system of evaluation of the medical care was working in France.

A very discrete and mild control over utilization has been organized by the Social Security Administration, mostly based on a certification for admission. In the near future the global budget system is expected to destroy the incentive for overutilizations and abuses.

The Control of Hospitals

There is a regular control of hospitals in France. An initial accreditation is given by the minister of health, following the advice of the National Committee for Health Equipment.

This authorization classifies the hospital into a category of institution, enabling it to provide care that will be reimbursed by the social security.

Utilization of services is supervised by a special body of inspectors called "Praticiens-conseils de la Securité Sociale." These physicians number about 4,000, belong to the Social Security Administration, and come from all sectors of medicine. Because their positions are high paying, they are highly sought after. The overall professional reputation of this body of inspectors, however, is often questioned by the hospital doctors whom they are supposed to control. Their task consists of giving their approval to the full reimbursement (*prise en charge*) of any costly procedure or prolonged stay in the hospital. This system is cumbersome and sometimes causes delays since the authorization must be given before the act is performed. A new mechanism of computerized a posteriori approval is currently being tested on the basis of a "provisional length of stay" compatible with a probable diagnosis.

Apart from this system, which involves only the Social Security Administration, there is a control over the adequacy and the general conformity of the institutions with regard to standard of care. This control is imposed by the Medicins inspecteurs de la santé, a body of civil servants who belong to the ministry of health. These physicians are placed under the authority of the DDASS. They number about 300 and are not as well paid as the Praticiens-conseils, thus there is a dramatic scarcity of such inspectors and many positions stay unfilled, especially in remote areas. Their task is to survey the current activities of the different institutions. They work at random or when an incident or an accident occurs. In fact, they have very little time to organize any systematized control. At the national level, the Inspection General des Affaires Sociales (IGAS) represents a body of high-ranking inspectors, the majority of which are not physicians but administrators. They can give an expert opinion upon request or when an important issue is addressed. Every year the IGAS publishes a "special report" that is supposed to be the state of the act in a given area. For example, the 1980 report dealt with professionals in health, the 1979 report focused on the institutions of health, and health prevention services were the topic of the 1978 report.

On the administrative side, a periodic audit of hospitals, selected at random, is carried out by the Cour des Comptes, an independent body of finance experts who have jurisdictional power over the whole French administration.

EFFORTS TO CUT EXPENSES

In 1975 the oil crisis drew attention to the deficit in the health care budget. At that time social security was placed under the jurisdiction of the minister of health. Before this change the operation of health services had been separate from the source of resources, with little or no coordination between them. The continuous discrepancy between the growth rate of health care expenditure (and the corresponding rate of the insurance premium) and the stalling growth rate of the national economy was considered by the government as a source of potential problems.

The first response of the minister of health and social security was to advocate voluntary efforts to stem the growth of expenditure and to state that a limit would be determined on the proportion of "mandatory participation" demanded of the citizen. The actions that followed were of a more serious nature. Perhaps the most important action taken was the placing of a limit on the number of students entering medical schools. As noted earlier, steps were taken to contain costs in the pharmaceutical area by modifying the payment scheme and by trying to influence physician prescribing patterns.

In July 1979, after five years in government, Minister of Health and Social Security S. Veil resigned from her position. Together with Secretary of State J. Farge, the newly appointed minister, J. Barrot, consecrated efforts to find a solution to the persistent deficit in the health budget. An "emergency plan" ensued, which intended to link the future growth rate of health expenditure to the growth rate of the general economy. To achieve this goal, the government passed a series of *decrets*. The first of these gave to the minister of health the power to close down hospital beds. The second was intended to accelerate the decrease in the quota of students entering medical schools. Another, which stirred a very bitter controversy, aimed at forcing the *mutuelle* (private insurance) that covers co-payments to leave a small amount of the health bill to the consumer, thus making patients more cost-conscious. Although the principle of leaving some of the costs to the consumer was already embodied in the 1946 law that created the French social security, this decree was never implemented because the *mutuelles* succeeded in raising a strong enough wave of protest.

When the Socialist government came into power in May 1981, the newly appointed minister of national solidarity, Nicole Questiaux, made it clear that she "was not interested in accounting in the social sector." For one year the government acted as though there was no longer a financial crisis. A sizeable number of new jobs were created in the hospitals, and new heavy equipment (scanners, for example) were authorized. This era of welfare did not last more than one year. Minister Questiaux was forced to leave the government in June 1982, and a new minister, Monsieur Beregovoy, made a public statement upon taking office that the deficit of the social security would be solved by a drastic cutting down of expenses. Among the proposed measures were a cutback in certain services. A flat rate of co-payment to partially cover food and board in the hospital has been installed, as well as a special tax on alcohol and tobacco that will directly benefit the social security.

The most important proposed change, however, is the withdrawal of a fee-for-service system to reimburse the hospital; this is to be replaced by a global budget system. A deadline for the implementation of the new policy has been set at January of 1984.

PUBLIC HEALTH

In theory, public health is the responsibility of the ministry of health; however, there has always been discussion of this matter since in many instances the social security finances the public health programs. But the Social Security Administration is now placed under the responsibility of the ministry of social affairs and national solidarity, a newly created agency, and is separate from the ministry of health.

The history of the relationships between the administration of public health and the Social Security Administration has always been complex and full of conflict, at the local as well as the central level. Until March 1977 Social Security was a branch of the ministry of labor; this was so because the health risks insurance was considered a part of the fringe benefits that workers were entitled to. This separation between service providers and payers, however, paved the way for a high inflation in the sector, since neither the prescriptor of services nor the beneficiaries of them were cost-conscious.

In 1977 President d'Estaing reorganized the government and created one single and comprehensive ministry of health and social security, which was given a prominent ranking in the cabinet. This department was placed under the authority of Madame S. Veil, who stayed in office for more than three years—the longest period a health minister has lasted in office in the past twenty years.

Veil, a former lawyer, became very popular by proposing a law that legalized abortion in France. Bitterly attacked by her own political majority, she was thus supported by the opposition. She also started campaigns against cigarette smoking and alcoholism, and initiated legislation to control the safety and effectiveness of drugs. She left office in 1979 and was followed by Jacques Barrot and Secretary of State for Social Security Jean Farge. New public health programs were not among the priorities of this cabinet, which was committed mostly to reducing the escalating rate of health expenditures. However, special emphasis was placed on the fight against alcoholism, with the public announcement by President d'Estaing of a ten-year plan, which was given a special budget in 1980.

In May 1981 the ministry of health and social security was once again separated. The ministry of national solidarity was given the highest prestige and power, and received responsibility for social security. The ministry of health kept authority over hospitals and public health programs, and control of pharmaceuticals and medical research went under the responsibility of the ministry of research (which merged later with the ministry of industry). The ministry of education kept control of medical education.

Madame Questiaux, the new minister of national solidarity, announced when she came into office that she "was not interested in accounting"—meaning that she did not want to follow her predecessor's policy of cutting down public expenses, noticeably in health and for social matters. But she was not followed on that stand by the government and was forced to leave the cabinet after one year in office.

The new minister, P. Beregovoy, immediately established a plan to control the health expenditures, but basically this turned back to budgetary policy, limiting the acquisition of new equipment and the expansion of public jobs to a minimum. This brutal change started a crisis between the ministry of health and the newly appointed minister of social affairs, until President Mitterand forced the two ministers to make a public reconciliation in front of the press. The real implication of the divorce between the administrations of health and of social security, however, is the weakening of the health administration. Since most of the decisions taken by the ministry of health have budgetary implications, the Social Security Administration and the ministry of budget have the power to veto them, a situation which has arisen very often.

The ministry of health thus has very limited powers: its budget is almost entirely dedicated to "mandatory expenses" that comprise long-term programs such as those for maternal and child care, health education and prevention, rehabilitation, mental health, and others. Ninety percent of the 1981 health ministry budget was allocated to long-term budgeted programs, for which the minister has no choice but to continue. The remaining 10% is the only real budget that the ministry is free to allocate. In 1982 a sizeable portion of it, 200 millions francs, was placed on local programs for prevention through the creation of four pilot regions that were considered underserved: North, Languedoc-Roussillon, Center, and Alsace. In these regions a committee for the promotion of health, comprised mostly of trade union representatives, and consumers' associations were formed to encourage public health programs at the local level. No format for working nor requirements were imposed on these committees; they are free to choose their own rules.

Among the long-term mandatory public health programs, the most important are the following:

Sanitation and environment control. The ministry of health prepares the regulations on environmental hygiene in association with the ministry of environment. These regulations relate to safety of drinking water, recreational waters, improvement of sanitary conditions, housing standards, safety of foods, and poison control. The control of hygiene is, in principle, a responsibility of the commune, but the administration for implementing the programs is organized at the level of the department.

Communicable disease prevention. There are four compulsory immunizations in France: tetanus, diphtheria, poliomyelitis, and tuberculosis. There is also a network for prevention of tuberculosis and of sexually transmitted diseases.

Maternal and child health. Prematernal, maternal, and child care programs are entirely free: during her pregnancy, a woman (married or single, French or foreign) is entitled to seven prenatal examinations. The delivery is supported by social security, in public hospitals as well as in private clinics. A "maternity record" is then opened, which becomes the source of epidemiological information at the same time that it allows coverage by social security. During the postnatal period, 6,800 clinics for infants can give care free of charge. The budget for these Protection Maternelle et Infantile centres is supported by the ministry of health. About 7,000 physicians, 700 social workers, and 2,300 midwives are engaged in such a program. Recently, priority has been given to new activities, such as epidemiological research, training of personnel, family planning, and health education.

School health. Since 1945 there has been a school health service that provides systematic surveillance of children at the four key steps of their development (4, 7, 10, and 14 years). This service, composed of about 1,200 physicians, 2,500 nurses, and 1,500 social workers, was in a state of underdevelopment until the Left came to power in 1981. The new minister made clear his commitment to the development of the school health service by creating new positions in the areas that were particularly underserved. However, the mere increase in the number of practitioners did not change the conditions of the existing corps, which is almost entirely composed of women with relatively low salaries.

Health care for the elderly. Apart from the ordinary acute hospital level of care, old people have access to long-stay institutions, day-care centres, and home care services that are aimed at underloading the hospitals and providing better and more suitable care. A special secretary of state has the full responsibility for the promotion of health and social services for old people.

Mental health services. The major feature in the mental health program in France is the sectorisation, started in 1970 and aimed at providing services in the communities for mental patients, thus avoiding hospitalization. This system, which is supported in part by the hospitals, has shown its success over the past seven years. The new Socialist government has announced that it will start to close about 20,000 hospital beds in psychiatric institutions.

CONCLUSION

Under the pressure of political change the different medical professions were forced to waver between making services more accessible (especially in the public sector) and protecting liberal medicine. A subtle balance between public and private initiative has been so far preserved in almost all types of service and does not seem to be doomed by the new Socialist government, although the health sector was placed under the responsibility of a Communist minister.

In mid-1982 the government published the *Charte de la Santé* which is supposed to state all the political orientations in the health domaine. In the ambulatory care sector, it guarantees independence and freedom to private practitioners. It announces also that new experiences, like the health community centres will be encouraged. In the hospitalization sector, priority will be given to the "general hospitals," nonteaching hospitals. A reform in the hospital professions is scheduled on the basis of a unique statute for all salaried, full-time staff physicians. Finally, the *Charte* insists on the necessity to control health expenditures, saying that "the health system must be accountable to the nation. Any wasted money is a precious resource that is lost for the community, and also hinders efforts to heal someone somewhere . . . ."

In order to achieve the objective of control, the French government will develop instruments for evaluation, in the public as well as in the private sector, and will implement a budgetary policy for the hospitals. There have been few concrete changes in the functioning of the system; as already mentioned, the only major decision that has been made is the withdrawal of the authorization for full-time doctors to see private patients in the public hospitals. However, various other projects are currently underway and will undoubtedly raise some controversies next year. The most important reforms currently under discussion (which will then be presented under the form of a law) deal with the following issues: (1) emergency care, (2) postdoctoral training, (3) mental health, and (4) research administration. A new style of management has also emerged, which is characterized by a major participation of consultants from the trade unions and other associations.

The future of these reforms is hard to tell. A large majority of the medical community was far from being satisfied by the former government. The French health care system relies very much on a tacit compromise between state intervention and liberalism, and is thus very sensitive to any political instability. In October 1982 an impressive demonstration was organized by the doctors' association, displaying a large dissatisfaction with the current government. In December 1982 a new plan for placing a new budgetary policy for hospitals was accepted with a certain indifference, three months before an expected change in the cabinet composition.

Despite a major change in its political orientation, the French health system has not undergone any fundamental change in its structure and is working in conditions that are undoubtedly comparable to those that prevailed prior to the 1981 elections. This is a sign of stability and solidity, but it is also a sign of relative conservatism and traditionalism, two characteristics that could in the long run change drastically: the majority of the physicians will be under thirty-five years old in 1990, and their number is going to be excessive. Will the new structure in the health professions bring an end to what some people now refer to as the golden era, when there were no limits to the expansion in the sector? The majority of the French are pessimistic on that subject, as are most people in European countries.

Table 1 Population by age and sex, 1 January 1978, France

	Years			
	Less Than 20	20 to 64	Over 65	Total
Males	8,440,075	14,745,784	2,864,568	26,050,427
Females	8,077,959	14,574,100	4,479,030	23,131,089
Total				53,181,516

Table 2 Live births, marriage rate, birth rate, fertility rate, and life expectancy, 1980, France

Population	53,713,000
Live births	800,400
Marriage rate	6.2/1,000 inhabitants
Birth rate	14.9/1,000 inhabitants
Average number of children per woman (fecundity rate)	1.95
Life expectancy at birth	
Males	70.1
Females	78.3

Table 3 Infant mortality and neonatal mortality for selected years, France

Age	1960	1965	1970	1975	1980
Under 1 year	27.1	21.9	17.2	12.6	9.8
Under 28 days	—	27.7	22.5	16.7	13.5

Table 4 Infant mortality for six most common causes, 1979, France

	Males	Females	Total
Perinatal mortality (under 28 days)	1,224	883	2,107
Birth defects	845	683	1,528
Sudden death and dehydration	534	348	882
Accidents and poisoning	408	264	672
Infectious diseases	110	86	196
Respiratory diseases	92	69	161
Undefined causes	309	219	528
Total	3,522	2,552	6,074

Table 5 Fifteen leading causes of death, 1979, France

Causes	Deaths
Total	532,388
Cardio-vascular diseases	199,164
Cancer and malignant tumors	126,253
Accidents, poisoning, or violent deaths	49,959
Digestive track diseases	35,973
Respiratory diseases	31,452
Nutrition, metabolism diseases	13,214
Nervous system diseases	12,714
Genital and urinary system diseases	9,615
Old age and senility	8,724
Mental disorders	7,127
Infectious diseases	6,700
Sudden death	2,556
Congenital defects	2,349
Blood and immune system diseases	2,552
Perinatal mortality	2,107
Muscle and bone diseases	1,725
Skin and subcutaneous diseases	1,638
Pregnancy and delivery complications	92
Undefined causes	10,307

Tables 6 and 7 Reasons for admission to general hospitals, 1977, France

	Males	Females
Infectious diseases	2.6	2.2
Malignant diseases and tumors	6.6	5.0
Alcoholism, liver cirrhosis	4.1	1.4
Nervous system diseases	3.2	3.6
Cardio-vascular diseases	12.3	12.4
Respiratory diseases	8.4	5.8
Digestive diseases	8.9	8.7
Senility	10.1	10.2
Delivery	—	10.3
Urinary and genital diseases	5.5	7.3

NOTE: Rate per 100 patients admitted.

Table 8 Persons active in the major health occupations, France

	1980 Total	Rate Per 100,000 Population	% Increase From 1975 to 1980
Dentists	30,321	56.6	+3.2
Pharmacists	36,491	68.1	+2.7
Midwives	9,382	85.0	—
Nurses			
RN	176,889	330	+5.9
Total	245,994	459	+4.4
Physiotherapists	34,572	64.5	+3.0
Other professions	16,497	—	—

SOURCE: Conseil de l'Ordre.

NOTE: There are also about 300,000 people employed in the Social Security Administration and 200,000 persons in health-related industry.

Table 9a Medical schools and medical students (3 final years) 1982, France

School and Location	Students
Paris	
Bichat	758
Bobigny	357
Broussais	491
Cochin	497
Créteil	603
Bicêtre	465
St. Louis	752
Necker	582
Ouest	569
Pitié	652
St. Antoine	686
Total	6,412
Province	
Amiens	424
Angers	384
Besançon	410
Bordeaux	1,353
Brest	279
Caen	391
Clermont-Ferrand	418
Dijon	438
Grenoble	640
Lille	1,421
Limoges	391
Lyon	1,551
Marseille	1,562
Montpellier	917
Nancy	947
Nantes	503
Nice	446
Poitiers	350
Reims	424
Rennes	558
Rouen	559
St. Etienne	274
Strasbourg	952
Toulouse	971
Tours	523
Antilles	60
Total	17,146
Grand Total	23,558

Table 9b New medical graduates in France

	1960–1969	1975–1979	1980–1988
Average new graduates per year	2,617	8,605	8,687
Average increase per year	1,800	6,858	5,375

Tables 10 and 11 Physicians by type of practice, 1980, France

Type of Practice	Physicians	% of Total
Exclusive private	42,579	39
Private and part-time salaried	17,358	16
Exclusive salaried (hospital)	15,797	14.5
General practice	47,993	44
Specialty	51,262	47
Noncuring	9,830	9
Total	109,073	
Women	20,962	

SOURCE: Conseil de l'Ordre.

Tables 12 and 13 Information not available.

Table 14 Hospitals by type of ownership and number of beds, 1980, France

Type of Hospital	Institutions	Capacity in Beds
Public sector		
University hospitals	28	—
General hospitals	496	—
Local hospitals	349	—
Total acute care	873	272,367
Long-term care	—	20,190
Specialized care (mental)	—	122,967
Total	1,038	415,524
Private sector		
Proprietary	1,622	106,261
Nonprofit	823	75,365
Total	2,445	181,626
Grand total	3,483	597,150

SOURCE: CREDOC.

Tables 15, 16, and 17 Information not available.

Table 18 Health expenditures: percentages by types of care, selected years, France

Year	Hospital	Ambulatory Care	Drugs and Other Medical Goods
1960	40.6%	36%	18.7%
1965	43.0	33	20.5
1970	49.5	31.4	16
1975	53.3	30.8	12.8
1978	54.7	31.4	11.3
1980	50.4	19.1	20.5

Table 19 Health expenditures by type of expenditure and source of funds (in percentages), France

	Public Funds		Social Security	Mutual Aid Voluntary Funds	Out-of-Pocket Personal Expenses
	Central	Local			
Hospitals	2.8%	2.4%	86.8%	1.3%	6.7%
Ambulatory care	.9	.3	57.9	6.3	34.6
Drugs and other medical goods	1.3	.6	55.3	6.7	36.1
Total	1.9	1.5	71.3	3.8	21.5

Table 20 Information not available.

Table 21 Average annual increase of health expenditure compared to different indexes, France

	1960–1970	1970–1979
Population	1.06	−0.57
Volume per person	7.67	6.82
Relative price	0.73	−0.72
Relative value	9.60	6.67
General price index	4.04	9.21

Health Services in the Federal Republic of Germany

*Siegfried Eichhorn**

INTRODUCTION

The area of the Federal Republic of Germany (the FRG) including West Berlin, in 1980 had about 61,658,000 inhabitants. The ratio of males to females was 48:52%. In 1979 there were 5.6 marriages, 9.5 births, and 11.6 deaths for every 1,000 inhabitants. The infant mortality rate was 13.6. Children below the age of six comprised 5.7% of the population; 12.8% were children from six to fifteen years; 65.8% were persons of employable age, from fifteen to sixty-five; and 15.7% were persons sixty-five or older.

Producing roughly 200 million working hours daily, a gross national income of 1,193.3 milliard DM (Deutsche marks) per year is raised by about 26 million working people. In order to safeguard the public welfare, as well as to guarantee the rights of the individual, the FRG is established as a democratic and social federal state. This federalism depends on the principle of not concentrating all power in the federal authority, but allowing the eleven states (*Länder*) with their districts and communities to participate in the political life.

The economic system of the FRG works by the rules of market economy and has the following characteristics: sound and legal competition; social security of the individual by a number of social measures—labour protection, protection of the working class against sickness, safeguards against incapacity and unemployment, provision for the aged, promotion of vocational and advanced training, wide dispersion of property, family and health care; regulative economic policy in the sense of business promotion and control with regard to a favourable combination of price stability, economic growth, degree of employment, and international competition; financial politics as an element of security of the social net; formation and safeguard of property.

Within the FRG's whole economy, the health care system consists of all of the institutions and persons which are supposed to promote, support, and restore the health of the population. Because the system is a vital component of the society's infrastructure, it is

*The author gratefully acknowledges the assistance of Dipl.-oec. Barbara Schmidt-Rettig and Agnes Machozek.

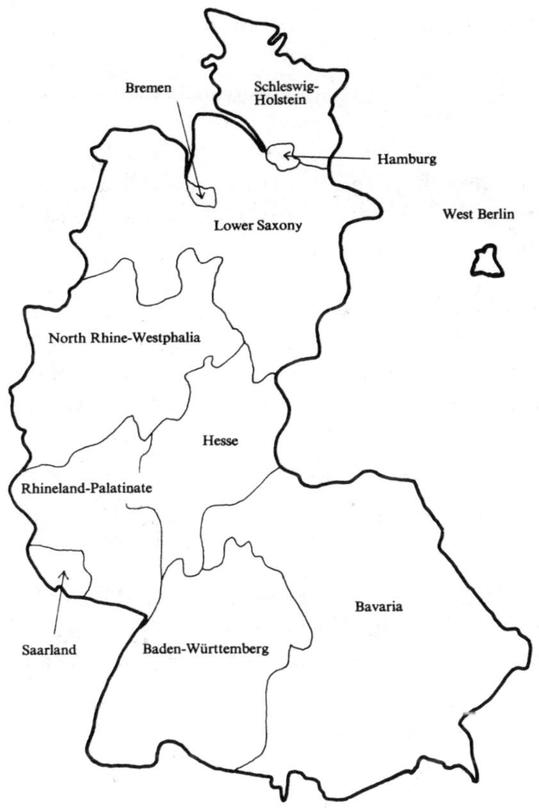

primarily financed by public funds. The government is responsible for seeing that medical services are offered to the entire population on as equal terms as possible. Even so, the state has left the provision of all kinds of medical care to private initiative and to voluntary and nonprofit self-help organizations; it only acts as offerer of medical services in cases where voluntary self-help and private initiative will not be sufficient (*Subsidiaritätsprinzip*).

Among the suppliers of medical services, there is a variety of private doctors and other health personnel, hospitals as well as other medical institutions, which are supported either by local authorities or by one of the more than ten different voluntary associations. Moreover, there are many professional organizations—the general medical councils, the dentists' and pharmaceutical societies, and a number of professional associations for other health personnel—that supply medical services, as well as numerous societies for the promotion of certain areas of social health care. On the demand side of health services, the free choice of one's own doctor or hospital is an important feature of the federal German health care system. This principle is based on the knowledge that a solid and independent relationship of confidence between the patient and his doctor is a necessity for modern preventive medicine as well as for successful diagnosis, therapy, and rehabilitation. The health insurance system is another determining feature on the side of demand. Nearly 93% of the population enjoy the benefit of the social sickness funds; 5 to 6% (soldiers, prisoners, and receivers of national assistance, for example) have other legal rights for health services; the remaining 1 to 2% are privately insured. The social health insurance is composed of a number of autonomous sickness funds, while private sickness insurance is guaranteed by several independent private sickness funds.

Consequently, the structure and organization of the federal German health care service are based on the principle that, in a modern state, administrative authorities on the one hand and the voluntary associations and private individuals on the other have to cooperate for the benefit of the health of the individual as well as that of the whole nation. The state thus sees its health-political task as providing a solid basis that will ensure the health of the people, and, consequently, give them the chance for free development of their own personalities.

The federal ministry for youth, family, and health and the federal ministry of labour and social affairs are the appropriate authorities for the legislative tasks concerning health care services. These activities consist of measures against dangerous and contagious diseases—hygiene; admission to professions within the health care system; provision of pharmaceutical services—business with toxicants; protection at trade with food stuffs, necessaries or luxuries; hospital care, medical engineering in hospitals, hospital financing; health provision and education, and rehabilitation; preventive medicine; establishing regulations for doctors' charges; health insurance; promotion of health care research; international health services.

The states of the FRG (*Länder*) are responsible for the implementation of the federal laws and have the right to adopt their own legislation (as long as it does not conflict with the federal legislation). The states also supervise the public health service.

MEDICAL CARE

Supply of Medical Services

The federal health care system can be divided into four large areas: ambulatory medical (outpatient) care, hospital (inpatient) care, social health assistance, and public health service. Within these areas the following functions can be differentiated: health education, preventive medicine, primary medical care, specialized medical care for outpatients and for inpatients, rehabilitation, inpatient care and home care of the aged and needy, and other medical welfare measures (e.g., general public health services). In principle medical efficiency and the effectiveness of the whole range of medical and nursing care for the people depend to a critical extent on whether and how far all of these individual areas are integrated into a complete system or act independently from each other.

Typical of the present form of medical organization in the FRG is the separation as regards organization, personnel, and finances of the various stages of care, above all the division between inpatient treatment and the treatment of nonhospitalized patients. One striking feature is that hospital facilities are virtually limited to the treatment of inpatients; hospital activities in the outpatient fields are of very little significance. The following facts clarify the present situation:

Physicians in Germany are divided into two distinct categories in which membership is almost mutually exclusive. Members of one category practice in, and are salaried employees of, hospitals and other institutions. Members of the other category are self-employed, working in independent private practice (*freie Praxis*), providing ambulatory care in the community. Physicians working in private practice are, in numbers, about equally divided between general practitioners and specialists.

It is the duty of doctors in private practice to take care of nonhospitalized patients, either as general practitioners or as specialists. With few exceptions, hospitals are not licensed as institutions to provide ambulatory care or to treat nonhospitalized patients. Specialists among the hospital staff are only consulted for ambulatory care if there is no appropriate specialist in private practice in the area concerned.

Hospitals are limited to inpatient care. Facilities for semihospitalized care, as well as the outpatient work for the hospitals, are insignificant.

The functions of health education and preventive medicine were originally restricted to the public health service. Today, however, that service can no longer cope with the comprehensive duties involved, particularly as it has too few doctors and many areas suffer a lack of adequate facilities and sufficient equipment. Consequently, a great deal of preventive medicine today is carried out by doctors in private practice.

The majority of medical rehabilitation measures financed by social health insurance schemes are carried out in general hospitals for inpatients, while those measures financed by pension insurance schemes are carried out in their own hospitals. The responsibility for occupational and social rehabilitation is with the local authorities.

Inpatient care for the aged and for those needing nursing service is in the hands of either the local authorities or the voluntary associations. The latter predominate. The local health authorities are responsible for financing. Conditions are similar for home care (however, home care is not sufficiently developed).

All other measures of health welfare—primarily, health inspection, hygiene measures, special welfare services (for example, for those suffering from tuberculosis or venereal diseases, the physically handicapped, the incurables, and the drug addicts)—are the responsibility of the public health service.

Physicians' Services

The total number of practicing physicians in 1979 was 135,711; 60,512 (44.6%) were working in private practice, 62,827 (46.3%) were chiefly occupied in hospitals, and 12,372 (9.1%) were working at authorities and public-law entities or were otherwise medically occupied. It should be mentioned that 24,672 physicians did not work as doctors. Approximately 4.3% of the doctors in private practice are at the same time also working in hospitals (*Belegärzte*).

At the end of 1979, 62,695 (46.2%) of working physicians were specialists; general practitioners came to 73,016 (53.8%). All not-specialized doctors working in hospitals—38,106 (28.1%) of all working physicians—were in training programs. Of all specialists, 32,789 (52.3%) were working in private practice; 25,516 (40.7%) were working in hospitals; and about 4,388 (7%) were working in public health services, in administration, or in research.

Over the last twenty years there has been an obvious improvement in the availability of medical services, which is reflected in the ratio of doctors to population:

1960: 1 medical practitioner to 703 inhabitants
1970: 1 medical practitioner to 612 inhabitants
1980: 1 medical practitioner to 442 inhabitants

As to physicians in private practice, the development ratio is:

1960: 1 physician to 1,858 inhabitants
1970: 1 physician to 2,332 inhabitants
1980: 1 physician to 1,028 inhabitants

The age structure of the doctors shows that 24% are younger than 34 years, 17% are 35 to 39 years old, 20% are 40 to 49 years old, 15% are 50 to 59 years old, 10% are 60 to 65 years old, and 14% are 66 years or older.

All physicians are united in general medical councils (*Ärztekammern*), which are public bodies—that is, organizations with compulsory membership and compulsory contributions. The general medical councils are organized on a regional basis; the largest regional unit is the *Land* medical council. Since the *Länder* cover almost all medical questions, there is no single federal union of the *Länder* medical councils in the form of a public body. The Federal Medical Council represents only a voluntary working team of the *Land* medical councils. The medical councils are concerned with the cooperation of colleagues, including professional jurisdiction, questions of postgraduate and continuing education, and adherence to medical ethics.

In addition, there are a series of other medical organizations. Since these organizations are unofficial and are free from government influences, they can represent medical professional interests without inhibitions. They include the Association of Physicians of Germany (*Hartmannbund*), an association of free or private practicing doctors, an association of the leading hospital physicians, an association of physicians with employee status and in the civil service (*Marburger Bund*), and a professional association of practitioners. The medical faculties of the universities are united in the Western German Medical Faculty Assembly, and the individual medical branch representatives at the universities belong to unions which are more or less closed.

All these official and nonofficial associations are represented by a board of directors of the German Medical Assembly, which is the general representative body of the Federal Medical Council. This assembly meets once a year, when the aims and ideas of the German medical profession are submitted to the public and the government, and current questions regarding health and hospital care, as well as health and social policy, are discussed.

It would be foolish to deny that the practical influence of decisions taken by physicians has of late been reduced. Improved information and communication have drawn attention to the relation between physician and patient. In addition, the increasing technicality of medicine lessens the personal relation between physician and patient, and also reduces the willingness of the individual and the public generally to accept without criticism all health-related decisions made by the physician. As a result of this development, the extraordinarily dominant position of the physician in society has been somewhat weakened. Judging by present trends, in the long run the power of the official and unofficial medical associations will be reduced to that of comparable associations in other professions.

Ambulatory Medical Care

The main part of ambulatory services in the areas of prevention, diagnosis, and therapy are provided by the physicians in free (private) practice; hospital physicians are involved only to a small degree. An approximate quantitative picture of the scope of ambulatory medical services is given by a periodic microcensus enquiry of the public, which shows that during a four-week period, 20% of the population was sick for at least one day; 92% of these have had medical treatment and 14% were treated in the hospital.

The ambulatory sector of the health care system is responsible for (1) preventive medicine (registration of risk factors, risk indicators); (2) health provision advisory service/ early recognition of diseases; (3) diagnosis in case of sickness, to the extent that hospital care is not necessary (survey of case history; diagnosis supported by chemical or physicial evidence); and (4) therapy, to the extent that hospital care is not necessary (somatic, psychotherapeutic, socialtherapeutic).

Organization—Solo and Group Practice

Ambulatory medical services are divided into solo practice and group practice. Solo practice is predominant, but in the last twenty years group practice has advanced. However, comparing this development with that in other industrial states, group practice in Germany made only modest gains against solo practice, the reason being mainly the fear that group practice might be the first step towards nationalization of the health service; therefore, solo practice resisted group practice development. Although the social-political discussions on this subject at times were quite passionate, more and more group practices were started during the later years. Compared to solo practice, a group practice can offer a greater range of services, more continuous medical care for the patient, lower costs, and a higher efficiency in running a practice.

Medical cooperation in the field of ambulatory medical care advanced with the joint use of equipment for technical laboratory diagnosis in the late 1950s. The installation of the first mechanized analysis equipment at first seemed to make modern laboratory diagnosis possible for the physician in solo practice; economically, however, it did not work out. Consequently, the laboratory partnership (*Laborgemeinschaft*), being a greater economic unit, was a logical solution to let physicians in solo practice also participate in the benefits of modern technical laboratory diagnosis.

Parallel to these technical applicance groups (*Apparategemeinschaften*), group practice developed. Married couples, both physicians, would not see the necessity of running two practices; doctors who were parents wanted their children to enter the practice; young physicians did not want to renounce the advantages of team work as it is practiced in hospitals. In this way solo practices of the same disciplines—as well as those of different or complementary disciplines—amalgamated into one organization. In 1960 there were about 45,000 doctors in solo practice, 114 laboratory partnerships, and 163 group practices; in 1976 there were about 53,000 doctors working in ambulatory medical care, 3,900 laboratory partnerships, and approximately 4,000 group practices. Altogether in 1976 there were approximately 11,000 physicians working in group practices—about 20%. Group practice within the area of ambulatory medical care had gained a large importance, especially considering that more than 16% of all free practicing doctors were in laboratory partnership.

The trend towards group practice is also reflected by the annual net increase of newly settled practices. During 1970 to 1976 these settlements averaged 10.7%. On the other hand, the annual net increase of physicians in laboratory partnerships improved by 33.6%, in group practices by 26.3%. The undeniable advantages of group practice (economical labour supply of qualified personnel, greater efficiency of technical capacities, improvement of scientific knowledge through more intensive contacts, better conditions for personnel on stand-by duty, substitution during illness or vacation) are the reasons that of recent years more and more doctors have chosen to work in group practices. The associations of doctors in free practices estimate that in 1980 about 30% of the medical doctors were working in group practices. Furthermore, it is predicted that by 1990 about 65% of all doctors in private practices will be working in group practices and, independent from this, about 40% of all doctors still in private practice will participate in laboratory partnership.

Comparative studies of several group practices for 1976 regarding output, costs, income, and turnover show the following:

On an average 4,945 patients were treated in solo practices; the total turnover amounted to 297,579 DM; the margin was 50.4%; and the pretax profit was 149,800 DM.

On an average 3,723 patients were treated annually in group practices; the total turnover amounted to 262,521 DM; the margin was 54.4%; and the pretax profit was 142,700 DM.

Consequently, doctors in group practices treated only three-fourths of the number of patients as comparable solo practices. Therefore, solo practices have higher turnovers, which, however, are partly balanced through the higher margin the group practices gain, owing to the advantages of economic cooperation. Owing to the higher margin, quite a number of group practices even obtain a higher profit than corresponding solo practices, although they have a smaller total turnover.

Financing

Instead of being paid by their patients (who would be refunded by the health insurance fund), doctors in private practice are paid by the physicians' organizations, which receive the money from health insurance funds. Physicians in private practice must join an association of sickness funds physicians (*Kassenärztliche Vereinigungen,* or KVs). Altogether there are eighteen KVs in the German *Länder.* At the federal level, there is a *Kassenärztliche Bundesvereinigung* (KBV). Membership in the KV is a requirement for having the right to treat a patient from the sickness fund.

The outstanding characteristic of the KVs is the enormous range of both rights and responsibilities with which the statute has endowed them, either by themselves or jointly with the sickness fund. For many purposes the KVs have to establish joint commissions (*Ausschüsse*) with the sickness funds at both the federal and *Land* levels. It is the KVs, for example, which are legally responsible for assuring that sickness funds members have available to them at all times the ambulatory care to which they are entitled. They are required to draw up plans in cooperation with the sickness funds to ensure that physician's care is available, including emergency and "covering" services. They are required to draw up medium- and long-term staffing plans to meet expected demands for physicians' services. The KVs are, in fact, legally responsible to the sickness funds (and the latter in turn are legally responsible to their members) for assuring that individual physicians fulfill their obligations to the funds and their contributors. On the other hand, the KVs represent the interests of individual physicians vis-à-vis the funds.

According to a 1960 decision of Germany's Supreme Constitutional Court, the constitutional right to exercise one's profession independently makes it obligatory for the KVs to accept all qualified physicians as members: neither the KVs nor the sickness funds can limit the treatment of contributors to a closed panel of physicians. Patients are free both to choose and change physicians. Thus, despite the high degree of structuring and regulation of the system at the level of institutions and associations, the individuals on both sides—contributors/patients and doctors—are unrestricted in an important sense, or at least have certain rights guaranteed.

Finally, and very importantly, the KVs are responsible for disbursing to the individual physicians the total monies they receive from the sickness funds. Individual physicians have always been paid on a fee-for-service basis by their KVs. Until the 1960s the funds paid the KVs on the basis of the number of the funds' members who consulted KV physicians, that is, on a capitation basis. Since the mid-1960s, however, the KVs have received money calculated on the basis of the total services rendered by individual physicians, a method considered by many people to be a contributory cause of the "cost explosion." The previous capitation system was not as cost inhibiting as it might seem; the capitation fee could be increased when morbidity or wage levels rose.

Connected to the task of disbursement to individual physicians, the KVs administer a two-tier review system (a review board and an appeals board) to ensure the "economic soundness"—that is, cost effectiveness—of the services rendered by the individual physician. (Under the principles laid down by the statute, patients are entitled to "adequate, effective, and economically sound" medical attention.) In principle and purpose, this review system somewhat resembles the PSROs in the United States, with an important difference being that the sickness funds and the appropriate association of sickness funds physicians are equally represented on the review commissions.

The list of services for which physicians are paid, as well as the definition of those services and their relative values, are negotiated federally. The federal statute governing the insurance sickness fund regulations (RVO, or *Reichsversicherungsordnung*) does not require that the formulae and principles determining the sum of money that is to be transferred from the sickness funds to the associations of sickness fund physicians (KVs) be the same as the formulae and principles used to distribute funds from the KVs to the individual physician. Both issues are subject to negotiation. Thus, the parties might agree—as was indeed the case up to 1965—that the sickness funds would pay the KVs on a capitation basis (according to the number of members enrolled, or *Kopfpauschale*), or on the basis of the number of sickness certificates issued (*Fallpauschale*), or—as has been the case since the 1960s—on the basis of the aggregated value of services rendered. But the KVs have always paid the individual physician on a fee-for-service basis.

Patients do not register with a physician; hence, a capitation payment system to individual physicians is not possible. Remuneration of individual physicians through a standard fee for each sickness certificate issued—i.e., on the basis of number of cases treated (*Fallpauschale*)—was very unpopular with the majority of physicians and is now prohibited by the new law. The system of remuneration adopted by the parties must take into account the kind and extent of the services rendered, but also makes sure that there will not be "an excessive expansion of the activity of physicians."

Payment to individual physicians by their state-level physicians' association (KV) has generally been on a fee-for-service basis and continues to be so. To determine the fees to be paid, two steps are involved that may or may not be fused: (1) the establishment of a list or catalog of services and (2) the value to be attached to those services. The catalog of services used by the funds (i.e., their definition and their description) has for some time been negotiated at the federal level by all parties concerned. Until 1977 the *Ersatzkassen* (substitute sickness funds) did this quite independently both of the RVO-Kassen and of government authorities, in negotiations with the Federal Association of Sickness Fund Physicians (KBV). The KBV agreements always use a government schedule, the "Official

Services Catalog" (*Amtliche Gebührenordnung für Ärzte, or GOÄ*), as the basis for their catalog of services and their monetary values.

Over the years a joint commission has revised both the list and the relative monetary value of services, sometimes quite dramatically. It has done so in order to influence utilization patterns and take changing costs and technology into account. Thus, in 1971 the value of home visits was raised to encourage their use. In 1975 the value of all laboratory services was lowered *en bloc* to take into account the growing utilization of automatic equipment that had resulted in overuse and large profits.

However, until 1977 the centrally negotiated relative monetary values, though expressed in monetary terms, constituted only a base line on which state-level negotiations took place between each of the separate RVO fund associations (*Landesverbaende*) and the KV of that state, to establish the actual level of monetary values. Indeed, until that year actual final agreement was a matter for each local fund. Thus, except in the case of the substitute funds, only the list and the description of services were definitely settled at the federal level, and by all RVO-funds together.

This pre-1977 pattern of negotiations, in which the KV of each state arrived separately at monetary agreements with the various statutory funds, contributed to the health cost explosion. It permitted the KVs to begin negotiating and to settle, first with those funds in those states where they were likely to obtain the largest increase. This would be with funds which, because of the membership income and health status, were affluent enough to be able to afford a large increase. These agreements would then be used for leverage against other types of funds, and in other states, in a kind of "whipsaw" tactic well known in this type of negotiation.

In 1977 a cost containment law was passed which was innovative because it specified (1) that there would now be a single catalog and description of services for both RVO and *Ersatzkassen,* and (2) that the list would be expressed in relative point values, which would also henceforth be common to all funds, both RVO and *Ersatzkassen.* The new catalog and point system is known as the "unitary evaluation measure" (*einheitlicher Bewertungsmaßstab*). However, the actual monetary value of each service and of each "point" can still be different between funds and states. "Whipsawing" is therefore not eliminated, although there is now greater pressure for uniformity.

The most important regulations to contain costs among physicians in free or private practice are: (1) the control of physicians' remuneration and the new structures created to do so; (2) incentives and other measures to decrease the demand for services; (3) measures to control expenditures for prescriptions; and (4) various other mechanisms designed to control expenditures. The amount of reimbursement the sickness funds transfer to the KVs henceforth must be negotiated and contractually agreed upon at the level of the states. When renegotiating this total amount (*Gesamtvergütung*), the parties must take into account changes in the average insurable wage, the "income orientated outcome policy." This means that the expenditures of the sickness funds have to be coordinated with the receipts. Therefore, the income of the individual doctor is limited by the total amount the KVs and the sickness funds are reimbursing. If the fees charged by doctors in private practice for services rendered exceed the total fee amount, the KVs cut the relative point value, thus limiting the total income of the doctors.

Both partners—the sickness funds and the KVs at the federal level—must annually make recommendations concerning appropriate increases in total remuneration. In doing so, they take into account insurable wages, practice costs, and working time, as well as kind and number of services needed as determined by medical advances.

Further measures for cost containment were the limitation of particular services (e.g., in the area of laboratory diagnostics), increased control by the KVs of the medical-technical services covered, the limitation on total expenditures for prescriptions, and other cost-decreasing changes in rights to services (e.g. provision of household help, provision of nursing care, rest and recuperation, dental technical services).

In order not to make cost containment a static statute but a constant scheme that adapts to the actual circumstances, a Concerted Action Conference was instituted. The setting up of this annual top-level conference was among the most notable innovations of this new law. The conference is convened by the minister of labor and social affairs, and its participants consist of representatives of the associations of sickness funds (*Ersatzkassen* and RVO) and the associations of physicians, dentists, and pharmacists, of the pharmaceutical industry, hospitals, trade unions, employers, the states, and associations of municipalities and counties, as well as of other government ministries. Its tasks are to make recommendations concerning the appropriate changes in the total compensation available for physicians and dentists, and ones concerning the total sums to be spent on prescriptions; recommendations that would stimulate the effectiveness, efficiency, and rationalization of the health system (obviously a broad charge); and recommendations to develop basic medical and economic information and data to help formulate policy.

Primary Care

In the FRG, primary care medical services represent the most frequent symptoms or diseases for which neither a specialist nor a hospital would normally be consulted. However, primary care has to initiate and coordinate all further medical care, if necessary, via a specialist or a hospital.

In the German health care system, most primary care is provided by the general or family practitioner. However, because a patient can consult a specialist directly, without having first seen his family doctor, specialists also provide primary care to a certain extent. The role of the specialist in primary care has been documented by KV studies, which show the different percentages of services the particular groups of specialists provide in primary care: ophthalmologists 20%, surgeons 50%, gynaecologists 50%, ENT (ear, nose, and throat) specialists 20%, dermatologists 30%, internists (internal medicine) 80%, paediatricians 90%, lung specialists 10%, neurologists 40%, orthopaedic surgeons 30%, urologists 10%.

The increasing importance of medical technology involving both specialized equipment and personnel, and the increased costs which result, are the reason why diagnostic facilities and services are more and more centralized, either in diagnostic centers or at hospitals with highly qualified staff and appropriate technical capacities. With the increasing concentration of medical care at medical centers and hospitals, the limited range of work and the professional isolation of primary care physicians increase. This development is the main cause for the worldwide reputation of the family doctor as a "second-class doctor," with the result that the number of family doctors working in primary medical care decreases. However, given developments in the health field in terms of increasing knowledge and technology and the new emphasis on preventive medicine, primary care becomes increasingly important. The family doctor is the first point of contact between the individual patient and the entire system of medical care. The professional knowledge and the personal empathy of the family doctor are determining factors in seeing that individual patients are guided to the appropriate level of health care. His decisions primarily determine what kind of measures have to be introduced. It is he who has to decide whether primary care is sufficient or whether special medical outpatient or inpatient care is required.

Recognizing the importance of the position of the family doctor, the FRG is currently attempting to reform primary care by (1) higher quality of medical services (improvement of training and further education for physicians, especially with a view towards primary care—improvement of cooperation and communication within the area of primary care), (2) the securing of regionally proportional medical services (intensification of contingency planning), and (3) economic efficiency of diagnostic and therapeutic services (promotion of group practices and technical equipment groups).

Patient Access to Care

The usual way to enter the German health care system is for a patient to consult a doctor working in an independent practice of ambulant care. In case of illness, all social-insured patients must go to a doctor who is member of the KV. They are not obliged to consult a certain doctor (e.g., a general practitioner) but are free to go either to a general practitioner or to any specialist. Apart from instances where some hospital doctors are members of the KV and therefore are permitted to have patients in ambulant care, social-insured patients normally are not allowed to consult hospital doctors directly. When a hospital stay becomes necessary, a doctor in an independent practice has to transfer the patient to the hospital and hospital physicians take over; in other words, there is a sharp division between medical care in the ambulatory area and the hospital area.

In case of illness, the patient normally consults his family doctor, who usually is a general practitioner. He is responsible for regular medical care for acute and long-term diseases. If in the course of the treatment special tests and attendances should become necessary, the family doctor will refer the patient to a qualified KV specialist in independent practice. Only when no such appropriate specialist in independent practice is available may the patient be referred to a hospital doctor, provided this doctor is a member of the KV and therefore is permitted to treat ambulatory social-insured patients. After this special treatment, the specialist refers the patient back to his family doctor. Depending on the type of special treatment, the patient may be referred back and forth to other specialists, a circumstance which is quite a burden for the patient. On the other hand, the continuation of doubtful treatment and repeated diagnostic tests may raise the costs considerably.

The sharp division between ambulant care in independent practices and inpatient treatment leads to a kind of "referring-chain" for the patient (family doctor—one, two, or more specialists in independent practices—hospital—specialist or family doctor). This fragmentation of medical care has negative consequences on the effectiveness as well as on the efficiency of the German health care system and is a main weak point of the German system.

Ambulatory Care Planning

Since 1977 the KVs together with the sickness funds have been investigating present and future needs for ambulant medical care in order to prevent a deficit in this area and to eliminate existing deficits. The reason for these investigations was—as in most of the other industrial countries—that the municipal areas had an excessive supply of medical care while rural districts were experiencing a deficit; still, the medical problems were basically similar, although some specialties were found to be represented adequately in rural areas. The planning bases for primary care are areas with populations of approximately 5,000, for medical care by specialists, 50,000 to 120,000 population. Following are the approximate physician to population ratios considered necessary for adequate medical care:

Specialists	Ratio
General practitioner	1: 2,400
Eye specialist	1:24,500
Surgeon	1:47,500
Gynaecologist	1:16,000
Dermatologist	1:41,000
ENT specialist	1:30,000
Internist	1:10,000
Paediatrician	1:25,000
Neurologist	1:50,000
Orthopaedic surgeon	1:37,000
Radiologist	1:60,000
Urologist	1:66,000

The KVs are able to assist physicians who are willing to set up private practice in as far as they are able to interest them in going to areas with insufficient medical care (for example, by providing real estate and by warranting credits for furnishings and medical equipment). Each general practitioner and specialist has to take charge of the emergency service over the weekend and beyond the regular working hours from Monday until Friday according to a schedule set up by the KVs. In cases of emergency, especially when accidents occur, patients may at any time—even during the normal working hours on weekdays—consult the emergency department of a hospital. If hospitalization is not necessary, the patient will be transferred to a doctor of his own choice in an independent practice for further treatment.

HOSPITALS

German hospitals, like all Western hospitals, date back to the early Christian hospitals and monastic infirmaries. They were homes for invalids and injured persons, and for old people having no family nor means of support. Because the doctors were rather inefficient, nursing ranked before medical care. Charity towards helpless persons was the motivation behind these activities.

Information on hospitals in German-speaking regions can be found in church and municipal archives dating back more than 1,000 years. At first, as in other European countries, hospitals and churches were linked, the hospitals being an annex of a church or chapel. Medieval hospital care originated in the monasteries; from the ninth century onwards, it took place in the chapter-infirmaries in the towns. From the eleventh century, as a consequence of the Crusades, the Orders of Knighthood (hospital orders) strongly stimulated their development. Hospitals then were remarkably well equipped and for a long time they served as example and incentive to medieval nursing care. It was only when the citizens became conscious of their importance and started to live Christian lives as individuals that civil hospital orders came into existence, which allowed the citizens to influence nursing by taking responsibility for it.

Characteristically, the towns then handled everything that happened within their own walls. Therefore, they tried to care for those people who depended on others for help because of illness, age, or other reasons. It was due to this attitude, as well as to the citizens' pride, that even small towns possessed well-equipped hospitals. These institutions were no longer attended by nursing communities belonging to an order, as during the Middle Ages, but by salaried municipal nurses of both sexes. This system, which originated in the Reformation countries, prevailed until the beginning of the nineteenth century. The word "hospital" was already being used; it meant the buildings in which "curable sick persons were accommodated, fed, nursed, and cured."

While persons with all kind of diseases shared the same room in the medieval infirmary, a hospital was recorded for the first time in the eighteenth century as having twelve different sickrooms in order to give each type of disease a room of its own. Hence, there was often a division into medical and surgical wards, into rooms for external and internal diseases, as well as wards for pregnant women and contagious patients.

This is the beginning of the modern hospital system in Germany. Physicians used the hospitals as a place for therapy, research, and training. The patients were attended by doctors together with the nursing associations. Hospitals became therapeutic centres. The state grew more aware of their important role in maintaining the population's health. Prussia put the hospitals under state authority in the General Land Law of 1794, anticipating similar measures in other countries. By introducing compulsory health insurance in 1883, Germany legally included hospital care in the social security system for its citizens. Because hospital services originated in the isolated and uncoordinated hospitals and nursing homes of the Middle Ages, the type and number of hospital beds were not regulated by federal, state, or local authorities. At the beginning of the twentieth century, a variety of small hospitals were built on the initiative of public and voluntary hospital owners. The type and number of hospital beds were determined almost exclusively by the individual hospital owners and doctors; consequently, there is no lack of hospital beds today and, in fact, there exists an oversupply. However, there is a disproportionate regional distribution and grouping of specialized beds as well as of facilities for diagnosis and therapy.

Beds, Performances, and Staff

The 3,286 hospitals in the FRG (including West Berlin) in 1979 had a total of 712,055 beds; that is an average of 11.59 hospital beds per 1,000 inhabitants. This ratio of hospital beds to population varies between 10.23 in Niedersachsen (Lower Saxony) and 12.84 in Bremen, and 18.05 in West Berlin. There are even greater regional differences in the number of hospital beds within the various states. These regional differences, however, do not allow any definite conclusion to be drawn about regional needs because some of the hospitals are of more than local importance (university hospitals, larger municipal hospitals, and special hospitals, such as tuberculosis sanatoria). The regional differences in the total number of beds are partly balanced through the imposition of the various catchment areas, mainly within the various states. The overall bed/population ratio is very high by international standards, despite a small decrease since 1975, and some policy makers in West Germany refer to the existence of a "bed mountain." The ownership of hospitals in the FRG has not been affected by the prevailing social insurance system. The institutions continue to be owned by regional and local authorities, voluntary associations, and, to a small extent, profit-making organizations.

Of all hospital beds, 52.2% are in public hospitals; 35.4% in private nonprofit voluntary hospitals, and 12.4% in private profit-making hospitals. Public hospitals are financed by the federation, the *Länder* (e.g., university hospitals), the local authorities, or even by the statutory boards. In general, the private nonprofit, voluntary hospitals are run (owned) by charitable organizations of the church or by free welfare organizations. Private profit-making hospitals are owned by one or several private persons, generally medical physicians, and belong in the field of business enterprises.

Public and private nonprofit hospitals do not require government licenses since they are not business enterprises. Profit-orientated private hospitals need licenses, which are granted to the owners personally. All hospitals, regardless of the type, are subject to government supervision, which is executed by the local boards of health; psychiatric hospitals are subject to special supervision. However, the local health officers have no significant influence on the running of hospitals, except for general police interests in case of danger.

At present there is no *legal* obligation in the FRG for the provision of hospitals, such obligations being only partly incorporated into some of the state acts. However, there are special regulations for the provision of epidemic beds. Thus, there is a limited amount of compulsory construction of hospitals. The local authorities are obliged by regulations to provide hospital beds only for the control of contagious diseases. The social health insurance institutions must provide hospital beds for the medical treatment of casualties. The *Land* welfare organizations must provide appropriate accommodation for the treatment and nursing of indigent and psychopathic persons and the disabled. The provision of general hospital beds is left largely to local authorities and to private nonprofit organizations. The state acts only as supplier of hospital services, or asks local authorities to do so, in cases where voluntary self-help and private initiative are not sufficient. To a larger extent than in most other European countries, hospital beds in Western Germany are provided by private nonprofit organizations. The responsibility for general hospitals is borne by various bodies; for example, hospitals are run by religious communities, parishes, secular associations, and others. Those operating private profit-orientated hospitals are mostly members of the medical profession.

The *Länder* confine themselves to providing beds for psychiatric and disabled persons, while the Federal Republic only provides hospitals for disabled ex-servicemen. The interest of the social insurance institutions in public hospitals is only important in the cases of hospitals concerned with tuberculosis, rehabilitation, and prevention.

There has been a steady decline in the proportion of publicly owned hospital beds, from 63% in 1938 to about 52% in 1979. The share of the private, nonprofit, charitable sector increased from 31% in 1939 to 37% in 1952, but has since declined to about 35% in 1979. The private profit-making sector has been expanding since 1952 and has increased its share of hospital beds from 5% then to about 12% in 1979. During the postwar era an upward trend in the total supply of beds began, which lasted until the 1975–1978 period. The highest rates of growth in the number of beds occurred during the 1960s. From 1975 the number of beds in public and private charitable hospitals fell and, despite a further increase in the number of private profit-making beds, the total number of beds also declined. This movement was in accordance with government policy to reduce the number of beds. It may be premature, however, to attribute this fall to the capital expenditure controls introduced in 1972.

Looking at the classification of hospitals by bed capacity, the main emphasis is on hospitals of 200 to 300 beds (16.5% of all beds). These are followed by hospitals of 100 to 200 beds (15.5% of all beds) and by hospitals with 300 to 400 beds (12.5% of all beds). Of all beds 17.9% are in hospitals with more than 1,000 beds—university hospitals, larger municipal hospitals, tuberculosis sanatoria, mental hospitals, and homes, for example. In public hospitals, 51.2% of the beds are in establishments with 500 or more beds; in voluntary hospitals, the concentration lies with hospitals between 200 and 500 beds (53.4% of hospital beds); and in private hospitals, about 62% of all beds are in institutions having up to 250 beds. It is remarkable that of late about 20% of all private hospital beds are in hospitals of the 200 and 300 bed category. This is attributed to the erection of new "practice-clinics." An interesting point is that, compared to previous years, the number of beds has decreased in smaller hospitals and has increased in larger ones. Most surprising is the increase in the number of beds in hospitals with 200 to 500 beds. The average bed capacity (216 beds) is one of the problems in the FRG. Almost 40% of all hospitals have less than 100 beds. The optimal average bed capacity would be 350 to 500 beds. That would mean the FRG would need about 1,700 hospitals instead of 3,286.

Of all hospitals 45.4% are general hospitals, each having several medical departments (e.g., surgery, internal medicine, gynaecology/maternity, and departments for throat, nose, ear, and eye diseases). Specialized hospitals, accounting for 55.6% of hospitals, are specialized either in the treatment of certain kinds of diseases or groups of diseases (e.g., surgical hospitals, lying-in hospitals, orthopaedic hospitals), or in special methods of treatment (e.g., observation hospitals, sanatoria). Sixty percent (60%) of the hospital beds are in general hospitals, 40% in specialized hospitals. It is usual to distinguish between hospital beds for general or acute hospital services and special hospital services. Hospital beds for tuberculosis, for cripples and addicts, for psychiatric cases and chronic diseases are considered special hospital services. They are characterized by a longer than average stay and are, as a rule, of supraregional importance. The bed/population ratio for special hospital services amounts to 3.8 per 1,000 inhabitants. General hospitals are characterized by a short average stay and are mostly of limited regional importance. The bed/population ratio for general hospital services is 7.8 per 1,000 inhabitants.

University hospitals are fully integrated into the general hospital service. In this connection they fulfill two tasks: supraregional highly specialized hospital care, and medical education and medical research. In 1980 there was a total of sixty-one university hospitals, of which fifty-four were university general hospitals and seven were university special hospitals (primarily for psychiatry and neurology), having a total of about 40,000 beds. University hospitals are run quite independently, usually de facto controlled by the corresponding university medical school, although ultimate ownership is by the state government. Because of the increasing number of students, it is no longer possible to carry out the one-year bedside training of medical students only at university hospitals. For this reason all university hospitals have affiliation agreements with some regional general hospitals in their immediate neighbourhood, which are called "academic teaching hospitals."

Approximately 11.3 million inpatients are treated annually, and the number of hospital days amounts to about 219.7 million. For each 1,000 inhabitants there are 185 hospital admissions and 3,580 hospital days each year. Every hospital bed is occupied for an average of 300 days per year; the average occupancy thus comes to 82.2% and the average length of stay is 20.1 days. The general hospital service shows an average length of stay of about 15.2 days. The average number of patients treated under the general hospital service is 156 per 1,000 inhabitants. This number has increased constantly during the past years. In 1960 the figure was about 110. Since 1970 the number of patients treated by hospital services has steadily increased (21.6%). The reasons for this increase are, to a great extent, the change in age structure of the population (a higher average age) and higher morbidity, both of which lead to more frequent hospital stays. During the same period, the number of hospital days has slightly decreased (0.5%). The increase in the number of hospital patients and the decrease in hospital days from 1970 to 1979 resulted in a decrease in the average hospital stay by 3.54 days, or 14.8%. The average occupancy rate has decreased by 4.5% in the same period.

During the last decade (1970–1980) there has been a corresponding increase in hospital services and in the number of hospital personnel. Actually, the diverse professional groups show the following increments and percentage increases: hospital doctors from 41,589 to 70,038 (68.4%); nursing personnel (including auxiliary nursing personnel) from 161,607 to 269,951 (67%); nursing students from 49,544 to 68,539 (38%); personnel working in departments for diagnostics and therapy from 37,720 to 61,295 (63%); personnel working in hospital pharmacies from 2,617 to 4,531 (73%); and personnel working in supply services and administration from 208,450 to 239,226 (15%). The total number of hospital personnel has increased from 521,451 to 742,161 (42%).

Hospital Financing

In the past, the sickness funds took over all of the costs for the hospital stay for all social-insured patients. The hospital was reimbursed in the form of a global comprehensive day rate. As a result of this financing system, nearly the whole population had the right to hospital care and insured persons could demand optimal care in the hospital without having to consider the cost of the stay.

Beginning in the 1950s hospital costs in the FRG, as in all Western countries, began to rise sharply. If these rising costs were fully refunded to the hospitals by the social sickness insurance, it would be necessary to increase contributions by the insured. To prevent this, the federal government issued regulations in 1954 limiting the amount of the daily rate. The difference between the actual costs and the insurance reimbursement for daily rates was covered by unsystematic contributions from the owners or public authorities, as well as by private contributions or withdrawals from the hospitals' real assets. This, in turn, brought about chronic hospital deficits that were estimated to have reached over 10% of the total expenses. Naturally enough, hospitals were extremely dissatisfied and blamed both the social health insurances and the government for these losses. Substantial deficits accumulated which threatened the hospitals'—particularly the voluntary hospitals'— very existence. In 1971 hospitals had an annual deficit of more than 1,000 million DM.

Finally, after much political wrangling, the federal government in 1972 adopted a law intending to safeguard the financial position of hospitals and regulate the daily charges that could be levied by hospitals on health insurance. The new hospital financing law is based on cost reimbursement principles. The costs incurred by an individual hospital are reimbursed fully for services as long as the hospital operates effectively and economically. The aim of the new law is to divide hospital costs between operating costs directly incurred by the individual patient—staff costs, medicine, food, etc.—and investment costs—in legal terms, the cost of building and equipping a new hospital and of depreciation. The latter are normally called "providing costs" (*Vorhaltungskosten*). Operating costs are now charged in full to sickness funds; investment costs are provided by public authorities (federal, state, and local governments) out of taxation. In 1973 this basic hospital financing law was supplemented by federal government regulations concerning costing and pricing of operating costs (*Bundespflegesatzverordnung*).

Federal, state, and local authorities make reimbursements, one-third each, for the costs of building and equipping a new hospital—not including the cost of the building site. Per-bed costs for different types of hospitals are determined by the states as an upper limit for reimbursable investment costs. The hospital is reimbursed for depreciation each year by a lump sum per bed. The amount of global depreciation charges is thereby dependent on the bed prices for new hospital buildings. Costing and pricing of operating expenses are regulated in the *Bundespflegesatzverordnung;* all services for patients are accounted for and priced proportionally according to the number of days of hospitalization. The sickness fund is charged a global comprehensive daily rate (*Pflegesatz*) for each day an insured patient is hospitalized, a rate which covers all necessary and economically justified operating costs for all general services. For additional services (single room, television, extra food, treatment by a doctor of one's free choice, etc.) patients are charged directly. Private patients who are not socially insured pay the same daily rate as is charged for an insured patient. Generally, the 70,000 physicians working in hospitals are paid a salary that has been negotiated collectively between their organization and the appropriate association of hospitals. However, physicians in charge of clinical departments derive a predominant part of their total income from private fee-paying patients.

Price regulations permit the following methods for determining costs: (1) Costs not incurred directly by inpatient treatment (outpatient department, training and research, auxiliary service, etc.) are eliminated. This is done either by deducting part of the bill or by estimating costs incurred. (2) Costs are determined for general services using estimated cost functions and eliminating any additional services. In doing so, most hospitals take as a basis the "expenditure" incurred for this calculation but not the actual "costs."

The daily rate to be paid by sickness funds is negotiated with regional groups of hospitals or with the individual hospital. The agreed-upon rate is submitted to an official of the state government (*Pflegesatzbehörde*). If that official does not approve the negotiated rate, an alternative is negotiated between the two parties. The state official has the power to make the final determination of the daily rate.

Losses incurred during one period can be brought forward to the next if an external cost efficiency audit determines that the losses were not caused by the hospital's negligence.

Hospital Planning

The main reason for splitting the financing of hospital services into two parts (investment costs and depreciation costs paid out of taxation, and operating costs paid by the patients or their sickness funds) was not a financial one but rather is based on the need to intensify, qualify, and improve regional hospital planning. For medical and economic reasons, it is not advisable to provide certain special equipment and specialist beds everywhere, in view of the comparatively low demand in some areas; rather, it is best to concentrate beds and equipment in a few central places. It therefore is not sufficient when calculating bed demand to determine only the extent of the demand for hospital services in a specific area. It is just as important to distribute the equipment and specialist beds correctly among the various types of hospitals (basic service, regular service, central service) in order to achieve an optimal hospital service for the population and a well differentiated and graduated hospital network.

Previously there was no governmental regional planning in the FRG. Planning was left to the individual hospitals and to the regional planning groups of several hospitals. Until 1972 the voluntary compliance of the various hospitals within this network of general hospital service was not systematically supervised and supported by the government. In cases of financial applications, the states subsidized from 30% to 90% of the construction of new hospitals with public funds. The health authorities as a rule examined the question of need and suitability of the proposed hospital in relation to the whole network of hospital service. In order to coordinate the regional distribution of hospital beds, a new law not only regulates the financing system but also the regional hospital planning. Since 1973 each state is responsible for drawing up a hospital plan that gives a very general estimate of the necessary number of hospital beds and their regional distribution; this should assure equitable hospital care for the entire population. The plans of individual hospitals must fit into the framework of the regional hospital plan. Hospitals cannot get money from the state to finance depreciation of an existing hospital or to finance the investment cost for a newly planned hospital if they are not included in the regional hospital plan. It should be mentioned that in all these matters of regional hospital planning the state (*Land*) works together with the state hospital association and the state associations of the sickness funds. Thus, both associations participate in the state regional hospital planning activity.

State hospital laws specify the details as to the financing of the investment costs and the regional hospital planning. These state hospital laws are not unified federally but differ from state to state.

As a result of the autonomous position of the states, there are considerable variations in the endowments of hospital care resources. Regarding the distribution of hospital beds between the different states, the bed/population rate (number of hospital beds per 1,000 inhabitants) showed wide differences in 1965, ranging from 3.97 in Bremen to 11.05 in Rheinland-Pfalz and Baden-Württemberg (except West Berlin with 14.58). In 1980 the bed/population rate was 10.23 in Niedersachsen and 12.84 in Bremen. These figures suggest that government regulation of capital expenditure in the hospital sector since 1972 has not had any impact yet. It should also be noted that from 1965 to 1980 some states have moved from being relatively underprovided to being relatively overprovided, and vice versa. Of the regions that were relatively deprived in 1965, only Niedersachsen and Nordrhein-Westfalen had below average bed/population ratios in 1980.

MEDICAL EDUCATION

Medical education and training are regulated by the Registration Order for Physicians and consist of: (1) at least six years of study in the science of medicine at a university or college with, during the sixth year, a 48-week period of practical training at a university hospital (or, if its training capacity is exhausted, at another hopsital); (2) education in first aid; (3) two months of nursing service; (4) four months of clinical experience; and (5) two examinations: the medical preliminary examination and a medical examination which must be passed in three stages. The examinations—except the third stage, which includes a verbal part—consist of multiple choice questions. After all have been passed, the appropriate regional medical authority grants registration as a medical doctor, which entitles the holder to practice medicine without restriction in the FRG and West Berlin. Upon completion of training, however, most medical doctors spend several years as an assistant doctor or head physician at a hospital, with the intention of either advancing in general medicine to become a general practitioner or to become a specialist by undertaking added appropriate training.

The general practitioner, or family doctor, is irreplaceable in the medical care of the population. He is competent to treat cases when neither hospital treatment nor the consultation of a specialized physician is necessary. As opposed to former generations, young doctors nowadays do not consider the profession of the family doctor as the ideal. They aspire rather to advanced training in specialized areas in order to work either in a hospital or in their own specialized practice.

Advanced training and the activities of a specialized physician are governed by the state medical councils (*Landesärztekammern*). Medical doctors can advance and specialize in the following fields: general medicine; anaesthesiology; industrial medicine; ophthalmology; surgery, which branches into vascular surgery, paediatric surgery, plastic surgery, thoracic and cardio-vascular surgery, and accident surgery; dermatology and venereology; gynaecology and obstetrics; ENT diseases; internal medicine, which includes endocrinology, gastro-enterology, haematology, cardiology, pulmonary and bronchial diseases, and nephrology; paediatrics, which includes infant cardiology and psychiatry for children and young people; laboratory medicine, including medical microbiology; pulmonary and bronchial diseases; oral and featural surgery; neurosurgery; neurology; nuclear medicine; public health care; orthopaedics; pathology, including neuropathology; pharmacology; psychiatry; radiology, including radiotherapy; forensic medicine; and urology.

Before a doctor can practice in one or more of the advanced medical branches, he must complete the prescribed advanced training for the specialty and pass a prescribed examination. The respective *Landesärztekammern* officially certify individuals as specialized physicians.

Relatively few doctors practice in the theoretical fields of medicine (e.g., pathology, hygiene, pharmacology); others work in the pharmaceutical industry, as full-time medical referees for sickness funds, with insurance companies and so forth, or as industrial physicians. The only group of physicians who are in an exceptional position are those in the public health care. Only they, before being employed, have to complete a special course at an academy for public health care and pass an examination for the medical civil service.

The title "Dr. med.," which most doctors bear, is dependent on preparing a dissertation and on passing a verbal examination. The title is granted by the Faculty for Medicine. Members of countries of the European Economic Community can obtain official recognition as physicians without difficulty; consequently, they have the same legal rights as German doctors. Persons who cannot obtain automatic recognition as physicians in Germany—for example, foreigners not originating in EEC countries—may practice only upon special permission.

There were 24,596 applicants for the study of general medicine in winter 1977–78; only 5,761 (23.42%) could be admitted due to enrollment limits. Because sufficient study places are lacking, they are disposed on the basis of a selection system that considers the qualification of the student as well as the result of an examination he has to pass.

In the FRG there are twenty-seven universities with medical faculties. No fees are charged by the universities; rather, medical education is financed by the federal government and the *Länder*. Medical students finance their personal costs by private money, scholarship, or by means of a loan.

Continuing Medical Education

The medical councils of the *Länder,* being public-law entities, have issued vocational regulations specifying that physicians are obliged to undertake continuing education. There are no further legal instructions on how to fulfill this obligation. The continuing medical education of physicians is organized and implemented by the Federal Medical Council and the medical councils of the *Länder.* They offer continuing education in the form of conferences, courses, and congresses. The scientific societies also make an important contribution to the further education of the physicians. They primarily appeal to the specialized doctors in their own special branch. It is estimated that annually about 65 to 70% of the doctors in the FRG take the advantage of such continuing medical education.

THE NURSING PROFESSION

History of Nursing

Nursing was initially considered to be just another charity organization, but in the wars of 1864, 1866, and 1870–71 the care of the sick and wounded gained so much importance that the idea of public nursing became quite popular.

The proper training of the nursing staff became more and more important as medical science progressed. This was particularly true in surgery—especially after antisepsis and asepsis had been introduced. Over time many public hospitals established nursing schools. After six or twelve months of training, mostly given by assistant medical directors, a hospital internal examination was given.

At the turn of the century large public hospitals started to establish their own sisterhoods of nurses. At the same time the number of free sisters, or "wild sisters," as they were called by the associations, grew rapidly because there was a great demand for trained nursing personnel, especially in the large towns. Shortly after 1900, Agnes Karll founded the Association of German Nurses in Berlin, which offered its members help at finding employment and obtaining reasonable insurance, and advice on questions concerning employment or legal rights. Even before the First World War there were attempts to improve the working conditions of hospital nurses. For example, problems relating to regular working times and shift work were examined.

From 1900 to 1910, Prussia advocated uniform training of nursing personnel. However, recommendations for three years of training were not accepted, given the need for nurses. In 1907 the public (national) examination was introduced in Prussia, to be given after completion of a one-year course at a nursing school. During the next ten years most of the other countries introduced similar requirements.

In 1934 the NS-Sisterhood was established as a party-political organization for nurses. In 1939 the following organizations existed: the National-Socialistic Sisterhood (NS-*Schwesternschaft*); the National League of Free Sisters and Nurses; the Sisterhood of the German Red Cross; *Diakoniegemeinschaft,* a league of the head offices of Protestant nursing orders and sisterhood unions; and *Caritasverband,* a league of the head offices of Catholic nursing orders and sisterhood unions.

In 1938 the federal law (*Reichsgesetz*) for the Order of Nursing Care was issued, which regulated the admission for training, the training process, and certain affairs of professional nursing care.

The Present Situation in Nursing

The Law for Sick-Nursing (*Krankenpflegegesetz*) specifies that everybody who wants to practice as "nurse," "ward sister," "male nurse," or "nurse's assistant," either in sick care or in children's care, needs special permission. The law also states the conditions under which this permission is granted, refused, or withdrawn.

Sister, Nurse/Male Nurse

To secure permission, a student must now complete a three-year course of instruction and pass an examination. The examination is taken before an official board that is chaired by a medical civil servant of the responsible authority. It consists of both verbal and written sections. Upon passing the exam, a license is issued by the responsible authority. Some senior nurses and others may take advanced training in anaesthesia, intensive care, surgery service, psychiatry, or in district health care.

Children's Nurses

Registration requirements for training in infant sick care are the same as for general sick care. Training is held at a public nursing school and lasts three years. The programs emphasize the special factors relating to problems and care of children.

Female and Male Nursing Assistants

These personnel must complete a one-year course at a public nursing school and pass an examination to receive a license.

SOCIAL WELFARE SERVICE

The social welfare service is a paramedical institution assisting the ambulant medical care patient in the domestic area. It is the task of the welfare service to offer comprehensive help in sickness care, care for the elderly, and family and domestic care. Sickness care by the social welfare service is always requested in those cases where hospital stay is advised but is either not feasible or is avoidable. Also, the welfare service—with partly voluntary helpers—assists those seeking advice on social questions.

Potential supporters or sponsors of the social welfare service may be the associations of public welfare, the churches, and the communities. Agreements on reimbursement of costs are made between the sponsors and the sickness funds.

Sickness Care

The social welfare service is not allowed to render any medical assistance; this is, according to the RVO (federal insurance regulations), unconditionally reserved to the physicians. Consequently, the offer of performance of the welfare service may only include those functions of domestic sickness care which can be left to the nursing personnel. The nurses do their jobs in the patients' homes and are responsible for their work. At the same time, however, they are supporting the attending doctor, because nursing a patient is inseparably connected to medical treatment. This is particularly evident in ambulant and hospital treatment and care. Here it is the doctor who is in command of the diagnostic or therapeutic measures—for example, giving certain injections; dispensing medicine; dressing wounds; monitoring temperature, pulse, respiration, and blood pressure; observing and controlling patients; and other things.

The nurse in the social welfare service is a little more independent in the performance of her duties; however, the social welfare service does not infringe upon the doctor's prerogatives whatsoever. The social welfare nursing personnel change dressings, attend wounds, give injections, change catheters, give enemas, treat decubitus ulcers, give irrigations, provide inhalations, and provide similar nursing services.

Medical Control

The sickness care provided by the social welfare service may only be given upon medical orders and under constant medical control. The doctor is responsible for his instructions and for the medical supervision of the welfare service personnel. The nursing staff of the service, however, is not considered the doctor's auxiliary health personnel. It bears sole responsibility for the correct performance of the care ordered by the doctor, who will not be held liable for mistakes made by the nursing staff in executing his orders.

HEALTH COSTS AND HEALTH INSURANCES

Health Costs

In 1980 the cost for health services amounted to 200,520 million DM. That total corresponds to 13.44% of the gross national product and about 41% of the total social budget (DM 403,477 million in 1978). Prevention and medical assistance account for 64.4% of the total cost; 58.4% went for medical services in the area of ambulatory care and hospital care; 30.6% went for services occurring as a result of an illness (professional and social rehabilitation, loss of income, pensions owing to unemployment, or incapability to work); 1.5% went for training of health personnel and health research; and miscellaneous expenditures account for another 3.7%. The total cost for health services is financed as follows: 14.3% from taxes, 43.7% sickness insurance, 7.4% pension insurance, 3.1% accident insurance, 4.4% private sickness insurance, 18.8% employer, and 8.3% private households.

The block of expenditures for direct medical services in the ambulatory and hospital care sector is composed as follows: fees for doctors and dentists in private practices 28.4%; drugs, dressings, aids and appliances, and artificial teeth 31%; hospital care 35.1%; and inpatient prevention and rehabilitation services 5.4%.

Since 1970 the total cost of health services has risen from 70.337 billion DM to over 200 billion. Feeling is widespread that this explosion has reached its limit. Whatever method of financing health care is used, either taxation or insurance, the money must come from current real resources. The federal government and most sectors of the population are becoming more and more convinced that the health system which demands contributions of 12% from all wages and salaries must be stabilized if the internal economy and the competitiveness of the German industry on the world market is not to suffer perilous consequences.

World War II left Germany with many of its hospitals destroyed and with massive shifts in its population, particularly refugees from Eastern Germany, Poland, and Czechoslovakia. There was, therefore, an undisputed need to rebuild and to build a large number of hospitals. By the 1970s the FRG had 3,500 hospitals, with about 710,000 beds. This meant, for a population of about 61 million, a bed density of nearly 12 per 1,000. When, by the mid 1970s, beds and costs increased more and more, there was a general outcry that too many beds had been built and, in fact, a "bed mountain" of about 50,000 to 70,000 beds was freely discussed. As experienced in other countries, however, there has been strong resistance to any substantial reductions and closings of hospitals; nevertheless, in the last few years approximately 20,000 beds have been closed. It is fully understood that real savings in hospital expenditure cannot be made by closing down individual beds, but only by shutting down, completely, wards and general hospitals.

The first efforts to deal seriously with the problem of health care costs were seen in 1975. After long discussions in 1977, the minister for labour and social order made a cost containment law which attempted in a variety of ways to curb the seemingly uncontrolled spiral of rising costs. The basic underlying principle was to effect a stabilization—or, better expressed, an equilibrium between financial input from the contributions of the insured and costs—by making increases in health care expenditure dependent on an equivalent rise in employment income. This also forms the basis for calculating social insurance contributions, the so-called income-conditioned expenditure policy.

The main instrument of this new trend in health policy is the "Concerted Action." This is a kind of corporate advisory parliament where seats are given to all organizations representing health care interests—the associations of doctors, insurance funds, pharmacists, and dental surgeons, to name a few. Hospitals as such are not formally affected by the new law, but they nevertheless take part in the sessions of the new body on a voluntary basis. Concerted Action meets twice a year and is expected to agree upon the size of the increases of doctors' fees, pharmacists' charges, and so on, which should not be exceeded in the next year.

The second instrument of the cost containment measures is the restriction on the range of services paid by the sickness funds (petty payments—for example, some routine medicine—are taken out of the service catalogue of the sickness funds; some services—for example, course of baths—are harder to obtain; while others—obtaining dentures, for example—have to be paid partly by the patient).

It seems that between 1977 and 1979 the objective of the cost containment law was broadly achieved in that cost increases were kept in line with the rise in wages and salaries. No increase in the contribution rates to the health insurance funds was necessary to avoid a substantial deficit. In 1980, however, a critical situation arose: costs substantially exceeded employment income and, thereby, the receipts of the insurance funds. The government attempted, first of all, to curb hospital costs, considered by many to be the decisive cost factor. Moreover, realizing that the Concerted Action may have lost its force, the government was also attempting to tighten the control of ambulatory care expenditure, in particular, medical fees, the price of medicines, and the cost of technical dentistry. After long negotiations between the states, the associations of the sickness funds, the hospital associations, and the different associations of physicians and dentists, two new cost containment laws came into force at the end of 1981: the cost containment supplementary law and the hospital cost containment law.

The following items are part of the service catalogue of the new cost containment supplementary law: (1) A check on the expenditures in certain sectors of the health care system by means of direct measures (e.g., reduction of fees for technical dentistry and prolongation of the price agreements for dressings, aids, and appliances). (2) Measures for improving efficiency of health production (e.g., introduction of a price list for pharmaceuticals; improvement of integration and communication between the different health sectors, especially between the care inside and outside of the hospital; limitation of hospital stays to six days in cases of confinement). (3) Improved the cost consciousness of the insured patients (most importantly, by increasing the insured person's share for the costs of dental services and by increasing charges for prescription drugs, dressings, aids, and appliances).

The main target of the hospital cost containment law is to strengthen the self-administration of the associations of hospitals and sickness funds. The steps to be taken are: (1) Direct participation of the regional hospital associations and the regional associations of sickness funds in the procedures to draw up the state hospital plans. (2) Introduction of the principle of bargaining for determining daily rates. The regional associations of the hospitals and the sickness funds agree upon the amount of the daily rate, which then must be approved by the government. (3) Agreement by the federal associations of the hospitals and the sickness funds on the principles of hospital planning as well as on the principles and standards for effective and efficient hospitals, especially for the staff requirements (*Personalbedarf*). (4) The regional associations of hospitals and sickness funds to install audit committees for controlling the effectiveness and efficiency of hospitals; furthermore, they form an arbitration committee to judge cases where the hospitals and sickness funds hold differing opinions. (5) Inclusion of the hospital sector in reaching agreements, that expenditures in the hospital field have to be guided by the income situation of the sickness funds. It must, however, be noticed that, in principle, the inclusion of the hospitals in these agreements does not affect the cost-covering principle. The sickness funds must continue to compensate hospitals for necessary and economically justified treatment costs.

As a supplement to the hospital cost containment law, the regulations for costing and pricing hospital services are to be changed to create more incentives for effectiveness and efficiency. The hospitals, on one hand, will keep economically obtained surpluses and, on the other, must bear losses if they are caused by the institution.

In the long run, containment of health care costs is possible only by transferring less demanding functions in capital and personnel from the hospital to other areas of the total health care system, primarily to semi-hospitalized, outpatient, and primary care. A solution can be found only by integrating specialized medical care inside and outside the hospital. The best way would be a personnel integration: when the patient is transferred from ambulatory care to hospital care or vice versa, he or she continues to be treated by the same specialists. Under an integrated plan, the doctors in primary care would refer the patients to the hospital or to a group practice for specialized treatment, and there it would be decided whether the specialized diagnosis and treatment should be carried out on an ambulatory, semi-hospitalized, or inpatient basis. In this way, the preliminary diagnosis and follow-up treatment could be organized largely on an ambulatory or semi-hospitalized basis. The main advantage of integrating specialized medical care would be increased medical efficiency and economy.

Social Insurance

The character, organization, and structure of the German health security system are determined by "social insurance." A special form of social security in which insurance principles and the needs for social adjustments are brought together, social insurance is distinguished by its compulsory character. It arises from the Social Insurance Acts of 1881 and includes insurance for sickness, accident, pension, unemployment and unemployment relief, children's allowances, and pensions for farmers.

Social Sickness Insurance

The cornerstone of the German health care system is the social sickness insurance with its network of sickness funds (*Krankenkassen*).

The basic insurance principle. The sickness insurance is based upon compulsory insurance. According to present law, all who are employed, have been employed (retired persons), are trained for employment, or are temporarily unemployed are compulsorily and automatically insured. Manual workers are insured irrespective of the size of the wage packet, but nonmanual workers are insured only if their salary is below a certain amount, a figure which will vary from time to time (at present it is 3,525 DM per month). However, employees whose salary exceed this limit are entitled to continue their insurance voluntarily.

Organizational structure. There are eight types of statutory sickness funds (GKVs) and within these types there are many individual funds. The eight types are subdivided into two major categories: six state insurance regulation funds (RVO-*Kassen*) and two *Ersatzkassen*.

The RVO-*Kassen* are regulated in detail by the 1911 *Reichsversicherungsordnung* (federal insurance regulations). The RVO regulations have been revised many times, most recently by the 1977 and 1981 cost control laws. The *Ersatzkassen* (one for nonmanual and one for manual workers) permits large numbers of white-collar, as well as some blue-collar workers, to enroll in these funds instead of contributing to one or the other of the RVO funds.

The administration of the sickness insurance appears extremely decentralized, being in the hands of about 1,300 separate and intensely autonomous sickness funds for different categories of employees, localities, etc. This provides a fair amount of choice for the insured. In particular, the individual funds are free to determine—within regulated limits—the amount of the contributions they are levying. At present these compulsory contributions average about 11.37% of earnings up to the prevailing maximum. One-half of this amount is paid by the employer, who, under recent changes of the law, has to make similar contributions to the voluntary insurance of the more highly paid employees. For the unemployed and retired, contributions are made by the respective public insurance funds. There is no subsidy given by either federal government or regional authorities to the sickness insurance.

Kind and amount of insured and insurance services. The total number of insured persons is 35.4 million: 20.6 million are obligatorily insured, 4.5 million are voluntarily insured, and 10.3 million are retired. The sickness insurance includes approximately 93% of the population of the FRG and includes the family members of those who participate in the insurance (about 23 million). The other 7% are those who are entitled to a total or partial refund of their treatment costs by the state or the welfare authorities (because of different legal claims for medical treatment) and those patients who take out private insurance.

The cash benefits and services provided by sickness insurance are very comprehensive indeed. They include coverage for: (1) the prevention and early detection of illness; (2) comprehensive medical and hospital services for the curing of illness, and comprehensive provisions for rehabilitation; (3) income maintenance, namely sick pay; (4) financial and medical assistance during pregnancy and delivery; (5) help with the regulation of pregnancy and with legal sterilization and legal abortion; (6) help with the maintenance of households that have children in need of care and with the continuation of farming operations; and (7) financial benefit in the case of death of the insured or coinsured. The specific cash and service benefits that make up the above seven categories fall into two types, according to statute: a list of benefits and services, determined and revised by statute, which the funds must offer their members (*Regelleistungen*); and cash benefits and services that they may offer (*Mehrleistungen*)—whether to do so or not is decided by the contributors (doing so, of course, increases the contribution rate). Any benefit or service that is neither on the list of required ones nor on the list of optional ones may not be offered. Over time, the list of required benefits and services has increased substantially, leaving very few optional ones. Consequently, little room has been left for the funds to compete with each other on this basis. Another consequence has been, of course, a rise in contribution rates.

Characteristic of the sickness insurance in Germany is the service principle (*Sachleistungsprinzip*). As far as ambulatory care is concerned, the sickness funds provide their members with quarterly valid "sickness certificates" (*Krankenscheine*), which entitle the patient to consult any doctor who is working in private practice and is a member of the KV. The doctor is then paid for his services by the sickness fund via the KV. The sickness funds formally agree to pay the costs of hospital treatment by issuing a cost-paying certificate (*Kostenübernahmeschein*).

The total expenditure of the sickness insurance was 85.7 billion DM in 1980, representing about 21% of the whole social budget. Of the total expenditure, 32.73 billion DM (38%) was for ambulant medical services (doctors' fees 15.36 billion DM, prescription fees 12.56 billion DM, medical aid and appliances 4.81 billion DM); 25.34 billion DM (30%) was for hospital services; 12.86 billion DM (15%) was for dental care; and 6.67 billion DM (7.8%) was for income maintenance (sick pay). It should be noted that there are no copayments for doctors' fees or hospital costs that the insured has to pay himself. For prescription charges or the prescription of glasses the insured must pay 20% of the cost for prescriptions—20% but not more than 4 DM. The sickness fund indeed pays the total dentist's fee for artificial teeth, but only 60% of the dental technical services.

Administration. By far the largest number (about 50%, or 16.5 million people) of all members (35.4 million people) are in the *Ortskrankenkassen* funds (OKs). There were 270 OKs in 1980. These local funds are intended first and foremost for the main body of blue-collar workers. However, they also provide a "safety net" for anyone else who is entitled to be insured, or who has to be insured, and either cannot or does not want to belong to one of the seven other kinds of funds. Because OK members are drawn heavily from the ranks of the lower-paid strata of manual occupations, equal contribution rates yield lower absolute contributions per member when compared with similar rates for contributors to other sickness funds. This means that the OKs have to spend less per member to keep in financial balance. The OKs, therefore, have had to keep the services they offer to their members (and the payment per service they offer to physicians) closer to the statutory minimum and below the level of competing *Kassen,* especially that of the *Ersatzkassen.* This, in turn, has made the OKs unattractive. Indeed, they have lately had to expand the list of their services, and their expenditures per member—and contribution rates—have increased correspondingly.

Company-based funds (*Betriebskrankenkassen*) numbered 850 in 1976 with a total of about 4.3 million members. In addition, there are 156 funds for different crafts (*Innungskrankenkassen*) with a sum of 1.8 million members; 19 funds for 860,000 persons engaged in agriculture; one for miners (*Bundesknappschaft*) with 1 million contributors; and one for sailors with 61,000 contributors. These six, the RVO-Funds, are supplemented by the two *Ersatzkassen:* one group for white-collar employees (19 million contributors in seven relatively large funds); the second for blue-collar employees (430,000 members in 8 funds).

The underlying governing principle of the funds is the right of the insured, above all, to be in control of the funds, either exclusively (as in the case of the huge *Ersatzkassen*) or, more usually, together with the other contributing party, the employers. This principle applies also to the control of retirement funds and workmen's compensation funds. The actual mechanism of governance and control consists of an assembly of representatives, which approves the statutes and by-laws, the contribution rates, and some of the services to be offered, and elects the fund's boards of directors. Germany's trade unions play the key role in the funds as consumer representatives. German employers also are active in the funds, but understandably somewhat less so than the trade unions.

A final, and important, organizational characteristic of the funds is the way they are organized into *Landesverbaende* (associations) at the level of the *Land* (state)—or into major divisions where the *Land* is large—and at the federal level (*Bund*). Thus, there is a *Bundesverband der Ortskrankenkassen* (BdO) and *Bundesverbaende* for each of the other types of funds, except for the seafarers (since there is only one of these). It is these associations at the *Land* level, or just below it, and the federal associations that increasingly do the negotiating or at least the recommending, depending on what the issue is.

Accident and Pension Insurance

Other branches of the social insurance that finance certain medical services are the accident insurance and the pension insurance.

The accident insurance must compensate the injured, his next of kin, or his dependants following an accident. This is done either by restoring the employee's fitness for work and relieving the consequences of the accident, or by paying money to the injured, his next of kin, or his dependants. According to the law, all employed people must be insured against occupational accidents. The accident insurance is divided into several trade cooperative associations (*Berufsgenossenschaften*). Each branch of trade and industry has its own trade cooperative association which provides accident insurance, including pensions, for workers and employees on the basis of employers' contributions. The total expenditures of the trade cooperative associations for medical services amount annually to approximately 5.5 milliard DM.

The preservation, improvement, and restoration of the capability for gainful work falls within the scope of the pension insurance, as do output measures to improve the health standards of the insured population and the granting of pensions (for retirement and because of incapability to earn one's own living). These pensions may be paid not only to the insured but also to their next of kin. All employees and trainees are required to have this type of insurance.

The pension insurance for manual workers is provided by the single *Land* insurance institutions; pension insurance for nonmanual workers is centrally provided by the Federal Insurance Institution for Employees. The medical services are financed through the premiums (contribution fees) that the insured and their employers bear at equal rates (a certain percentage of the wage or salary); in 1980 this was 16.2%.

The total expenditure of the pension insurances for medical services in the field of prevention and rehabilitation amounts to approximately 13.5 milliard DM.

Private Sickness Insurance

The private sickness insurance includes all private insurance companies that insure people against loss of income or special costs associated with illness. The field of the private sickness insurance (PSI) can only be seen in connection with the social sickness insurance. The benefits of the PSI include: insurance of sickness costs, hospital day pay insurance (coverage of the hospital bill regardless of cost), hospital supplementary insurance for financing additional, optional services (e.g., one-bed room, telephone, television, and treatment by a doctor of one's choice), and insurance for income maintenance, that is, day pay insurance. In 1980 the members of the Association of the Private Sickness Insurances showed 7.691 million people insuranced for sickness costs; 5.994 million for hospital day pay insurance; 4.306 million for supplementary insurances; and 1.596 million for insurance against loss of income. There are about 40 such private insurance companies in the FRG.

The private insurance for sickness costs is under the greatest pressure from the social sickness insurance. That more population groups are included among the obligatorily insured and that authorization for voluntary insurance has expanded has considerably restricted the group of people who are exclusively entitled to private insurance. The civil servants, who in case of illness are refunded by their authority up to 80%, represent the largest privately insured group. On the other hand, only one-third of the self-employed are privately insured.

Those branches of the PSI that add to the benefits of the social health insurance (hospital insurance for supplementary hospital services and day-pay insurance—the latter being important in those cases where the voluntarily insured do not receive any further salary after the six-weeks term has expired) have been most capable of development. With regard to the further development of the social security, the following alternatives are being discussed as possible future tasks of the PSI: (1) extension of the social sickness insurance to the entire population—the PSI covers the remaining gaps in medical care and insures supplementary services; (2) preservation of the status quo concerning the allotment of basic insurance to social sickness insurance and private sickness insurance—with the expansion of the private supplementary insurance; and (3) intensification of competition between the social sickness and private sickness insurances by making the general sickness insurance more like the system of private sickness insurances.

PUBLIC HEALTH

The public health services deal with the public tasks in the field of medical care and the investigative activities connected with them. The *Länder* are responsible for organizing the public health services, as are the local authorities. The administrative organization for these services varies according to the size of the respective *Land.*

Local Public Health

Under the 1934 Law for Unification (standardization) of the Health Services, the local authorities must establish a local health board to be responsibile for the direction of public health services. In the *Länder* Baden-Württemberg, Bayern (Bavaria), Rheinland-Pfalz (Palatine), and Saarland, the local health boards are governmentally directed, that is, the *Land* maintains professional and administrative supervision. In the *Länder* Hessen, Niedersachsen (Lower Saxony), Nordrhein-Westfalen (Northrhine-Westfalia), and Schleswig-Holstein, the boards are integrated into local administration, so that the *Land* only has the professional supervision. The "*Länder*" Berlin, Hamburg, and Bremen are subject to special regulations.

The local authorities (cities and rural districts) are the lowest administrative health authorities. It is the duty of the local health boards to implement the general state requirements to secure and to improve the health of the population. In this connection, they must provide medical services in the following fields: (1) Health supervision (observation and evaluation of the population's health status; health planning; hygienic instructions; health education; and control of circulation of drugs and poisons); (2) Tasks of regulation and supervision of the professions and the organization of public health (controlling the persons employed in the health sphere; supervision of the organization of public health and professional assistance in health planning, e.g., of hospitals, chemists' shops, blood donation, lifeguard service); (3) Hygienic duties (control of epidemics with preventive inoculations; environmental hygiene, i.e., food, housing, school, and business hygiene); (4) Health support—social hygiene (eugenic care including marriage counseling; general health education, instruction, and guidance; health care in schools; mother and child welfare; welfare for tuberculosis patients, venereal patients, physically handicapped persons, addicts, and others who are in need of care; promotion of hygiene and exercises); and (5) Official inquiries and opinions—expert opinions (official, judicial, and confidential).

State Public Health

At the level of the *Länder,* the tasks of the public health services are carried out by the health department of the *Land* ministry. The *Land* health department is the supreme health authority responsible for the professional supervision of all public health care in its *Land,* including local health boards. Supervision of social insurance—including sickness insurance, trade health service, veterinary medicine, and food control, as well as all further tasks relating to health care—are among the responsibilities of the *Land* ministry.

The federal structure of the FRG requires considerable coordination among the states in health care. Attending to this purpose, the Conference of the Ministers of Health serves as the institutionalized structure for cooperation of the supreme health authorities of the states among themselves and with the federation. Besides the state ministers of health, other members of this conference are the federal minister for youth, family, and health affairs as well as the federal minister for labour and social affairs. The Conference of the Ministers of Health aims at an informal policy of coordination between the states and the federation (*Bund*) in the area of health care. Its tasks are to agree on the execution of federal and states laws, to discuss drafts of bills concerning health care, and to reach an agreement on questions relevant to health care.

The Association of the Leading Medical Officers of the States (*Arbeitsgemeinschaft der leitenden Medizinalbeamten der Länder*) prepares the agenda for the Conference of the Ministers of Health. This association consists of the heads of the health departments of the state ministries, with participation by the federal minister for youth, family, and health affairs, and deals with and coordinates legislative questions and matters relating to the execution of laws in health care; it also advises the federal minister who is responsible for health and hospital care.

Further joint institutions of the *Länder* relating to health and hospital care are the Institute for Medical and Pharmaceutical Examination Questions, Mainz (*Institut fur medizinische und pharmazeutische Prüfungsfragen, Mainz*), whose tasks include preparation of the governmental medical and pharmaceutical examinations for physicians and pharmacists, as well as scientific research in the field of examination methodology; and the Academy for Public Health Care (*Akademie für öffentliches Gesundheitswesen*), which is responsible for the education and advanced education of doctors, dentists, and other professions in the field of public health care, and for scientific research in public health care.

In addition, there are the following interregional investigation institutions and other special services in public health care:

The boards of health support the public health departments in the field of prevention and control of infectious diseases and environmental hygiene by means of analysis (microbiological, parasitological, serological, radiological, hygienic analysis) as well as by advice on water supply works, purification plants, refuse disposal units, disinfection plants, and so on. In the FRG there are 49 such boards of health, with about 1,200 special personnel, more than 200 of them being physicians.

The chemical and food control boards aim at safeguarding the population from health dangers in connection with food, tobacco products, cosmetics, and utensils. They also protect the food consumer from deceiving or confusing information concerning the quality of goods. For this purpose, chemical analysis and expert judgements on food, cosmetics, and other similar substances are carried out, as well as inspections of the manufacturing firms which produce them. There are 46 such boards in the FRG, with about 1,400 special personnel, 450 of them being food analytical chemists.

The duty of the forensic medical services is to provide expert judgement based on medical, physical, and psychiatric information in court for trial in cases of custody, guilt responsibility, etc.—to assist the administration of justice. There are special institutions for forensic medical services in the federal German states of Bavaria, Berlin, Hamburg, Northrhine-Westphalia, and the Saarland. In the other federal states, the boards of health and the university institutes take care of the forensic medical services.

Federal Public Health

The federal ministry for youth, family, and health and the federal ministry for labour and social affairs share the tasks for public health care at the federal level. Both ministries place emphasis on advising the federal Diet and the federal government regarding health political issues.

There is also the Federal Board of Health, which is responsible for research work in the field of public health services, provision of statistical data, supervision of business with narcotics, and maintenance of a register for drugs; the Federal Health Council, which is composed of seventy-seven nonprofessional members from scientific and professional associations, local institutions for public welfare, etc., and assists the federal government in drafting health legislation; and the Federal Centre for Health Instruction, which is responsible for developing the principles governing the content and methods of health education, and for the planning and execution of special information measures regarding specific topics of health instruction.

The Future of Public Health

Although the public health service is often called the third pillar of public health care (along with ambulatory care and hospital care), its effectiveness and efficiency is not highly regarded in the FRG, neither by the medical doctors' professional organizations nor by the population. One has to realize that, from the quantitative aspect, the staff situation of the public health services is extraordinarily deficient and will even be getting worse in the near future due to the age structure of the doctors currently employed. The reasons for the shortage of doctors are the present scope of work (much administration—little medical work) and the low pay—in comparison to other medical professions. From the medical point of view, the poor image is augmented by insufficient equipment, lack of adequate premises, and frequent bureaucratic behaviour of those employed in public health care.

The widespread sceptical attitude towards the public health services is verified by the fact that important tasks (health education, prophylaxis, consultation work, advice for socially problematic families) are not completely fulfilled but are partly transferred to doctors in private practice. In addition, the lack of cooperation and communication has particular negative consequences. On one hand, this lack results in unnecessary work; on the other hand, valuable information gets lost which, among other things, could be the basis for initiatives of the boards of health.

Ideas for reform of the public health services tend to provide for one health board per 300,000 inhabitants, being composed of four sections:

Section 1: Administration—supervision of health, information, and documentation—electronic data processing—epidemiology—health education—planning;

Section 2: Food supplies—environmental hygiene—epidemic hygiene;

Section 3: Centre for juvenile health—centre for special prophylaxis and after-treatment—dental centre;

Section 4: Centre for disabled persons—psychiatric centre.

It is, however, a fact that the real problem of the public health services—the lack of physicians—cannot be solved just by better planning and organization. It also requires improvements in education and further training, as well as a comprehensive pay reform.

Table 1 Population by age and sex, Germany

	1979				1980			
	Number (Thousands)		%		Number (Thousands)		%	
Age	Male	Female	Male	Female	Male	Female	Male	Female
All ages	29,317.1	32,122.3	100.0	100.0	29,481.0	32,176.9	100.0	100.0
Under 6	1,799.3	1,716.5	6.2	5.3	1,815.2	1,726.8	6.2	5.4
6 to 15	4,017.6	3,830.1	13.7	11.9	3,820.4	3,640.6	13.0	11.3
15 to 18	1,619.0	1,530.0	5.6	4.7	1,657.6	1,555.0	5.6	4.8
18 to 21	1,528.3	1,446.1	5.2	4.5	1,578.6	1,487.9	5.4	4.6
21 to 45	10,815.6	10,224.2	36.7	31.9	10,917.6	10,283.5	37.0	32.0
45 to 60	5,191.6	5,917.2	17.7	18.4	5,315.8	5,893.0	18.0	18.3
60 to 65	890.4	1,350.2	3.0	4.2	964.1	1,467.4	3.3	4.6
65 and over	3,455.3	6,108.0	11.8	19.0	3,411.7	6,122.8	11.6	19.0
Median age	34.2	39.4			34.4	39.7		

SOURCE: *Statistisches Jahrbuch 1981 für die BRD,* S. 60; *Statistisches Jahrbuch 1982 für die BRD,* S. 60.

NOTE: Data are estimates of resident population as of 31.12.1979 and 31.12.1980.

Table 2 Live births, birth rates, and fertility rates, Germany

Year	Births	Birth Rate	Fertility Rate
1980	620,657	10.1	46.7
1979	581,984	9.5	44.3
1978	576,468	9.4	44.5

SOURCE: *Statistisches Jahrbuch 1980 für die Bundesrepublik Deutschland,* S. 71; *Statistisches Jahrbuch 1981 für die Bundesrepublik Deutschland,* S. 72; Statistisches Jahrbuch 1982 für die Bundesrepublik Deutschland, S. 67, 71.

NOTE: Rates on an annual basis. Birth rates per 1,000 population and fertility rates per 1,000 women aged 15 to 44.

Table 3 Infant mortality rates by age, selected years, Germany

	Under 1 Year	28 Days to 1 Year	Under 28 Days
1950	55.3	20.8	34.5
1960	33.8	9.9	23.9
1965	23.8	5.4	18.4
1967	22.8	5.0	17.8
1969	23.2	5.3	17.9
1970	23.4	5.0	18.4
1971	23.1	5.2	17.9
1972	22.4	5.7	16.7
1973	22.7	6.4	16.3
1974	21.1	5.8	15.3
1975	19.7	5.9	13.8
1976	17.4	5.5	11.9
1977	15.4	5.2	10.2
1978	14.7	5.4	9.3
1979	13.6	4.9	8.7
1980	12.7	4.8	7.9

SOURCE: *Statistisches Jahrbuch 1973 für die BRD,* S. 55; *Statistisches Jahrbuch 1977 für die BRD,* S. 360; *Statistisches Jahrbuch 1979 für die BRD,* S. 378; *Statistisches Jahrbuch 1982 für die BRD,* S. 67, 386.

NOTE: Rates per 1,000 live births.

Table 4 Infant mortality rates by selected causes, selected years, Germany

Causes of Death[a]	1960	1965	1970	1971	1972	1973	1974	1975	1976	1977	1978	1979	1980
Total, under 1 year	33.8	23.8	23.4	23.1	22.4	22.7	21.1	19.7	17.4	15.4	14.7	13.6	12.7
Natural causes deaths (1–799)	—	23.3	22.7	22.3	21.5	21.5	19.9	—	16.3	14.5	13.7	12.7	11.9
Infective and parasitic diseases (001–139)	—	0.2	0.6	0.7	0.8	0.9	0.9	—	0.8	0.8	0.7	0.5	0.5
Alimentory deficiency, other metabolic diseases, and disturbances of immunity (260–279)	—	—	—	—	—	—	—	—	0.1	0.1	0.2	0.1	0.1
Pneumonia (480–486)	—	—	0.8	0.7	0.6	0.6	0.5	—	0.4	0.3	0.4	0.4	0.3
Congenital anomalies (740–759)	—	4.1	4.0	4.2	4.1	4.3	4.0	—	3.8	3.6	3.4	3.3	3.1
Special diseases of early infancy (760–779)	—	—	15.2	14.6	13.9	13.4	18.2	—	9.4	8.1	7.4	6.4	5.8
Accidents (E800–E999)	—	0.6	0.9	1.0	1.1	1.4	1.2	—	1.1	1.0	1.0	0.8	0.7

SOURCE: *Statistisches Jahrbuch der Bundesrepublik Deutschland,* 1982, S.67, 386; 1981, S. 382; 1980, S. 370; 1979 S. 378; 1978, S. 378; 1977, S. 360; 1976, S. 88; 1975, S. 88; 1973, S. 74; 1972, S. 62; 1971, S. 55; 1967, S. 76.

NOTE: Rates per 1,000 live births.

[a]Numbers from the International Classification of Diseases 1979, 9th revision.

Table 5 Death rates for twelve selected causes of death, selected years, Germany

Cause of Death[a]		1968 Rank	1968 Death Rate	1968 % of Total Deaths	1977 Rank	1977 Death Rate	1977 % of Total Deaths	1978 Rank	1978 Death Rate	1978 % of Total Deaths	1979 Rank	1979 Death Rate	1979 % of Total Deaths	1980 Rank	1980 Death Rate	1980 % of Total Deaths
All causes	(001–999)		1,216.4	100.0		1,148.1	100.0		1,179.3	100.0		1,160.0	100.0		1,156.0	100.0
Tuberculosis	(010–019)	12	10.4	0.9	11	4.4	0.4	11	4.1	0.3	11	3.5	0.3	11	3.1	0.3
Malignant neoplasms (digestive)	(150–159); (197.4–9)	3	103.6	8.5	3	101.3	8.8	3	100.7	8.5	3	97.8	8.4	3	97.9	8.5
Malignant neoplasms (respiratory)	(160–163); (197.0–3)	4	37.3	3.1	4	43.2	3.8	4	44.6	3.8	4	43.0	3.7	4	44.1	3.8
Diabetes mellitus	(250)	7	27.6	2.3	6	27.1	2.4	6	27.5	2.3	6	23.4	2.0	6	22.2	1.9
Ischemic heart disease	(410–414)	2	156.7	12.9	1	221.8	19.3	1	230.8	19.6	1	203.8	17.6	1	109.8	18.1
Cerebrovascular diseases	(430–438)	1	178.7	14.7	2	159.9	13.9	2	166.0	14.1	2	167.5	14.4	2	165.8	14.3
Influenza	(470–474)	11	10.5	0.9	12	1.1	0.1	12	2.1	0.2	12	1.4	0.1	12	0.8	0.1
Pneumonia	(480–486)	5	31.4	2.6	9	21.7	1.9	7	24.0	2.0	7	22.4	1.9	8	20.7	1.8
Liver cirrhosis	(571)	9	24.1	2.0	5	27.6	2.4	5	27.6	2.3	5	27.5	2.4	5	26.6	2.3
Decrepitude	(794)	6	29.9	2.5	10	10.5	0.9	10	10.7	0.9	10	10.8	0.9	10	10.6	0.9
Accidents	E810–E82[illegible])	8	26.8	2.2	7	23.7	2.1	8	23.1	2.0	9	20.9	1.8	9	20.3	1.8
Suicide	(E950–E95[illegible])	10	20.5	1.7	8	22.7	2.0	9	22.2	1.9	8	21.5	1.9	7	20.8	1.8
All other causes			558.9	45.9		483.1	42.1		495.9	42.1		516.5	44.5		513.3	44.4

SOURCE: *Statistisches Jahrbuch der Bundesrepublik Deutschland,* 1980, S. 366; 1982, S. 382.

NOTE: Rates per 100,000 population

[a]Numbers from the International Classification of Diseases 1979, 9th revision.

Table 6 Average length of stay (in days), Germany

Hospitals	1977	1978	1979	1980
All hospitals	20.8	20.3	20.1	19.7
Hospitals of acute patients	15.8	15.5	15.2	14.9
General hospital	17.3	16.7	16.1	15.5
Hospital of internal diseases	21.6	20.0	20.5	20.4
Childrens' hospital	15.3	14.8	13.5	12.7
Hospital of surgery	13.9	13.4	13.2	13.1
Accident hospital	25.0	23.7	22.6	21.7
Orthopaedic hospital	31.3	29.4	28.1	27.0
Hospital of gynaecology and obstetrics	9.6	9.2	9.0	8.7
Other special hospitals	14.9	14.3	14.4	14.3
Special hospitals	58.7	57.2	53.7	53.1
Tuberculosis	72.2	66.4	63.6	60.1
Psychiatry	190.4	176.7	167.2	159.8
Neurology	39.7	41.6	38.6	37.8
Psychiatry and neurology	139.6	136.5	128.1	123.4
Rheumatism	30.3	28.4	29.4	29.1
Chronic patients	244.5	219.0	165.8	170.8
Sanatoria	30.1	30.4	28.9	29.9
Other special hospitals	38.5	39.0	38.5	38.2

SOURCE: *Statistisches Jahrbuch 1979 für die BRD,* S. 381; *Statistisches Jahrbuch 1980 für die BRD,* S. 373; *Statistisches Jahrbuch 1981 für die BRD,* S. 385; *Statistisches Jahrbuch 1982 für die BRD,* S. 389.

Table 7 Information not available.

Table 8 Major and allied health care workers, Germany

Professions and Occupations	1960			1970			1980		
	Number Active	% Distri-bution	Rate Per 100,000 Population	Number Active	% Distri-bution	Rate Per 100,000 Population	Number Active	% Distri-bution	Rate Per 100,000 Population
All professions	121,000	100.0	225.1	166,702	100.0	275.7	210,786	100.0	341.8
Physicians	74,603	61.7	138.8	105,976	63.6	175.3	139,431	66.1	116.1
Dentists	30,594	25.3	56.9	31,262	18.8	51.7	33,240	15.8	53.9
Veterinarians	—	—	—	8,598	5.2	14.2	9,441	4.5	15.3
Pharmacists	15,803	13.1	29.4	20,866	12.5	34.5	28,674	13.6	46.5
All occupations	129,459	100.0	358.1	288,216	100.0	476.7	377,898	100.0	612.8
Healing practitioner	2,573	1.3	4.8	2,732	0.9	4.5	6,654	1.8	10.8
Nursing	130,617	67.9	243.0	199,457	69.2	329.9	262,711	69.5	426.0
Midwives	9,303	4.8	17.3	6,857	2.4	11.3	5,566	1.5	9.0
Maternity care	674	0.4	1.3	832	0.3	1.4	579	0.2	0.9
Masseurs and medical bath attendents	10,337	5.4	19.2	13,862	4.8	22.9	20,610	5.5	33.4
Remedial gymnasts	4,008	2.1	7.5	5,978	2.1	9.9	10,924	2.9	17.7
Occupational therapists	—	—	—	775	0.3	1.3	2,895	0.8	4.7
Medical technologists	15,887	8.3	29.6	27,194	9.4	45.0	30,049	8.0	48.7
Pharmacological assistants	15,312	8.0	28.5	26,144	9.1	43.2	32,314	8.6	52.4
Dietitians	1,338	0.7	2.5	2,259	0.8	3.7	3,337	0.9	5.4
Disinfectionists	2,410	1.3	4.5	2,126	0.7	3.5	2,259	0.6	3.7

SOURCE: *Statistisches Jahrbuch der Bundesrepublik Deutschland,* 1962, S. 86, 87; 1972, S. 66; 1982, S. 387.

Table 9 Operational schools, medical students enrolled by sex, and medical school graduates by sex, 1980, Germany

		Women	
	Total	Number	%
Medical schools (universities)			
Medicine	27		
Dentistry	20		
Medical students	78,289	27,168	34.7
Medicine	68,773	24,783	36.0
Dentistry	9,516	2,385	25.1
Medical graduates	5,387		
Medicine	4,576		
Dentistry	811		

SOURCE: *Deutscher Hochschulführer,* 51. Ausgabe, Stuttgart: Verlag Raabe 1981, S. 42,44; *Statistisches Jahrbuch 1982 für die BRD,* S. 356, 360.

Table 10 Physicians and physicians per 100,000 population, selected years, Germany

Year	Active Physicians	Total Population (Millions)	Physicians Per 100,000 Population	Population Per Physicians
1952[a]	68,135	50.0	136.3	733.7
1960	79,350	55.4	143.1	698.6
1965	85,801	59.0	145.4	687.8
1970	99,654	60.7	164.3	608.6
1971	103,910	61.3	169.5	590.0
1972	107,403	61.7	174.2	574.2
1973	110,980	63.0	176.2	567.5
1974	114,661	61.1	187.8	532.5
1975	118,726	61.8	192.0	520.8
1976	122,075	61.5	198.4	504.0
1977	125,274	61.4	204.0	490.1
1978	130,033	61.3	212.0	471.6
1979	135,711	61.4	221.2	452.1
1980	139,431	61.6	226.5	441.6

SOURCE: *Statistisches Jahrbuch der Bundesrepublik Deutschland,* 1982, S. 50; 1973, S. 34; *Ausgewählte Zahlen für das Gesundheitswesen 1980. Statistisches Bundesamt 1982* (Reihe 1, Fachserie 12: Gesundheitswesen), S. 48.

[a]Saarland excluded.

Table 11 Physicians by speciality, activity, and place of practice, as at 31 December 1980, Germany

Specialty	Total Physicians	Patient Care: Total	Patient Care: Non-Hospital-Based Practice	Patient Care: Hospital-Based Practice	Administration and Research
Total physicians	139,431	127,241	62,029	65,212	12,190
General practice	74,817	66,918	28,268	38,650	7,899
Specialties	64,614	38,052	33,761	26,562	4,291
Anaesthesia	3,536	3,367	194	3,173	169
Ophthalmology	3,391	3,354	2,954	400	37
Surgery	6,260	5,939	1,456	4,483	321
Paediatric surgery	123	122	11	111	1
Accident surgery	700	685	160	525	15
Gynaecology and obstetrics	7,296	7,169	4,867	2,302	127
Oto-rhino-laryngology	2,911	2,863	2,338	525	48
Dermatology & Venereology	2,136	1,996	1,657	339	140
Internal medicine	16,625	15,227	9,307	5,920	1,398
Gastroenterology	314	312	97	215	2
Cardiology	323	317	73	244	6
Pulmonary diseases	1,232	897	517	380	335
Paediatrics	5,022	4,506	3,051	1,455	516
Neurology and psychiatry	4,856	4,416	1,930	2,486	440
Laboratory medicine	749	579	287	292	170
Mouth and jaw surgery	385	370	228	142	15
Neurologic surgery	257	254	22	232	3
Orthopaedics	2,890	2,781	2,102	679	109
Pathological anatomy	596	429	69	360	167
Pharmacology	223	104	6	98	119
Radiology	2,821	2,697	1,178	1,519	124
Urology	1,968	1,939	1,257	682	29

SOURCE: *Statistisches Bundesamt* (Ed.): Berufe des Gesundheitswesens, 1980. Stuttgart-Mainz, 1982 (Gesundheitswesen, Fachserie 12, Reihe 5), Seite 9.

Table 12 Average net income from medical practice by specialty, 1979, Germany

Medical Practice	DM[a]
Total	151,763
Total one-man practice	157,995
General practice	150,995
Internal practice	160,105
Paediatrics	124,117
Gynaecologist	138,956
Ophthalmologist	172,868
Oto-rhino-laryngologist	132,818
Orthopaedic	240,656
Radiologist	192,057
Neurologist	183,366
Dermatologist and venereologist	179,888
Group practice	151,080

SOURCE: *Kostenstruktur bei Ärzten,* Zahnärzten, Tierärzten 1979; *Fachserie 2: Unternehmen und Arbeitsstätten,* Reihe 1.6.1; *Statistisches Bundesamt* (Hrsg.); *Stuttgart: Verlag Kohlhammer 1981,* Seite 20–23.

[a]Rate of representation was 2.3%. Dates based on question blanks.

Table 13a Hospitals and beds by hospital size, Germany

Type of Hospital (in Beds)	Hospitals		Beds	
	1970	1980	1970	1980
0–24	375	233	5,603	3,550
25–49	554	392	20,184	14,477
50–99	746	588	52,663	41,665
100–149	473	444	57,193	52,890
150–199	359	377	61,560	65,499
200–299	454	499	107,828	117,671
300–399	251	267	84,935	91,738
400–499	122	157	53,262	68,526
500–599	72	72	38,716	38,707
600–799	68	83	46,334	56,204
800–999	32	35	28,765	30,960
1,000 or more	81	87	126,211	125,823
Total[a]	3,587	3,234	683,254	707,710

SOURCE: *Statistisches Jahrbuch 1972 für die Bundesrepublik Deutschland,* S. 67; *Statistisches Jahrbuch 1982 für die Bundesrepublik Deutschland,* S. 388.

[a]In 1970 there were 12 hospitals without beds and 1980, 5 hospitals without beds.

Table 13b Hospital admissions, average daily census, and occupancy rate by type of hospital, Germany

Type of Hospital	Admissions (in Thousands)		Average Daily Census (in Thousands)		Occupancy (%)[a]	
	1970	1980	1970	1980	1970	1980
All hospitals	8,859	11,175	605	602	88.5	84.9
Hospitals for acute patients	7,882	9,770	397	398	86.8	83.3
General hospitals						
Without demarcated special sections	433	175	22	8	84.9	83.5
With demarcated special sections	6,492	8,579	327	348	87.0	83.5
Hospital of internal diseases	146	184	11	10	89.2	85.7
Childrens' hospital	185	184	10	6	84.8	73.4
Hospital of surgery	208	226	9	8	85.9	84.8
Accident hospital	31	38	2	2	97.3	97.1
Orthopaedic hospital	53	85	5	6	91.3	84.9
Hospital of gynaecology and obstretics	237	191	7	5	83.0	80.2
Other special hospitals	96	109	4	4	80.3	81.1
Separate hospitals	977	1,405	208	204	92.0	88.1
Hospital of tuberculosis	83	38	24	6	86.6	78.9
Hospital of psychiatry	66	117	53	52	100.5	90.7
Hospital of neurology	18	21	2	2	93.4	85.4
Hospital of psychiatry and neurology	95	120	59	41	98.0	88.8
Hospital of rheumatism	46	54	4	4	94.7	93.4
Hospital of chronic or geriatric patients	9	20	9	9	94.5	95.6
Sanatoria	580	803	47	66	82.6	85.3
Other special hospitals	79	232	9	24	78.1	88.6

SOURCE: *Statistisches Jahrbuch 1972 für die Bundesrepublik Deutschland,* S. 68; *Statistisches Jahrbuch 1980 für die Bundesrepublik Deutschland,* S. 373; *Statistisches Jahrbuch 1982 für die Bundesrepublik Deutschland,* S. 389.

[a]Nursing days multiplied by 100 and divided by beds and 365.

Table 14 Hospitals and beds by types of ownership or sponsorship, Germany

	1979		1980	
	Hospitals	Beds	Hospitals	Beds
Total	3,286	712,055	3,234	707,710
Owner-/Sponsorship				
Public	1,195	371,504	1,190	370,714
Free, nonprofit	1,113	252,396	1,097	248,717
Private	978	88,155	947	88,279

SOURCE: *Statistisches Jahrbuch 1982 für die Bundesrepublik Deutschland,* S. 388.

Table 15 Nursing homes and nursing home beds, 1979, Germany

Type of Institution	Institutions	Beds
Home for the aged	3,762	286,233
Nursing home, geriatric	624	109,953
Multi-sectional institution	1,365	—[a]
Homogeneous institution	142	8,866[b]
Total	5,893	405,052

SOURCE: *Gesellschaftliche Daten, Reihe: Berichte und Dokumentationen,* Band 20. Press- und Informationsdienst der Bundesregierung (Hrsg.) Bonn, 1979

[a]The beds in multi-sectional institutions are distributed as follows:
Home for the aged people—92,087 beds
Nursing home, geriatric—50,287 beds.

[b]The beds cannot be divided into institutions.

Table 16 Adjusted expenses per inpatient day in community hospitals, 1978 to 1980, Germany

Groups	1978		1979		1980	% Change
	Expense	% Change	Expense	% Change	Expense	1978 to 1980
All	151.10	9.02	164.73	9.48	180.34	19.35
Part-time consultant hospitals[a]	79.48	31.33	104.38	−0.29	104.08	30.95
Hospitals						
With up to 1 demarcated special section	99.16	3.97	103.10	14.36	117.91	18.91
With up to 2 demarcated special sections	127.24	10.96	141.18	9.40	154.45	21.38
With up to 3 demarcated special sections	139.14	10.33	153.52	9.87	168.67	21.22
With up to 4 demarcated special sections	146.19	9.56	160.17	9.50	175.38	19.97
With up to 6 demarcated special sections	154.40	8.75	167.91	9.17	183.31	18.72
With up to 8 demarcated special sections	168.89	6.96	180.64	8.82	196.57	16.39
With up to 11 demarcated special sections	172.10	7.48	184.97	9.77	203.04	17.98
With more than 11 demarcated special sections	215.17	11.64	240.21	9.51	263.05	22.25

SOURCE: *Deutsche Krankenhausgesellschaft: Auswertung der Selbstkostenblätter,* 1978, 1979, 1980 (S. 34, 35, 35).

[a]Without part-time consultants expenses per inpatient day.

Table 17 National health expenditures: amount and per capita amount by major source of funds and percentage of Gross National Product, selected years, Germany

	1970	1972	1974	1975	1976	1977	1978	1979	1980
National health expenditures (billions)	70.337	94.479	123.648	137.241	146.289	155.285	169.350	183.496	200.520
As % of the GNP	10.36	11.42	12.53	13.26	13.00	12.93	13.12	13.12	13.44
Sources of funds									
Public expenditures	9.871	12.949	16.836	18.345	19.292	20.538	22.909	25.371	28.590
Statute health insurance	24.411	35.461	51.015	60.000	65.517	68.735	73.550	79.468	87.572
Office for securing life annuities	6.663	8.437	10.737	11.516	12.016	12.729	13.052	13.585	14.750
Statute accident insurance	2.520	3.095	3.800	4.453	4.815	5.121	5.485	5.857	6.270
Private health insurance	3.616	4.320	5.563	6.131	6.698	6.911	7.349	8.046	8.815
Employer	17.315	22.007	24.928	25.467	26.005	28.061	33.373	35.685	37.783
Private expenditures	5.941	8.210	10.769	11.329	11.946	13.190	13.632	15.484	16.740
Per capita expenditures	1,159.70	1,531.96	1,992.59	2,219.69	2,377.48	2,529.07	2,761.43	2,986.64	3,252.24
Sources of funds									
Public expenditures	126.75	209.97	271.31	296.71	313.53	334.50	373.55	412.95	464.39
Statute health insurance	402.48	574.99	822.11	970.42	1,064.78	1,119.46	1,199.31	1,293.45	1,422.43
Office for securing life annuities	109.86	136.80	173.03	186.26	195.28	207.31	212.83	221.11	239.58
Statute accident insurance	41.55	50.18	61.24	72.02	78.25	83.40	89.44	95.33	101.84
Private health insurance	59.62	70.05	89.65	99.16	108.86	112.56	119.83	130.96	143.18
Employer	258.49	356.84	401.71	411.89	422.63	457.02	544.18	580.82	613.71
Private expenditures	97.95	133.12	173.54	183.23	194.15	214.82	222.28	252.02	271.91
Percentage distribution of funds	100.0	100.0	100.0	100.0	100.0	100.0	100.0	100.0	100.0
Public expenditures	14.03	13.71	13.62	13.37	13.19	13.23	13.53	13.83	14.26
Statute health insurance	34.71	37.53	41.26	43.72	44.479	44.26	43.43	43.31	43.67
Office for securing life annuities	9.47	8.93	8.68	8.39	8.21	8.20	7.71	7.40	7.36
Statute accident insurance	3.58	3.28	3.07	3.24	3.29	3.30	3.24	3.19	3.13
Private health insurance	5.14	4.57	4.50	4.47	4.58	4.45	4.34	4.38	4.40
Employer	24.62	23.29	20.16	18.56	17.78	18.07	19.71	19.45	18.84
Private expenditures	8.45	8.69	8.71	8.25	8.17	8.49	8.05	8.44	8.35

Addenda									
Gross National Product (billions)	679.0	827.2	986.9	1,034.9	1,125.0	1,200.6	1,290.7	1,398.2	1,491.8
Population (thousands)	60,651	61,672	62,054	61,829	61,531	61,400	61,327	61,439	61,656
Annual percentage changes									
National health expenditures		34.32	30.87	10.99	6.59	6.15	9.06	8.35	9.28
Public expenditures		31.18	30.02	8.96	5.16	6.46	11.54	10.75	12.69
Statute health insurance		45.27	43.86	17.61	9.20	4.91	7.01	8.05	10.20
Office for securing life annuities		26.62	27.26	7.26	4.34	5.93	2.54	4.08	8.58
Statute accident insurance		22.82	22.78	17.18	8.13	6.36	7.11	6.78	7.05
Private health insurance		19.47	28.77	10.21	9.25	3.18	6.34	9.48	9.56
Employer		27.10	13.27	2.16	2.11	7.91	18.93	6.93	5.88
Private expenditures		38.19	31.17	5.20	5.45	10.41	3.35	13.59	8.11
Gross National Product		21.83	19.31	4.86	8.71	6.72	7.50	8.33	6.70
Population		1.68	0.62	−0.36	−0.48	−0.21	−0.12	0.18	0.35

SOURCE: *Statistisches Bundesamt (Ed.): Ausgaben für Gesundheit 1970 bis 1980,* Stuttgart-Mainz, 1982 (Gesundheitswesen, Fachserie 12, Reihe S. 2), S. 29.

Table 18 National health expenditures by type of expenditure and source of funds, per capita amounts, and percentage distribution, 1980, Germany

Type of Expenditure	Total	Public Expenditures	Statute Health Insurance	Office for Securing Life Annuities	Statute Accident Insurance	Private Health Insurance	Employer	Private Expenditures
Total (Million DM)	200,520	28,590	87,572	14,750	6,270	8,815	37,783	16,740
Preventive and care measures	11,916	6,918	2,471	260	364	3	1,900	—
Health care service	4,097	1,682	255	260	—	—	1,900	—
Health care & early recognition	1,355	117	874	—	364	—	—	—
Other care measures	6,464	5,119	1,342	—	—	3	—	—
Treatment	116,857	10,561	73,496	3,467	1,496	5,781	5,316	16,740
Ambulatory treatment	31,936	1,296	21,172	1	544	1,734	1,716	5,473
Inpatient treatment	42,001	8,992	26,935	—	906	2,632	1,939	597
Sanatorium treatment	6,634	86	494	3,396	24	—	458	2,176
Drugs & medical sundries	36,286	187	24,895	70	22	1,415	1,203	8,494
Rehabilitation	61,350	8,202	7,612	10,539	3,232	1,198	30,567	—
Professional & social rehabilitation	4,595	4,291	—	180	124	—	—	—
Rehabilitation for livelihood (diseases & invalidity)	56,524	3,875	7,515	10,276	3,103	1,198	30,557	—
Other rehabilitation	231	36	97	83	5	—	10	—
Education & research	2,909	2,909	—	—	—	—	—	—
Nonsplittable expenditure	7,488	—	3,993	484	1,178	1,833	—	—
			Per Capita Amount					
Total	3,247.3	463.7	1,420.3	239.2	101.7	143.0	612.8	271.5
Preventive and care measures	193.3	112.2	40.1	4.2	5.9	0.0	30.8	—
Health care service	66.4	27.3	4.1	4.2	—	—	30.8	—
Health care & early recognition	22.0	1.9	14.2	—	5.9	—	—	—
Other care measures	104.8	83.0	21.8	—	—	0.0	—	—
Treatment	1,895.2	171.3	1,192.0	56.2	24.3	93.8	86.2	271.5
Ambulatory treatment	518.0	21.0	343.4	0.0	8.8	28.1	27.8	88.8
Inpatient treatment	681.2	145.8	436.8	—	14.7	42.7	31.4	9.7
Sanatorium treatment	107.6	1.4	8.0	55.1	0.4	—	7.4	35.3
Drugs & medical sundries	588.5	3.0	403.8	1.1	0.4	22.9	19.5	137.8

Rehabilitation	995.0	133.0	123.5	170.9	52.4	19.4	495.8	—
Professional & social rehabilitation	74.5	69.6	—	2.9	2.0	—	—	—
Rehabilitation for livelihood (diseases & invalidity	916.7	62.8	121.9	166.7	50.3	19.4	495.6	—
Other Rehabilitation	3.7	0.6	1.6	1.3	0.1	—	0.2	—
Education & research	47.2	47.2	—	—	—	—	—	—
Nonsplittable expenditure	121.4	—	64.8	7.8	19.1	29.7	—	—
			Percentage Distribution					
Total	100.0%	100.0%	100.0%	100.0%	100.0%	100.0%	100.0%	100.0%
Preventive and care measures	6.0	24.2	2.8	1.8	5.8	0.0	5.0	—
Health care service	2.0	5.9	0.3	1.8	—	—	5.0	—
Health care & early recognition	0.7	0.4	1.0	—	5.8	—	—	—
Other care measures	3.2	17.9	1.5	—	—	0.0	—	—
Treatment	58.4	36.9	83.9	23.5	23.9	65.6	14.1	100.0
Ambulatory treatment	16.0	4.5	24.2	0.0	8.7	19.7	4.5	32.7
Inpatient treatment	21.0	35.5	30.8	—	14.4	29.9	5.1	3.6
Sanatorium treatment	3.3	0.3	0.6	23.0	0.4	—	1.2	13.0
Drugs & medical sundries	18.1	0.7	28.4	0.5	0.4	16.1	3.2	50.7
Rehabilitation	30.6	28.7	8.7	71.5	51.5	13.6	80.9	—
Professional & social rehabilitation	2.3	15.0	—	1.2	2.0	—	—	—
Rehabilitation for livelihood (diseases & invalidity)	28.2	13.6	8.6	69.7	49.5	13.6	80.9	—
Other rehabilitation	0.1	0.1	0.1	0.6	0.1	—	0.0	—
Education & research	1.5	10.2	—	—	—	—	—	—
Nonsplittable expenditure	3.7	—	4.6	3.3	18.8	20.8	—	—

SOURCE: *Statistisches Bundesamt (Ed.): Ausgaben für Gesundheit 1970 bis 1980,* Stuttgart-Mainz 1982 (Gesundheitswesen, Fachserie 12, Reihe S.2), S. 29.

Table 19 Information not available.

Table 20 Percentage of population covered by private health insurance, selected years, Germany

Year	Members of Social Health Insurance	Persons with Private Health Insurance		Persons with Private Additional Health Insurance (In Thousands)	Persons with Private and Private Additional Health Insurance	
		Number (In Thousands)	% of Population		Number (In Thousands)	% Population
1980	35,260	4,800	13.61	3,700	8,500	24.10
1975	33,493	4,200	12.54	—	—	—
1970	30,646	5,800	18.93	2,740	8,540	27.87
1965	28,739	6,600	22.97	—	—	—

SOURCE: *Statistische Jahrbücher für die Bundesrepublik Deutschland,* Statistisches Bundesamt, Wiesbaden. *Die private Krankenversicherung,* Zahlenbericht 1980–81. Statistisches Bundesamt, Wiesbaden, Fachserie 13, Reihe 1, "Versicherte in der Kranken- und Rentenversicherung." *Bundesarbeitsblatt,* Der Bundesminister für Arbeit und Sozialordnung, Heft 3 (März 1981).

Health Services in Japan

Masami Hashimoto

INTRODUCTION

Japan's health system is complex. It serves over 115 million people within four main islands covering an area of 377,435 square kilometers, slightly smaller than the state of California, with a span of some 3,000 kilometers long. More than 67% of the land is covered by mountains and forests; the remainder is divided into residential and industrial areas on the one hand, and cultivated land on the other. As a result, the country is heavily overpopulated. Distinct seasonal climatic changes are observed in all parts of the country. The people are ethnically homogeneous and speak one language. Illiteracy presents no problem.

Japan has been called the most rapidly changing society in the world, and this is true in many areas. In the health field, for example, during the three decades after the Second World War, the nation's health scene changed drastically, beginning with the challenge of nationwide epidemics such as typhus, smallpox, and cholera, through the battle against tuberculosis, and then on to the problems of chronic degenerative diseases and environmental pollution episodes.

The country, however, has been also called a dynamic society without change, and this too seems true. For example, the delivery of medical services depends heavily on private medical practitioners along with a nationwide social health insurance scheme.

The modern health system in Japan evolved during the past 100 years in response to the country's pressing social needs and demands of each period. It bears many similarities to its original models in the Western countries, but there are also many notable differences. To truly understand the health system of a country, it is essential to note the character of the social, cultural, and political contexts within which the system evolved. It is some 2,000 years since Japan's unification. Mainly due to the natural milieu and geographical setting, an insularity in the Far East, Japan's culture has been highly self-centered and closed off from the rest of the world, especially the West. However, situated at a meeting point of East and West, the people of Japan have shown a unique aptitude for learning foreign cultures and ideas, and for adapting them to their own cultural milieu. Japan acquired from sixth-century Chinese culture its writing system, Buddhism, and medicine; the sixteenth-

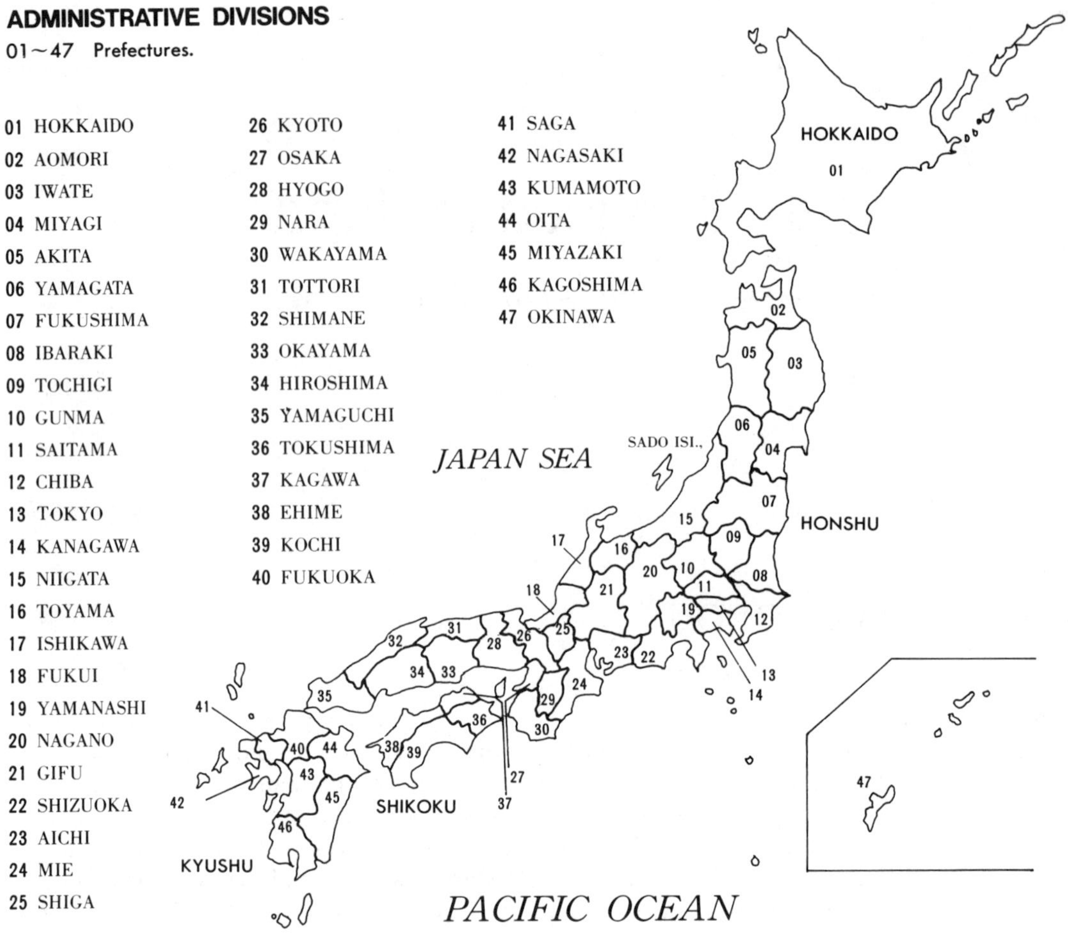

century Portuguese cultural influence came in through Catholicism and elements of Western medicine, and Dutch medicine, especially that after the seventeenth-century.

In 1867 there was a short, sharp civil war known as the Meiji Restoration: an alliance of powerful landowners, young samurai, and mercantile capitalists overthrew the feudal system. The Meiji era (1868–1912) represents a most brilliant period in the history of Japan: within only a few decades, a modern nation with up-to-date industries, political institutions, and social patterns was established. Leaders of the new government eagerly sought to adopt the institutions of Western countries which then seemed best suited to the modernization of the country—for example the British navy and merchant marine, the army system of Prussia, and the American business methods. The government decided in 1870 to adopt the German medical system, which was then considered the most advanced in Europe; this remained a strong influence until the end of the Second World War. Meiji leaders also selected the Prussian political system as a model because of its strong central government based upon well-developed industries. It seems, however, that they carried this out without fully understanding the underlying philosophy of Western democracy.

In 1874 a medical code (ISEI) which heralded the start of modern medical and public health administration of the country, was enacted. The ISEI covered medical, public health, and pharmaceutical administrations as well as medical education, a licensing system for medical practice, and other areas. During the succeeding decade, a transfer from traditional medical methods to Western methods—substantially, the German method—was completed.

In 1889 a constitution was promulgated which set up a constitutional monarchy, and a highly centralized nation was established, aimed at "a wealthy nation and strong army." Afterwards, however, the country became involved in the Sino-Japanese War (1894–95) and the Russo-Japanese War (1904–5), which were accompanied by an industrial revolution. By the end of the First World War (which the country joined under the provisions of the Anglo-Japanese Alliance of 1902), Japan was recognized as one of the world's major powers.

After the war, however, the country underwent a series of depressions, sustaining serious damage especially from the world depression; the resulting social tension was exploited by extremists, and the political parties lost power steadily, being replaced by a military clique. After the outbreak of the China Incident in 1937, the country became ever more deeply involved in war, leading finally to surrender in 1945. Thus, only eighty years after the Meiji Restoration, with its attendant great hopes of modernization and democratization, the country had to start again. World War II brought almost complete destruction of the old system with the loss of nearly two million people and about one-half of the land area.

After the Second World War, Japan was occupied by foreign forces for the first time in its history. During the occupation period, which lasted until April 1952, the country carried out a democratic social reform with strong support from the U.S. occupation authority. It was a second turning point in Japanese history, and the new constitution became the cornerstone of its new era. Promulgated on November 3, 1946 and effective on May 3, 1947, the new constitution differs in three essential points from the Meiji Constitution: (1) the emperor is the symbol of the state and of the unity of the people. Sovereign power now rests with the people; (2) Japan renounces war as a sovereign right; and (3) fundamental human rights are guaranteed as eternal and inviolable.

As the basis of the nation's health, article 25 of the constitution declares that the promotion and improvement of public health, together with social security and social welfare, are the responsibilities of the nation.

The Diet is the highest organ of state power and the sole law-making body. It consists of the House of Representatives with 511 seats and the House of Councillors with 252 seats. Executive power is vested in the cabinet, which consists of the prime minister and not more than twenty ministers of state. The cabinet is collectively responsible to the Diet. The judiciary is completely independent from the executive and legislative bodies.

The country is divided into forty-seven prefectures, including the metropolis of Tokyo. Local administration is conducted at the levels of prefectual, and city, town, and village governments, each level with its respective assemblies. The prefectural governors and city, town, and village mayors, as well as the members of the local assemblies, are elected by the registered voters of the districts. The powers of these units are specified by the Local Autonomy Law (1947).

MEDICAL PRACTICE

Physicians and Their Distribution

The ratio of physicians to population grew steadily during the last decade due to a national policy (1970) to increase the number of medical schools which aimed at a target ratio of 150 physicians per 100,000 population. It is estimated that by 1990 the ratio will fall somewhere around 185 physicians per 100,000 population. At the end of 1980 there were 156,235 physicians in Japan. The number increased 6,006 (4.0%) from the previous year, and the physician/population ratio became 133.6 per 100,000. Of these physicians, 148,815 (95.2%) were in medical practice; the numbers in nonclinical teaching or research, and health administration were 3,664 (2.3%) and 2,099 (1.3%), respectively.

Of the physicians in clinical practice, 65,114 (43.8%) were owners of medical facilities—for example, hospitals or clinics—and 83,701 (56.2%) were employed in medical care facilities. Women physicians comprised 9.9% of the total practicing physicians.

The geographical distribution of physicians is uneven. For example, at of the end of 1980, as compared with the national average of 127.3 physicians per 100,000 population in clinical practice (95.2% of all physicians), several higher prefectures showed about 180 and several lower prefectures showed as low as 70. The specialty distribution is also uneven. The shortage of physicians in the fields of public health, as well as in the basic medical sciences, has become serious in recent years. For example, about 60% of the posts of full-time physicians of public health centers were continuously vacant. To secure health center physicians, the ministry of health and welfare provided a special scholarship grant, but the effectiveness has been doubtful. On the other hand, from the beginning of the 1970s, three medical schools were established to cope with the shortage of physicians in rural or remote areas, mining and other industries, and the Defense Agency: the Local Autonomy Medical College, the Industrial Medical College, and the Defense Medical College. It is still too early to evaluate these efforts.

Private Practitioners

Throughout the history of medical practice in Japan, the role played by private practitioners has been significant. Even today—despite establishment of a nationwide social health insurance scheme in 1961 which led to a form of socialization of the medical services in that they are now available on demand—the delivery of services still depends heavily on the private sector.

The private practitioner in Japan is not a general practitioner. Typically, a private practitioner spends five years or more in a medical school or university (after completion of six years of medical education) to get the higher academic degree of "Doctor of Medical Science," which roughly corresponds to a Ph.D. in the Western system. This degree is also a valuable status symbol for private practitioners. At the same time, despite a long-standing debate, there is no nationally recognized or formal system of specialty training and registration. Therefore, the private practitioner in Japan may properly be called an expert. However, a new trend is beginning to emerge: in recent years academic societies in medical science have established their own systems of specialty training and registration. Currently, there are fourteen academic societies that started in this direction;

internal medicine, medical radiology, general surgery, dermatology, and neurology are just several.

Solo practice is overwhelmingly prevalent among private practitioners; group practice is still in the experimental stage, appearing sometimes, for example, in new towns. Meanwhile, hospitals in the country are predominantly "closed systems," that is, staffed by full-time salaried medical staffs and almost always closed to private practitioners in the district. Recently, however, the Japan Medical Association has been encouraging the establishment of local medical association hospitals, i.e., hospitals established and utilized by a local medical association, aimed at the promotion of effective community medicine. The number of these hospitals is increasing steadily and there are now 160, including those under construction and planned ones; about 50 are presently in operation. Generally, these provide inpatient medical services, medical examinations, and health screening (preventive programs) by private practitioners.

Private practitioners are most influential in the community, and national health policy has in turn been quite favorable to them. Local medical associations, which are composed mostly of private practitioners, form the Japan Medical Association (JMA), which currently includes about 90% of those in active practice. Founded at the beginning of this century, the JMA is the most powerful medical group in the country. A voluntary professional organization (not a trade union) organized at the national, prefectural, and local levels, it exerts considerable influence on national medical policies and also pursues various professional as well as academic activities.

Currently there are no formal data as regards the working hours and estimated incomes of the various medical specialties. Generally speaking, however, private practitioners in the country are working hard: according to a recent survey on a nationwide sampling of private practitioner clinics conducted by the JMA, the average working hours (including participation in community health programs by a practicing private practitioner) are 216 hours per month, that is, 54 hours per week in 1978. According to the same survey, an average yearly income figure for 1,500 private clinics showed a total (gross) medical income of 69,420 thousand yen. Clinic and other professional expenses averaged 42,170 thousand yen, thus yielding an average net income of 27,250 thousand yen. The private physician's income is considerably high in general, compared to other professional people.

Patient Access to Care

There were 76,730 general clinics in 1979 throughout Japan; that figures at an average of 66.1 clinics per 100,000 population, or 1,514 people per clinic. Of these clinics, nearly 60% were practitioner offices with examining rooms, but about 40% had 19 or fewer patient beds, for a total of 283,490 beds. A Japanese hospital has 20 or more beds. It should be noted that private clinics in Japan are equipped with fairly elaborate equipment for diagnosis and treatment and, as mentioned before, most of the private practitioners have become expert in some area of clinical medicine.

Thus, for most of the Japanese people, accessibility to and availability of medical care are fairly well assured. When a person desires some kind of medical care, the common route is to call his or her "home doctor's" office, but there is no restriction on choosing another doctor or facility. A person who wants to receive medical care is free to go to any clinic or hospital and simply present the health insurance membership card. Practically all medical care facilities are under the health insurance program. Needless to say, this pattern is very convenient for patients, but it is an expensive system and one which easily results in abuse of medical care. Moreover, there still remain problems such as doctorless remote districts and difficulties in getting medical care on holidays and at night.

It should also be noted that in Japan the pattern of dispensing drugs is quite different from the prevailing one in the Western countries, namely, separation of medical and pharmaceutical practices. Efforts had been made by the government since the beginning of the Meiji era for a separation; finally, in 1951 the Diet passed a new law amending the related laws for this purpose. However, the traditional pattern is still prevalent in the country, mainly because a large part of a physician's income comes from prescriptions under the present payment system by various health insurance programs. At the same time, there is an expectation among Japanese people that all drugs should be prescribed and supplied by the physician.

Primary Care Physicians

Private practitioners in modern Japan have played an essential role in the delivery of medical care services. More than 75,000 clinics provide primary medical care to the patients in their communities; most are owned and operated by private practitioners who typically are experts trained for more than five years after graduation from medical school at a teaching hospital in some area of clinical medicine. In general, medical school teaching hospitals and large public hospitals have highly specialized full-time medical staffs. In the outpatient departments of these hospitals, primary medical care is also provided.

Recently, emergency medical care has drawn considerable citizen attention, and prefectural and municipal governments are making efforts, with the support of the ministry of health and welfare, to establish an emergency medical care system including medical care on holidays and at night. The transportation of emergency patients is currently handled by the fire stations in the district concerned, and in these areas, too, the private sector plays a significant role.

Following the Alma-Ata Declaration in 1978, the subject of primary health care (PHC) has been discussed more frequently by various health-related professional groups. But, as is common in the Western countries, the understanding of PHC by the medical profession seems to be that of primary medical care. Primary care has become, however, a priority for the medical profession, and the JMA and the ministry of health and welfare together have been sending medical staff from national hospitals to the United States for training in primary care.

HOSPITALS

Hospitals and related systems in Japan have notable peculiarities compared with the systems in the Western countries, mainly due to their historical and cultural background. The first Western-style hospital was established in Japan in 1557 A.D. in Bungo (presently Oita) by Portuguese Jesuit Louis Almeida. However, because of the prohibition of Christianity by the Toyotomi administration and a policy of isolationism by the succeeding Tokugawa administration for a period of over 200 years, the study of Western ideas, including medicine and medical practice, was possible only through a small window in

Nagasaki by Dutchmen who were often oppressed by the administration up to the end of the Tokugawa era. The Yojosho Hospital in Nagasaki, which was established in 1861 by Dutch navy medical officer J.L. Pompe van Meerdervoort, heralded the start of a first modern Western-style hospital with 120 beds. Subsequently, a great interest to study Dutch spread among the young Japanese generation.

At the time the Meiji government decided to adopt Western medicine officially, the only Western medical care facilities were public hospitals attached to medical schools. It was from these hospitals that physicians were sent out to national and prefectural hospitals, which were then the only medical care facilities in those communities. To become the director or chief of staff of these hospitals was the prime objective of the young physicians who were being sent there by the professors of the medical schools. It should be noted that the Japanese traditionally regard public institutions as superior to private ones, and this has been responsible for the development of private clinics mainly staffed by graduates of private medical schools rather than public medical schools. As noted already, public hospitals were operated on the basis of a "closed system," having very little contact with private practitioners.

The concept of hospitalization in Japan has traditionally been different from the Western hospitalization concept. Specifically, there are no "acute" hospitals in the country at the present time. Patients with chronic illnesses, who would be in nursing homes in the Western societies, have always been treated in Japanese hospitals or clinics as inpatients. This has resulted in a much longer average length of stay in general hospitals—thirty-seven days in 1980—as compared with the Western nations. As noted later, that nursing homes in Japan are still very weak is mainly due to the above sociocultural tradition. Another peculiarity in the hospital system is the lack of a formal referral system between clinics and hospitals, and in turn competition between clinics and hospitals, particularly small hospitals.

Hospitals are classified into four groups: general hospitals, tuberculosis hospitals, mental hospitals, and communicable disease hospitals. They are also classified by sponsorship into national, local government, public service corporative, individual, and so on. In 1980 there were 9,055 hospitals with 1,319,406 beds, as compared with 8,294 hospitals with 1,164,098 beds in 1975. Thus, during the last five years the number of hospitals and beds have grown by 9.2% and 13.3%, respectively.

In recent years tuberculosis hospital beds have decreased notably, and general and mental hospital beds have greatly increased, reflecting the changing disease patterns in the country. The Medical Service Law (1948) presently provides detailed licensing regulations for hospitals, which must have 20 or more beds. Although clinics can have up to 19 beds, the law specifies that their managers shall endeavor not to accommodate any patient for more than 48 hours, except in cases where there is an unavoidable necessity in medical consultation. Consequently, there is almost no essential difference between clinics and small hospitals in the services they provide. In 1979 the hospital beds ratio per 100,000 population was 1,092.8. Of these, 727.4 were general beds, 259.0 mental, and 79.0 tuberculosis. Adding the clinic beds of 283,490, however, the bed ratio per 100,000 population would be some 1,326—which is more than that of the United States.

General Hospitals

In 1979 the 7,749 general hospitals in Japan had a total of 1,026,619 general hospital beds, the average number of beds per one hospital being 132. Of these hospitals, 2,120 (27.9%)

had 50 to 99 beds, 962 (12.4%) had 100 to 149 beds. Thus, 3,082 (40.3%) of the nation's general hospitals had fewer than 150 beds. Individuals and private medical service corporations sponsored 67.5% of all general hospitals; the remaining group (32.5%) were publicly sponsored. There seems to be no essential difference among these general hospitals except that public hospitals are usually larger and have more advanced equipment and facilities. In 1979 the number of full-time personnel per 100 beds was 11.5 medical doctors, 0.6 dental doctors, 1.9 pharmacists, 38.9 nurses, 8.9 technicians, and 20.6 others. Thus, for every 100 beds there were 82.2 personnel.

General hospital beds are typically classified in three categories: (1) private room for one patient who is required to pay additional for this type of accomodation; (2) semi-private rooms, which usually have three to six beds, and (3) ward beds, that is, large rooms with many beds. This last type is a carry-over from the old charity hospitals, and is rapidly on the decline.

Special Hospitals

There are traditionally four types of special hospitals in Japan: mental, tuberculosis, communicable disease, and leprosy. In 1979 there were 966 mental hospitals with 223,066 beds; 48 tuberculosis sanatoria with 5,268 beds; 21 communicable disease hospitals with 1,386 beds; and 16 leprosy sanatoria with 12,742 beds. By sponsorship, medical service corporations (52.2%) and individuals (34%) are dominant among the mental hospitals; individuals (31.3%) and medical service corporations (29.2%) among the tuberculosis sanatoria; city, town, and village governments (95.2%) among the communicable disease hospitals; and the ministry of health and welfare (81.3%) among the leprosy sanatoria.

In addition to the traditional special hospitals, since the 1960s there has been a trend to establish high-level medical centers for special diseases or categorical areas by the ministry of health and welfare and by prefectural and large municipal governments. At the national level, for example, the National Cancer Center is the central medical institution for research and treatment of cancer, and the National Cardiovascular Disease Center is the central medical institution for research and treatment of cardiovascular diseases. Meanwhile, many prefectures established prefectural cancer centers or adult disease centers, and several larger prefectures and municipalities established child medical centers or maternal and child medical centers.

Medical School Teaching Hospitals

The original structure and character of medical school teaching hospitals in Japan were established by teaching hospitals attached to medical schools earlier in the Meiji era. At that time, due to the official adoption of German medicine as a substitute for long-standing Chinese medicine, the urgent task of these teaching hospitals was the education and training of Western-style physicians at a quick pace. Consequently, physician-centered treatment and medical services became highly dominant instead of patient-centered ones. At the same time, these teaching hospitals were strongly influenced by the German hospitals, particularly the German university hospitals, as evidenced by the great power and freedom enjoyed by the directors or chiefs of each therapeutic unit. This resulted in a lack of cooperation and coordination among various clinical and specialty units in a hospital—which we now recognize as essential for effective hospital care. It might be noted that this milieu of the early university teaching hospitals remains to some degree in the national university medical school teaching hospitals and other large scale public hospitals even today, despite the change of medical policy from the German system to American after the Second World War.

In April 1981 there were 104 teaching hospitals attached to universities or medical colleges: 44 national, 11 public, and 49 private teaching hospitals. In addition, there were 6 teaching hospitals attached to the medical research institutions that were also parts of universities or medical colleges. Sponsorship of the national medical school teaching hospitals is by the ministry of education, science, and culture. Generally, teaching hospitals of medical schools are large facilities, the average number of beds being 486, with highly advanced, sophisticated equipment for diagnosis and treatment. These hospitals are primarily aimed at medical education, the training of undergraduate as well as graduate medical students.

In addition to the medical school teaching hospitals mentioned above, the ministry of health and welfare designated 176 teaching hospitals as of April 1981 for the residency training of newly qualified physicians. This total was made up of 42 general hospitals and 4 mental hospitals at the national level, 86 general and 6 mental hospitals of prefectural and other public hospitals, and 37 general hospitals and 1 mental hospital in the private sector.

Hospital Licensure and Inspection

Based on the Medical Service Law (1948), permission to establish a hospital must be secured from the prefectural governor, except, of course, for national hospitals. The law sets the standards for a hospital such as regards the structure, equipment, and number of staff. These standards must be met not only in order to open a hospital but also to ensure that the levels for appropriate medical services are met by hospitals already in operation. Medical care inspectors from the prefectural government periodically inspect the hospitals.

During the last two decades, following the establishment of a nationwide social health insurance scheme, national medical policy has emphasized the quantitative strengthening of medical care facilities and medical manpower. In recent years, however, where these quantitative requirements have been met, the quality aspects of medical care have drawn the attention of citizens as well as of the medical profession. There has been no formal quality check system of medical care such as peer review or the PSRO systems in the United States. This seems mainly due to the traditional emphasis among the medical profession in the country for professional freedom and individual professional independence. Recently, a new trend began to establish a committee for quality assurance among the prefectural medical associations, for example, in Hiroshima, Osaka, Shizuoka.

Hospital Finance and Policy

Medical care services are supported primarily by the social health insurance scheme. As will be described in more detail later, payment for medical practice is based on a "fee-for-service" pattern and is calculated by a "point system," which is based on the monthly bills submitted to the Social Insurance Medical Care Fee Payment Fund. Here even university hospitals are no exception.

Investment expenditure of nationally owned hospitals is financed by the national government, while maintenance and current expenditure by medical care fees is paid by the social insurance carrier with partial liability by patients. Conditions for publicly owned hospitals are similar to the national hospitals, with substitution of the prefectural or municipal governments for the national government. Among privately owned hospitals, most of which are proprietary, there are public loan schemes for capital investment: the Medical Care Facilities Financing Corporation and the Pension Welfare Service Public Corporation finance private medical facilities by long-term loans at low interest. These corporations choose and screen the recipients of loans on a priority basis according to policy guidelines set up by the government. The amount of the financing arranged by the Medical Care Facilities Financing Corporation in 1980 was some 830 billion yen. The Pension Welfare Service Public Corporation provided 22.8 billion yen that same year for medical care facilities. As with the national and public hospitals, maintenance and current expenditures of private hospitals are financed by the social insurance carriers and the patients.

Generally speaking, the sponsoring body has considerable influence over hospital policy. However, the legal requirements already mentioned and the "self-paying financial rule" basically limit the activities of a hospital. This rule provides that the whole expenditure of a hospital should be covered by the medical services income of the hospital. For private hospitals, the investment cost is included. It should be noted that a number of local hospitals are carrying out active, continuing community health programs in addition to inpatient and outpatient care, but in these cases the additional community health services are mostly conducted at the financial self-sacrifice of the hospital by the enthusiastic leadership of senior medical staff. Competition between hospitals is considerable, particularly after the application of the "self-paying" financial rule to the local governmental hospitals in 1966, when private hospitals and local governmental hospitals became highly competitive. This resulted in a decreased number of public hospitals due to serious financial deficit.

In 1979 national medical care expenditures increased 9.5% from the previous year. It is estimated that the contributing factors were increases of the number of patients (2.5%) and of the contents of medical care (7.0%). The cost of hospital care has risen notably in recent years, and for the rise in hospital costs and in health costs generally, three factors would be noted. The first is a demographic change, particularly an unusually fast increase of elderly persons in recent years. The second factor is new medical technology and new services due to the advances in science. The third factor is inflation, namely rising costs of food, fuel, and so forth, which reflect most immediately on the salaries of personnel.

Hospital abuse is a very complicated, difficult problem to judge mainly because of the peculiarities of the hospital system. A basic issue relating to hospital abuse would be unusually long general hospital stays—37 days in 1980. This is three to four times longer than the stays in the Western countries, and results from the peculiar pattern of hospitalization in Japan, as already mentioned.

It should be noted that in contrast to the trend in the Western countries, the number of general hospitals and their beds is increasing steadily despite the already high bed to population ratio in the country. Still, there has been no legal restriction or control on establishment or extension of hospitals, except for the public hospital control designated in the Medical Service Law in 1962. Hospital planning based on such a procedure as "certification of need" in the United States is most urgently needed in Japan.

Unfortunately, there is no formal information in the country as regards surgical waiting lists.

MEDICAL EDUCATION

Historical Overview

As mentioned, in 1870, soon after the Meiji Restoration, the new government decided to adopt the German system as the official medical policy, and in 1874 the ISEI was enacted. Since then, the official career of Western medicine in the country has a centennial history. But, it should be also noted that before the official adoption of Western medicine there had been a history in Japan of Chinese medicine for over 1,000 years.

In the sixth century A.D., the Chinese culture with Buddhism and the writing system was brought to Japan via Korea. The Shitennoji, the oldest hospital in Japan, was an outgrowth of Buddhism. During the Nara and Heian periods, from the eighth to twelfth century, medical care was exclusively for the Imperial Family, and all medical men were employed by the Imperial Court. After the eighth century, a sort of medical education system was carried out exclusively by the fund of the Imperial Court. Generally, however, the character of the Chinese medicine was strongly influenced by Buddhism and was highly philosophical and abstract.

Western medicine was introduced to Japan by the middle of the sixteenth century. At that time the Portuguese Catholic missionaries had arrived in the southern part of the country, bringing with them some aspects of Western medicine together with Christianity. Afterward, however, the Tokugawa era (1600–1867) took a policy of isolationism for a period of over two hundred years (1639–1858), and foreigners were forbidden to enter the country with the exception of Dutch and Chinese traders at the limited spot of the Nagasaki harbor. But from this small window, Dutch medicine passed into the country and had a notable impact.

In 1774 a historical event took place which heralded the starting point of modern medicine in Japan. This was the translation of the Dutch edition of a German anatomy book, published by two young Dutch-studying Japanese scholars who were motivated by an observation of a dissection of a human body; the scholars immediately noted that their traditional anatomy teaching in Chinese medicine was very different from this new experience. Afterward, a number of medical doctors from Western countries came to Nagasaki; among the most eminent figures were Philipp Franz von Siebold, who stayed in Japan for six years from 1823, and J.L.C. Pompe van Meerdervoort, who came to Japan by government invitation in 1857 and left in 1862. From the school established by Dr. Pompe, a number of notable leaders in the field of medicine emerged. Meanwhile, around the middle of the nineteenth century, Dutch-studying medical scholars organized private Dutch-studying schools; among them was the notable Teki-Juku founded by Koan Ogata in Osaka, from which many eminent leaders in the Meiji Restoration appeared. In 1849 smallpox vaccine was imported by a Dutch physician, and as a result of efforts by Dutch-

-studying Japanese scholars, the Vaccination Center in Edo (now Tokyo) was established in 1858, which is the origin of the Tokyo University Medical School of today.

Adoption of the German system as Japan's official medical policy lasted as a strong influence in every field of medicine, including medical education and research, and social health insurance. In 1871 two German physicians came to Daigaku-Toko (presently the Tokyo University Medical School) by the invitation of the government. They introduced the German system and reorganized the traditional medical education system, instituting a three-year premedical education period with a succeeding five years of medical education. At that time lectures were often given in German. The Tokyo University Medical School started in 1877, and the Kyoto University Medical School, the second school, was established in 1897.

During the 1870s and 1880s, many German physicians came to Japan to teach medicine, and many younger Japanese medical scholars went to Germany to study. In 1875, on the occasion of the medical practice examination, the government required that all physicians should study Western medicine. Traditional Chinese medicine was not prohibited, though it was allowed only for physicians trained in Western medicine. Chinese medical practitioners then constituted a majority of physicians; for example, in 1874 80% of all physicians practiced Chinese medicine, while only 20% were trained in Western medicine. But, under strict governmental policy, Chinese medicine quickly lost its official position. To cope with a serious shortage of the regularly educated physicians in Western medicine, many medical schools were started and offered a shorter period of education.

Before World War II there were seven Imperial University medical schools in Japan and schools in Korea and Taiwan. Besides these schools, a number of Igaku-Senmon-Gakko schools, providing shorter periods of medical education, existed. During the war the number of Igaku-Senmon-Gakko increased to 51 in order to cope with the shortage of physicians resulting from the war.

Medical Education in the Postwar Period

After the Second World War, based upon the new constitution and under the powerful guidance of the U.S. occupation forces, the national health system was reorganized as part of the overall social reform. Medical education was no exception. The postwar period may properly be called a period of American influence. In 1947 the Fundamental Law of Education and the School Education Law were enacted as the basic structure and principle for the educational system of the new era. Thus, based on the so-called six-three-three education system—i.e., after 12 years of general education—six years for medical and dental education (university or college) and four years for other disciplines were set. As a result, 23 of the Igaku-Senmon-Gakko schools were closed and the rest were leveled up as medical colleges; therefore, the prewar difference between the Imperial University Medical School and Igaku-Senmon-Gakko was eliminated. Furthermore, in line with the U.S. pattern, a system of internship (one year) and national medical examinations were introduced in 1946.

Thus, an applicant for medical education must graduate from a senior high school and successfully pass an entrance examination for medical school. Afterward, he or she must take two years of premedical course work, followed by four years of medical education. Then, to achieve a license to practice medicine, the student must pass the national medical examination, which is administered by the ministry of health and welfare. The national medical examination initially came after completion of a one-year rotating internship; however, the internship system produced many problems, particularly related to the social and financial status of the medical graduates. The internship system was finally abolished in 1968. In the same year the Medical Practitioners Law was amended to recommend that graduates of medical schools undergo graduate residency training for more than two years immediately after acquiring the license to practice. The residency training would be carried out in the hospitals attached to a medical school and hospitals designated by the minister of health and welfare. Currently, more than 80% of the newly licensed physicians receive this residency training and 80% of them are being accepted by the medical school teaching hospitals. In 1975 the second workshop on medical education supported by WHO was held in Japan for those teachers in medical schools and in hospitals designated for residency training.

At the end of 1981 there were 80 medical schools in Japan with a total yearly enrollment of 8,360 students. Sponsorship of these schools is: 42 national schools (4,560 students), 8 public schools (660 students), 29 private schools (3,040 students), and one Defense Agency medical school (100 students). The target set by the government of at least one medical school in each prefecture is now fulfilled.

Nearly 30% of the medical students are sons or daughters of medical practitioners. Following the establishment of many private medical schools during the last decade, in contrast to the national and public schools, these schools drew widespread attention because of their high cost. In many cases, students were required to pay a large amount for admission. It might also be noted that the number of medical school graduates who failed the national medical examination came to over 2,000. These trends have become major problems, and solutions are urgently needed.

Graduate and Continuing Education

In 1957 a new program, a doctor course in medical science, was introduced in the medical schools as an integral part of the establishment of advanced, graduate education system in universities and colleges. The doctor course in medical science lasts four years. For graduates of medical school there is an entrance examination and a required knowledge of two foreign languages.

In recent years the JMA has been conducting various programs of continuing education for medical practitioners through television, radio, meetings of various academic societies, training seminars, and similar methods. Such continuing education is not mandated, however, and currently there is no formal reexamination of medical practitioners to continue in practice. The Institute of Public Health conducts graduate education programs together with continuing education programs for the various health professions, including physicians. Since 1980, in addition to the traditional one-year Diploma in Public Health course, there has been a two-year course leading to a Master of Public Health, and a succeeding three-year course leading to Doctor of Public Health.

Foreign medical school graduates from other countries are required to pass the national medical examination in order to practice medicine in the country. There are about 1,000 foreign physicians in Japan, who practice mostly in remote, rural districts. Most came from Korea or Taiwan and received their medical education and license in Japan before the Second World War.

NURSES AND OTHER NONMEDICAL HEALTH PERSONNEL

As noted earlier, medical care has been carried out mainly by the private sector, with not only nurses but also all other nonmedical workers trained predominantly as assistants to the physician, strongly oriented to the curative side of health care.

Nurses, Midwives, and Public Health Nurses

Nurses are more established occupationally than midwives or public health nurses. Indigenous midwives practiced in the Edo era (1603–1867), although it was not until 1899 that the national government provided the first Midwives Regulation, twenty-five years after the ISEI established the education and licensing system for physicians. Regulations for clinical and public health nurses did not arrive until 1916 and 1941, respectively.

Before World War II, education for nurses consisted of two years of professional training after graduation from a secondary school. After the war, the professional education system for nursing improved significantly. The Public Health Nurses, Midwives, and Nurses Law (1948) dictated that the nursing education system be based on a three-year course with recruitment of students from among the senior high school graduates. This basic course can be followed by public health nursing or midwifery training, each running at least six months. An assistant nurse training course and the so-called upgrading course—a two-year session whereby assistant nurses may be raised to the status of nurses (a three-year night school version is also available)—has been added since 1948.

This 1948 version of the nursing education curriculum was revised in 1968, and new curricula for the preparation of public health nurses and midwives followed in 1971. The current approach is distinguished by the strengthening of liberal arts subjects and the systematic transition to nursing. In addition, the conventional array of special subjects, which had been so closely patterned after the requirements of the individual divisions of medical examination and treatment, has been overhauled so that students are initiated to four major fields of nursing: general, adult, motherhood, and infantile nursing.

Currently, problems in nursing education are: (1) the coexistence of various types of nursing educational institutions, which tend to generate a gap between them; (2) the establishment of nursing schools depends heavily on private medical care facilities, and this has led to severe financial limitations since they are not covered by the School Education Law; and (3) as for the nursing instructors, the current law provides no special standards other than possession of a nursing license and clinical experience.

Currently, there are no health occupations such as the physician assistants or nurse practitioners of the United States. From the community health or primary health care point of view, a most important professional group is the public health nurse. A basic policy for strengthening the education and work of public health nurses is very much needed.

Other Nonmedical Health Occupations

After the war, various nonmedical health occupations emerged as a result of the progress in the medical sciences and the advances in technology. In addition to the prewar occupations—dental technicians, x-ray technicians, dieticians, etc.—new occupations emerged, such as dental hygienists, radiology technicians, laboratory technicians (professional level), occupational therapists, physical therapists, and so forth. A basic common problem among these nonmedical health occupations is the fact that their education and training systems still depend on special training schools apart from the formal education system that is based upon the School Education Law. The resulting shortage of facilities, poor staffing, and financial provisions, compared with formal schools under the School Education Law, is noteworthy.

NURSING HOME AND COMMUNITY HEALTH AGENCIES

Mainly due to the traditional hospitalization pattern in the country, nursing homes, which are now very popular in the Western countries, are not well developed in Japan. At present, there are principally three kinds of residential facilities for the aged: homes for the aged, nursing homes, and homes for the aged with a moderate fee. Of these, the first has a fairly long history from the prewar periods, and the second and third ones are postwar institutions.

Homes for the aged are for those sixty-five years and over who have difficulty in being cared for and nursed in their own homes because of their physical or mental conditions as well as for environmental or economic reasons. Of the costs for the administration of these homes, 80% is borne by the national government, 20% by the prefectural, municipal, town, or village governments, which have their welfare offices in their respective areas and are also responsible for patient placement.

Nursing homes accommodate those "bed-ridden" aged. The financial aspect of their administration is the same as with homes for the aged except that those who can afford to pay are requested to meet the cost, the amount of which is decided according to the economic status of the client. The placement of patients is made through the local welfare offices.

Homes with moderate fees are divided into two types. In type A the meals are provided, whereas in type B the residents have to cook for themselves. National subsidy is given for the cost of the administration of these homes, but type A residents are required to pay about 23,700 to 26,700 yen and for type Bs the approximate upper limit is fixed as 18,000 yen per month. In 1978 the numbers of these facilities and total capacity were: 714 homes for the aged with 55,482 beds; 938 nursing homes with 71,352 beds; and 143 moderate fee homes for the aged with 8,952 beds.

The welfare office is the comprehensive, first-line organ for social welfare administration and services, and it carries out not only various aid programs for the needy, activities of care, and fostering and rehabilitation as stipulated by the relevant laws, but also other overall activities related to social welfare. The total number of the welfare offices was 1,140 as of June 1975, 343 of which were established by prefectures, 793 by cities and metropolitan Tokyo wards, and 4 by towns and villages. The total number of full-time staff of the welfare offices was 51,128 persons as of June 1975.

As of May 1975 there were also 402 welfare centers, established to provide a variety of welfare services to the population. There also were child guidance centers, providing a number of child welfare services, established in some 152 prefectures and large municipalities. Recently, a small number of day care facilities and ambulatory rehabilitation facilities have been developed by local governments.

HEALTH INSURANCE AND HEALTH COSTS

Social Health Insurance Scheme

Background. In 1922 the Health Insurance Law, the first social insurance program in Japan and in the Asian region, was enacted to cover laborers working in the places covered by the Factory Law or the Mining Law. Enforcement of the law was delayed until 1927 because of a series of socioeconomic and natural disasters. When the program finally started, the insured numbered only 1.9 million. Following this law, in 1938 the National Health Insurance Law was enacted, covering farm, forestry, and fishing people. Since then, government efforts have been made continuously to improve and promote health insurance programs; finally in 1961 the national goal of universal coverage had been achieved by an entirely revised National Health Insurance Law.

There are now in Japan three major schemes for medical care security, and they are an integral component of the social security scheme. The first, and the core of the system, is the social health insurance scheme covering the whole population of the country. The second is the medical assistance scheme, based on the Daily Life Security Law (1950). The law provides for public assistance, subject to a means test, to all needy persons. This scheme consists of aid for livelihood, education, housing, medical care, maternity, occupation, and funeral. All aid, except medical care, is provided in cash. The third major scheme is the public medical care scheme for selected diseases or disorders. There are presently thirteen such programs based on the laws, for example, the Tuberculosis Control Law (1950), the Mental Health Law (1950), the Maternal and Child Health Law (1965), the Old People's Welfare Law (1963), and so forth.

Classification of the programs. Medical services are supported, for the most part, by health insurance. The health insurance programs in the country can principally be divided into two categories: health insurance for employees and their dependents, and the national health insurance program for others. The former category is subdivided into several programs. One is the government-managed health insurance (*seikan-kempo*), the insurance carrier being the government. Another is the society-managed health insurance (*kumiai-kempo*), which is established for each specific type of large enterprise through a special health insurance society for the employees of the enterprise. There are also insurance programs for specific groups of workers—the seamen's insurance program, the day laborers' health insurance program—and four types of mutual aid association insurance programs such as for civil servants.

The national health insurance program for other citizens is managed by the primary local authorities (cities, towns, and villages) throughout the country. These programs also include specific national health insurance associations that are organized exclusively for a profession or trade. (Table 20 shows the coverage of social health insurance scheme by program as of March 1979.)

Benefits. Generally, the benefits include physician and dentist services in the hospitals and clinics for diagnostic procedures and treatment including medication, surgical operations, and hospital care and services. Preventive examinations and normal delivery are not included in the benefits. There are also cash benefits for absentees from work due to sickness, injury, or childbirth, from the fourth day of disablement for at most six months, providing allowances equal to 60% of his or her standard remuneration.

Because of the differences in financial conditions, the degree of partial liability borne by the beneficiaries varies between the programs. The benefit rate for the beneficiaries in the employees' health insurance programs is 100% except for a small partial liability for the first medical consultation and for the first month when hospitalized. Expenses for a private room, for special denture material, or for a private nurse are excluded from the benefits. The benefit rate for dependents covered by the employees' health insurance program managed by the government was raised from 50% to 70% in 1975. With the national health insurance program, the benefit rate has been 70% for both householders and dependents since 1968. Many associations provide fringe benefits in with the association health insurance, in addition to the legal benefits, such as a partial liability benefit for dependents.

Since 1973 the partial payment by the patient and dependent has been subsidized by the government in the case of tuberculosis and mental diseases; where the dependent's payment exceeds 39,000 yen a month, that patient is entitled to reimbursement matching the amount in excess of 39,000 yen as "special payment for the expensive medical care" (*kogaku-ryoyohi*). This became a benefit to members of the national health insurance program in 1975. In addition, if patients are aged 70 years or older, they get free medical service from their primary local authority with a slight income limitation. Any insured person who wants to receive medical service is free to go to any hospital or clinic and present their membership card. Practically all medical facilities are under health insurance programs.

Finance and contribution. Health insurance is supported by contributions and subsidies from national or local governments. As a rule, the premium of the employees' health insurance is shared on a 50–50 basis by employee and employer, and the amount is determined by multiplying the wage of the insured by a fixed rate. In the government-managed health insurance, the rate was raised to 8% of a standard remuneration in February 1978. The rate of the association-managed health insurance varies among associations, but it is generally low as compared to the government-managed health insurance.

In the national health insurance, most insurers collect premiums from their members as an object tax under the Local Tax Law. Since 1959 the liability of the National Treasury in connection with the medical care benefit of the national health insurance has been provided for in law. The national subsidy is presently about 45% of the medical care benefits. Because of continuing deficits, the liability of the National Treasury in the government-managed health insurance has also been provided for in law since 1973. The national subsidy rate is now 16.4% of the medical care and the selected cash benefits.

Payment method and cost control systems. In the early stage of health insurance in Japan, a contract was made between the insurers and a medical association determining a yearly sum per capita, but in 1948 the present fee-for-service payment system was adopted according to a recommendation of a U.S. medical mission.

Thus, at the end of each month, each participating hospital or clinic makes a bill for the services rendered based on the flat fee schedule determined by the minister of health and welfare. The fee scale is called the "point system"; each act of medical practice is given a certain point score, and a fee is computed by multiplying the point score by the unit cost. The unit cost at present is 10 yen. The bill is submitted to the Social Insurance Medical Care Fee Payment Fund, which pools the money from each program, and the bill is checked by a medical consultant before payment. Unnecessary treatment is sometimes checked here and deleted, which often brings complaints from participating hospitals and clinics. Currently, the average rejection rate by the fund's Board of Audit stands at 0.8% of total payment.

In order to determine the fee schedule, the minister of health and welfare requests the recommendation of the Central Social Insurance Medical Council, which consists of six representatives of insurers, six representatives of providers (for example, physicians, dentists, and pharmacists), and three representatives of the public interest. Today, treatment under health insurance is almost free from restrictions, and practically no drugs, clinical tests, or surgical operations are excluded from use if effective. For example, renal dialysis, kidney transplant, pace-maker implants, and CT scans are approved under health insurance. However, there is continuous tension between the ministry of health and welfare and the Japan Medical Association focusing on the standard medical fee. The major complaints are that the point system is too low, that there are restrictions on the use of some new drugs and technology which physicians wish to administer, and that all physicians receive the same payment regardless of qualification or experience.

National Medical Care Expenditure

During the last two decades there has been a notable increase in national medical care expenditure. This figure includes the costs covered by health insurance, including accident insurance, public medical care, and the sum paid by each patient directly. Therefore, the figure excludes expenses for health examinations, maternity care, vaccination, corrective eyeglasses, artificial limbs, and treatments by a massagist, acupuncturist, or moxibustioner (a trained certified technician who cauterizes with moxa, originally introduced from Chinese medicine as a healing art against neuralgia, etc.). Since 1955 the national medical care expenditure has increased from a baseline of 100.0 to 470.0 in 1965; 2,712.7 in 1975; and 4,201.8 in 1978. During these periods, the proportion of funds provided by social insurance increased from 43.7% in 1955 to 72.7% in 1978, and the proportion of payment by patients decreased from 34.9% in 1955 to 11.7% in 1978.

The ratio of the national *medical care* expenditure to GNP rose from 2.69% in 1955 to 3.42% in 1965, responding to the attainment of a nationwide social health insurance scheme, and continued to increase up to 1973. However, a revision of the point system was made due to the increase in wages and prices after the energy crisis, and was accompanied by the new medical care policies mentioned earlier. All of these factors contributed to the unprecedented annual increase of national medical care expenditure by 35.8% in 1974, which came to 3.95% of GNP. The GNP growth was abruptly slowed after the energy crisis, but the trend of increasing medical care expenditure did not change. Thus, in 1978 the national medical care expenditure increased 17% over the previous year, and showed a sum of 10,000.4 billion yen, which represented 4.78% of GNP, or an average expenditure of 86,900 yen per capita.* Such a situation led to arguments in favor

*There is no all-inclusive health expenditure figure in Japan, as distinct from medical care. The amounts of the items such as public health, casual medical supply purchases, medical research, etc. are very small compared to the national medical care expenditure.

of limiting free medical care for the aged and increasing the share of the cost to be borne by the patients.

In the 93rd Diet in 1980 a reform bill of the Health Insurance Law was approved after two years of hot discussion. The main revisions of the law were: (1) improvement of the benefit rate for hospitalization of dependents from 70% to 80%; (2) increase of the partial liability by the insured in the cases of first medical consultation, and for a period of a month per day when hospitalized, from 600 yen to 800 yen, and from 200 yen to 500 yen, respectively; (3) lowering the starting point of the *kogaku-ryoyohi* for indigents from 39,000 yen to 15,000 yen; and (4) increase of the upper limits of the premium rates, from 0.8% to 0.91% for the government-managed health insurance and from 0.9% to 0.95% for the society-managed health insurance.

PUBLIC HEALTH

Historical Overview

As mentioned, the modern public health administration of Japan has evolved during the last 100 years in response to the pressing social needs and demands of each period. The pattern of public administration was introduced from the Western European countries and has evolved on the basis of the Meiji Constitution of 1889. Consequently, its long-standing pattern of strict legislative character is based on relevant administrative laws and stresses "line" much more than "staff" organization. The public health administration, started by the enactment of the ISEI in 1874 and oriented by the Meiji Constitution, was solely the responsibility of governmental agencies up to the end of the Second World War, in contrast to the medical care delivery scheme which was heavily dependent on the private sector.

During the first half of the Meiji era, the pressing health problems were outbreaks of acute infectious diseases such as cholera and smallpox. The public health administration became highly centralized and legal control oriented. After 1893, local public health administration was brought under the jurisdiction of the local police administrations, and this lasted to the end of the Second World War. In the latter half of the Meiji era, Japan underwent its industrial revolution, and environmental sanitation became an urgent task of the government. However, because of financial difficulties and repeated wars during the period, the provision of basic sanitary facilities was delayed for a long time. The Taisho era (1912–26) was marked by growing social tension under a series of economic and natural disasters. This period saw a change of disease pattern, from acute infectious diseases to socially rooted chronic infectious diseases, such as tuberculosis. Although there were continuing wars and increasing pressure from the military clique, various health laws were nonetheless enacted to cope with the changing disease pattern.

In 1938, in response to the social situation, the ministry of health and welfare was established. (As regards public health, it should be noted that the first Health Center Law was enacted in 1937; also, the Institute of Public Health and rural and urban health training centers were established by a grant from the Rockefeller Foundation in 1938.) Immediately after the war, based upon the new constitution, the national health system was reorganized. This was done with powerful support from the U.S. occupation authority under an extremely depressed national economy accompanied by inflation, shortage of food, and nationwide epidemics. The government made all efforts to reorganize and strengthen the national health system by legislation and by establishing the nationwide health center network in particular. Thus, a most notable change in the demographic pattern, "from high birth-death to low birth-death," occurred during the first postwar decade. From the beginning of the second decade, urbanization and industrialization were accelerated, and an improvement of the social health insurance scheme for the whole population was achieved in 1961.

Since then, the country has undergone a drastic socioeconomic change accompanied by rapid growth in the GNP, heavy chemical industries, information technology, and so forth. The improvement of life expectancy at birth and the decrease in the birth rate resulted in an aging of the population and changing disease patterns. The third decade was marked by serious pollution episodes and a great awakening of the people to the importance of environmental and community health.

Outline of the Present Status

Under the central government there are 47 prefectures including Tokyo Metropolis, and some 3,200 primary local authorities—that is, cities, towns, and villages, each with local government units and elected assemblies. These local governments conduct local public administration with the local autonomy power designated by the Local Autonomy Law of 1947.

There are usually four levels of general health administration in the country: central government; prefectural government; prefectural health center; and city, town, and village government. Currently, thirty large municipalities designated by the Health Center Law (1947) are required to establish their own health centers in place of prefectural governments.

Public health administration is principally divided into three categories: general health administration, school health administration, and industrial health administration. Of these, school health administration is highly decentralized in contrast to the highly centralized industrial health administration; general health administration falls somewhere between these two extremes. There are presently more than 100 national laws relating to medical and health matters. Many of them were enacted after the war, and some were enacted by amendments to prewar legislation. Some are very old, for example, the Infectious Disease Prevention Law (1897) and the Leprosy Prevention Law (1907). There are 9 laws on disease prevention, 25 on environmental health, 11 on public health, health administration, and health statistics, 14 on medical care and medical personnel, 9 on pharmaceutical affairs, and a number of other laws relating to health—laws on social welfare, social health insurance, and so forth. There are many orders and regulations for implementation of these national laws, made by the cabinet or a related ministry. Within the above-mentioned legal framework at the national level, enactment of local regulations or rules are made by the local governments under the terms of the Local Autonomy Law (1947).

The fiscal year begins on 1 April and ends on 31 March in the following year. At the national government level, the annual general account budget for each ministry or agency is designated in the standard budget, which includes the national subsidy rate that is based in turn on the relevant national law. In the fiscal year 1981 the national subsidy amounted to 14,058 billion yen, and this figure stood at 31% of the total general account budget of the central government. Of these subsidies, the largest category is the social security scheme, which amounts to some 5,000 billion yen under the jurisdiction of the ministry of health and welfare. The total general account budget of the local government budget has been some 30% larger than the national government general account budget in recent years. Local government income consists mainly of local taxes (about 30% of the total revenue), equalization grants from the national government, national subsidies, and local government bonds.

Ministry of Health and Welfare (Koseisho)

Established in 1938, the ministry of health and welfare has various missions to serve the people of Japan in protecting their health and promoting welfare. The ministry is composed of nine bureaus (public health, environmental health, medical affairs, pharmaceutical affairs, social welfare, children and families, health insurance, pension, and war victims' relief), two departments (statistics and information, and water supply and environmental sanitation), and one separate agency, the Social Insurance Agency. In addition, the ministry has some affiliated research institutes: the Institute of Population Problems, the Institute of Public Health, the National Institute of Mental Health, the National Institute of Nutrition, the National Institute of Health, the National Institute of Hospital Administration, and the National Institute of Hygienic Sciences. Of these, the Institute of Public Health, established by the donation of the Rockefeller Foundation in 1938, is the only comprehensive education and research institution at the graduate and postgraduate level in the country. The principal roles of the ministry are: (1) health and medical service—taking measures for the prevention and treatment of various diseases, improvement of environmental health, adequate provision for medical care facilities, training of health and medical manpower, quality control over pharmaceutical preparations, and control of narcotics; (2) social welfare service—taking measures to provide a minimum standard of living for the indigent people, giving aid to the disabled people and widowed families for facilitating their eventual self-support status, helping to provide adequate care and protection of children, and taking measures for the serious problem of the aged population, which will be further accelerated in the future; and (3) social insurance—administration and implementation of various health insurance and pension schemes to relieve the economic burden on individuals in the case of sickness, old age, invalidity, etc. In addition to the above, the ministry is giving aid to war-bereaved families as well as atomic bomb sufferers. It also directly administers its own national hospitals and sanatoria including highly specialized institutions such as the National Cancer Center and the National Cardiovascular Disease Center. Each bureau of the ministry conducts the research necessary to carry on its work. For example, the Medical Affairs Bureau provides cancer research grants, and the Pharmaceutical Affairs Bureau provides research grants for the development of drugs. In addition, the ministry's Office of Planning and Evaluation and Office of Science and Technology have their own research grants, namely, for health and welfare administrative services, and for medical technology, and special ministerial research grants for large scale nationally needed subjects.

The ministry regularly conducts a number of health statistical analyses and nationwide health-related surveys. The results are published annually by the ministry, the principal reports being: (1) *Data on the Medical and Health Services Demand:* (a) on revealed demand (surveys based upon the reporting system)—surveys on communicable diseases, food poisoning, patients, the government-managed health insurance, medical care assistance, and medical care benefits of the national health insurance; vital statistics; reports on hospitals, national hospitals, and national sanatoria; (b) on potential needs and demand (surveys based upon interviews)—surveys on national health and national nutrition, basic survey on health and sanitation, basic survey for health and welfare administration, and special surveys on the selected diseases (tuberculosis, mental disease, cancer, cardiovascular disease, etc.); and (2) *Data on the Medical and Health Services Supply:* surveys on medical care facilities and on health manpower (physicians, dentists, pharmacists, public health nurses, clinical nurses, midwives, and other allied health personnel), reports on the national health administration activities and on the health center operation, statistical report on eugenics and maternal protection, school health statistics, industrial health statistics, guideline of the local equalization grant scheme, statistics of the local government finance, etc.

Prefectural Governments and Health Centers

The organizational structure of prefectural government is designated by the Local Autonomy Law. The number of health-related divisions are four to eleven, according to the population size of prefectures. Each prefectural government has a department or bureau responsible for health administration in order to carry out its health programs in compliance with the national policies and programs directed by the ministry of health and welfare.

All prefectural governments have a local (prefectural) health laboratory that assists their health centers by performing various laboratory tests and investigations on diseases. There are currently twenty-one local health laboratories established by large municipalities besides those at the prefectural level. Prefectural government also has a mental health center that both assists mental health consultation in the usual district health centers and provides counseling services for complicated and difficult cases.

As mentioned before, based upon the Health Center Law (1947), all prefectural and 30 large municipal governments must establish health centers aiming at one for every 100,000 population, for the improvement of public health in each health center district. The health center is financed by local and national governments. As of April 1980, there were 855 health centers throughout the country; of these, 655 were prefectural, 144 were municipal, and 53 were in metropolitan Tokyo. The health centers are classified into five types: U (urban), UR (urban-rural), R (rural), and L (large area with small population). In addition, an S type is responsible for small areas with less than 30,000 population. According to this classification, there were 275 U, 98 UR, 320 R, 128 L, and 34 S health centers as of April 1980.

The health centers serve as the community health service agencies as well as the district health administration units. As of April 1980 these were staffed by 1,203 physicians, 1,271 veterinarians, 7,313 public health nurses, 1,461 x-ray technicians, 1,773 laboratory technicians, 1,168 nutritionists, 890 health statisticians, 556 health educators, 5,586 food and sanitary inspectors, 1,160 meat inspectors, and 4,925 administrative service personnel.

During the first decade after the war—when urbanization and industrialization were hardly noticeable due to the destruction of the war, and health activity of cities, towns, and villages was very weak—health centers contributed remarkably to the improvement of community health, especially in communicable disease control, maternal and child health, nutrition, tuberculosis control, food and sanitary inspection, public health nursing, health education, and so on. Afterwards, however, particularly since the 1960s, the country underwent drastic socioeconomic changes, and there have been notable shifts in community health needs and demands due to the changes in disease patterns and different modes of living of the people. To cope with these changes, the ministry of health and welfare has promoted since 1960 "integrated health planning" (*kyodo-hoken-keikaku*) at the primary local authority level, accompanied by a new classification and some reorganization of health centers. The health and welfare ministry subsequently developed a plan to reform the existing health center network, based on a report from a ministerial advisory committee in 1977 to establish the "health and medical services area"—that is, up-to-date health units of secondary level within each prefecture—and most of the existing health center districts have been noted to be adequate to this level of area.

The functions and programs of the health centers are: control of communicable diseases (including preventive vaccination); control of tuberculosis; control of venereal diseases; control of other diseases (e.g., trachoma, parasitic diseases, degenerative diseases, etc.); promotion of mental health, and maternal and child health (health guidance for pregnant women, nursing mothers, and babies and infants, medical guidance for handicapped children, mother's classes, and others); consultation on the eugenic protection; dental hygiene; improvement of nutrition; food, milk, and meat sanitation; rabies prevention; maintenance of environmental sanitation (in houses, hotels, public bathhouses, theaters and other such entertainment facilities, laundries, barber shops, beauty parlors, garbage and waste disposal facilities, water supply facilities, sewage and graveyards); matters concerning environmental pollution, medical affairs (concerning the Medical Service Law, the Medical Practitioner's Law, etc.), pharmaceutical affairs (concerning the Pharmaceutical Affairs Law, etc.), public health nursing, medical social service, health laboratory service, health and vital statistics, and health education for the public.

City, Town, and Village Governments

In April 1981 there were 3,255 (646 city, 1,991 town, and 618 village) primary local authorities throughout the country. On the average, each prefectural health center thus had 3 to 4 primary local authorities in its district. (In the cases of the health centers established by large municipalities, the situation is somewhat different in that each health center district is a part of the larger city.)

At the city, town, and village level governments, there is a division or section responsible for health, and usually public health nurses are employed. The primary local governments carry out various community health programs—health screening against tuberculosis, medical examination for people over 65 years of age, preventive vaccination, etc.—based upon the relevant laws, in addition to the basic environmental services such as water supply, refuse and nightsoil disposal, and so forth. Furthermore, in recent years most of the primary local authorities developed on a voluntary basis such programs as health screening for cardiovascular diseases, cancer, and so on.

All primary local governments are also required by law to establish and run a national health insurance program; in many cases, medical care facilities, including hospitals, are established by the local national health insurance body and provide medical services directly to the inhabitants. "Integrated health planning" by city, town, and village governments has been encouraged by the ministry of health and welfare since 1960, and this sort of community health planning with citizen participation has become popular among the local authorities in recent years.

In the 1978 fiscal year the ministry of health and welfare inaugurated a new national health policy, "national health development," which provided some national grants to each primary local government for the promotion of health development efforts aimed at comprehensive, continuing health care for all inhabitants. At the same time the ministry introduced a new plan, as an integral part of the above policy, to establish small-scale community health stations throughout the country with some national subsidy. About 300 stations are currently established at the primary local authority level. Associated with these community health facilities are some 700 maternal and child health centers at the primary local government level.

Health Planning

Mainly due to the traditional public administrative milieu of the country, categorical health planning by respective administrative units had been predominant at all levels of government for a long time, as evidenced in tuberculosis control and maternal and child health. There was a planning process on a categorical basis: (1) assessment of present status, (2) problem identification, (3) priority setting, (4) providing policy formulation, legal basis, and budget making, (5) national and local implementation, and (6) evaluation. During the 1960s, however, social demand for comprehensive planning grew as a result of drastic socioeconomic changes accompanied by demographic alterations, urbanization, heavy chemical industrialization, technological innovation, and so on. Under such a socioeconomic situation, the National Double Income Plan of 1960 (a ten-year socioeconomic development plan) played a significant role to promote overall socioeconomic development plans at various levels of local governments. Within this framework, health planning has been developed gradually.

At the local level, however, it is worth noting that since 1960, integrated health planning at the primary local authority level has grown steadily, with an increasing participation of the people in the respective communities. In 1969 the local governments were requested by the Local Autonomy Law Amendment to develop a "principal vision" or long-range goals as the guideline for a socioeconomic development plan for each local authority. Afterwards, medium-term development plans were formulated at the primary local authority level, with a health sector plan as a part of these plans. Currently, a popular pattern of the planning at this level is to organize advisory committees composed of members of the local medical association, health-related professionals, and members of voluntary organizations, and often representatives of schools, social welfare agencies, and health centers concerned, and so forth. At this level, the planning process commonly used is composed of seven steps: (1) community health survey, (2) community health diagnosis, (3) technical planning, (4) administrative planning, (5) health education, (6) community health organization, and (7) evaluation. The principal role of the health center concerned is to provide data, technical advice, and assistance to the committee and in turn to the primary local authorities.

Recently, regional (prefecture and large city) health planning started gradually with some national grants for organization of advisory committees for this purpose.

Grass-Roots Organizations and Community Participation

The traditional grass-roots organizations are highly popular both in rural and urban communities, for they are helpful in contributing to daily community life. These organizations are voluntary in character, and generally collect small membership fees on a household basis, carry out various programs (for example, recreation, community festivals, and sanitation), circulate notices from the relevant local governments, and so forth.

In addition to these multipurpose citizen organizations, there are commonly diversified organizations, groups, and circles such as women's associations, clubs for the aged, children's associations, PTAs, and so on.

After the war, the people actively participated in various community primary health care programs. This community health action was based at first in the field of environmental sanitation, particularly with vector control campaigns against serious outbreaks of epidemics. This pattern of citizen participation then grew steadily in various community health programs, for example, in maternal and child health, family planning, tuberculosis control, parasite control, and nutrition. From the end of the 1950s through the 1960s these interested citizens received technical guidance from their health centers. At present, many primary local governments nominate voluntary health leaders or communicators for the promotion of community health.

Under the above-mentioned conditions, many different kinds of volunteer associations have been organized, aimed at the improvement of the community's health. For example, in Osaka prefecture there are voluntary women's associations for health in every city, town, and village, and a prefectural federation was organized with some 200,000 members in 1954. Every prefecture now has some kind of federation of the voluntary health associations in cities, towns, and villages located in their area.

Thus, there is a growing trend of city, town, and village health planning which started in 1960 and was encouraged by the ministry of health and welfare. As noted, the ministry introduced a new national health policy of "community health development" in 1978. It seems too early to evaluate this new health policy, but undoubtedly, with an active citizen participation in community health programs, there are hopeful signs for the sound improvement and promotion of the nation's health in the future.

CONCLUSION

Japan's health care system is indeed complex. It bears many similarities to Western systems but at the same time many peculiarities due to its sociocultural background. The country adopted a nationwide social health insurance scheme in 1961, and medical care services are now primarily supported by the health insurance scheme based on the fee-for-service pattern. The delivery of medical care services is highly dependent on the private sector. The ratios of hospital beds to population and of medical manpower to population are high, and there are 80 medical schools with an annual enrollment of 8,360 students.

During the three decades after the Second World War, Japan made remarkable strides in the area of its nation's health, and in recent years life expectancy at birth increased and the infant mortality rate dropped; Japan's statistics in these two areas are among the best in the world. However, the country is now undergoing an extremely difficult new era, due to the aging of its population at an unusually high tempo and hard financial conditions at both the national and local government levels. Consequently, a new department on health care for the aged was established in 1983 in the Bureau of Public Health. The objective is to introduce a new system for the well-aging of the adult people, in addition to the medical service program for the aged.

Japan is extremely poor in natural resources but fortunately has well-educated people throughout the country who are increasingly concerned with community health; also, most private practitioners actively participate in community medicine. Community participation and involvement in health have been noticeable since the Second World War.

From the institutional point of view, the basic problem in the current system is the gap between the curative, preventive, and social welfare components. The new well-aging scheme will play an important part in overcoming this problem in the coming ten years.

Bibliography

Bowers, J.Z. *Medical Education in Japan.* New York: Harper & Row, 1965.

Broida, J.H., and N. Maeda. "Japan's High-Cost Illness Insurance Program—A Study of Its First Three Years, 1974–76." *Public Health Reports* 93 (March–April, 1978).

Fuse, S. "Ishi no Rekishi" (A history of physicians in Japan). *Chuko-Shinsho,* no. 534, Chuo-Koron-Sha, 1979.*

Hashimoto, M. "A Case Study on Health Planning Methods in Japan—Comprehensive Community Health Planning." *Bull. Inst. Publ. Health,* vol. 26, nos. 3–4 (1977).

Hashimoto, M. "Health Care and Medical Systems in Japan." *Comparative Medicine East and West* VI, no. 3 (1978).

Hashimoto, M. "The Professional Education and Training of Non-medical Health Personnel in Japan." *Social Science and Medicine,* vol. 12A, Pergamon Press, 1978.

Hashimoto, M. "Studies on the Development and Future Demand/Supply of Health Manpower in Japan." *Bull. Inst. Publ. Health,* vol. 29, no. 1 (1980).*

Hashimoto, S., K. Kiikuni, et al. *Health Services in Japan.* Tokyo: Japan Convention Service Inc., 1977.

Japan Medical Association. "National Medical Care." *Almanac, 1966–1981. Shunju-Sha, Tokyo.**

The Japan of Today. Tokyo: International Society for Educational Information, 1980.

Jonas, S. "Japan Strain Under Complex Health System." *Hospitals,* J.A.H.A., vol. 49, 1975.

Katabami, J., et al. "A Survey of Physician Activities." *Bull. Inst. Publ. Health,* vol. 30, no. 1 (1981).*

Kosei-Tokei-Kyokai. *Kokumin Eisei no Doko* (Trends in the nation's health). 1981.*

Ministry of Health and Welfare. *Health and Welfare Services in Japan.* Tokyo: Yoshida Finance and Social Security Law Institute, 1977.

Nursing in Japan. Tokyo: Japanese Nursing Association, 1977.

Ohmura, J. "Analysis of Factors Affecting the Needs and Demand for Medical Care." *Social Science and Medicine,* vol. 12, no. 6A, Pergamon Press, 1978.

Social Insurance Agency. *Outline of Social Insurance in Japan.* Tokyo, 1980.

Story, R. *A History of Modern Japan.* Baltimore: Penguin, 1967.

Sugaya, A. "Nihon no Byoin" (Hospitals in Japan). *Chuko-Shinsho,* no. 600, Chuo-Koron-Sha, 1981.*

Takemi, T. "The General Practitioner in Japan." *World Medical Journal* (January–February, 1971).

* Written in Japanese only.

Table 1 Japanese population by age and sex, 1980

Age	Number (Thousands)		%	
	Male	Female	Male	Female
All ages	57,120	59,092	100.0%	100.0%
Up to 4 years	4,343	4,157	7.6	7.0
5 to 9	5,099	4,869	8.9	8.2
10 to 14	4,552	4,334	8.0	7.3
15 to 19	4,196	3,976	7.4	6.7
20 to 24	3,901	3,853	6.8	6.5
25 to 34	9,922	9,804	17.4	16.6
35 to 44	8,695	8,742	15.2	14.8
45 to 54	7,529	7,657	13.2	13.0
55 to 64	4,438	5,608	7.8	9.5
65 and over	4,445	6,094	7.8	10.3
Median age	32.4	34.3		

SOURCE: Prime Minister's Office, *Census Report.*

Table 2 Live births, birth rates, and fertility rates, Japan

Year	Births	Birth Rate	Fertility Rate[a]
1979	1,642,582	14.2	0.84
1978	1,708,643	14.9	0.86

SOURCE: Ministry of Health and Welfare, *Vital Statistics.*

[a]Net reproduction rates per one woman aged 15 to 49.

Table 3 Infant mortality rates by age, selected years, Japan

Year	Under 1 Year	28 Days to 11 Months	Under 28 Days
1950	60.1	32.8	27.4
1960	30.7	13.7	17.0
1965	18.5	6.8	11.7
1970	13.1	4.4	8.7
1971	12.4	4.1	8.2
1972	11.7	3.8	7.8
1973	11.3	3.9	7.4
1974	10.8	3.7	7.1
1975	10.0	3.3	6.8
1976	9.3	3.0	6.4
1977	8.9	2.8	6.1
1978	8.4	2.7	5.6
1979	7.9	2.6	5.2

SOURCE: Ministry of Health and Welfare, *Vital Statistics.*

Table 4 Infant mortality rates by selected causes, selected years, Japan

Causes of Death	1955	1960	1965	1970	1975	1979
Total, under 1 year	39.8	30.7	18.5	13.1	10.0	7.9
Pneumonia and bronchitis	9.4	8.5	3.6	1.7	0.9	0.4
Gastro-intestinal diseases	3.4	2.3	1.0	0.5	0.2	0.2
Immaturity, unqualified				1.3	0.8	0.5
Other diseases of newborn	16.2	12.5	6.9	1.1	0.7	0.1
Congenital anomalies	2.1	1.9	2.0	2.0	2.1	2.0
Birth injuries; asphyxia of newborn; unspecified	1.1	—	1.8	1.9	1.7	2.5
Accident	1.0	0.8	0.7	0.6	0.5	0.4
All other causes	6.6	4.7	2.5	4.0	3.1	1.8

Source: Ministry of Health and Welfare, *Vital Statistics.*

Note: Because of the changes in disease classification in 1968 and 1979, data are not strictly comparable.

Table 5 Death rates for the 13 leading causes of death, Japan

	1960			1970			1979		
Causes of Death	Rank	Death Rate	% of Total Deaths	Rank	Death Rate	% of Total Deaths	Rank	Death Rate	%of Total Deaths
All causes		756.4	100.0		691.4	100.0		597.3	100.0
Cerebrovascular diseases	1	160.7	21.3	1	175.8	25.4	1	137.7	23.1
Malignant neoplasms	2	100.4	13.3	2	116.3	16.8	2	135.7	22.7
Diseases of heart	3	73.2	9.7	3	86.7	12.5	3	96.9	16.2
Pneumonia and bronchitis	5	49.3	6.5	6	34.1	4.9	4	28.5	4.8
Senility	4	58.0	7.7	5	38.1	5.5	5	25.5	4.3
Accidents	6	41.7	5.5	4	42.5	6.2	6	25.3	4.2
Suicide	8	21.6	2.9	9	15.3	2.2	7	18.0	3.0
Cirrhosis of liver	12	9.7	1.3	10	12.5	1.8	8	14.2	2.4
Hypertension	11	16.2	2.1	7	17.7	2.6	9	14.0	2.3
Nephritis and nephrosis	10	16.5	2.2	11	8.9	1.3	10	8.0	1.3
Diabetes mellitus	13	3.4	0.5	13	7.4	1.1	11	7.0	1.2
Tuberculosis	7	34.2	4.5	8	15.4	2.2	12	5.8	1.0
Gastro-enteritis	9	21.2	2.8	12	8.3	1.2	13	3.5	0.6
All other causes		150.3	19.9		112.4	16.3		77.2	12.9

Source: Ministry of Health and Welfare, *Vital Statistics.*

Table 6 Information not available.

Table 7 Information not available.

Table 8a All active major and allied health care workers: 1960, 1970, and 1980, Japan

Year	All Health Professions	Physicians	Dentists	Pharmacists	Public Health Nurses	Midwives	Registered Nurses	Veterinarians
				Number Active				
1960	389,303	103,131	33,177	60,257	12,796	55,436	105,800	18,706
1970	441,813	118,990	37,859	79,393	14,007	31,559	139,229	20,776
1980	645,337	156,235	53,602	116,056	17,957	25,867	248,165	27,455
				% Distribution				
1960	100.0	26.5	8.5	15.5	3.3	14.2	27.2	4.8
1970	100.0	26.9	8.6	18.0	3.2	7.1	31.5	4.7
1980	100.0	24.2	8.3	18.0	2.8	4.0	38.5	4.3
				Per 100,000 Population				
1960	311.1	110.4	35.5	64.5	14.0	60.9	116.2	20.0
1970	427.7	114.7	36.5	76.5	13.6	30.7	135.5	20.2
1980	520.1	133.6	45.8	99.3	15.4	22.1	180.2	23.7

SOURCE: Ministry of Health and Welfare, *Annual Survey of Physicians, Dentists, and Pharmacists;* Ministry of Health and Welfare, *Annual Report on National Health Administration.*

Table 8b All active major and allied health care workers: 1960, 1970, and 1980, Japan

Occupation	1960	1970	1980
Dieticians (registered)[a]	—	801	1,696
Occupational therapists[a]	—	305	857
Physical therapists[a]	—	1,082	2,517
Clinical laboratory technicians[a]	—	—	26,827[b]
Sanitary laboratory technicians[a]	4,980	15,984	2,443[b]
Radiology technicians[a]	—	6,411	13,821
Speech pathologists and audiologists[a]	—	—	647
Licensed assistant nurses[c]	70,065	164,464	263,439
Dental hygienists[c]	1,390	5,804	18,775
Dental laboratory technicians[c]	7,701	8,722	19,684
X-ray technicians[c]	6,147	6,211	4,142

SOURCE: Ministry of Health and Welfare, *Annual Survey of Physicians, Dentists, and Pharmacists;* Ministry of Health and Welfare, *Annual Report on National Health Administration.*

[a]Basic educational preparation at least baccalaureate level.
[b]These figures are not comparable due to an institutional change during the 1970s.
[c]Basic educational preparation less than baccalaureate level.

Table 9 Operational medical schools, medical students enrolled by sex, and medical school graduates by sex for the academic year 1978 (April 1978–March 1979), Japan

Number of operational medical schools	76[a]
Total medical students	48,704
Women medical students	6,084 (12.5%)
Total medical graduates	6.309
Women medical graduates	733 (11.6%)

SOURCE: Ministry of Education and Culture, *Basic School Survey.*

[a]There were by 1981, 80 medical schools with an annual enrollment of 8,360 students.

Table 10 Physicians, population, and physician/population ratios, selected years, Japan

Year	Total Physicians	Total Population (Millions)	Physicians Per 100,000 Population	Population Per Physician
1950	76,446	83.2	91.9	1,088
1960	103,131	93.4	110.4	934
1965	109,369	98.3	111.3	899
1970	118,990	103.1	114.7	866
1971	123,178	104.4	117.3	848
1972	125,302	105.7	116.7	844
1973	126,327	108.1	116.2	856
1974	128,455	109.4	116.7	852
1975	132,479	111.3	118.4	840
1976	134,934	112.4	119.3	833
1977	138,316	113.5	121.2	821
1978	142,984	114.5	124.1	801
1979	150,229	115.5	129.4	769
1980	156,235	116.2	133.6	744

SOURCE: Ministry of Health and Welfare, *Annual Survey of Physicians, Dentists, and Pharmacists.*

Table 11 Physicians by specialty and activity, 31 December 1980, Japan

Specialty	Total Physicians	Major Professional Activity					
		Patient Care			Other Professional Activity		
		Patient Care Total	Office-Based Practice	Hospital-Based Practice (Full-Time)	Teaching or Research Other Than Clinical Medicine	Administration and Public Health	Others
Total physicians	156,235	148,815	70,395	78,422	3,664	2,099	1,657
Internal medicine		24,571	6,827	17,744			
Respiratory		467	19	448			
Gastroenterology		946	123	823			
Cardiovascular disease		968	35	933			
Pediatrics		7,342	2,475	4,867			
Psychiatry		1,349	60	1,289			
Neurology		203	22	181			
Neurology (internal medicine)		463	9	454			
General surgery		10,406	563	9,843			
Orthopedics		5,418	781	4,637			
Plastic surgery		280	12	268			
Beauty surgery		11	8	3			
Brain-neurological surgery		2,025	11	2,014			
Respiratory surgery		92	—	92			
Cardiovascular surgery		347	—	347			
Pediatric surgery		236	33	203			
Obstetric-gynecology		8,422	3,697	4,725			
Obstetrics		28	4	24			
Gynecology		240	112	128			
Ophthalmology		6,182	3,887	2,295			
Otorhinolaryngology		4,767	2,936	1,831			
Broncho-oesophagus		15	—	15			
Dermatology		2,460	869	1,591			
Urology		1,909	79	1,830			

Table 11 *Continued*

Specialty	Total Physicians	Major Professional Activity					
		Patient Care			Other Professional Activity		
		Patient Care Total	Office-Based Practice	Hospital-Based Practice (Full-Time)	Teaching or Research Other Than Clinical Medicine	Administration and Public Health	Others
Venereal diseases		8	6	2			
Anal		125	86	39			
X-ray therapy		125	6	119			
Radiology		1,508	43	1,465			
Anesthesia		1,645	15	1,630			
General practice		1,633	1,447	186			
Internal medicine and related specialties		33,493	23,906	9,587			
General surgery and related specialties		10,412	6,591	3,821			
Internal medicine and surgical specialties		19,375	15,567	3,808			
X-ray Therapy and Radiology		9	4	5			
Others		1,014	91	923			
Unknown		321	69	252			

SOURCE: Ministry of Health and Welfare, *Survey on Physicians, Dentists, and Pharmacists,* 1980.

NOTE: Specialty reported by individual practicing physician on the occasion of annual survey on physicians by the ministry.

Table 12 Information not available

Table 13 Hospitals, beds, admissions, average daily census, and occupancy rate, by type of hospital, Japan

Type of Hospital	Hospitals		Beds (Thousands)		Admissions (Thousands)		Average Daily Census (Thousands)		Occupancy (%)	
	1970	1979	1970	1979	1970	1979	1970	1979	1970	1979
Total in Japan	7,973	8,800	1.062	1,092	5,648	6,783	854	1,037	81.6	83.0
Psychiatric	896	966	178	223	142	154	253	306	104.3	102.3
Communicable Disease	35	21	2.8	1.4	4.2	0.8	1.4	0.5	6.1	2.3
Tuberculosis	160	48	24.4	5.3	18.4	6.1	120	54	66.2	57.3
Leprosy	14	16	13.2	12.7	0.2	0.2	9.0	8.8	68.3	67.3
General	6,868	7,749	836	1,027	5,482	6,622	471	667	80.3	80.9

SOURCE: Ministry of Health and Welfare, *Hospital Report*, 1979.

Table 14 Hospitals by type of ownership or sponsorship, 1979, Japan

Ownership or Sponsorship	Hospitals					
	Total	Psychiatric	Communicable Disease	Tuberculosis	Leprosy	General
Total	8,800	966	21	48	16	7,749
National	450	3	—	1	13	433
Ministry of Health and Welfare	255	3	—	—	13	239
Ministry of Education	58	—	—	1	—	57
Other	137	—	—	—	—	137
Public	1,366	51	21	11	—	1,283
Prefecture	300	38	1	7	—	254
City, town, village	773	11	20	4	—	738
Red Cross	98	—	—	—	—	98
Kosei-Ren[a]	116	1	—	—	—	115
Other	79	1	—	—	—	78
Social insurance organization	141	—	—	1	—	140
Public corporation	359	63	—	6	2	288
Medical service corporation	2,734	507	—	14	—	2,213
School corporation	69	1	—	—	—	68
Company	87	1	—	—	—	86
Other corporation	239	12	—	—	1	226
Individual	3,355	328	—	15	—	3,012

SOURCE: Ministry of Health and Welfare, *Survey on Medical Care Facilities,* 1979.

[a]Federation of Agricultural Welfare Corporations

Table 15 Nursing homes and nursing home beds, Japan

Type of Nursing Care and Related Homes	Homes			Beds		
	1963	1973	1978	1963	1973	1978
Home for the Aged	673	890	939	47,024	67,770	71,060
Nursing Home	1	350	799	80	26,503	61,515
Home with Moderate Fee	16	82	164	1,082	5,352	10,036
Total	690	1,322	1,092	48,186	99,625	142,611

SOURCE: Ministry of Health and Welfare, *Survey of Social Welfare Institutions.*

Table 16 Information not available.

Table 17 National medical expenditure: amount and per capita amount by major source of funds and percentage of Gross National Product, selected years, Japan

	1979	1975	1970	1965	1960	1955
National medical expenditure (billion yen)	10,951	6,478	2,496	1,122	410	239
As % of the GNP	4.92	4.27	3.32	3.35	2.53	2.69
Sources of funds (billion yen)						
Government	1,382	847	282	147	45.1	27.9
Social health insurance	8,305	4,793	1,732	744	241.5	118.5
Employees' insurance	4,971	3,026	1,134	518	172.1	95.2
National health insurance	3,066	1,628	536	202	59.8	18.8
Others	268	278	62	24.8	9.6	4.5
Direct patient pay	1,264	838	482	231	122.9	92.3
Per capita expenditures (thousand yen)	94.3	57.9	24.0	11.4	4.4	2.7
Sources of funds						
Government	11.9	7.6	2.7	1.5	0.5	0.3
Social health insurance	71.5	42.8	16.7	7.6	2.6	1.3
Employees' insurance	42.8	27.1	10.9	5.3	1.8	1.1
National health insurance	26.4	15.3	5.2	2.1	0.6	0.2
Others	2.4	1.4	0.6	2.5	0.1	0.1
Direct patient pay	10.8	7.5	4.6	2.3	1.3	1.0
Percentage distribution of funds	100.0	100.0	100.0	100.0	100.0	100.0
Sources of funds						
Government	12.6	13.1	11.3	13.1	11.0	11.7
Social health insurance	75.8	74.0	69.8	66.3	59.0	49.6
Employees' insurance	45.4	46.8	45.4	46.1	42.0	39.9
National health insurance	28.0	25.1	21.5	18.0	14.6	7.9
Others	2.5	4.2	2.5	2.2	2.3	1.9
Direct patient pay	11.5	12.9	19.3	20.6	30.0	38.7
Addenda						
Gross National Product (billion yen)	222,702	149,501	73,046	32,814	16,207	8,865
Population (thousands)	116,133	111,940	103,720	98,275	93,419	89,276
Annual % change						
National medical expenditures	9.5	20.4	20.0	20.0	13.0	11.0
Government	5.5	16.4	21.6	20.6	12.8	5.7
Social health insurance	10.4	22.0	21.1	21.3	16.9	11.2
Employees' insurance	8.9	20.7	21.5	19.9	13.8	9.8
National health insurance	13.2	24.5	20.0	25.0	29.7	19.0
Others	6.9	21.7	23.0	21.0	−0.4	4.7
Direct patient pay	8.1	16.2	16.1	11.1	8.7	12.3
Gross National Product	7.7	20.4	15.8	13.1	19.1	13.3
Population	0.8	1.7	1.1	1.1	0.5	1.1

SOURCE: Ministry of Health and Welfare, *National Medical Expenditure,* 1979, 1975, 1970, 1965, 1960, and 1955.

Table 18 National medical expenditure by type of expenditure and source of funds, per capita amount, and percentage distribution, 1979, Japan

Type of Expenditures	Total	Government	Social Insurance	Patient
Total amount (in million yen)	10,951,000	1,381,800	8,304,900	1,264,300
Hospital inpatient services	3,948,200	818,500	2,881,100	241,000
Hospital outpatient services	1,773,800	155,200	1,358,600	260,000
Clinic inpatient services	455,900	56,200	346,800	52,900
Clinic outpatient services	3,526,000	315,000	2,742,500	486,900
Dental services	1,131,300	25,900	893,900	211,600
Pharmacy services	115,500	11,000	93,000	11,500
Per capita amount (yen), total	94,288	11,890	71,512	10,887
Hospital inpatient services	34,038	7,039	24,886	20,794
Hospital outpatient services	15,275	1,332	11,728	22,427
Clinic inpatient services	3,960	487	3,004	4,573
Clinic outpatient services	30,361	2,711	23,456	41,915
Dental services	9,712	226	7,723	18,181
Pharmacy services	1,037	95	787	980
Percentage distribution, total	100.0	100.0	100.0	100.0
Hospital inpatient services	36.1	59.2	34.8	19.1
Hospital outpatient services	16.2	11.2	16.4	20.6
Clinic inpatient services	4.2	4.1	4.2	4.2
Clinic outpatient services	32.2	22.8	32.8	38.5
Dental services	10.3	1.9	10.8	16.7
Pharmacy services	1.1	0.8	1.1	0.9

SOURCE: Ministry of Health and Welfare, *National Medical Expenditure,* 1979.

Table 19 Table not applicable.

Table 20 Coverage of social health insurance by program as of 31 March 1979, Japan

	Total (Thousands)	Insured (Thousands)	Dependent (Thousands)	%
Total population	114,511			100.0
Employees' insurance	70,420	30,560	39,860	61.3
Government-managed health insurance	29,715	13,815	15,900	25.9
Society-managed health insurance	26,961	11,077	15,884	23.5
Day laborers' health insurance	568	349	219	0.5
Seamen's insurance	681	222	459	0.6
Mutual aid association	12,495	5,097	7,398	11.1
National health insurance	44,508	—	—	38.7

SOURCE: Ministry of Health and Welfare.

Health Services in the Netherlands

Harmen A. Tiddens,
Joep (P) Heesters, and
Joost (M) van de Zande

INTRODUCTION

With 14.2 million inhabitants and a land area of 33.929 km^2, the Netherlands is a densely populated country. The greater part of the land is used for agricultural purposes. The remaining 35% is used for residental purposes, industry, and woodland; in addition to this, 8% is constituted by water, one of the characteristic physical elements of the Netherlands.

The form of government in the Netherlands is a constitutional monarchy. The head of the Dutch state is Queen Beatrix, who is vested with symbolical rather than actual power. Within the political system, which is drawn up according to the principles of parliamentary democracy, legislation and policy come about as follows:

By means of voting, usually once every four years, the population determines the distribution of the 150 seats in the Second Chamber. In the recent elections of 1982 the Social Democratic party (the PvdA) became the largest party, with 47 seats, followed by the Christian Democratic party (the CDA), the Conservative party (the VVD), and the Liberals (D'66). The other eight parties each have a very limited number of seats. The four largest parties then proceed to consultations for the purpose of forming a government. Dutch political practice is always that a cabinet is formed in which the Christian Democrats decide to cooperate with the Social Democrats or the Conservatives. Although the government, under the leadership of the prime minister, holds the actual power, the First and the Second Chambers exert a strong measure of control on its activities and policy proposals. The First Chamber, which numbers 75 seats, is chosen by the members of the 11 provincial states.

As was the case with all highly industrialized countries in the world, the Netherlands entered a period of serious economic reversal upon the oil crisis of 1973. In the period of 1970 to 1980 unemployment among the total working population, which consists of more than 4.7 million persons, climbed from 0.9 to 4.7%. In the beginning of 1982 the Netherlands had 470,000 registered unemployed persons, nearly 10% of the working population.

In spite of this possibly temporary recession, the Netherlands is one of the most prosperous countries in the world. In 1980 a gross national product of more than 330 billion guilders and a net national income at market prices of nearly 300 billion was realized. This yielded an average per capita income of 21,000 guilders.

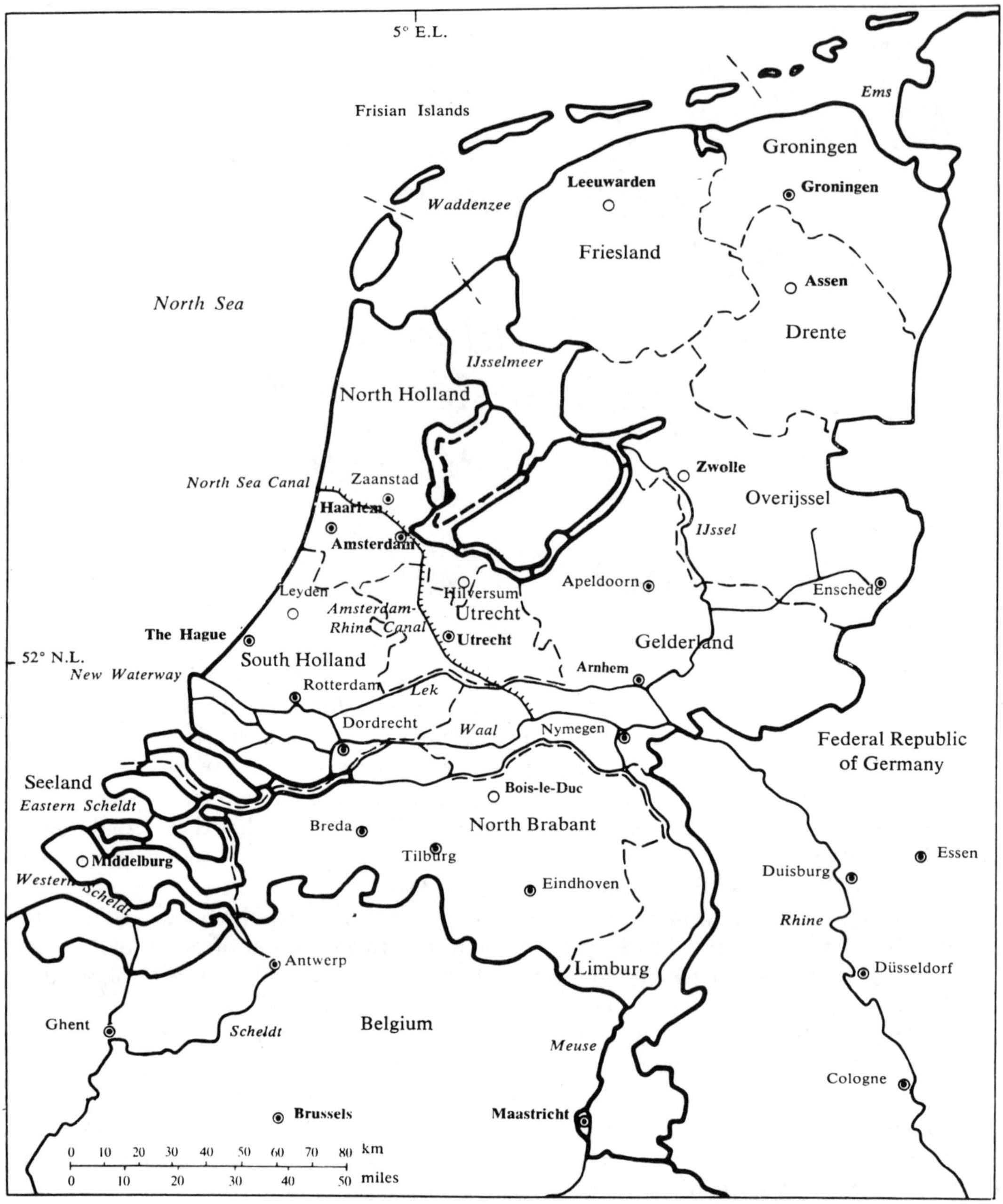

The distribution of the working population according to sectors in which income is earned reflects the high level of development of the Netherlands: 6% of the working population is employed in agriculture and fishery, 21% in industry and the exploitation of minerals, 20% in trade, 7% in transport and communication, and 22% in the service sector. The welfare state, which evolved in the Netherlands after the Second World War, involves an extensive system of social facilities in the areas of social relief, disability, unemployment, old age grants, and sickness insurances. These facilities guarantee the individual a basic income in the case of serious and unforeseen circumstances.

The consequence of the effort of the Dutch society to create an exceptionally good system of social facilities was that in 1980 the collective costs and premium pressure on the national income had climbed to nearly 60% If these facilities are to be maintained at the level which has become customary in past years, the government will be faced with a serious problem. As a consequence of declining income combined with a rapidly increasing number of unemployed persons, the need to economize has become unavoidable.

Aims toward economization in the health care sector will also need to be applied, as price developments in this policy area show a strong tendency to rise. In 1975 the total costs of health care was 17,038 billion guilders; in 1980 it increased by 61% to 27,774 billion. In addition to the price component in this rise, which is mainly brought about by inflationary processes, a clear volume (numbers, quality) component is to be observed.

The Dutch system of health care has some striking characteristics. The first of these is the high quality of its facilities. Both the training of all personnel who are employed in the system and the material facilities, in the form of buildings and apparatus, meet the highest standards. In the creation of this system, private initiative played a determinant role, the force and value of which have hardly diminished up to the present.

In addition, the scientific level of medical treatment is mainly focused on the curative aspect, and rapid developments and changes here are noteworthy. The fact that the Netherlands is a highly industrialized rich society is confirmed by the demographic morbidity and mortality rates.

In recent years the birth rate has fluctuated around 12.5 per 1,000 inhabitants, with a perinatal mortality of around 11.3 per 1,000 neonatals. The total mortality of the Dutch population is 8 per 1,000, the major causes of death being coronary and arterial diseases, various forms of cancer, and traffic accidents. Life expectancy at birth in 1979 was 72.4 years for men and 78.9 years for women, and it is assumed that this life expenctancy will increase further. The striking aspect of these figures is that the difference in life expectancy between the sexes remains large. It is possible that survival chances of men in the age group 30 to 64, the group which carries the greatest risk with respect to the three most important causes of death mentioned, will increase as a consequence of continued campaigns in the framework of health information and education.

The ageing of the population leads to an increasing need for geriatric facilities. In the coming decade the society will have to meet this need both quantitatively, in the form of expansion of the number of institutions and beds, and qualitatively, for instance, by expanding the medical specialism in geriatrics.

HISTORICAL DEVELOPMENT OF THE DUTCH HEALTH CARE SYSTEM

The General Situation in the Netherlands in the Nineteenth Century

Until far into the late nineteenth century, the state of health of the Dutch population was positively deplorable. This situation was the consequence of the following factors:

Only at a very late stage did the Industrial Revolution, which had taken place in England during the eighteenth century, find a footing in the Netherlands. As a result, the Netherlands long retained its primarily agricultural character. Partly due to the natural limitations of the agricultural area, a sharp population increase resulted in a wave of urbanization. Since there was little investment in industrial production capacity, no employment was created in this sector. A pauperized urban proletariat, which existed under the most unhygienic conditions with all of the epidemiological consequences, was the result.

Creation of Legislation

Around the middle of the nineteenth century, the distress among the population was such that the pressure exerted on government to take measures for its relief became extremely strong. The Dutch Medical Society, founded in 1849, played a key role here. In 1865 this pressure resulted in the first form of systematic legislation in the Netherlands. Prime Minister Thorbecke designed a legal framework of four acts in which both the practice of medicine and medical supervision by the state were regulated. These acts were the Medical Practice Act, the Pharmacological Practice Act, the act governing the conditions for being granted competency to perform as physician, pharmacist, etc., and the Act Governing the State Supervision of Health Care. Execution of the first three acts was placed in the hands of a state committee, and this immediately resulted in the central regulation of medical training. In the Act Governing the State Supervision of Health Care, the provincial inspector, a physician appointed and paid by the Crown, was accorded a central position.

The acts of 1865 constituted the impulse for one of the most specific characteristics of the Dutch system of health care: the government delegated various jobs to the municipalities. Because of the lack of funds, the latter were, however, not in a position to fulfill their tasks. The result was that the citizens themselves were obliged to develop the necessary health facilities. The resulting privately organized health care, in short the private initiative, continues today to fulfill a central role in the system. The various religious groups (Catholics, Protestants) founded their own charity institutions and societies and collected their own funds. Ultimately, this resulted in a fragmented set of facilities.

The second half of the nineteenth century witnessed rapid social, technological, and scientific developments. The Health Act of 1901 created the following four authorities for the state supervision of health care: the Central Health Council, the central authority, consisting of the four chief health inspectors and three nominated members; four chief health inspectors operating at the national level; provincial health inspectors; and health committees for municipalities with more than 18,000 inhabitants, with the function of keeping a check on hygiene and the quality of health care facilities.

In practice, this construction did not operate efficiently. There were especially complaints regarding the central authorities; therefore, government decided to change the set-up. The Health Act of 1919 altered the position of the Central Health Council to that of an advisory body, called simply the Health Council, which, invited or uninvited, could inform the minister regarding matters of interest in the area of health care. In the Health Act of 1933, for reasons of economy it was decided to dissolve the health committees. The structure of state supervision of health thus became extremely simple. In 1941, during the

German occupation (1940–45), the Sickness Funds Decree was issued. This proved to be very important for the Netherlands because it led to the institution of the Sickness Funds Council in 1948.

The following institutions were established by the Health Act of 1956: (1) the Central Council for Public Health, which advises the minister on matters of a general and organizational nature; (2) the provincial health councils, which stimulate, advise, and coordinate at a provincial level; and (3) the Health Council, which continued in its original form except that its advisory function clearly assumed a scientific nature. This act in fact provided the basis for the present system of legislation.

Current Legislation and Authorities

The present welfare state came gradually into being in the postwar Netherlands. An important consequence of this for health care is that the government must play a different role. Legislation—the primary function of which was to safeguard health care facilities that were operated on private initiative and by independent professionals—had to be expanded and changed. Over the years government thus enacted and implemented a large amount of new legislation. The main characteristic of this development is the transition from a system of care which is in principle based on charity, to a legally determined *right* to health care for each individual citizen, for which the government is responsible. Important aspects which can be distinguished in the legislation are:

The practice of medical and paramedical professions. This practice is regulated by the Medical Disciplinary Act of 1928, the Medical Practise Act of 1865, and the Paramedical Professions Act of 1963. In order to harmonize this part of legislation, a bill governing the professions in individual health care (BIG) is being prepared. This bill will regulate uniformly *all* professions in individual health care by means of a system for guarding against the unauthorized use of professional titles; this supersedes the system used until now for protecting the use of professional titles.

Social insurance. This consists of: the Sickness Fund Act of 1964 (ZFW), an employees' insurance; the Exceptional Medical Expenses Act of 1968 (AWBZ), a national insurance for the costs of admission and stay in the hospital from the 366th day, and in nursing homes and other institutions for physically and mentally handicapped persons from the first day; and the bill for a national health insurance, which resulted from plans of the Den Uyl Cabinet (1973–77). Because of the strong effects of the proposed measures on the distribution of income, political resistance was so heavy that the plans were shelved for an indefinite period. The heightening of the financial costs for government as a consequence of such a national insurance also played a role.

Financing. The Hospital Tariffs Act of 1965 indicated the Central Agency for Hospital Tariffs (COZ) as the central executive body. The COZ was a civil authority, its main duty being the representation of all social organizations concerned with the fixing of tariffs. Its field of work included: general and special hospitals, psychiatric hospitals and institutions for the mentally deficient, nursing homes, other institutions recognized under the AWBZ, the "Cross Organizations" (home help and health advice), and ambulance services. In practice this meant that the COZ assessed the costs of the institutions with the guidelines it had drawn up. These guidelines were decisions taken by the board of the COZ that were applicable to one or more categories of institutions. Consequently, the COZ was more concerned with evaluating the cost calculations of the institutions than with regulating tariffs in a narrower sense. The guidelines were implemented after approval by the minister of health and environmental hygiene and the Sickness Fund Council.

The Health Care Tariffs Act, introduced on February 7, 1982, regulates the fixing of all fees in the field of health care. One of the changes is the substitution of the Central Agency for Health Care Tariffs (COTG) for the COZ. The main task of the COTG, a public body which consists of independent experts, is to streamline and introduce uniformity into the fragmented and confused system of fees and tariffs. Contrary to past procedures, the COTG is responsible for the *complete* system of fees and tariffs. The procedure followed up to the present has not been very clear. The level of fees of the independent contractors in health care (specialists, general practitioners, physiotherapists, etc.) was regulated by separate authorities: on the one hand, by the Sickness Fund Council for people insured under the Sickness Fund Act and the AWBZ; on the other hand, for privately insured patients by the minister of economic affairs on the basis of the Price Act. The COTG is composed of chambers in which all parties concerned with arriving at tariff agreement (doctors, pharmacists, sickness funds, etc.) are directly represented.

In short, the procedures for arriving at tariff agreements are: (1) the central government fulfills a regulatory role in the development of general guidelines; (2) the COTG draws up specific guidelines advised by the chambers; (3) guidelines are ultimately approved by the government; and (4) the government then issues definite directives which may, for instance, consist of maximation of the tariffs.

Organization. The Health Act of 1956 regulates the Health Council, the Central Council for Public Health, the provincial health councils, and the state supervision of health.

The Hospital Facilities Act of 1971 regulates the tasks and composition of the Commission on Hospital Facilities. The purpose of this act is to draw up a national hospital plan under which fall all general and special hospitals and other intramural facilities mentioned in the act. It was hoped that this plan would provide the possibility for centrally regulating the volume of facilities.

The Revised Hospital Facilities Act of 1979 envisages adapting the overcomplicated structure of the national plan. The principle is to draw up provincial hospital plans as indicated by the minister on the basis of national guidelines. New to the act is the possibility that the minister may close down superfluous institutions.

The Health Care Facilities Act (WVG), which recently has been passed in the Second and First Chamber, regulates the quantitative and qualitative aspects of health care. It relates not only to intramural facilities—as was the case with the Hospital Facilities Act—but also to the consequences of policy measures for the extramural sector. The goal of this bill is to arrive at optimum attunement of intramural and extramural facilities; organizationally, the bill leads to the conversion of the Central Council for Public Health into a National Health Council with adapted duties and composition. Key concepts are planning, regionalization, and decentralization of tasks of the central government to provinces and municipalities. It is rather difficult to realize planning in the Dutch set-up, since health facilities are mainly controlled by private initiative. Consequently, it is extremely difficult for government to assume an initiatory and planning role. Regionalization may serve as an aid in the planning process by the creation of health regions, within which the cohesion between intra- and extramural facilities must be effected. The planning process proceeds gradually on the basis of national guidelines.

Decentralization implies the transfer of duties from a central level to provincial and regional levels. An important issue of this policy is that local authorities are better informed regarding specific local problems and thus can operate more effectively. As a result, the demands of the population for further democratization of policy with respect to health care will be satisfied.

It is clear that the legal framework for policy with respect to the extramural sector must be explicitly regulated in the WVG. By drawing up a policy for the establishment of independent professionals, for example, an integrated facilities plan would become possible. Whether the above-mentioned policy proposals will be realized in the 1980s remains questionable. As a consequence of the economic recession, the financial ability of the central government to set up extremely expensive decentralization projects has become very limited.

Schematic overview of laws.

	Existing	Future
Facilities	Revised Hospital Facilities Act of 1979	Health Care Facilities Act of 1982
Tariffs	Health Care Tariffs Act of 1982	
Financing	Sickness Funds Act of 1964 Exceptional Medical Expenses Act of 1968	

Creation of the System of Sickness Funds

The origins of sickness funds are found in the Middle Ages, when the guilds played a central role. These (craft) guilds were associations which furthered the collective interests of their members, craftsmen, artisans, and small traders, and provided aid to these members, who were all master craftsmen. To be able to fulfill this service, "boxes" were instituted; these were funds which upon payment of a contribution, provided financial assistance in the case of sickness or death of a craftsman.

At the beginning of the seventeenth century it became possible for hired workers to form their own guilds. The resulting workers' "boxes" were the real precursors of the present sickness funds. In addition to grants in cash, it was also possible to obtain grants in kind in the form of services of the doctor, surgeon, or apothecary, who were usually employed by the boxes. Payment of the doctor and apothecary was on the basis of a fixed amount per year or per registered member (capitation fee). Besides this, over the years the boxes became increasingly open, so that they became accessible to greater sections of the population. During the Napoleonic occupation (1795–1813) the guilds were abolished; however, the need for the services which they had provided continued to exist and was even intensified by the general pauperization and the commencing industrialization.

In addition to the mutual boxes, insurance companies grew up on a commercial basis, the so-called societies, which offered insurance not only for medical aid but also for sickness allowances and funeral costs. The enormous proliferation of boxes and societies that took place during the nineteenth century involved large risks, not only for the insured persons but also for the providers of aid. In order to arm themselves against this risk, the latter group, especially the doctors with practices in the cities, formed their own sickness funds, and certainly not only for idealistic motives. Doctors in rural areas followed, setting up the doctors' funds. By paying contributions, the patient was insured for medical aid and sometimes medicines.

In addition to the doctors' funds, at the end of the nineteenth century sickness funds were set up and administered by the insured persons themselves, and industrial sickness funds, set by employers for their personnel, came into being. The physicians, united in the Dutch Medical Association (KNMG), viewed this as a serious threat to their power, both financially and with respect to authority and autonomous functioning. Consequently, in the beginning of the twentieth century the KNMG resorted to the institution of "Society Sickness Funds," which replaced the doctors' funds. A new aspect in the organization of these funds, in addition to the doctors, the insured persons were also represented on the boards.

The history of sickness funds is marked by strong contrasts of interests and conflicts. Especially the KNMG, with the society sickness funds on the one hand and the Dutch trade unions with mutual sickness funds on the other, was not able to arrive at uniform regulations. Moreover, it is important to stress the distinction between "sickness funds insurances" and "sickness allowance insurances" in the Dutch system of social insurance. Policy motivation in this context is that insurance for medical care is of importance for the *whole* population under a certain level of prosperity, while sickness allowance insurance is particularly relevant to the working part of the population that loses income in the case of sickness. A further consequence of this distinction is that the doctor is able to focus his loyalty primarily on the patient. The independence of his decisions is guaranteed since the duty of controlling disability for work rests with the executive bodies of the social insurance.

The Health Insurance Act of 1913, which was only implemented in 1930, is based on this division and lays down that only employees who are registered with a sickness fund can claim sickness allowances. This condition was, however, only implemented for the first time during the German Occupation (1940–45). On 1 November 1941 the Sickness Fund Decree was introduced, the most important elements of which were: (1) compulsory insurance for employees and their families if their income was lower than the wage limit for the Sickness Allowance Act then in force; (2) supervision, which rested with a commissioner appointed for this purpose (this person was later assisted by an advising committee for the sickness funds); and (3) an admission regulation for sickness funds, entrusted with the implementation of the insurance.

In 1940 there were 650 sickness funds, which insured 50% of the population in a most divergent manner. On the basis of the admission regulation, this number was later reduced to 204 approved sickness funds. As a consequence of mergers, over the years a further decrease in numbers has taken place. In 1980 a total of 62 recognized funds remained. The result of this regulation was a uniform and extensive packet of facilities for all compulsorily insured persons, based on payment of premiums in accordance with financial capacity and dependent upon payment of 50% by the employer. The wage limit was set at the same level as that for the Sickness Allowance Act, which resulted in a considerable increase in the number of insured persons.

In addition to the compulsory sickness fund insurance, the voluntary form continues to exist. This is intended for people who are not compulsorily insured and have an income lower than the wage limit for compulsory insurance. In 1947 the limits of both forms of sickness fund insurance were set at the same level and the packet of facilities offered was harmonized.

In 1949 supervision of sickness fund insurances was altered by the act governing the Sickness Fund Council. The duties of this Sickness Fund Council are to advise the minister on matters relating to the sickness funds insurance and the AWBZ, including the task of advising on premium payment levels. Besides this main function, the council must also administer the General Revenues, the Revenues for Old Age Sickness Fund Insurance, and the General Fund for the Exceptional Medical Expenses; supervise the management and administration of sickness funds and of executive bodies of the AWBZ; and approve agreements between sickness funds and independent contractors (doctors, pharmacists, etc.). The thirty-five members of the council—which may be supplemented by four extra members for matters relating to the AWBZ—represent an equal number of Crown employers, members, employees, representatives of the sickness funds, and professionals in health care.

In 1957 a third form of sickness fund insurance came into being: the old age sickness fund insurance. This is intended for persons sixty-five years of age and older whose income does not exceed the income limit. The limit in 1982 was 27,541 guilders. With this form of insurance the premium covers the whole family, the height of the premium being dependent on income. This premium is levied on the basis of five income groups. The deficit which comes about in this insurance, as a consequence of the fact that insured persons pay only part of the total costs, is borne by the government and the compulsory sickness fund insurance.

The Sickness Fund Decree imposed by the Germans was superseded by the Sickness Fund Act of 1964. With this act, unification of the existing sickness fund legislation became a fact.

The Present Sickness Fund System

Since sickness funds are civil bodies with a legal function, they can differ widely in the manner in which they are administered.

Until 1976 there were four organizations to which sickness funds could belong. These cooperated closely in the Joint Council of Sickness Fund Organizations. In 1976 it was decided that these organizations should unite in a central body, the Association of Dutch Sickness Funds (VNZ). In addition to its representative function, the VNZ reaches agreements with groups of providers of health care and health care institutions, maintains contact with government, and manages the National Sickness Fund Information System (LISZ).

The output of the LISZ constitutes the basis of national statistics. Moreover, this data serves an important function as a policy instrument for regional sickness funds in consultation with hospitals and specialists.

Private Health Insurances

The part of the population not covered by one of the three sickness fund insurances (approximately 30%) is privately insured.

The history of private insurance is much more recent than that of sickness funds. In addition to the societies mentioned before, around 1920 local associations were established that provided insurance against costs resulting from admission to a university hospital. Following this example, various insurance companies included hospital costs in their policies. The Sickness Fund Decree of 1941 accelerated this development. This decree laid down that in the future, hospital costs would fall under sickness fund insurance—which had not been the case up to that time. A person insured with a sickness fund had only been able to insure himself against these costs by means of supplementary insurance.

The result of this expansion was that in 1945 the sickness funds instituted their own health insurance companies so that they would still be in a position to insure clients who, as a consequence of an increase in income, exceeded the limit of compulsory or voluntary insurance. A unique aspect of this insurance was that persons who had formerly been insured with the sickness funds were admitted to this health insurance without any form of selection and on normal conditions. This nonselection for people who exceeded the wage or income limit of the sickness funds insurances was taken over by private insurances in the 1950s.

The private health insurance companies that are united in four organizations cooperate in the National Consultation Committee for Private Health Insurance Companies (KLOZ). The functions of this body run parallel with those of the VNZ, the difference being that the KLOZ does not make any agreements with the organizations of providers and of health care institutions. This form of insurance is based on the restitution system, whereby the insured person pays the provider, and later is refunded the amount, either partly or in full, by his health insurance (see figure 1). The sickness funds system, on the other hand, rests on provision in kind whereby the provider receives the fee directly from the sickness funds (see figure 2).

In addition to individual insurance, collective private health insurance is also encountered. This form is on a voluntary basis, but the fact that the premium is low, partly as a consequence of the employer paying part of the premium, lends a strong impetus to collective insurance. The private health insurance for civil servants, operated by statutory public insurers, is, however, a compulsory collective form.

A peculiarity of private insurance is the possibility of being insured for a higher class in the hospital than third class, the sickness fund class. For people with a sickness fund insurance it is possible to take out a supplementary insurance that makes them eligible for a higher class. A person insured for a higher class receives more privileges when admitted to a hospital. Besides this, the specialist fee for these patients will be higher.

The health insurance companies, which operate both on a for-profit and a nonprofit basis in various legal organizational forms, are supervised by the Insurance Chamber. This chamber controls mainly the solvency of the insurers and keeps check of whether guidelines relating to reserves are adhered to.

The Exceptional Medical Expenses Act

Sickness funds and admitted private health insurances are charged with execution of the Exceptional Medical Expenses Act, the AWBZ. This act regulates a national insurance that covers the costs of medical treatment as well as nursing and other care in the case of serious or prolonged illness or disability.

I = insured person
C = insurer
H = provider of aid
P = premium
F = fee
S = service

Figure 1

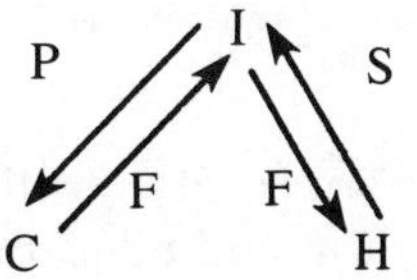

Figure 2

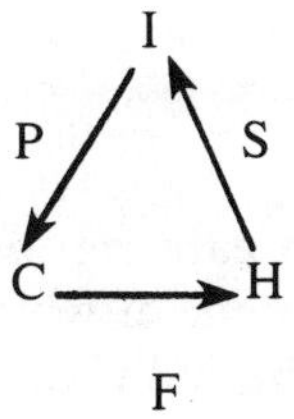

Operation of this law extends to all residents of the country plus workers who are not residents but do fall under Dutch income tax regulations; not covered are residents who fall under foreign income tax regulations. The packet offered by the AWBZ, which has been laid down by an Order in Council, covers: the stay in a hospital after the 365th day, the first 365 days being covered by the sickness fund insurance or the private health insurance; the stay in a nursing home from the 1st day; the stay in an institution for the mentally deficient from the 1st day; medical homes for children (facilities for children under the age of 15 with physical or mental handicaps, intended for temporary sojourn); medical day nurseries (multidisciplinary treatment centers for physically handicapped children); institutions for people with disabilities of the sensory organs (the deaf and blind); "The Village" in Arnhem (treatment and residential center for 375 physically handicapped persons); a number of unregistered institutions (the "homes"); and day centers and substitute homes for handicapped persons.

The AWBZ further serves to finance: ambulatory mental health care (by the units described later), the "Cross Organizations"—home help and health advice services at local, provincial, and national levels, and various other services (vaccination programs, services for persons placed under medical supervision by court order, day nursing in nursing homes, etc.).

In order to receive services under the AWBZ, one must apply to one of the executive bodies. The executive body must determine that an individual is eligible for AWBZ services before the patient is placed in an institution recognized by the AWBZ. This implies that there has to be a contract between the institution and the executive body.

The institutions maintain contacts with the executive bodies via a sickness fund that also regulates medical supervision. Payment of the bills from the institution takes place through the Central Administration Office, a joint agency of the executive bodies.

Supervision of the operation of the AWBZ rests with the Sickness Fund Council, which also controls the General Funds for Exceptional Medical Expenses. The central government pays premium receipts and a government contribution into this fund. Premium receipts for 1982 are estimated at 5.69 billion guilders and the government contribution at 1.76 billion. In addition to these sources, the act permits the possibility of levying a personal contribution in cases where an insured person receives nursing and other care. This contribution depends on the level of income. Account is taken of a basic amount over which no contribution is paid, as well as a maximum contribution. The idea behind the levying of this contribution is that if a person spends a long time in a health care institution, there is a saving in food, housing costs, and washing, which, in the majority of cases, benefits only family members or heirs. The total of these personal contributions for 1982 is estimated at 0.6 billion guilders.

THE SUPPLY OF HEALTH CARE

Classification of the System

Health care can be classified in three ways: (1) positive health care, the most important instrument of which is health information and education—the main goal of this care is to help the individual in achieving and maintaining a good state of health; (2) preventative health care, which aims at timely prevention of illness; and (3) curative health care, the goal of which is the effective curing of illnesses. Partly as a consequence of the policy goals on the structure of the health care system formulated in a 1974 policy proposal, this typology has been concretely applied via a classification into *echelons*. The four echelons are defined as follows:

The *basic echelon* is concerned with extramural and preventative treatment. The goal strived after—namely, maintenance of the highest possible level of public health—can be realized by means of general and specific care. The former finds expression in health information and education, the combating of infectious diseases, technical hygienic care, and quality control of foodstuffs and elements that are harmful to the environment. Specific care relates to consultation bureaus for babies and toddlers, the combating of venereal diseases, school and university health care, school dental care, and occupational health. Important roles of the basic echelon are concentrated in the district health services (DGD) and the municipal medical and health services (G.G. & G.D.) which, in addition to the above-mentioned duties, are also responsible for the regulation of ambulance services, first aid in the case of accidents, and sometimes mental health care.

The *first echelon* encompasses all nonspecialized extramural and curative facilities. A criterion of this echelon is its direct accessibility. The role of the general practitioner is exceptional in the whole health care system; the GP occupies a "gate-keeper function," which implies that, in principle, all referrals to other echelons take place via him.

Others who may be included in the first echelon are dentists, pharmacists, physiotherapists, midwives, and district nurses. Access to these persons is either direct (dentist, midwife) or indirect—after referral by the GP (physiotherapist, pharmacist). In recent years there has been a definite tendency towards the formation of mono- and multidisciplinary teams in the form of group practices and health centers.

The *second echelon* encompasses all specialized facilities, both for inpatient and outpatient care, with the exception of rehabilitation centers. In addition to the hospitals (general, special, and university hospitals), which fulfill a specifically somatic-curative function, this echelon also includes psychiatric institutions that use short-term treatment methods (such as the psychiatric departments of general hospitals) and institutions with prolonged treatment methods. It also encompasses ambulatory mental health care. An important role in this second echelon is played by the medical specialist who treats the patient both in the hospital and as an outpatient.

In conclusion, the *third echelon* encompasses facilities for permanent and long-term intramural and extramural care. In addition to rehabilitation centers, this includes institutions for the mentally deficient and nursing homes for mentally disturbed old people and somatically ill people.

By means of this functional classification, in 1974 a first step was taken toward streamlining and attunement of the supply of facilities.

Hospitals

The way the present hospital system functions dates back to the nineteenth century. During this period, a radical change took place in the traditional system of care that had operated up to this time, which had been highly dependent on the church. This dependency found expression in the location of hospitals and almshouses, which were often situated near a monastery, where care for the sick rested mainly with the clergy. The Christian charitable impulse to create facilities for the sick is clearly evident in the manner in which hospitals are run today. In view of the legal regulation that hospitals may not function on a for-profit basis, the legal status of the institutions which have derived from private initiative is that of foundations or societies. The religious background is reflected in the ownership of hospitals: of a total of 231 recognized institutions in 1980, 60% were either Catholic- or Protestant-sponsored; the remaining hospitals were nondenominational.

In addition to this ideological difference, hospitals may be subdivided according to function. The most usual typology is the following: (1) In *general* hospitals *at least* the following basic specialties are present: internal medicine, surgery, gynaecology and obstetrics, ophthalmology, otolaryngology, neurology, anaesthesia, and radiology and roentgenology. At the end of 1980 there were 176 general hospitals with 60,364 beds. (2) In *special* hospitals, treatment is focused on specific complaints or particular categories of patients; examples of these institutions are rehabilitation clinics, childrens' hospitals, and asthma clinics. In 1980 hospitals of this type encompassed 47 institutions with 6,092 beds. Government policy is aimed at gradually decreasing these facilities, with the exception of childrens' hospitals and rehabilitation centers. (3) Until now *university* hospitals have fallen under the competency of the minister of education and sciences. In addition to the primary function of providing the practically oriented component in medical training, the 8 university hospitals with a total of 6,760 beds also fulfill the role of central hospital for the region in which each is situated. Medical scientific research is also an important function of these hospitals.

Tendencies in the Hospital System

As a consequence of the important role played by private initiative in the creation of intramural facilities, there is a real danger that it will hardly be possible to coordinate and regulate the supply of facilities. The rapidly increasing prosperity of the 1960s, together with sociocultural factors like breaking away from the church and disintegration of family ties, resulted in a sharp rise in the demand for ultramodern and extremely costly treatments and cures.

The resulting expansion in supply of health care—which partly found expression in an increase in the number of hospital beds from 55,000 in 1960 to 74,000 in 1970, a 35% increase compared with a population increase of 13%—had to be checked in view of the financial consequences. As noted earlier, legislation with respect to hospitals took the form of the Hospital Facilities Act and the Hospital Tariffs Act. With the aid of the first of these, government was in a position to draw up planning policy for hospitals at both national and regional levels. Taking account of specific factors, such as the structure of the regional population, government policy is now aimed at a reduction in the number of beds to 3.7 per 1,000 inhabitants. The aim is to meet this norm in the near future.

The total number of days spent in hospitals by all patients taken together has decreased in recent years. Important factors in this framework are the average length of stay in hospital and the number of admissions. A decrease visible in the first of these factors has had a stronger effect than the increase in the number of admissions; this is obvious from quantitative data that shows a further decline in the occupancy rate of the hospitals. One factor which may be responsible for the changes in hospital data is the construction year of the building. A newer hospital often coincides with a high medical-scientific and technical level of facilities. Moreover, working in (relatively) modern hospitals with up-to-date apparatus may result in more efficient care and treatment methods. The Dutch hospital system in general consists of modernized hospital "campuses" with a qualitatively high level of care that mainly concentrates on curative treatment of acute diseases.

Government, in close cooperation with representative bodies such as the Dutch National Hospital Council, concentrates mainly on limiting the present capacity. In coming years the number of hospital beds will be reduced by a minimum of 6,000; in addition, there will be closer supervision of the total amount made available for investments in new hospitals and the renewal of old hospitals.

Organization of the General Hospital

A distinction can be made between an open and a closed hospital. In an open institution, the patient is free in the choice of specialist, who in turn has free access to the hospital. In a closed hospital, however, there is a contract with a team of specialists, the members of which treat patients to the exclusion of all other specialists. As a consequence of the nonprofit character of a general hospital, the legal status is always that of either a foundation or a society.

As a result of this, the policy-making body at the top takes the form of a governing board, which is organized by means of cooperation or election in a meeting of members. This governing board is the highest body in the organization and appoints the board of management and the heads of services, and draws up contracts with specialists. Especially in larger hospitals, the board of management often consists of three persons—an administrator, a director of nursing, and a medical director. Though the attention of each is primarily focused on a certain section of the organization, the total board of management is responsible for policy in its entirety. Separate from the management is the level of medical staff, which includes all specialists who work in the hospital whether they operate as independent professionals under contract with the governing board or as employees of the hospital.

The house staff, which encompasses all nonspecialized doctors who are employees of the hospital and work under the supervision of a specialist, constitute a separate level.

Hospital Tariffs and Financing

As was previously mentioned, the Central Agency for Health Care Tariffs (which replaced the Central Agency for Hospital Tariffs in 1982) plays an extremely important role in the determination of the tariffs.

The tariffs charged by hospitals can vary from an all-out to an all-in tariff. In the case of an all-out tariff, only the costs of general and nursing care of the patient are included, so that all other services are charged separately. Normally, the hospital tariff does not include specialists' fees; these are declared separately. The way in which hospital costs are covered depends on contracts with the sickness funds. Depending on the income of the insured person, the hospital bill will be paid by the sickness fund or (directly or indirectly) by the health insurance company.

Psychiatric Institutions and Institutions for the Mentally Deficient

Psychiatric hospitals can be subdivided into general psychiatric institutions, of which there are 42 with a total of 23,000 beds, and special psychiatric hospitals, of which there are 28 with a total of 1,500 beds.

The nature of treatment in general psychiatric institutions has altered considerably in the past decade. The duties of government in the area of intramural mental health care rest on obsolete legislation in the form of the Mental Illness Act of 1884. As a consequence of considerable delay in preparation, only in 1980 has a bill been designed to supersede the Mental Illness Act, namely, the bill governing special admissions to psychiatric hospitals. However, the delay in legislation has not determined the quality of psychiatric treatment. This treatment is, in fact, of the highest level. The change which has come about in intramural care is that the emphasis in treatment has shifted from long- to short-stay. Macro figures illustrate this by showing that in spite of the drastic reduction in the number of available beds—partly as a consequence of the resolve to reduce the number of beds to 1.5 per thousand inhabitants—the number of admissions has nearly doubled in a period of ten years. The total number of days spent in psychiatric hospitals by all patients collectively has decreased considerably, while the average number of admissions per bed has doubled.

An important reason for the shortening of the length of hospital stays is the "hospitalization syndrome," which implies that patients who have spent a long time in institutions on account of mental problems cannot, or only with great difficulty, fit back into society. Resocialization of the patient becomes extremely difficult since he or she prefers the safe isolation of the institution. The construction of small-scale, well-equipped, and centrally located modern psychiatric hospitals greatly increases the possibility for resocialization of the patient. Moreover, it is evident that this means a more humane approach and way of treatment for the patient.

The above principles have led to a reduction in the average length of stay in an institution from a few years in the 1950s to three or four months in 1980.

Intramural care for the mentally deficient encompasses nursing and general care in homes specially designed for this purpose. These may be subdivided into clinical centers, the large institutions; medical-orthopedagogic institutions, limited to treatment of children; and homes which offer possibilities for treatment. The differences between these forms lie in the duration of care and treatment, which is permanent in the clinical centers, and the possible degree of integration into society. Modern mixed forms have evolved into the "phase houses" which form part of an institution, where children can function more independently in an ordinary residential neighborhood, and the "external pavilions," in which mentally handicapped children can function more independently with guidance.

Under the AWBZ, there are a total of 142 recognized institutions for the care of the mentally deficient, with approximately 29,000 beds.

Nursing Homes

As a consequence of the ageing of the population, the demand for institutions where especially older and very old people can be permanently looked after and treated has increased considerably since the 1950s. In 1961 there were 30 nursing homes with 6,400 beds; as a consequence of the introduction of the AWBZ in 1968 and the resulting alteration in financing, this number had climbed to 215 homes with 24,500 beds in 1970. At the end of 1980 there were 323 nursing homes with a total of 46,343 beds.

Nursing homes can be divided into three types. (1) There are homes for somatically ill patients, in which treatment is aimed at reactivation, general care, and terminal nursing. There are 162 such institutions with 18,000 beds. (2) There are institutions for mentally disturbed old people. Characteristically, patients in these nursing homes suffer disturbances in the psycho-social balance, resulting in serious behavioral abnormalities. The cause of this is mostly old age; therefore, these patients are in general called psycho-geriatrics. There are 79 institutions with 11,000 beds in this category. (3) There is a combination of the two forms, with both somatic and psycho-geriatric departments. In this category there are 82 institutions with more than 17,000 beds.

Since by far the majority of old people admitted to these homes remain there for lengthy periods, the nature of such an institution is primarily that of a home rather than of a hospital.

One of the problems in the psycho-geriatric area is that while the main goal of the nursing home is reactivation of old people, in practice the function of these institutions is the care of patients with chronic complaints of a terminal character. A possible and not too often applied solution might be found in the day center linked to a nursing home, which aims at combating or lessening functional disturbances of patients in the area of activities of daily life (ADL). In 1980 the number of places available was 1,030 with a potential need of 2,700—a clear indication of a shortage.

The fact that people live to an increasingly older age will certainly call greater and more intensive attention to the health care system. All things being equal, the level of facilities, which in recent years has been vastly expanded, adapted, and modernized, will be insufficient in the future. In this context, one should not only consider curative and intramural facilities; very often help for the aged could also take place extramurally. The extramural care for the elderly who live in residential neighborhoods should thus be proportionately increased.

Other Intramural Facilities

A specific type of facility which, in principle, cannot be placed in the category of intramural treatment is constituted by: (1) day centers for the handicapped, in which mentally and physically handicapped people, who live at home, receive occupational and physical therapy during the day, five days a week. There is a growing need for such semimural facilities, of which the development from 6,800 places in 1975 to 9,650 in 1980 bears witness, and (2) substitute homes for handicapped persons, whereby the pupils live in dwellings in city neighborhoods under the guidance of a staff. Here, too, figures point to a growing demand for these facilities: 4,560 places in 1975, 7,580 in 1980.

The remaining intramural facilities which should be mentioned are medical childrens' homes—a total of 20 with more than 1,100 places; medical day centers for toddlers—23 institutions with 1,400 places; institutions for people with sensory handicaps—13 institutions with approximately 1,800 places for people who are deaf, hard of hearing, blind, or have defective sight.

Extramural Health Services

Ambulatory Mental Health Care

Partly thanks to the decrease in taboos surrounding mental health problems, the way has been cleared for an extensive network of ambulatory facilities. In the 1970s there was a considerable expansion of institutions that operate in the marginal area of social (well-being) work and health care or that concentrate on specific psycho-therapeutic problems.

Within the organized ambulatory mental health care (AGG), the following services can be distinguished:

The Social Psychiatric Service (SPD) is primarily aimed at preventing admission of patients to intramural psychiatric institutions. The SPD is illustrative of the idea that psychiatric patients should function in the society as long as possible.

The Medical Bureau for Pedagogic Problems (MOB) provides psycho-social help for the youth and family by means of multidisciplinary treatment of a psychiatric or pedagogical nature.

The Bureau for Marriage Counselling and Family Problems (LGV) is an extension of social work; its main task is to provide solutions in seriously dislocated interpersonal relations, such as in the case of an unsuccessful marriage.

The Consultation Bureau for Alcohol and Drugs (CAD) concentrates on persons with addiction problems. In the past this function was mainly limited to the treatment of alcoholics, but in the future the CAD will also play a key role in the reception and treatment of the country's 10 to 15 thousand heroin addicts. Close consultation is sought with municipalities in this difficult problem area.

The Social Pedagogic Service fulfills an important role in meeting the needs of the mentally handicapped. The Youth Psychiatric Service (JPD) concentrates on psychiatric problems among adolescents. The Institute for Multidisciplinary Psychotherapy (IMP) provides for the patient a prolonged and intensive treatment with a nonclinical form of psychotherapy.

The above-named services, which mainly operate in the form of foundations, encompass a total of 118 different institutions with approximately 3,600 staff. Financing falls under the AWBZ. Coordination of organizations and attunement of the various areas of work to each other is placed increasingly in the hands of the regional institutes for ambulatory mental health care (RIAGG).

The main task of the RIAGG is to channel patients who have been referred by the GP or social workers to the most suitable form of assistance. The long-term intention is that the independently functioning SPDs, IMPs, and MOBs will disappear.

Another recent development is the increasing demand for a psychiatric department in the general hospital—a semimural facility, for both inpatient and outpatient treatment, with a limited number of beds where psychiatric patients can be treated for short periods.

The "Cross Organizations": Organizations for Home Help and Health Advice

The work of the "Cross Organizations" is a very specific branch in the health care system for which it is difficult to find a counterpart in other countries. The origin of these organizations dates from the last decade of the nineteenth century. Partly on the initiative of a state health inspector, the need for a preventative and aid authority materialized. In accordance with common practice, three organizations evolved from private initiative, each with a specific signature and operating separately—the White-Yellow Cross (Roman Catholic), the Orange-Green Cross (Protestant), and the Green Cross (nondenominational). As a consequence of increased separation from the church by the population, and in anticipation of a change in the way of financing in 1980 whereby a personal contribution was maintained but the AWBZ became the main financer instead of central government, a merger between the organizations came about. The Cross Organizations operate at three levels, local, provincial, and national, and serve 75% of the total population, who become members of a local organization by means of paying a contribution.

The work of the Cross Organizations encompasses many areas. The local organizations operate from a district center by means of district nurses and nursing assistants who take care of people by: providing aid to mothers and advice on hygiene (inclusive of trained aid to general practitioner or midwife in the case of home deliveries, and care of the mother and newborn at home; supplying articles on loan for home nursing; offering the necessary nursing, care, guidance, and information in connection with sickness, convalescence, invalidity, old age, and death.

The services thus encompass both nursing and care facets, and curative and preventative elements. The work of the local Cross Organizations is coordinated at a provincial level. The National Cross Organization functions as policy-maker and consultation partner.

Municipal Medical and Health Services and District Health Services

The municipal medical and health service (G.G. and G.D.) fulfill an important role in extramural health care. Its duties, which are mainly in the field of positive health care and at the preventive level, can vary widely per institution. Generally speaking, these services can be subdivided into: general health care, in which the emphasis is on prevention of infectious diseases, providing care for vulnerable groups, cooperating in admission policies, furnishing homes for old people, nursing homes, health information, and health education; youth health care, which includes care of school children of both ordinary and special education institutions; occupational health, which includes the provision of medical examination of municipal staff and of first aid courses; mental health care, school psychiatric aid and social-psychiatric care for adults and children; and ambulance services. The thirty-five GG and GDs are financed by the municipalities.

The duties of the district health services (DGDs), of which there are twenty-four, are identical to those of the municipal bodies. As the name implies, a DGD provides joint public health care for a number of municipalities.

MEDICAL EDUCATION AND MEDICAL PRACTICE

Basic Medical Training

A Short Historical Overview

The founding of the University of Leyden in 1575 marked the first form of organized scientific education in the Netherlands. From that year the possibility existed to train as a physician within the faculty of medicine by completing courses in clinical and basic subjects like anatomy and botany. The other provinces soon followed the examples of Holland and Zeeland. The University of Groningen was founded in 1614, the University of Utrecht in 1636.

The best and most important faculty of medicine, however, continued to be that of Leyden. Inseparably linked with this faculty is Herman Boerhaave (1668–1738), who in a short time raised the level of medical education enormously. The national and international fame of the brilliant physician Boerhaave is evident from the large number of translations of his books. Essential in Boerhaave's method is the mechanistic system whereby he found a solution to the conflict between the chemiatric and iatrophysic schools. Boerhaave's natural scientific methodology resulted in the founding of the university clinic.

Thorbecke's act of 1865 brought an end to the uncoordinated and unregulated developments in the training of physicians. From this year on there were fixed requirements with respect to university education and examinations. There were at the time four medical faculties: Leyden, Utrecht, Amsterdam, and Groningen. The title of doctor could be used only by authorized persons, but the one who had achieved this title obtained a professional monopoly.

The rapid development in the field of medical science in the twentieth century led to the appearance of the medical specialist. In order to guarantee control of both training and quality, in 1933 the Dutch Medical Association instituted the specialists' registers. A significant change in medical training came about in the 1960s. By changing the academic statute in which the conditions and guidelines with respect to scientific education are laid down, a completely new curriculum design came into being in 1968. By this means the faculties obtained a greater degree of autonomy in the specific design of the six-year program that constitutes the basic training for a physician.

Present Training

To be admitted to the scientific training as a physician that is offered by eight medical faculties—Leyden, Amsterdam (two universities), Utrecht, Nijmegen, Groningen, Rotterdam, and Maastricht—the student must have graduated from grammar school with a certificate which includes the subjects of mathematics, physics, chemistry, and biology. The average age for beginning such a course of study is eighteen. As a consequence of the limited training capacity in the various medical faculties, in 1972 it was decided to fix a quota for the number of students to be admitted. This implies limitation of the number of first-year students to approximately 1,900 per annum.

Selection is carried out by means of (weighted) ballot procedures among all the applicants, the number of which is many times the number of available places. Attunement of the number of students to training capacity and not to future need for physicians is one of the principles that is at the moment under critical consideration. Training officially covers six years and is concluded with a final examination that confers the degree of "basic doctor" and permits practice in residency training programs. During this period, theoretical-practical training is given. As a consequence of criticism of the too one-sided somatic and curative approach to the patient in traditional training, a different curriculum design was developed at the medical faculty of the University of Limburg, which was founded in 1973. Here the emphasis shifted from viewing the individual simply as a somatic entity to an approach where he or she was viewed as a psycho-social entity; the program has a strong emphasis on problem-based learning.

Training of the General Practitioner

After basic medical training, a physician may specialize as a GP by means of taking a postgraduate course lasting one year. During this period the young physician assists an established GP in his practice, by which means he gains an intensive knowledge of the most prevalent somatic and psycho-social sickness syndromes. Those GP institutes which are linked to the medical faculties play an important role in this postgraduate training.

Since 1973 the GP training is concluded by the physician being enrolled in the relevant register. This takes place automatically on request, so that no further examinations are called for. The suitability of the GP has already been assessed during his period as assistant to an established GP and the postgraduate training.

The number of registered GPs is on the rise: from 4,809 in 1975 to 5,556 in 1981. As a consequence, the average number of patients per GP has declined from 2,828 in 1975 to 2,536 in 1981. Taking into account the most recent population forecasts of the Central Bureau of Statistics and alternative estimations of the average size of a practice (2,000, 2,200, and 2,400 patients), the future demand for qualified GPs points to a surplus of GPs that will become even greater if no measures are taken with respect to policy on the establishment of GPs, reduction of the size of practices, and limitation of training capacity.

Role of the GP

The GP plays a central role in the Dutch health care system on account of the "gate-house function" that is ascribed to him. This means that a patient must first consult a GP before consulting a specialist, except in acute cases. The GP thus has a determinant role in the referral of patients to other echelons.

The institution of the postgraduate GP training has led to an increase in the status and quality of GPs. Along with this can be observed a clear shift towards teamwork. The number of group practices (mono-disciplinary teams of at least three doctors who have the same professional address) increased from 36 in 1975 to 72 with a total of 247 GPs in 1981. An increase can also be observed in the number of health centers, which are multidisciplinary associations with a minimum of one GP, one district nurse, and one social worker, who operate at the same address. This number has risen from 34 in 1975 to 96 with a total of 319 GPs in 1981.

Government policy with respect to first echelon of care, as laid down in *The Outline of First Echelon Health Care* of 1980, seeks to strengthen the role of the GP. In future the GP should have more say in indicating what laboratory, x-ray, or other examinations he considers necessary for the patient. The specialist, losing some of his autonomy, would then operate on a more consultative basis with the GP.

The development toward a decreasing number of GPs who operate independently and an increasing number who work in teams—group practices, health centers, and partnerships—is clear. Of the 5,556 GPs in 1981, 59.4% worked independently and 40.6% operated within some form of team; in 1978 these percentages were 66.5 and 33.5, respectively. Government stimulates the quantitative growth of teamwork by means of financial regulations and special forms of subsidy. The result of this will undoubtedly be a further increase in the number of health centers and group practices.

The Medical Specialist

The second alternative open to a newly qualified physician is to specialize. The average duration of the specialization phase is 4.6 years, the trainee gaining clinical experience by working in the intramural sector. If at the end of this training period the requirements of the speciality are met, he or she is entered onto the relevant specialist register of the Specialists' Registration Commission (SRC), an executive body of the Dutch Medical Association (KNMG). The SRC also selects supervisors of training and training institutions by means of inspection committees.

The KNMG is the most important representative body of physicians. In addition to its representative function in the various consultative bodies in the health care system, it works to further the material interests of its members (GPs, specialists, and physicians employed by various authorities) in consultations with government, sickness fund organizations, etc., with respect to tariffs and fees. It also exerts control on the correct behavior of the physician in accordance with medical science and ethical norms. This control runs parallel to the regulations of the Medical Disciplinary Act. To this end the KNMG has developed a form of jurisdiction of its own, namely, medical disciplinary law. In addition, the KNMG attempts to further medical scientific developments and advance public health.

The specific interests of the various professions among physicians are furthered by the National Organization of General Practitioners (LHV), of which 95% of GPs are members; the National Specialists' Organization (LSV), and the National Organization of Physicians in Employ (LAD). These three organizations operate within the KNMG. The registration of specialists is consequently a private regulation that is publicly accepted. The procedure that precedes the actual specialization phase is as follows:

The candidate informs the SRC which recognized specialist will act as supervisor and in which hospital, recognized for training, specialization will take place. If the SRC approves the application of the aspirant specialist, he can start his training. During the whole training phase, the progress of the specialist-in-training is annually assessed. The number of recognized specialties is 29, with 9,332 specialists in 1981, (in 1980, 8,939; in 1970, 5,460). A large number of these specialists work in the clinical fields of internal medicine, surgery, psychiatry and neurology, pediatrics and anaesthesia.

Functions of the Specialist

If the GP considers further examination or specialized medical aid to be necessary, he sends the patient to a specialist with a letter of referral. In principle, the patient is free to choose the specialist he would like to be treated by. A person insured with a sickness fund should see a specialist who holds a contract with his or her sickness fund.

The specialist examines the patient. Everything is then done to find the cause of the complaint in order to relieve the patient either by means of surgery or with the aid of medicines. The specialist endeavors to reduce to a minimum any possible risks to the patient. Because of rapid medical scientific developments in the past decade, many specialists in the same specialty have formed partnerships to facilitate cooperation.

The individual specialist has a contract with the governing board, while the salaried specialist has a contract of employment. A specialist may also establish a practice without binding himself to an intramural facility. The relationship between hospital and specialist has vast consequences for the cost of intramural health care. The hospital is interested in putting beds to maximum use because the number of staff (for example, nurses) is determined on the basis of the total number of days spent in hospital by all patients collectively. Meanwhile, the specialist, partly as a consequence of the necessity for eliminating risks, will be inclined to apply all the techniques he considers necessary. If he is an independent professional, the number of techniques also contribute to determining the level of his income. (It is worth noting that there is hardly a shortage of specialists, and in some specialties there is even a tendency toward a surplus.)

These processes have contributed to the rising costs of intramural health care. The demand for the introduction of a different system of financing than the existing one makes itself increasingly felt. Economization in intramural health care can, of course, be achieved by a limitation of the services performed and a lowering of the fairly high specialists' incomes.

Specialists who work in university hospitals (which fall under the ministry of education and sciences) usually receive a salary from the medical faculty. In other public hospitals, specialists in general also have a salaried job.

Status of the Specialist

Both the basic training of the physician and postgraduate training are of a high quality. The physician has a fairly high social status, which also finds expression in his large income and the awe in which the profession is held. The incomes of fourteen specialists who were surveyed in 1977 (in the context of the study of the van Mansvelt Commission) was estimated for 1980 and 1981 at 258,700 and 247,200 guilders, respectively. Since this data was given by the specialists on a voluntary basis, the estimation should be treated with some caution. By comparison: the gross modal income in 1981 was 35,000 guilders.

Characteristic of the profession is the fairly strong emphasis that is placed on curative treatment. The specialist obtains the necessary skills in the training phase of approximately 4.6 years. "Education permanente" offers the possibility of keeping knowledge and skills up-to-date. The physician himself decides whether or not he will participate in postacademic courses.

This set-up will soon be altered. The professional groups of both GPs and the various specialties have given the first impulse to systematic postacademic schooling by setting up a consultation body, Post Academic Medical Training (PAOG). This body is constituted of representatives of the medical faculties, the KNMG, and the ministries of welfare, health, and culture, and of education and sciences, and has as a goal to determine the structure and educational content of postacademic training for physicians.

As has already been pointed out, the specialist's primary loyalty is to the patient, who is usually treated both intramurally and extramurally by the same specialist. Within the hospital organization, specialists are united in the medical staff. This staff has important functions in consultation with the governing board and management on matters such as the acquisition of medical apparatus. In addition to this, within the medical staff, medical audit takes place.

The Specialist in Social Medicine

A third alternative for specialty training is to become a social medical specialist. Contrary to the norm with respect to other forms of specialization, the physicians who enter this form of training are mainly not newly qualified doctors; rather, they are physicians who have had experience as GPs or in a particular specialty.

During the training phase, the physician takes a basic course which concentrates mainly on the interaction between people and their environment. After this training has been completed with the necessary tests, the physician is entered in the register of recognized social medical specialists. The Registration Committee for Specialists in Social Medicine also is under the jurisdiction of the Dutch Medical Association.

The field of work covered by the specialist in social medicine encompasses the branches: labour and industrial medicine, youth health care, combating of disease, insurance medicine, and management in the health care sector. The first three forms accrue to basic health care and encompass both preventative and curative elements; consequently, the specialist in social medicine operates mainly in the area of public health. In 1981 there were 1,341 specialists in social medicine; in 1970, 1,029. It is expected that the demand for this profession will increase in the near future.

The Category of "Other Physicians"

The heterogenous category of "other physicians" includes qualified physicians doing postgraduate courses as GP or specialist, physicians in scientific education (as far as these are not registered as GPs, specialists, or specialists in social medicine), physicians in research institutions, nursing homes, and military service. In 1981 there were 10,758 physicians in this category; in 1970, 4,663.

The group of "other physicians" will increase in the future. Many doctors who have completed basic training will not be able to obtain a position to train as a specialist (or, even worse, having trained as a specialist, will not be able to find a job as a specialist), or having trained as a GP, to obtain a general practice. The still-existing shortage of specialists in social medicine can only to a limited degree absorb this surplus of physicians. It will be increasingly necessary for physicians to seek work outside of the traditional functions of GP and specialist. (At the moment less than 2% are employed in industry.) Moreover, the unemployed physician will cease to be an exception.

Controlling the Supply of Physicians

The policy measures which the ministry considers for controlling "medical over-population" are regulations governing the establishment of physicians, the control of jobs within intramural health care, recognition policy, policy regarding income and fees, and limitation of access to the profession. The last-mentioned instrument is, in fact, the most effective, at least if applied in time. Intervention is even now already too late. Of the supply of physicians for 1990, at the end of 1980, 92% were already either employed or in the "pipe-line." Considering the year 2000, this figure is 61%.

The quota of first-year medical students for 1980 is approximately 1,900, while 1,300 is estimated to be sufficient to meet demands in the year 2000.

Admission Policy With Respect to Foreign Doctors

On the basis of the regulations of the European Community, physicians from all member states must meet the same training requirements. This implies a free flow of doctors in member states. In 1980 the size of this stream was 85 specialists, physicians doing postgraduate courses, and other physicians who settled in the Netherlands for a longer period of time, as well as 185 European Community physicians who settled in the Netherlands for a short period.

Physicians from other parts of the world must apply to the commission governing the admission of foreign physicians, which may declare physicians fully qualified to practice in the Netherlands, admit them under restrictive conditions, or refuse them admission. In 1980, 30 applications fell under the first category, while 235 apply to the second category. These figures do not show great fluctuations.

Alternative Medicine

In recent years there has been considerable demand from the population for curative methods which differ from conventional medical scientific methods in the manner of diagnosis, treatment, and cure. This category encompasses, for example, Eastern methods of healing such as acupuncture, nature healing, and homeopathy. Someone who practices alternative medicine must be qualified in conventional medicine; others are forbidden from practicing medicine, so that persons who have been trained in special institutes are not recognized as physicians and are guilty of punishable behavior if they do practice medicine. Discussion continues around the question of alternative medicine, which encompasses approximately 2,400 practitioners.

Remuneration of GPs and Specialists

The GP receives payment for treatment to patients in two ways. For treatment of patients who are insured by sickness funds, the GP receives a capitation fee. The procedure followed is that the patient has himself registered as a patient of the GP of his own choice. On the basis of this registration, the GP provides medical aid in kind; the patient consequently pays nothing to the GP. The sickness fund pays the GP a fixed amount per registered patient. To this end, the two parties have a contract based on the Model Contract between the Sickness Fund Organization (VNZ) and the Organization of GPs (LHV), which must be approved by the Sickness Fund Council.

The gross fee of the GP is composed of the net fee, a contribution for the costs of the practice, and a pension contribution. The main characteristic of the capitation fee is thus that the GP receives a fixed amount per registered patient, irrespective of whether the patient requires his services or not. However, the size of the fee which the GP receives per patient is related to the number of sickness fund patients registered with him. Compensation for fixed costs of the practice is paid out to a maximum of 1,800 registered sickness fund patients.

In addition to patients insured with sickness funds, the GP also has private patients. These persons are treated on a fee-for-service basis, the GP being paid by the patient himself who, when he is insured against this type of help, will get a restitution from his health insurance. In this case, the GP is paid only if the insured person actually receives treatment. As a consequence of the large percentage of childbirths that take place at home, the GP has traditionally played an important role in providing obstetric services. Payment for delivery and pre- and postnatal care is on a "case" basis. On the average, the GP is annually in charge of approximately only four deliveries, the reason being that many GPs do not provide any obstetric services at all. Payment is based on the actual services rendered.

The specialist is paid on a fee-for-service basis except when salaried. In cases involving sickness fund insurance, there is a contract between the sickness funds and the specialists, in which ten categories of fees are distinguished. The sickness fund patient is free to choose from among all specialists who have a contract with his fund. The level of fees are determined in national consultation between the VNZ and the Organization of Medical Specialists (LSV). These must be approved by the Sickness Fund Council.

Fees for aid to privately insured patients must be approved by the minister of economic affairs. On the basis of the Price Act, a limit is usually placed on the maximum rise in fees.

The basis of sickness fund payment of the specialist is the referral, repetition, and consultation card system. The referral card is written by the GP when he refers the patient to the specialist. This card, like the other cards, represents a material value for the specialist and the sickness fund. The incomes of GPs and specialists are not made publicly known and thus must be estimated. On the basis of a normal practice of 1,800 sickness fund patients and 800 privately insured patients, the income of a GP may be calculated at 140,000 guilders, which was equivalent to an income, after deduction of taxes, of 51,300 guilders in 1977. As already mentioned, the income of a number of specialists was in the neighborhood of 250,000 guilders.

OTHER PROFESSIONAL GROUPS IN HEALTH CARE

Nursing Aids and Nurses

The occupation of nursing aid is intended for providing aid to people with lengthy illnesses. Consequently, the field of work covered by the nursing aid is mainly in the area of nursing homes, sanatoria, departments for the sick in homes for the elderly, or special departments of psychiatric institutions. Training is intramural and since 1980 is of 26.5 months duration. If the trainee is proven suitable by examinations and practical work, she then obtains competency to practice as a nursing aid. After this, the possibility exists for further training for guidance functions, or one may take a course for district nursing aid. Qualified nursing aids in the latter category work in the local Cross Organization (home help and health advice organization).

Development of the number of nursing aid trainees from 1976 to 1980 is as follows:

	1976	1977	1978	1979	1980
New pupils	7,349	6,919	7,019	7,150	6,000
Passed examinations	4,705	4,060	5,715	5,717	4,546
Total number of qualified nursing aids	33,674	38,534	44,249	49,966	54,512

The second main stream in the training system is training as a nurse. The student nurse may choose one of three forms of training:

The *nursing certificate A* involves a basic training of 3.5 years in a general hospital. The course encompasses theoretical and practical training, and is concluded with a state examination. Occupational possibilities of the qualified *A* nurse are both intramural and extramural in the area of social health care. Once the basic certificate has been obtained, there are various specialist courses which may be taken.

The *nursing certificate B* training concentrates on the care and nursing of psychiatric patients. The duties of the *B* nurse are mainly in the area of guidance and observation of the patient. The duration of training, which is also intramural, is three years. During this period the student is theoretically schooled in somatic, psychiatric, and general subjects, and obtains a practical training. The state-registered nursing certificate *B* offers the possibility of working professionally in intra- or extramural psychiatric institutions, in the psychiatric department of a general hospital, and so on. Postgraduate courses exist in the form of training courses as social-psychiatric nurse or sister tutor.

The *nursing certificate Z* can be obtained in six periods of 26 weeks of intramural training. This training qualifies a nurse to care for the mentally deficient. Each training period is rounded off with an examination, and the student obtains a certificate after successfully completing a final examination. The field of work to which this certificate gives access is mainly institutions for the mentally deficient.

These three possibilities for training are all intramural, so that the student already works in the institution during the period of training. In addition, the possibility exists for obtaining the Intermediate Occupational Training (MBO) or the Advanced Occupational Training (HBO) nursing certificate by attending extramural day courses. The MBO training takes three years and falls under the ministry of education and sciences. This legally recognized certificate authorizes the holder to work in all forms of health care. The HBO training takes four years and is also rounded off with an examination. Since 1980 the possibility exists for obtaining a university degree in social health. This course is given at the State University of Limburg in Maastricht. The future alumnae of this course can fill executive positions in health care.

Dentists and Pharmacists

From 1970 to 1980, the number of university-trained dentists rose from 3,205 to 5,346, an increase from 2.5 to 3.8 dentists per 10,000 inhabitants. This increase of trained dentists has consequently eradicated the shortage of dentists in the 1970s, despite the relatively great differences between the provinces in density coefficients—from 2.1 in Zeeland to 7.1 in Utrecht.

The number of university-trained pharmacists increased from 1,019 in 1970 to 1,529 in 1981. The figure for 1981 can be divided into 1,031 independent pharmacists, 303 assistant pharmacists, and 195 head and assistant hospital pharmacists. When interpreting these figures, account should be taken of the fact that there are more than 1,100 GPs who operate their own pharmacies. When these two categories are taken together, the total density coefficient of pharmacies comes to 1.5 per 10,000 inhabitants. For this profession, too, the saturation point has been reached, so that a limitation of admissions to the faculty and an establishment policy are essential.

Physiotherapists

Since 1969, when the "new style" of training physiotherapists was introduced, the Advanced Occupational Training (HBO) for the paramedical profession of physiotherapist has encompassed a training period of four years. Since the new curriculum was introduced, the twenty institutes which provide training have graduated 9,500 physiotherapists. In total, 14,632 physiotherapists, both old and new style, were included on the Register of Medical Professions of the Chief Medical Inspector.

The professional physiotherapist may establish his own practice or be employed in a salaried job. The former variant is extramural. The large group of newly qualified physiotherapists (in 1969, 172; in 1980, 1,330) constitutes a problem. In spite of the considerably increased medical consumption of physiotherapeutic treatment, both by sickness fund and privately insured persons, the supply of physiotherapists can hardly be absorbed. In order to forestall the threatening unemployment in this occupational group, it will be necessary to introduce both a system of control for the number of first-year students and an establishment policy as quickly as possible. Economy measures by sickness funds, especially in the area of physiotherapy, intensify this need.

Midwives

The three-year training in midwifery, which is provided by three institutes, encompasses theoretical and practical training that is concluded with examinations. Of the 898 midwives practicing in 1980, (in 1970 there were 775), 63% had their own practices; the remaining 37% functioned as assistants, substitutes, or workers in a clinic. The demand for obstetrical aid from midwives is determined by the custom that the majority of normal deliveries take place at home. The GP or the midwife is in charge of the delivery.

In 1970, 57% of all deliveries took place at home, 36% in a clinic. In the last decade this percentage has altered drastically. In 1980, 35% of deliveries took place at home and 61% in the clinic. By comparison with other countries, the percentage of home deliveries remains high. The fact that the number of midwives has increased in spite of the decreasing percentage of home deliveries must be ascribed mainly to the fact that nowadays GPs provide the necessary obstetrical assistance only sporadically.

It is expected that the demand for midwives will increase. On the one hand, this is a consequence of changes in demographic developments: the birth rate is rising for the first time in years, from 12.5 per 1,000 in 1979 to 12.7 per 1,000 in 1980; this is partly a result of the high birth rate of ethnic minorities and the slight general tendency to increased marital fertility. Furthermore, partly with a view to cost developments, policy is aimed at keeping the number of clinical deliveries to a minimum.

Other Occupational Groups

In the area of dentistry, oral hygienists with a paramedical status are encountered. The total number in this category is 550, the majority of whom work extramurally. In addition to physiotherapists, there are also paramedical therapists, who work according to the Mensendieck and Cesar methods. In 1981 these occupational groups, which consist mainly of women, counted 606 and 562 persons, respectively, registered with the chief medical inspector.

There were 2,206 dieticians registered with the chief medical inspector in 1981, also mostly women. Dieticians mainly work in institutions, in social health care, and in health information and education activities. Other professions with paramedical status which are worth mentioning are: orthoptists, radiodiagnosticians and therapeutic laboratory technicians, speech therapists, and occupational therapists.

COSTS AND FINANCING OF HEALTH CARE

Status and Function of the Financial Review *of Health Care*

It is of great importance to government to keep control of most developments in health care. One of the instruments developed to this end is the *Financial Review* of health care, an appendix of the estimates of the ministry of health and environmental hygiene, in which government formulates policy proposals for future years. The ministry of health and environmental hygiene was abolished in late 1982, and *health* came under the ministry of welfare, health, and culture. Important advisors in this framework are the Sickness Fund Council and the Central Council for Public Health.

From the quantitative data of the *Financial Review* (the sixth issue appeared in 1982), trends in the preceding period can be deduced. Up to the fifth *Financial Review,* which appeared in 1981, estimates for health care in the coming five-year period were drawn up, taking into account forecasts of the Central Planning Bureau and the consequences of government policy already implemented, which mainly consists of economization. In the sixth *Financial Review* such a forecast is lacking on the request of the minister of finance. However, it has been announced that medium-term problems will be dealt with in an "Autumn Memorandum." The sixth *Financial Review* consequently does not go further than a forecast for 1983.

In addition to a retrospective dimension, the *Financial Review* has retained only a limited prognostic dimension. Its goal, in addition to control of costs, is gradually to establish priorities in health care. The most important policy resolves of the sixth *Financial Review*

(1982) are a number of economizations amounting to 1,160 million guilders, which it is hoped can be achieved by: limitation of the increase of staff in the intramural sector by means of adaptation of staff guidelines and limitation of the number of independent professionals; limitations of the increase of personnel in the extramural sector—areas mentioned are dentistry, physiotherapy, ambulatory mental health care, and Cross Organizations; modification of incomes of staff and independent professionals; closing down of hospitals and hospital departments; less construction of new hospitals/less renovation; a general reduction of 2% in price compensation for expenditure on apparatus, etc.; limitation, price measures, and cost-sharing regulations with respect to medicines; limitation of the sickness fund packet; a higher personal contribution for persons admitted to an institution recognized by the AWBZ; a lower employer's contribution in the pension premium.

Development in the Costs of Health Care, 1977–80 and 1980–83

An important reason for the rise in the costs of health care is the fact that this is a very labor-intensive sector (approximately 70% of the total costs are labor costs) where possibilities for achieving an increase of productivity by mechanization and automation are almost nil. The increase in wage costs, for which industry is traditionally the price leader, thus hits health care extra hard. In addition to this, incomes in health care are, on the average, on the high side. Over time the rate of interest has also increased sharply, and health care operates for nearly 100% with loan capital. Building prices and the prices of medical installations rose very quickly. Until the present there was no question of a specific price of control for medicines.

Part of the rise of costs in the past was a consequence of a shift: costs were shunted from other sectors to health care. For example, many of the mentally deficient formerly remained at home or in other facilities outside of health care. Especially the introduction of the Exceptional Medical Expenses Act (AWBZ) exerted a very attractive influence. Before this time, for example, the Public Assistance Act (ABW) met many of the expenses.

Another factor is that the health care sector keeps many people alive. Since these people are, in general, not the strongest, they place relatively heavy demands on health care. In addition, the ageing of the population naturally plays an important role in rise of costs.

The increasing number of technological possibilities also constitutes an important costs-elevating factor. There are numerous innovations in health care: on the one hand, because a lot of new discoveries are made in this area and, on the other, because in this sector (as opposed to the profit sector) the "risks brake" hardly functions.

There has been, moreover, a change in the structure of households: the two-generation family (without the benefit of grandmother's advice)—having fewer contacts with neighbors and suppliers, and greater mobility—has become a common phenomenon. As regards lifestyle, it is important to note that smoking is on the decrease; the use of alcohol and drugs, on the other hand, is on the increase. The consequences of widespread and rapidly expanding unemployment of the youth could, seen in this framework, prove disastrous.

Mistakes in planning have also exerted an influence on costs; an example is the years of overcapacity in the hospital sector. Furthermore, the manner in which institutions and staff are financed has certainly not contributed to a limitation of the amount of treatment (misuse of financial incentives).

Table A Annual percentage growth of the costs per area of health care, 1977–80 and 1980–83

Area	Share of Costs, 1977	Average Annual Increase	Share of Costs, 1980	Average Annual Increase	Share of Costs, 1983
General practitioner	5.1	5.9	4.6	3.6	4.4
Dentistry	5.3	9.2	5.3	5.5	5.3
External treatment	1.9	17.3	2.4	5.4	2.4
Cross Organizations	1.8	10.3	1.8	9.2	2.0
Maternity nursing care	0.7	11.9	0.7	12.0	0.9
Ambulatory mental health care	1.2	14.4	1.4	8.1	1.5
Total extramural	16.0	9.9	16.3	5.9	16.5
Medicines, etc.	10.2	6.6	9.5	5.9	9.6[a]
Specialists' aid	6.7	8.4	6.4	2.4	6.0[a]
General, special, and university hospitals	33.5	9.3	33.7	5.9	34.0
Psychiatric institutes	6.5	7.7	6.0	7.0	6.2
Institutes for the mentally deficient	6.0	9.7	6.0	6.4	6.2
Nursing homes	10.0	10.4	10.3	5.2	10.2
Other institutions	3.0	11.5	3.2	6.6	3.3
Total intramural	58.7	9.5	59.2	5.9	60.0
Collective preventative care	2.6	9.2	2.6	6.7	2.7
Policy, administration, etc.	5.8	10.1	6.0	7.6	6.3
Decrease of excessive incomes of independent professionals	—	—	—	—	− 0.7
Closing down plan, 1983	—	—	—	—	− 0.3
Total	100 (21,289 billion)	9.2	100 (27,716 billion)	5.5	100 (32,556 billion)

[a]Exclusive of the effect of decreased excessive incomes of independent professionals.

Finally, over the years, the population has become less tolerant of all sorts of "inconveniences" which it would appear could be relieved medically. The more assertive patient nowadays claims a right to every care offered by the insurance packet.

Expressed as a percentage of the gross national product at market prices, the abovementioned costs developments imply an increase from 7.73% in 1977 to 8.34% in 1980.

More than one-half the total costs of health care derive from treatment in the intramural sector (see table A). Two factors play a determinant role in this connection: First, as a consequence of the labor-intensive nature of health care, wage and price increases in general are very important. Though government has taken steps toward modifying incomes in all income groups, incidental wage increases are at the root of the increase in wage costs. In addition, energy prices and the high level of interest brought about as a consequence of international circumstances and the size of the government deficit play a role.

As a second factor, the costs increase is a consequence of volume development. This concerns primarily capacity factors such as the size of staff and the number of available beds or places.

Consequently, in annual growth a price component and a quantity component may be distinguished. If we look only at the growth in volume, the figures are much lower.

Extramural Care

From volume growth figures in table B, it can be seen that the promise of reinforced primary health care included in the 1974 policy proposal on the structure of the health care system was, in fact, only realized in the area of ambulatory mental health care; GP

Table B Annual percentage growth per area of extramural care, 1977–80

Area	Price	Volume	Volume After Elimination of Population Growth (0.7 Per Annum)
GP, obstetrics	3.8	1.8	1.1
Dentistry	4.1	4.8	4.1
External treatment	7.2	9.4	8.7
Cross Organizations	6.4	3.7	3.0
Maternity nursing aid	7.3	1.9	1.2
Ambulatory mental health care	5.1	8.7	8.0

SOURCE: 5th and 6th *Financial Review*.

EXPLANATION PER CATEGORY OF TABLE B:

GPs: Increase in volume, mainly as a consequence of the reduction of size of practices (higher remuneration per patient).

Dentistry: Increase in volume, mainly as a consequence of an increase in the number of dentists and the expansion of the sickness fund packet.

Social health care: After correction for population increase, the increase in volume is 3.0% per annum for Cross Organizations and 1.2% per annum for maternity nursing care. For Cross Organizations, the increase in volume aimed at is 4%. In the area of maternity nursing care, the decrease in the number of births in recent years is compensated by a shift to extramural maternity nursing care as a consequence of changes in the insurance packet.

Ambulatory mental health care: The increase in the number of staff is 9.3% per annum (after correction for population growth 8.6% per annum).

Table C Annual percentage growth in the periods 1977–80 and 1980–83 of staff, beds (places), total number of days in institution, and the volume of other costs

Category of Institution	Size of Staff		Number of Beds		Total Days in Institution		Volume of Other Costs Per Day
	1977–80	1980–83	1977–80	1980–83	1977–80	1980–83	
Hospitals (including university)	2.4 (1.7)[a]	2.1 (1.5)	−0.5 (−1.2)	−0.5 (−1.1)	−0.9 (−1.6)	−1.1 (−1.7)	5
Psychiatric institution	2.1 (1.4)	2.1 (1.5)	−0.8 (−1.5)	0.7 (0.1)	−0.3 (−1.0)	−1.1 (−1.7)	2
Institution for the mentally deficient	3.2 (2.5)	2.9 (2.1)	1.5 (0.8)	0.9 (0.3)	1.4 (0.7)	0.7 (0.1)	2
Nursing homes	3.9 (3.2)	2.1 (1.5)	3.1 (2.4)	0.6 (0.0)	3.2 (2.5)	0.9 (0.3)	2
Day centers and family substitute homes	12.7 (12.0)	6.7 (6.2)	8.5 (7.8)	5.6 (5.0)	2.5 (7.8)	5.5 (4.9)	—
Total	2.5 (1.8)	1.0 (1.2)	1.3 (0.6)	0.7 (0.1)	1.4 (0.7)	0.6 (0.0)	

SOURCE: 6th *Financial Review*.

NOTE: For the period 1980–83, the "medium variant" of the population forecast made in 1980 by the Central Bureau of Statistics has been chosen: approximately 0.6% per annum.

[a]Between parentheses are figures after elimination of population growth.

Table C *Continued*

EXPLANATION PER CATEGORY OF TABLE C:

Hospitals: Annual increase of a number of characteristic variables in the period 1977 to 1980 (including university hospitals, excluding special hospitals).

	Inpatient	Outpatient
Admissions	1.9% (1.2%)[a]	
Average length of stay	−2.5%	
Number of outpatient visits		3.8% (3.1%)
Operations	1.5% (0.8%)	6.1% (5.4%)
Rontgendiagnostic examinations	0.0% (−0.7%)	0.0% (−0.7%)
Physiotherapy	4.1% (3.4%)	−6.6% (−7.3%)
Laboratory examinations[b]	9.5% (8.8%)	8.1% (7.4%)
Functional examinations	1.3% (0.6%)	7.1% (6.4%)

[a]Between parentheses are figures after correction for population growth.

[b]Exclusive of university hospitals.

Other categories: Developments in number of staff, number of beds, and total number of days spent in hospital reflect fairly adequately developments in capacity and occupancy.

Nursing homes: It is interesting to relate growth to the increase in the number of old people and especially the number of very old people (over 80 years). In the periods 1977 to 1980 and 1980 to 1983, this increase was as follows (between parentheses are figures after correction for population growth):

Period	1977–80	1980–83
Annual increase in number of persons over 65	2.1% (1.4%)	1.0% (0.3%)
Annual increase in number of persons over 80	3.8% (3.1%)	2.7% (2.1%)

assistance, Cross Organizations, and maternity nursing care hardly increased. There was, however, an enormous increase of "external treatment methods" (for 97% physiotherapy). This area was not indicated in the policy proposal as one to be promoted; increase in this area is thus probably the consequence of a *lack* of, rather than the *presence* of policy: the meek acceptance of the enormous increase in the number of physiotherapists. Judging from figures for 1983, it is to be expected that in the future, policy in this area will be adjusted.

Intramural Care

The division into price and volume components is much more difficult here as a consequence of the absence of uniform tariffs, the diversity of the staff who work in the various institutions, and the influence of cost components other than staff costs. Nonetheless, in order to obtain some indication of growth in volume in the periods 1977 to 1980 and 1980 to 1983, the annual volume increase is given in table C for a number of variables.

Financing of Health Care in 1980 and 1983

The financing of health care in the Netherlands in 1980 and 1983 is shown in simplified form in table 18a. As demonstrated by the financial scheme, the greater part of the costs of health care is financed by premium payments.

Higher costs, brought about mainly by the above-mentioned nominal costs components (salaries and interest), are consequently financed primarily by premium increases. The direct material role of government as financer of the health care system is subsidiary to that of sickness funds, private health insurers, and the AWBZ. The function of government rests more in the limitation of the increase of costs by wielding a restrictive wage and price policy, and by maintaining capacity guidelines in the form of, for instance, restriction of building and reduction of beds.

SUMMARY AND CONCLUSIONS

Both as regards financing of costs and initiation of new facilities, private initiative plays a central role in health care in the Netherlands.

In recent decades the government has attempted to get a greater grip on developments. To this end, various methods have been applied. One method is the issuing of policy memoranda, the first of which was the 1966 *Report on National Health Care,* which appeared under the authority of Minister of Social Affairs and Health Veldkamp. This report outlines a short- and long-term policy design in which public health is considered of great social importance. Under the influence of social developments, the necessity for internal and external democratization of the system of health care is emphasized.

Eight years later the 1974 policy proposal on the structure of the health care system appeared, under the authority of Under Secretary of Health Hendriks. Contrary to the

1966 report, this proposal placed emphasis on reduction of costs and streamlining of the supply of health care facilities. Policy lines developed to this end can be summarized with the concepts of echelonization and regionalization. The principle of echelonization, by which is meant functionally and qualitatively better attunement of the various forms of care to each other, has been further elaborated on *inter alia* the Outline of Primary Health Care and the Memorandum on Basic Health Care Services. The main element of the policy is the intensification of primary health care facilities by the extension of extramural care, in which the GP plays a central role. An attempt is made to put a brake on the cost explosion in health care, which is mainly brought about by treatment in the intramural sector, and to maintain the high quality of health care facilities that has been realized in the course of the years by, *inter alia,* improving relations between the first and other echelons. Regionalization of health care implies a decentralization of tasks from the central to provincial and local governments. Realization of this policy goal is hampered by the bad general economic situation.

A consequence of the health care policy followed has been the creation of relevant legislation. With the Health Care Tariffs Act and the anticipated Health Care Facilities Act, a legal framework will have been created in which the parties concerned can in the future arrive at an integral tariffs and facilities policy for health care as a whole.

It is essential in this connection that the participants collectively arrive at a new system. If government should desire to manipulate the entire system according to its own policy views, there would be the danger of (over) bureaucratization. On the other hand, persistence by the medical profession—that is, the specialists and their supporters—in demanding extremely high incomes and complete autonomy, can hardly be allowed to continue. In recent years a change has been observable in this professional group. A shortage of GPs and specialists has reversed into a clear surplus. This development will most probably lead to the institution of an establishment policy. With a view to this surplus, government should set a limit on the flow of students to para-medical training. Manpower planning for the health care sector must become a reality.

Finally, a gradual demarcation of priorities is of crucial importance. Costs developments cannot be kept under control if every medical-technological innovation can simply be introduced into health care facilities. Large investments exert a disproportionate amount of pressure.

The choice of a health care system that offers a high quality of care and is mainly focused on curative treatment should be submitted to discussion. One development that could possibly lead to changes is the increasing size of the group who choose alternative medicine and the so-called self-help groups. In addition to this, the fact that in medical training the patient is no longer viewed simply as an object of curative treatment, but also as a psycho-social entity, is important.

Short-term policy can only be aimed at counteracting stimuli which increase costs. In view of the percentage share of the various sectors, the amount of treatment given in the intramural sector is of great importance; reduction of this share by more outpatient care, for example, is essential. Possibilities for this are presented by the introduction of budget-financing and a different method of paying GPs and specialists. Because of the price-raising incentives which it engenders, the method of financing used up to the present should be adapted. In the background, social factors play a determinant role. As a consequence of the enormous increase in prosperity since the Second World War and the realization of the welfare state, extremely costly health care of the highest quality has become a matter-of-course right of the individual.

Public pressure for continuous improvement and renewal of existing treatment methods (for example, coronary surgery, research into cancer-combating drugs) is strong. There is vehement discussion to reinstate the link between use and costs, the "to-who benefits, pays" principle. Despite heavy social opposition, the introduction of cost sharing, for instance, for medicines and clinical treatment, where now the whole treatment is "free," will possibly be unavoidable.

The serious economic crisis makes it essential to demarcate priorities and to make fundamental and painful choices. All concerned must make a contribution in order to maintain the quality and solidarity necessary for the health care system.

Table 1 Population by sex and age, 1980, the Netherlands

	Male	Female
All ages	6,994,280	7,096,734
0	89,230	85,213
1	89,960	85,840
2	89,022	84,971
3	91,361	86,362
4	92,074	88,082
5–9	551,734	527,567
10–14	625,507	597,197
15–19	638,116	609,830
20–24	606,443	584,761
25–29	587,265	559,504
30–34	613,896	573,792
35–39	475,693	440,046
40–44	414,196	390,724
45–49	387,791	380,030
50–54	357,570	370,248
55–59	345,187	374,634
60–64	273,082	309,261
65–69	242,168	298,100
70–74	185,844	257,765
75–79	125,032	194,476
80–84	69,758	121,025
85 and over	43,351	77,306
	As a % of All Ages	
0–19	32.4	30.5
20–64	58.1	56.1
65 and over	9.5	13.4

SOURCE: Central Bureau of Statistics, *Statistical Yearbook.*

Table 2 Live births, birth rates, and fertility rates, the Netherlands

	1978	1979	1980
Live births	175,550	174,979	181,294
Birth rates	12.6	12.5	12.9
Fertility rates	1.58	1.56	1.59[a]

SOURCE: Central Bureau of Statistics, *Statistical Yearbooks.*

[a]The sum of all age-specific fertility rates.

Table 3 Infant mortality by age, selected years, the Netherlands

Year	Under 1 Year	28 Days to 11 Months	Under 28 Days
1950	26.6	8.8	17.8
1960	19.9	4.5	13.4
1965	14.5	3.1	11.4
1970	12.7	3.3	9.4
1975	10.6	3.0	7.6
1979	8.7	2.8	5.9
1980	8.6	—	—

SOURCE: Central Bureau of Statistics, *Statistical Yearbooks.*

Table 4 Infant mortality rates per 1,000 infants by six most common causes, the Netherlands

	Rates in		
Causes	1978	1979	1980
Certain conditions originating in the perinatal period	3.78	3.70	3.57
Congenital anomalies	2.93	2.77	2.68
Symptoms, signs, and ill-defined conditions	1.15	1.12	1.09
External causes of injury and poisoning	0.30	0.29	0.28
Diseases of the nervous system and sensory organs	0.32	0.23	0.22
Infectious and parasitic diseases	0.35	0.13	0.12
Other causes	0.93	0.49	0.97
All causes	9.76	8.73	8.93

SOURCE: Central Bureau of Statistics, *Statistical Yearbooks.*

Table 5 Estimated death rates per 100,000 population for leading causes of death, 1980, the Netherlands

Causes	Male	Female	Total
Infectious and parasitic diseases	4.8	3.9	4.4
Neoplasms	262.7	178.6	220.3
Endocrine, nutritional, and metabolic diseases and immunity disorders	9.4	15.2	12.3
Diseases of the blood and blood-forming organs	2.0	2.1	2.1
Mental disorders	1.8	2.5	2.2
Diseases of the nervous system and sensory organs	12.8	11.2	12.0
Diseases of the circulatory system	390.8	333.9	362.2
Diseases of the respiratory system	62.9	36.3	49.5
Diseases of the digestive system	26.7	28.7	27.7
Diseases of the genitourinary system	16.6	17.9	17.3
Complications of pregnancy, childbirth, and puerperium		0.2	0.1
Diseases of the skin and subcutaneous tissue	1.8	3.9	2.9
Diseases of the musculoskeletal system and connective tissue	2.5	4.7	3.6
Congenital anomalies	5.9	5.2	5.5
Certain conditions originating in the perinatal period	5.5	3.8	4.7
Symptoms, signs, and ill-defined conditions	43.4	32.3	37.8
External causes of injury and poisoning	51.8	34.5	43.1

SOURCE: Central Bureau of Statistics, *Statistical Yearbook.*

Table 6 Selected operative (surgical) procedures: number (in thousands) and average length of stay when performed in hospital, 1980, the Netherlands

Selected Operative (Surgical) Procedures		Number	Average Length of Stay (in Days)
010–059	Nervous system	10.03	20.4
060–079	Endocrine glands	5.06	16.8
080–169	Eyes	26.90	9.5
170–199	Ears	31.46	6.0
200–269	Respiratory system	104.00	5.5
300–369	Circulatory system	29.08	17.7
370–389	Blood-forming and lymphatic system	3.28	18.2
390–399	Breast	24.66	9.8
400–579	Digestive system	116.48	16.2
600–649	Urinary system	23.41	16.3
650–749	Genital organs	156.11	8.6
750–799	Gynaecological operations	42.41	9.0
800–889	Musculoskeletal system	135.74	16.8
890–909	Skin and subcutaneous tissue	31.15	13.1
	Total	739.74	11.9

SOURCE: Medical Records Foundation (SMR).

Table 7 Average length of stay in hospitals, 1979, the Netherlands

Diagnostic Categories	Males	Females	Total
Infectious and parasitic diseases	17.9	18.8	18.3
Neoplasms	19.3	17.9	18.5
Endocrine, nutritional, and metabolic diseases and immunity disorders	18.9	20.7	20.1
Diseases of the blood and blood-forming organs	16.4	18.9	17.8
Mental disorders	31.2	41.1	37.0
Diseases of the nervous system and sense organs	11.2	12.3	11.8
Diseases of the circulatory system	17.1	21.1	18.8
Diseases of the respiratory system	9.1	8.1	8.7
Diseases of the digestive system	14.5	17.6	15.9
Diseases of the genitourinary system	12.8	9.8	10.7
Complications of pregnancy, childbirth, and puerperium		9.2	9.2
Diseases of the skin and subcutaneous tissue	16.8	20.9	18.9
Diseases of the musculoskeletal system and connective tissue	13.6	19.0	16.2
Congenital anomalies	11.5	13.1	12.1
Certain conditions originating in the perinatal period	16.6	18.3	17.3
Symptoms, signs, and ill-defined conditions	12.1	13.6	12.9
External causes of injury and poisoning	15.8	20.7	17.9
All diagnoses	14.1	14.0	14.0

SOURCE: Central Bureau of Statistics, *Statistical Yearbook*.

Table 8 Estimated number of persons active in selected health field occupations, 1980, the Netherlands

	Persons Active	Rates per 100,000 Population
Dentists	5;346	38
Nursing aids	31,400	222
Nurses	47,700	338
Physiotherapists	14,632	103
Midwives	898	6
Dieticians	2,206[a]	15
Oral hygienists	550	4
Paramedical therapists	1,168[a]	8
Physicians	25,947	184
Pharmacists	1,463	10

SOURCE: C.J.N. van Brunschot, *Paramedische mankracht, een cijfermatig overzicht van enkele beroepsgroepen,* I.V.G. Tilburg.

[a]1981 data.

Table 9 Operational medical schools, medical students enrolled by sex, medical school graduates, and admissions by sex for 1979–80 and 1980–81, the Netherlands

	1979–80	1980–81
Medical schools	8	8
Total medical students	13,814	13,900
Women	4,376 (31.7%)	4,627 (33.3%)
Total medical graduates	1,558	1,432
Women	424 (27.2%)	402 (28.1%)
Total first-year students	1,387	1,410
Women	583 (42.0%)	628 (44.5%)

SOURCE: Central Bureau of Statistics, *Statistical Yearbooks.*

Table 10 Physicians and physician/population ratios, selected years, the Netherlands

Year	Physicians	Physicians Per 10,000 Population
1952	9,000	8.6
1960	12,809	11.1
1970	15,644	12.1
1975	20,200	14.9
1979	24,878	17.8
1980	25,947	18.4
1982	28,037	19.6
2000	39,000	24.9

SOURCE: Central Bureau of Statistics, *Statistical Yearbooks.*

Table 11 Physicians by specialty, 1980, the Netherlands

	Number
Physicians	25,947
General practitioners	5,468
Specialists	8,939
Allergology	14
Anaesthesia	596
Bacteriology	137
Cardiology	298
Cardiopulmonary—surgery	30
Clinical chemistry	13
Dermatology and venereology	287
Diseases of lung and tuberculosis	326
Diseases of mouth and surgery of jaw	5
Diseases of stomach and intestine	28
Internal medicine	1,305
Morbid anatomy	220
Neurosurgery	53
Obstetrics and gynaecology	545
Ophthalmology	404
Orthopaedics	228
Otolaryngology	377
Paediatrics	617
Plastic surgery	68
Psychiatry and neurology	1,578
Radiodiagnostics	199
Radiology and roentgenology	361
Radiotherapy	55
Rehabilitation	165
Rheumatology	72
Surgery	794
Urology	164
Public health physicians (registered)	1,302
Other physicians	10,238

SOURCE: The Van Mansveld Commission.

Table 12 Average net income of physicians by specialty, the Netherlands

Specialty	Inquired Income in 1977	Valuation 1980	Valuation 1981
Ophthalmology	220.2	197.5	178.7
Otolaryngology	213.7	272.4	277.6
Surgery	266.4	284.8	260.5
Orthopaedics	262.4	297.2	285.5
Gynaecology	251.6	250.2	237.0
Psychiatry and neurology	204.7	209.0	193.8
Dermatology	171.8	192.5	190.7
Internal medicine	230.4	242.2	235.5
Paediatrics	151.9	153.6	140.9
Cardiology	317.3	377.2	411.7
Radiology and röntgenology	352.9	370.4	339.6
Anaesthesia	216.5	248.7	235.5
Pulmonology	253.2	295.4	303.4
Urology	290.7	328.1	304.7
Average of inquiried (surveyed) specialties	240.0	258.7	247.2
Target income in negotiation with the government		184.5	181.5

Source: The Van Mansveld Commission.

Notes: Income after practice costs per specialist per specialty per 1,000 guilders. The reflected incomes per specialty are gathered from the incomes in solitary practice and group practice. The number of respondents from the 1977 inquiry (survey) is handled as a weighting factor.

Table 13 Hospitals by type, beds, admissions, discharges, deaths, nursing days, and occupancy of beds, 1980, the Netherlands

Type of Hospital	Institutions Recognized for AWBZ	Beds Recognized	Average Number of Beds Available	Admissions	Discharges	Deaths	Nursing Days	Occupancy of Beds in %
General hospitals	175	60,291	60,364	1,381,849	1,342,334	41,691	18,500,266	83.7
Academic hospitals	3	7,154	6,760	146,011	142,401	4,041	1,984,571	80.2
Categorial hospitals	47	6,221	6,092	58,056	57,031	1,172	1,817,535	81.5
Total	231	73,666	73,216	1,585,916	1,541,766	46,904	22,302,372	83.4

SOURCE: National Hospital Institute.

Table 14 Ownership and functions of Dutch hospitals, 1975

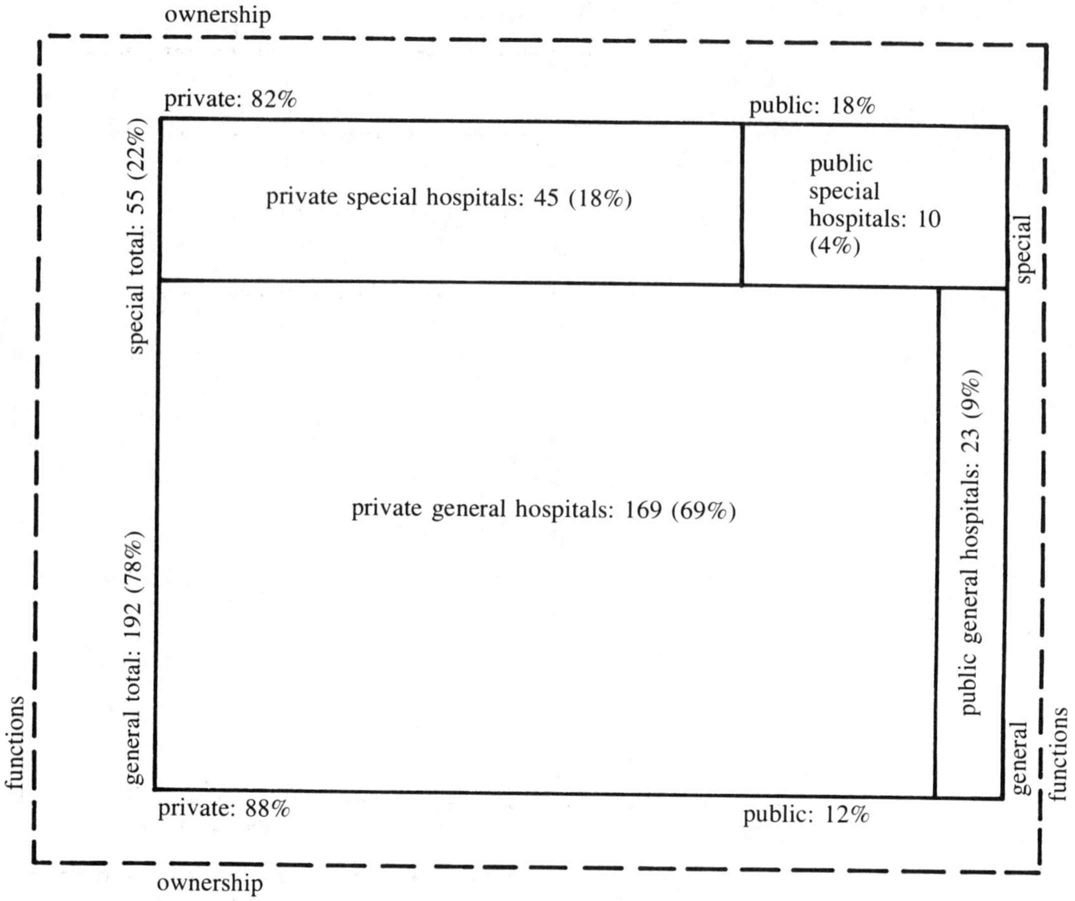

Total private (general + special): 213 (87%)
Total public (general + special): 33 (13%) - (incl. 8 academic [4%])

SOURCE: Geneeskundige Hoofdinspectie van de Volksgezondheid, 1978.

Table 15 Nursing homes and nursing home beds, 1980, the Netherlands

Nursing Homes	Institutions Recognized for AWBZ	Beds Recognized	Average Number of Beds Available	Admissions	Discharges	Deaths	Nursing Days	Occupancy of Beds in %
Homes for somatically ill patients	162	18,172	18,367	19,277	11,285	7,547	6,446,051	95.9
Home for the aged, mentally disturbed	79	10,948	11,136	4,659	1,638	2,845	3,946,697	96.7
Homes for both somatic and mental illness	82	17,223	17,278	15,017	7,901	6,385	6,129,442	97.1
Of which in								
Somatic wards		9,654	9.612	10,983	6,629	4,031	3,410,470	97.1
Psychiatric wards		7,569	7,666	4,034	1,272	2,354	2,718,972	97.2
Total	323	46,343	46,781	38,953	20,824	16,777	16,522,190	96.7

SOURCE: National Hospital Institute.

Table 16 Total costs of inpatient care, by type of expenditure and province, in general, university, and specialized hospitals (including health resorts), 1979, the Netherlands

	Groningen	Friesland	Drenthe	Overijssel	Gelderland	Urecht	N.-Holland	Z.-Holland	Zeeland	N.-Brabant	Limburg	The Netherlands
Personnel costs	310	154	104	367	623	502	1,295	1,304	93	666	387	5,605
Food	8	5	3	12	21	13	38	41	3	25	13	182
Expendable supplies	54	31	16	53	31	74	176	218	13	116	53	886
Depreciations	11	15	9	32	36	31	83	94	7	64	29	410
Interest	15	17	11	36	43	35	106	114	8	72	40	495
Sundry costs	35	20	8	43	90	67	177	191	13	98	42	785
Total	433	241	151	543	893	722	1,874	1,962	137	1,041	564	8,563
Running cost per inpatient day (guilders)	480	313	325	344	357	418	422	402	269	344	324	380

SOURCE: *Compendium 1979* and Central Bureau of Statistics.

NOTE: Figures in million guilders except "per inpatient day" costs, which are in guilders.

Table 17 Information not available.

Table 18a National health expenditures by type of expenditure and source of funds, per capita amounts, and percentage distribution, 1980, the Netherlands

Sources of Payment	Intramural	Specialist Aid	Pharmaceutical	Extramural	Collective Preventive Care	Policy Control	Total
In 1,000 guilders							
Sickness funds	6,605	923	1,552	2,114	—	733	11,927
Exceptional Medical Expenses Act (AWBZ)	6,530	—	—	770	—	130	7,430
Private insurance and household expenditures[a]	2,451	863	1,080	1,469	241	535	6,639
Government	624	—	—	157	425	262	1,468
Others	205	—	—	—	47	—	252
Total	16,415	1,786	2,632	4,510	713	1,660	27,716
Per capita (in guilders)							
Sickness funds	467	65	110	149	—	52	843
Exceptional Medical Expenses Act	461	—	—	55	—	9	525
Private insurance and household expenditures[a]	173	61	76	104	17	38	470
Government	44	—	—	11	30	19	104
Others	14	—	—	—	3	—	17
Total	1,160	126	186	319	50	117	1,959
Percentage distribution							
Sickness funds	40.3	51.6	59.1	46.7	—	44.4	43.0
Exceptional Medical Expenses Act	39.7	—	—	17.2	—	7.7	26.8
Private insurance and household expenditures[a]	14.9	48.4	40.9	32.6	34.0	32.5	24.0
Government	3.8	—	—	3.5	60.0	16.2	5.3
Others	1.3	—	—	—	6.0	—	0.9
Total	100.0	100.0	100.0	100.0	100.0	100.0	100.0

SOURCE: 6th *Financial Review* of the Dutch Health Care System.

[a]Including public insurance for civil servants.

Table 18b National health expenditures by type of expenditure and source of funds, 1980 and 1983 (estimated), the Netherlands

	Total Costs (by 1,000 Guilders)		Financer (By 1,000 Guilders): Sickness Fund		AWBZ		Private Insurance Company and Families[a]		Government		Other	
Type of Care	1980	1983	1980	1983	1980	1983	1980	1983	1980	1983	1980	1983
Intramural care	16,415	19,435	6,605	7,832	6,530	7,841	2,451	3,053	624	634	205	75
Specialist aid	1,786	1,952	923	1,000			863	952				
Pharmaceutical aid (including prostheses and material aid)	2,632	3,122	1,552	1,633			1,080	1,489				
Extramural care	4,510	5,359	2,114	2,496	770	1,015	1,469	1,712	157	136	47	61
Collective preventive care	713	866					241	294	425	511		
Policy, control, and other costs	1,660	2,067	733	928	130	163	535	660	262	316		
Total	27,716	32,801	11,927	13,889	7,430	9,019	6,639	8,160	1,468	1,597	252	136
Decrease of excessive incomes independent professionals		– 245		– 147				– 98				
Correction[b]			15	217	7	10	23	266	2	2	– 47	– 61
Total (According to *Financial Review*)	27,716	32,556	11,942	13,525	7,437	9,029	6,662	8,328	1,470	1,599	205	75
In percentage	100%	100%	43.2%	41.6%	26.8%	27.7%	24.0%	25.6%	5.3%	4.9%	0.7%	0.2%

[a]Inclusive of public insurance for civil servants.
[b]The total according to chapter 1 of the *Financial Review* and the calculation of the total on the basis of chapters 2 to 7 of this review shows a deviation.

Table 19 Information not available.

Table 20 Sickness fund insurance: persons covered in selected years, the Netherlands

Sickness Fund Insurance	1950	1955	1960	1965	1970	1975	1980
Compulsory	4,548,554	5,920,089	5,655,202	6,203,260	6,725,692	7,067,915	7,066,972
For the aged	—	—	665,966	678,904	858,021	1,000,399	1,079,960
Voluntary	2,461,965	1,985,571	1,815,381	1,778,195	1,512,337	1,514,796	1,559,002
Total	7,010,519	7,905,660	8,136,549	8,660,359	9,096,050	9,583,110	9,705,934

Source: Sickness Fund Council (ZFR).

Health Services in New Zealand

B. Joan Mackay

INTRODUCTION

The country of New Zealand lies in the South Pacific. It has three main and some smaller islands and it is over 10,000 kilometers from the west side of the United States, 2,000 from the southeast corner of Australia, and 7,000 from Southeast Asia. Its total area is almost 27 million hectares, about the same size as the British Isles. The climate is temperate and mean temperatures vary from about 15°C in the north to about 9°C in the south. January and February are the hottest months of the year, while July and August are the coldest. The terrain is largely mountainous. About 50% of the land is pasture and arable and about 26% is forest, either native bush or exotics. The standard of living is that of most developed countries, and the health and morbidity patterns are comparable.

New Zealand was initially settled by Polynesian migrants, the Maoris, before the fourteenth century. They named the country Aotearoa, the Land of the Long White Cloud, because of the observed phenomenon of the bank of low clouds that frequently covers much of the country. The first European to discover the land was Abel Tasman, in 1642, but Captain James Cook claimed it as British territory in 1769. It was not until 1840, however, that the first settlers landed in Port Nicholson, the harbour around which Wellington, the capital city, has grown. The Maori population at that time was thought to be between 200 and 300 thousand, but by the end of the century it had fallen to an estimated 42 thousand. This was attributed to the impact of the European on Maori culture and to the introduction of European diseases. In 1980 the estimated Maori population was 288,200 and 57% of these people were under twenty years of age. Over the last ten years the Maori population has increased about 2% annually, compared with 1% for the rest of the population. The total population of New Zealand now is a little over 3 million, with 13% belonging to minority cultures and 8.9% Maori; 80% live in urban areas and almost 73% in the North Island, including 94% of the Maori population.[1]

In the late 1930s and early 1940s New Zealand became known throughout the world for its advanced social welfare thinking. The early settlers, however, who were predominantly British, did not come with such considerations in mind; they had left the United Kingdom essentially to escape poverty and to obtain a better way of life in a new environment, but

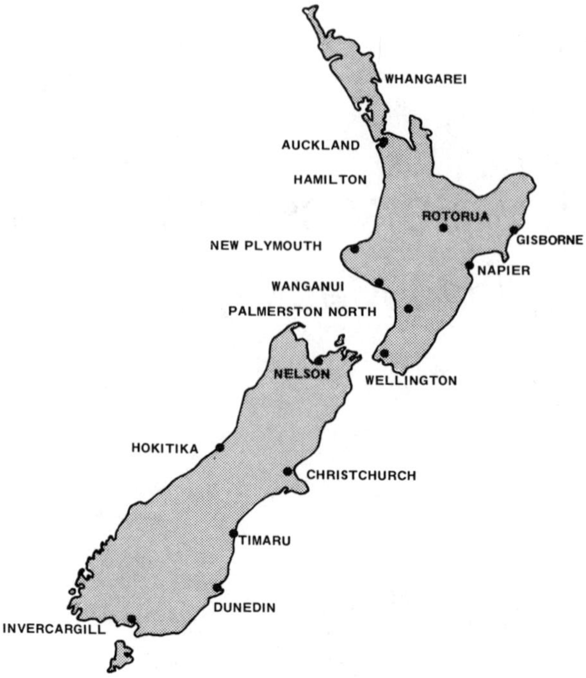

they brought with them their fundamental Scottish and English orientation. Their settlements were widely spaced around the country and, since communications were poor because of the difficulty of the terrain, they tended to develop their own schemes for self-help and community support. There were no wealthy philanthropists to assist, however, so it soon became evident that only the state had sufficient money or capacity to provide help when need was widespread. Thus, from an early stage the state participated in part, if not entirely, in the responsibility of providing health and welfare services. The settlers also brought the concept of what has been described as egalitarianism, by which they meant equalising upwards, and their hope was that everyone would move up into the middle classes. This egalitarianism was linked to humanitarianism, and both still constitute a strong influence in New Zealand today. As far back as 1846 Governor Grey built four small hospitals to meet the health requirements of Maoris and of sick and destitute Europeans.

It is probably not surprising, therefore, that the hardships of the Depression led to the 1938 Social Security Act and its revolutionary concept that the state should provide hospital and certain medical services on a universal basis at no charge to its citizens. Since that time there have been a number of modifications to the details of the act but no radical legislative reorganisation of it. There has been an evolutionary change, however, brought about in part because the right to charge the patient a fee was retained by the medical profession. Initially, no charge was made by the majority of doctors (or it was negligible compared with the benefit paid by the government), but with the passage of time the value of the benefit has diminished and a substantial proportion of the total fee is now paid by the patient.

Another somewhat revolutionary measure has been the passing of the Accident Compensation Act. This legislation abolished in New Zealand the action for damages at common law for personal injury suffered as a result of negligence, substituting a wide ranging scheme of monetary benefits and rehabilitative measures for all persons who suffer injury by accident, whether occurring at work or not. An injured person now receives earnings-related compensation equal to 80% of his or her preaccident earnings, with an upper limit in 1982 of $600.00 per week* and specified lump sums for permanent disability. The Accident Compensation Corporation (previously, the Commission) has responsibility for administering the act and it obtains its funds from various sources, including an occupational levy on all employers in the country.

These are only fragments of a complex health service that is provided for a relatively small number of unevenly distributed, multicultural people; for this service to be understood, it is important to consider its social, cultural, and political context.

New Zealand has a democratic parliamentary system of government based on that of its mother country, the United Kingdom. The early colony was granted dominion status and became self-governing in 1907, but it was not until 1946 that full constitutional independence was obtained. There is still one important link with Britain, however, and that is through the British monarch who is still the head of state of New Zealand. The country is politically stable, and free and regular elections for membership of the unicameral House of Representatives take place every three years. All New Zealand citizens over the age of eighteen are entitled to vote. There are two major parties, one of which functions as the government and the other as the opposition, the latter having the traditional, if unliked, role of watchdog. The rule of law is upheld by independent courts whose judges are appointed on a completely apolitical basis and are free of any control by the politicians. There is no written constitution, and British constitutional conventions tend to be considered by way of precedents. The executive of the House of Representatives is known as the cabinet and is made up of ministers in charge of various government departments. The Department of Health, for example, the central health authority, is responsible to the minister of health through the director-general of health, who is a medical practitioner and the principle officer of the department. The country is divided into eighteen health districts, each of which has a district office with a medical officer of health who is responsible for seeing that departmental policies are carried out. The medical officer of health does, however, have considerable statutory responsibility in his or her own right.

Alongside the system of central government, controlled by elected representatives, and a large public service, there is a complex system of local government. There are about 600 local bodies in total, all with elected members. Many of these have a single special purpose, such as the provision of a water supply, drainage, hospitals, or power, but others, about 200 in number, are territorial local authorities which have, among their other responsibilities, such basic health functions as the collection and disposal of refuse, the sanitary inspection of buildings, some duties in respect of water supplies and drainage, and the control of food premises. These are carried out in close conjunction with the Department of Health.

In addition to health districts, the country is also divided into twenty-nine hospital board areas, which are part of the local government system previously referred to. Their boundaries are not contiguous with health districts and the areas vary greatly in relation to the population served. The hospital boards are funded entirely from central taxation, although their members are locally elected.

From its very early days the state has been involved in the provision of hospital and

*All dollar references in this chapter are to New Zealand dollars. See conversion table in the Introduction.—ED.

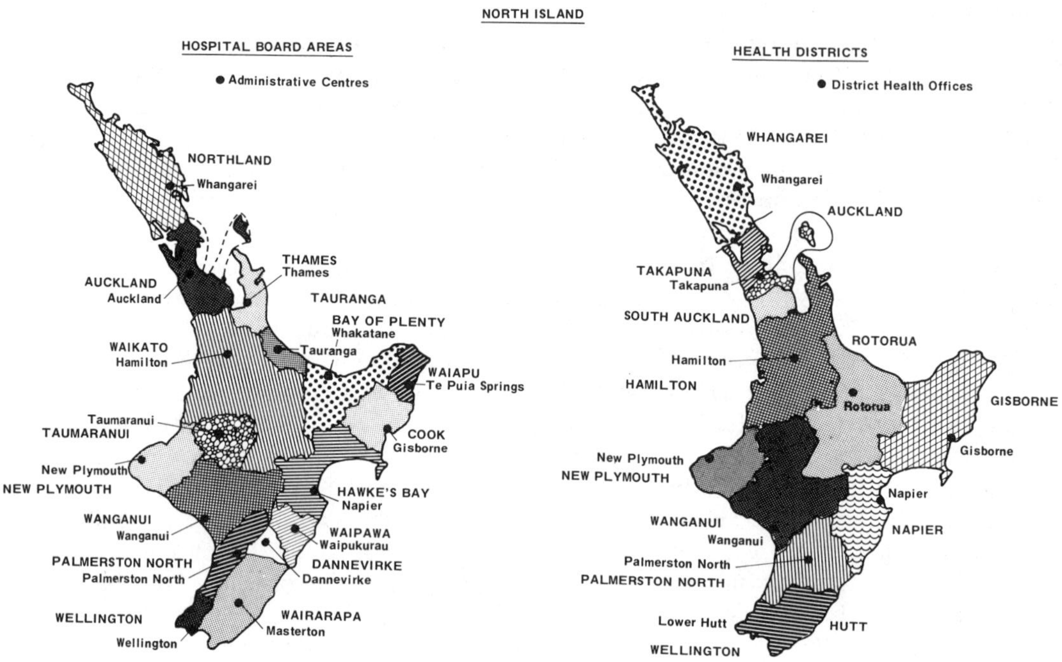
NORTH ISLAND
HOSPITAL BOARD AREAS
● Administrative Centres
NORTHLAND
Whangarei
AUCKLAND
Auckland
THAMES
Thames
TAURANGA
BAY OF PLENTY
Whakatane
Tauranga
WAIKATO
Hamilton
WAIAPU
Te Puia Springs
Taumaranui
TAUMARANUI
COOK
Gisborne
New Plymouth
NEW PLYMOUTH
HAWKE'S BAY
Napier
WANGANUI
Wanganui
WAIPAWA
Waipukurau
PALMERSTON NORTH
Palmerston North
DANNEVIRKE
Dannevirke
WELLINGTON
Wellington
WAIRARAPA
Masterton
HEALTH DISTRICTS
● District Health Offices
WHANGAREI
Whangarei
AUCKLAND
TAKAPUNA
Takapuna
SOUTH AUCKLAND
ROTORUA
Hamilton
HAMILTON
Rotorua
GISBORNE
Gisborne
New Plymouth
NEW PLYMOUTH
Napier
WANGANUI
Wanganui
NAPIER
Palmerston North
PALMERSTON NORTH
Lower Hutt
HUTT
WELLINGTON

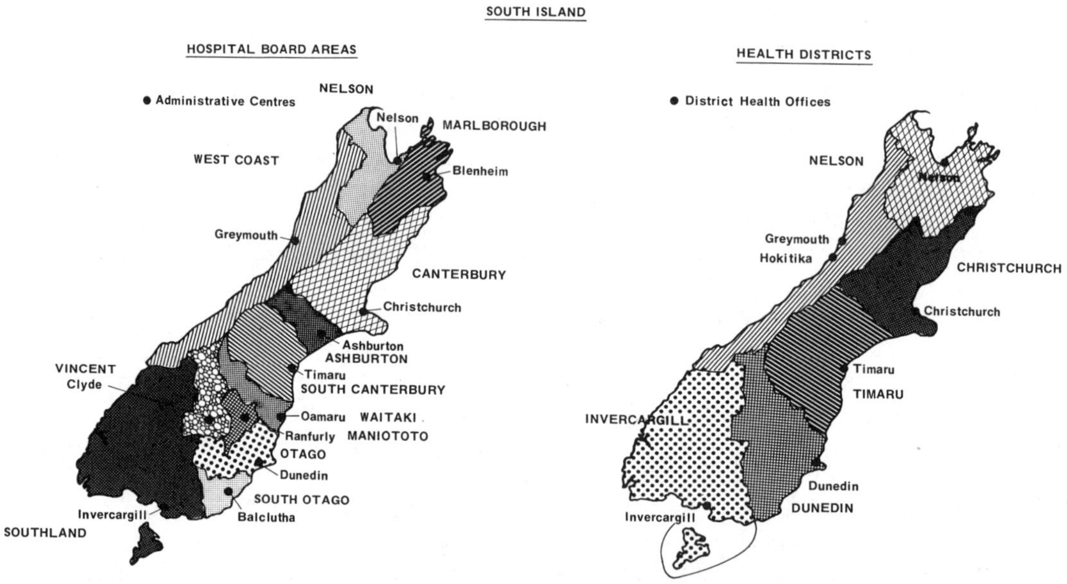
SOUTH ISLAND
HOSPITAL BOARD AREAS
● Administrative Centres
NELSON
Nelson
MARLBOROUGH
WEST COAST
Blenheim
Greymouth
CANTERBURY
Christchurch
Ashburton
ASHBURTON
VINCENT
Clyde
Timaru
SOUTH CANTERBURY
Oamaru
WAITAKI
Ranfurly
MANIOTOTO
OTAGO
Dunedin
SOUTH OTAGO
Invercargill
Balclutha
SOUTHLAND
HEALTH DISTRICTS
● District Health Offices
NELSON
Nelson
Greymouth
Hokitika
CHRISTCHURCH
Christchurch
Timaru
TIMARU
INVERCARGILL
Dunedin
DUNEDIN
Invercargill

community health services and has had a particular concern in the control of infectious diseases. It is of interest that the revolutionary concept of the 1930s—that health services should be available to and within reach of all New Zealanders—was supported by both the government and the opposition, differing only on the question of degree. Ultimately, the compromise was reached that a proportion of the services would be funded in total while for the remainder a charge would be made to the patient. Public hospitals and general practitioner obstetric services have thus remained free at all times. Another indication of compromise is that private hospitals have been partly subsidised by the state, so that they, too, have remained within reach of the average New Zealander should he or she wish to pay the additional cost involved. It is thus a very complex system of private and public funding in New Zealand, with private hospitals and patients both being subsidised by the state, and, undoubtedly, much of this has arisen as a result of that pragmatic approach which is such a major characteristic of New Zealanders.

A more recent development was an amendment to the Land & Income Tax Act in 1967 that made premiums paid for private health insurance deductible for the purposes of income tax. This made such insurance economical and attractive, and undoubtedly stimulated the development of voluntary private health insurance and private medical services.

In recent years the adverse change in the economic climate has conditioned a desire by the government to ensure that equity rather than equality is the basis for health benefits. This has been demonstrated in increased government subsidisation of health care for the elderly and of benefits for the young and for chronic sufferers of all ages. There also has been an increasing public and popular interest in health care, reflected in the phenomenally successful series of "telethons." The last of these 24-hour television marathons, held in 1981, raised over 5 million dollars, a huge sum for a population of 3 million. The telethon proceeds have on each separate occasion been devoted to a specific purpose—for example, for the disabled and for mental health—and are given to private and independent foundations to administer. Much of this money is then channelled to existing private and public health organisations.

Predictably, voluntary services are very much a part of life in New Zealand, but they, too, are generally heavily subsidised by the government. For example, a voluntary organisation known as the Royal New Zealand Society for the Health of Women and Children (the Plunket Society) is now responsible for the health of infants up to the age of five years, and about 86% of New Zealand's children are under the supervision of its nurses. A great deal of money is raised by the society and its branches, but the salaries of the Plunket nurses are paid by the government.

The fragmentation of some parts of the health service and the increase in medical specialisation has tended to conflict with economic and management constraints, with the result that politicians of both parties are now prepared to consider a major reorganisation of it. Two pilot schemes have been established, one in rural Northland and the other in urban Wellington, with the object of integrating those services provided locally by the hospital boards and those by the Health Department through its district offices. In addition, a mechanism is being devised to enable coordination of planning between the public, private, and voluntary sectors. The aim is to form a health board, but because this requires legislative change, which may be controversial, any legislation introduced is likely to be permissive in nature and not compulsorily applicable. Hospital boards will not be told what to do; instead, they will be given the right, if they wish to exercise it, to ask the minister for approval to amalgamate with the local district office of the Department of Health and to establish a new health board.

Since the members of each hospital board are elected by the local electors, there is a perhaps natural tendency on their part to resist any change that would bring Banquo's ghost to their board table in the shape of government appointees chosen for their special skills and attributes.

MEDICAL PRACTICE

In 1973 there were 3,444 active medical practitioners in New Zealand, and by 1980 the number had increased to 4,881—one physician for every 645 persons.

A medical school was established in 1857 by the Scottish settlers in Dunedin and until 1968, when 120 students graduated, it was the only one in the country.[2] In that year (1968) another school started in Auckland and 58 of its first students qualified in 1974. This school was set up in response to the fear prevalent in the late 1960s and lasting through the early 1970s that there would be a shortage of doctors in future years. By the end of the 1970s, however, the country was in economic difficulties and a zero trend in the population existed, so that a *surplus* of doctors was now feared. A medical manpower committee therefore recommended a cutback in the number of students entering the medical schools, and this brought about a reduction in intake of 12½% in 1980 and a further similar reduction in 1981.[3] The minister of health agreed to this step, however, only on condition that the medical profession itself introduce a scheme to ensure that those areas in the country which were known to experience difficulty in attracting doctors would not be allowed to suffer.

The basic medical qualification is the MB,ChB. New Zealand, however, has always had a significant number of doctors who received their training overseas. As many as 31.3% of practitioners in 1978 had obtained their initial medical qualification elsewhere, although this percentage will vary since on the average one-half of the incoming physicians depart within three years whilst a significant number remain and work in New Zealand.[4]

As a result of the fear of a surplus of doctors and because fewer New Zealand doctors are now going overseas permanently, there has been a necessary tightening of the controls on medical immigration. There are many possible explanations for the declining number of NZ doctors leaving, but the principal ones may be attributed to the current international situation, the difficulties of finding appointments overseas, and the simple fact that they find the life style in New Zealand more compatible and congenial than elsewhere.

The proportion of women in medical practice has increased quite dramatically in the last decade. Before 1970 only 10 to 15% of medical entrants were women, but by 1977 this had increased to 38% at Otago in Dunedin and 46% in Auckland, and the numbers are expected to increase steadily. In 1979, 14% of active medical practitioners were women.[5]

The majority of doctors are in private practice, either general or specialist, or have full-time or part-time appointments with hospital boards, the Department of Health, or the Accident Compensation Corporation.

Of the 1,823 doctors in general practice in 1980, over one-half were in solo practice, over one-third in group practice, and the remainder in health centres.[6] As well as working from their own rooms, some work in hospitals, both public and private, and home visiting is generally undertaken.

Specialists may be full-time hospital board employees, but the majority of them work part time in public hospitals and part time in private practice in their own rooms and private hospitals. In private practice they charge their patients a fee in addition to receiving the specialist fee-for-service provided by the state. However, if the patient's condition was due to an accident, all fees are paid by the Accident Compensation Corporation. A growing number of specialists are practising full time in public hospitals where they receive a salary and where their services attract no fee from the patient. Academic staff attached to the medical schools are also salaried, but they have the right to a small amount of private practice. Community medicine specialists work as hospital board administrators and as administrators and specialists within the Department of Health. In both cases they receive a salary. Doctors working in industry may be paid by the Department of Health or by the industry that contracts for their services.

A very high proportion of pathology work is done in private laboratories, particularly on referral from general practitioners. Most of this work is free to the patient. Smaller hospitals also make use of private pathology services and have their work done on a contractual basis. All the larger hospitals, however, have their own laboratory services. Similarly, x-ray examinations are heavily subsidised by the state, and many radiologists practise in private and claim the patient's benefit. Most acute medical care is given by the public hospital, but 16% of hospital beds are in the private sector.

For many years medical practitioners have been the highest earners in the professions, although there are signs that this is now changing. This has inevitably had an influence on recruitment to medicine: because the primary criterion for admission to the medical schools has been academic attainment, these schools have for many years taken the cream of the students.

Since the 1970s there has been a slowly increasing interest in general practice, and many young doctors are now choosing to enter this field of work. As entry is not controlled in any way, however, concern is being expressed that a possible surplus of doctors in the mid-1980s would move a majority into general practice and the resulting increased competition would cause a deterioration rather than an improvement of service to the public. The other major influence affecting practice has been the growth of private health insurance. Tax concessions and business-formed group schemes for workers have encouraged this and made it a major growth area, and, consequently, all forms of private medical practice have been stimulated.

The New Zealand Medical Association[7]

The New Zealand Medical Association is a limited company, the largest of its type in New Zealand, which has a membership of over 4,000 doctors, representing 81% of all practising doctors in the country.[8] All of its twenty-one divisions send delegates to a council that usually meets quarterly at its headquarters in Wellington. The association works through its executive and a number of committees, such as Central Specialists', Central General Practitioners', Central Education, Ethical, Medical Examination Fees, Maternity Benefits Negotiating, and the New Zealand Medical Journal Editorial.

The organisation is very powerful and uses its influence politically in many different ways. For example, it has representatives and nominees on many outside bodies and committees, such as the Medical Practitioners' Disciplinary Committee, the Board of Health and its specialist and technical committees, the Department of Health Poisons' Committee, the Nursing Education Review and Advisory Committee, the Nursing and the

Dental Councils, and the Opticians', the Chiropodists', and the Physiotherapy Boards. It is involved in the distribution of the funds of such bodies as the New Zealand Medical Education Trust and in research in the Traffic Accident Research Foundation. It would be accurate to say that no organisation or committee wishing to operate in the field of health would be complete without a representative or nominee of the New Zealand Medical Association.

The association has many statutory powers and responsibilities, most notably under the Medical Practitioners' Act 1968, which gives it control of standards of ethical behaviour over and above the right and duty of any corporate body to control the behaviour of its members. It is also concerned with disciplinary matters that may arise out of claims for state benefits and other such controversial issues, and it undertakes with the government any negotiations on behalf of the profession for the setting of fees.

The Colleges and Other Organisations

The colleges that have responsibility for specialists' training and for standards of medical care provided by their members in the specialties are the Royal Australasian College of Physicians, Royal Australasian College of Surgeons, Royal Australasian College of Radiologists, Royal College of Obstetricians and Gynaecologists, Royal College of Pathologists of Australasia, Royal Australian and New Zealand College of Psychiatrists, Royal New Zealand College of General Practitioners, Australasian College of Dermatologists, Faculty of Anaesthetists RACS, and a New Zealand College of Community Medicine.

The Medical Council is dealt with later in the "Control of the Medical Profession" section.

All specialists belong to their respective colleges. Recently, a determined attempt has been made to upgrade general practice and to align its college training requirements with those of the other colleges. The Royal New Zealand College of General Practitioners, with assistance from the government, has organised a family medicine training programme, culminating in an examination for membership of the college. The College of General Practitioners is still weak numerically but is experiencing considerable leadership.

The most recently established college is that of Community Medicine. The first part of its new training programme is an academic year of postgraduate study for the Diploma of Community Health. This course is held in Wellington and is followed by a further three-year training course for those wishing to become members of the college.

In addition to the colleges there are societies and associations, which are groups of doctors, specialists, and nonspecialists who are interested in a particular section of medicine, for example, the Obstetrical and Gynaecological Society, the Paediatric Society, and the New Zealand Medical Women's Association.

Primary Care Medical Practitioners

The title "Primary Care Medical Practitioner" refers in New Zealand to a general practitioner. There are many definitions of primary care but there is not a universally accepted one in the country; however, that which has been adopted in a pilot scheme to establish a health board in the Wellington region reads:

> Primary health care constitutes the first element of a continuing health process. It is a practical approach to making such health care accessible to all individuals and/or families in the community in an acceptable and affordable way, with their full participation and without necessity for referrals from any other point in the health care service. It should include preventive, curative, and rehabilitative services.[9]

Such a definition includes those doctors other than general practitioners who work in accident and emergency clinics, as medical officers in the Department of Health, in Family Planning Association clinics, and so on. Despite this definition, however, a primary health care medical practitioner is generally understood to be a general practitioner.

Demography

Between 1973 and 1980 there was an increase of 34.8% in active general practitioners. Consequently, the general practitioner workforce is relatively young, with only about 10% aged sixty-five years and over. In 1980 the number of general practitioners in active practice was 1,823 and the population per active practitioner was 1,727.

In 1971, 16 of the 118 graduates from medical school in New Zealand were women, but by 1980 the numbers had increased to 77 out of 233. General practice had 9.4% women in 1972 but 12.7% by 1979, and overseas graduates, both male and female, seem to have stabilised in the second half of the 1970s, with one-third of the male and one-half of the female general practitioners being overseas graduates.[10]

Distribution

Patients do not have to register with a particular doctor and any doctor can set up in general practice in any part of New Zealand. This has resulted in a degree of maldistribution between urban and rural areas and between the northern half of the North Island and the rest of New Zealand.

Obtaining and retaining doctors in rural areas has presented a number of problems. In some remote and difficult areas special arrangements for medical services were provided. These were designated "special areas," and at present are fifteen in number. Examples of these are isolated places such as the off-shore Chatham Islands and Hokianga in the North Island. The doctors in these areas have contracts with either the Department of Health or the hospital board to provide general medical services for one year; they are paid a salary and their services are free to the patients. Although they are, strictly speaking, independent contractors, their salaries are related to and increase with hospital board salaries; they have special leave arrangements; housing and heavy furniture are provided and the house is rent free. Loans are available for the purchase of a car if one is not provided. In some cases these doctors also dispense their own drugs.

In addition to the special areas, there are a number of rural areas in which, to provide an incentive for practitioners to work there, the government in 1979 made special loan finance available to local authorities who wished to build houses and set up surgeries for doctors. The government also introduced a practice nurse scheme in these areas, which has been so popular that pressure from the medical profession has caused it to be extended to urban areas. The nurse's salary is subsidised to 100% by the government or, alternatively, a 50% subsidy is paid plus a subsidy for each domiciliary visit, plus a car allowance. In 1979 about 900 practice nurses were employed by general practitioners but were paid wholly or in part by the government. A scheme was also introduced whereby hospital boards, as government agents, could provide health centres where this was desirable and requested by the medical profession. Fourteen of these were in operation in 1981, a number of them with practice nurses also provided by the hospital board.

In addition to these, the government has taken active steps to encourage general practice by establishing, on a fee-for-service basis, an entire series of general medical services benefits that vary according to the categories of patients and services; this gives travelling allowances and maternity benefits, and immunization benefits which are paid, whether the immunisation is carried out by the doctor or nurse, if the patient is under sixteen years and the immunization programme is approved by the Department of Health. Where doctors wish to try an alternative monetary arrangement to the usual general medical services scheme, special arrangements have been worked out for payment of fees instead of benefits. For example, a fee for a stated period of time is paid by the Department of Health for each person on the practice register of a medical centre. The fee is based on the annual national average for the general medical service benefit expenditure per head of the population. This is, in effect, a capitation fee for everyone on the register and is paid monthly, but over and above this the patient pays the doctor an additional fee. One health centre and one medical centre group practice are currently involved in such a scheme, their aim being to give total rather than episodic care. In addition, there are doctors employed as trainee registrars who work with established practitioners in a family medicine training programme in which trainees spend six months in an accredited training practice and six months in selected hospital posts. In December 1979 the intake was forty-five registrars and the number is increasing.

The Work of the General Practitioner

All general practitioners provide a service for sick persons. A few specialists, notably some specialist paediatricians, also give primary health care, but the majority of specialists will see only patients referred to them by a general practitioner. The payment structure of the state is such that a letter from the general practitioner to the specialist is necessary before the specialist benefit is payable, except in the cases of obstetrics, as explained below.

As in other parts of the world, an increasing amount of primary health care in New Zealand is being given at the accident and emergency rooms of public hospitals in the major cities. Also, psychiatric primary health care is available through the psychiatric outpatients' department at the request of the patient and not necessarily on referral from the general practitioner. With these exceptions, outpatients' clinics as a rule require a referral from the general practitioner.

Over 50% of all obstetrics is done by general practitioners, who can call on public hospital or private specialists as required. All general practitioner obstetric services are "free" to the patient and the fee is re-negotiated by the profession with the government at frequent intervals.

If a general practitioner believes the patient's condition warrants specialist care, it can be provided free through the public hospital system or, if desired, by state-subsidised private specialist care. Not all general practitioners practice obstetrics, however, and there are also patients who prefer to go to specialist obstetricians without being referred by their general practitioners and who are prepared to pay a fee in excess of the general practitioner state payment. If the patient has been referred, the obstetrician receives the specialist benefit; without referral, however, the obstetrician receives only the general practitioner benefit. General practitioners also make a significant contribution outside general practice to medical work such as community health and in the smaller hospitals away from the teaching hospitals.

Patient Access to Care

In the event of an accident, depending on its severity and the place it occurred, the patient might be taken to a local doctor who would either give the requisite care or refer him or her to the nearest Accident and Emergency Clinic of a public hospital. There are no such clinics in private hospitals. The whole costs would be met by the Accident Compensation Corporation, bearing in mind that treatment at a public hospital is free to the patient. If the accident occurred at work, the Accident Compensation Corporation would also pay earnings-related compensation in contradistinction to the means tested flat-rate sickness benefit from the Social Welfare Department, which would be available to people suffering personal injury other than by accident (for example, a recurrence of incapacity resulting from a long-standing back lesion). Many patients—whether because of accessiblity to care, the 24-hour service, or to prevent delay—would be taken directly to the hospital even though they could otherwise be treated by a general practitioner.

A sick person would normally go to his or her practitioner or, in some cases, the general practitioner would call at the home. There is usually very little delay in getting an appointment, depending on the urgency perceived by the patient and ascertained by the practice. If a routine examination or check-up is required, it is usually planned ahead with the patient.

Twenty-four-hour emergency medical care is provided by almost all practices, solo practitioners having arrangements with others similarly placed. Medical care is also given at major urban hospitals, although this is not encouraged; it seems that people living near the hospital, recent immigrants from the Pacific Islands who use hospitals in this way in their homelands, and people who do not wish to pay a medical fee are generally those who attempt to use the hospital for primary health care.

For a patient referred for pathological or x-ray investigation, services will be provided by private contractors and paid for entirely by the government in the case of the former, and in part in the latter. General practitioners may refer patients to public hospitals for x-rays in some cases, and then no fee is charged. Whether a patient goes to a public hospital or to a private radiologist depends on such circumstances as whether the pressure on the public hospital resources would lead to delay, if the hospital is inconveniently sited for the patient, or if the appointment system is not sufficiently flexible to suit the patients' requirements.

If the patient requires other specialist consultation, the general practitioner will, after discussion with the patient, refer him or her with the appropriate letter, either privately—in which case, although a specialist benefit is paid by the government, the patient will have to pay the balance—or to a hospital outpatient's department where no charge is made.

HOSPITALS

Hospital services are provided by a combination of state, private, and voluntary effort. Most hospital care is provided free to the patient by the government in modern, well-equipped hospitals that are run by hospital boards. There are 8 to 14 board members, who are elected locally every three years for each hospital district. The board is responsible for providing and maintaining hospital accommodation and health centres and medical, nursing, and such other services as the minister of health considers necessary. Hospital board districts, of which there are 29 in New Zealand, vary greatly in size both geographically and in population. In Auckland the population is over 800,000 while in Maniototo, the smallest area, it is a modest 2,500. Occasionally there have been attempts to introduce more rationally sized boards, but these have almost always proved politically impossible. Since 1958 all funding of public hospitals has come from the government; funding for private hospitals (of which there were 163 in 1979) is subsidised by the government in a number of ways, including a daily subsidy for all patients. This long-standing dual system of subsidised private and free public hospital care has existed since the early 1940s. In the 1979-80 financial year the cost to New Zealand taxpayers of all hospital services was $804.9 million, or about $258 per head of population. In 1981-82 the allocation to hospital boards was a staggering $933.6 million.[11]

There are 26,602 public and 5,164 private hospital beds—that is, about 84% in the public sector and 16% in the private. Successive governments have supported private (including voluntary) hospitals and have attempted by so doing to keep them financially within the reach of most New Zealanders. At present the daily benefit from the government differs for surgical, medical, and geriatric cases, but it is roughly equal to about 50% of the private fee charged; the balance is paid by either the individual or a combination of health insurance and individual payment. Health insurance membership fees may nowadays be met by the individual's employer. Surveys done by the health insurance groups have shown that the use of private hospitals is not restricted to any one sector of the population and that private hospitals may be chosen for convenience, to ensure the doctor of choice, or for the additional privacy involved. Whatever the reason, the patient obtains a government subsidy. The private hospital is regarded as an important part of the overall hospital system because it enables many of the simple procedures to be undertaken away from public hospitals and it is said to encourage specialists. By far the greater part of the training of health professionals, however, which is very costly in terms of time, money, and other resources, inevitably takes place in the public hospitals.

Although there are usually waiting lists for public hospitals, urgent cases are admitted without delay. The interpretation of such lists for nonemergency surgery is difficult, as investigation has shown that many of the names can be deleted for a variety of reasons. For example, a number of orthopaedic cases after a time refuse operation either because they have learned to live with their disability or have improved sufficiently to do so, and such an outcome is frequently anticipated at the time their names are put on the list. In addition, many patients will have received treatment privately because the government has kept this subsidised "private" care within easy reach of all New Zealanders. This may not continue to be so, as the country is facing increasing economic problems; the expansion of private health insurance is relevant to this context. In some specialties and in some geographic areas there are transient shortages of trained staff, and under these circumstances there may well be some delay in nonurgent specialist treatment. The increasing cost of superspecialties with high technology means that these are almost exclusively found in the public hospitals and major surgery, with very few exceptions, is always done there.

In addition to the usual inpatient accommodation, most general hospitals provide some outpatient services, the extent of which varies with the size of the hospital and local conditions. Normally, the patient is referred by the general practitioner for an appointment with a specialist at the outpatient department, but, as mentioned previously, psychiatric or accident and emergency patients frequently refer themselves.

The number of ageing people in the population has increased greatly in recent years, but the number of geriatric hospital beds, while also increasing, has not kept pace with the demand in many areas. In consequence, arrangements have been made whereby a public hospital that is short of geriatric beds may subsidise a private hospital which has such beds available.

In addition, religious organisations and other voluntary groups for many years have been active in assisting old people and have provided hospitals as well as homes for them. The government recognises this in a series of financial incentives, over and above other private hospital subsidies, by giving suspensory loans and staff subsidies. The minister of health is charged under the Hospital Act 1957 with providing and maintaining, through hospital boards, hospitals and hospital services, and with encouraging the provision and maintenance of private hospitals. The Department of Health advises the minister on, or can itself determine for the boards, the nature and standards of hospitals and associated services, the building requirements to provide these, and the levels at which the main professional staff groups are to be maintained. Furthermore, it can also determine the annual grants, the salaries, and the conditions of employment of about 60% of the staff and the measure of financial assistance, including loan finance to be given to private hospitals. The department licenses and supervises private hospitals, inspects the work of all hospitals, and is responsible for compiling financial and statistical data about them. The power and responsibility of central control is thus present in almost every aspect of the hospital service.

All of these functions and activities depend very greatly on the advisory mechanism that assists the Department of Health and the minister and upon which they are able to rely for much expert advice and assistance.

In addition to these traditional activities, a hospital board may provide a number of other services, such as community health, oncology and paediatric nursing, home dialysis, meals-on-wheels, home-help, laundry, social work support, and so on. Patient care is free, but some of the purely social services, such as home-help and meals-on-wheels, are subject to a moderate charge which is based on a means test.

Other Types of Hospitals and Services

Extramural Hospitals

An extramural hospital—a "hospital without walls"—refers to a system of hospital resources taken into the community. The quantum of such resources varies greatly. In Auckland, where the number of hospital beds has not kept pace with the population, there is a network of services including those provided by district nurses, physiotherapists, and social workers. Oxygen is supplied in the home, as well as "meals-on-wheels" and laundry services for appropriate patients.

Teaching Hospitals

The teaching hospitals are those connected with the medical schools at Dunedin and Auckland, and the clinical schools at Wellington and Christchurch. Considerable research takes place at these centres.

Mental Hospital Services

From the time of the early settlers until 1972, mental hospitals were the responsibility of the state and patients paid no fees. In 1972 their control passed to hospital boards with the exception of one private hospital, subsidised by patients' benefits, and one maximum security hospital for the criminally insane, which remained in the control of the Departments of Health and Justice. In total there are eleven psychiatric hospitals, but there are psychiatric beds in ten general hospitals as well as in outpatient clinics.[12] There are two sanatoria for alcoholics, and four hospitals and training schools for the mentally retarded.

Maternity Hospitals

The birth rate in New Zealand in 1980 per 1,000 mean population was non-Maori (European and all other races, including a growing number of migrant Polynesians from the South Pacific) 15.5 and Maori (people of one-half or more Maori ancestry) 22.25, giving a figure overall of 16.14. Approximately 99% of births took place in public hospitals or in the maternity unit of a general hospital. There are only 5 private maternity hospitals, which have a total of 29 licensed beds; the rest are public hospitals, most built since 1945, which are free of charge to patients, who are confined by the doctor of their choice. A small but increasing number of women are requesting delivery at "birth centres" or at home as an alternative to hospital confinement; in 1980, 382 (or .75%) of all births took place at home. The size of maternity hospitals varies greatly, ranging from 162 beds in National Women's Hospital in Auckland, the largest in New Zealand, to only 4 in Akaroa in the South Island.[13] The total number of beds available during the year ending 31 March 1979 was 2,714 in public hospitals, a rate of 9 per 1,000 mean population, and 111 in private hospitals, a rate too small to calculate.[14] Specialist obstetric and neonatal services are available in most areas. The National Women's Hospital in Auckland, established in 1947 in the prefabricated American Army Hospital in Cornwall Park but moved in 1964 to a custom-built hospital in Epsom, has provided a great stimulus to the development of intensive research and to a high standard of obstetric services.

Rehabilitation

To a greater or lesser extent, rehabilitation is undertaken at practically all general hospitals where physiotherapists, social workers, and occupational therapists are employed. Larger hospitals frequently have speech therapists, a clinical psychologist, a hospital rehabilitation officer, and their own orthopaedic workshops for the production of prosthetic appliances and surgical footwear. These larger hospitals have multidisciplinary teams, often in special units, for dealing with rheumatology, geriatric, and neurosurgical cases, while three have developed specialist rehabilitation units that provide a more comprehensive type of rehabilitation programme than can be provided in the physical medicine section of a general hospital.

Spinal injury units have been developed in Auckland and Christchurch (that is, one in the North Island and one in the South Island), where there is treatment for acute cases and provision for long-term stay, intensive rehabilitation, and sheltered workshop training.

The rehabilitation of geriatric patients, on the other hand, has been developed on a regional basis and is under the care of a regional geriatrician.

The early discharge of psychiatric and psychopaedic patients, a fairly recent development, has changed the approach to their rehabilitation. There is now a concentration on community support for psychopaedic patients, who are taught to live in the community rather than trained for a job—which almost by definition could be very vulnerable in adverse economic times.

Queen Elizabeth Hospital at Rotorua, the centre of a geothermal area in the North Island, has been developed as a centre for physical medicine and has a unit for the rehabilitation of cerebral palsy patients and those with developmental and neurological disfunctions. The hospital has outpatient and inpatient departments and extensive habilitation and rehabilitation sections, and has developed as a special hospital for sufferers from rheumatism.

Very few private hospitals undertake extensive rehabilitation programmes; however, the government has contributed funds to some private geriatric hospitals run by religious organisations and then has encouraged these institutions to provide appropriate rehabilitation facilities for their patients.

The rehabilitation work of the hospitals is very closely linked with the services of such government departments as Social Welfare, Labour, and Education and, of course, with the tremendous contribution made by voluntary organisations. These organisations are substantially subsidised by the Department of Health with salaries, loans, and buildings. A relative newcomer in this field is the Accident Compensation Corporation, which now has a specialist division for rehabilitation in medical matters and is very active in the broad field of rehabilitation following accidents.

Chronic Illness

In New Zealand there is one home for the very severely disabled, run by the Waipukurau Hospital Board. It is at once a home, a school, an extensive department for occupational therapy, and a sheltered workshop. By and large, the patients admitted have been regarded as impossible to maintain in the community, but it is of interest to note that, thanks to the excellent work done there, a number of them have been returned to the community. More recently, Laura Ferguson Trust Homes, named after the wife of a former governor-general, have been established in the main centres. For the less severely disabled, these homes develop and work closely with local hospital boards. Capital subsidies are available from the government.

Ambulance Services

Hospital boards are responsible for the provision of ambulance services. These are financed by the government and may be operated by boards but are usually run by a voluntary organisation, such as the Order of St. John or the Wellington Free Ambulance, which contracts to provide ambulance services and to train lay people in first aid and home nursing. Until recently most New Zealand ambulances were manned only by a driver and, if required, an assistant, who had to be obtained from voluntary lists of medical students or others with limited expertise—therefore, the majority of accident cases were usually attended only by ambulance people. The Ambulance Transport Advisory Board, which advises the minister of health on all matters pertaining to ambulances, was reorganised five years ago. The board is wedded to the concept that the ambulance should be regarded as an emergency ward and be appropriately staffed with trained people. They recommended that two men, who would work together as a team and be highly trained, should man each ambulance. A National Ambulance Officers' Training School was established in Auckland several years ago and a high standard set with basic training and an advanced paramedic course of three months' duration. It is intended that four instructors, all qualified advanced-care officers and employed by the school, will be stationed in Auckland, Wellington, Christchurch, and Dunedin. They will be available for consultation and will be improving the training in the regions. Ambulance planes and helicopters are used regularly in remote or inaccessible places by the Search and Rescue Organisation and for transporting patients to hospitals.

New Developments Associated With Cost Containment

Because of the economic climate in New Zealand, the 3.5% annual rise in real growth on health spending which has occurred over the past twenty years has had to be severely curtailed. After allowing for inflation, 0.5% growth will currently be funded by the government. In effect, with zero growth being aimed at, the government is looking at ways of restructuring the health services. As mentioned earlier, two pilot schemes, one at urban Wellington and the other in rural Northland, have been set up which plan the integration through a health board of the public-funded services provided by the Department of Health and the hospital boards. They also seek to coordinate the private, voluntary, and public sector planning of health services. As part of this reorganisation, a committee has reported on a new way of dividing up the money allocated to the hospital boards that is based on the current population figures adjusted for certain variables. In the past, allocations were made on population figures from many years before, and no account was taken of increases or shifts that might have occurred nor the needs of particular areas. The minister of health has made it quite clear that no hospital board will now be given authority—except in very exceptional cases—to provide extra public hospital beds where there is a surplus of suitable private beds already in existence. The unrestrained development of private hospitals is a difficult problem for hospital boards to cope with, but guidelines that have been issued to these boards over the past ten years, showing the number of beds they should provide and the constraints in the use of beds in excess of that, may go some way in providing a solution.

MEDICAL EDUCATION[15]

The first medical school in New Zealand, the Medical School of the University of Otago, was established in Dunedin in 1874 when a Dr. Coughtrey was appointed the first Professor of Anatomy and Physiology. There was little enthusiasm in either the university or the country as a whole for the establishment of such a medical school, and the fact that it was established was due entirely to the determination of James MacAndrew, superintendent of Otago Province. The school's first few years were very difficult; there was little, sometimes no accommodation, few, sometimes no students, and always very little money. Dr. Coughtrey resigned in 1876 and, again, thanks to the efforts of James MacAndrew, John Halliday Scott from Edinburgh was appointed in 1877 to the vacant chair. This could be identified as the real beginning of the medical school, as Dr. Scott was strongly supported by prominent Scottish medical professors. His influence on the students was such that the majority of them went from Otago to Edinburgh to complete their courses and thought of going nowhere else. The course began as a two-year study at Otago in preclinical subjects, after which the students went overseas to complete their qualification. In 1883 the senate of the University of New Zealand approved a four-year course and established the degree of MB,ChB (New Zealand).* Dr. Scott was named dean when a full medical school was established in 1885, and in its early years he was assisted by local doctors in giving instruction in the clinical school. He died in office in 1914 after thirty-seven years, by which time the annual intake of students had risen to 40. During the years of the 1914–18 war the school expanded, and by 1918 the faculty of medicine was the largest in the university. The number of students fell, however, from 365 in 1921 to 200 in 1927.

In 1924 the practice was introduced of sending senior students first to Christchurch and then to Auckland and Wellington for their clinical experience; this continued for a number of years. The school started to expand again in the 1930s and expansion continued through the Second World War, so that by 1945 the roll had climbed to 658. Now the biggest school in the Commonwealth, it had close contacts with the students in the faculties of dentistry, science, and home science, who attended certain lectures with medical students as did the students in the radiography and physiotherapy departments. By 1958 the school had expanded in buildings, staff, and research, and yet the rapid increase of the New Zealand population and the expansion of health services raised doubts about the number of doctors being produced. There were shortages of house surgeons throughout the country, and the difficulties of the medical school were increased by the newly introduced single block grant method of funding, which meant that its funds were included in the lump sum given to the whole university. The school was no longer being regarded as a national resource. Furthermore, the teaching hospitals were administered by an elected board on which there was no university representation. Since 1888 the Otago University had asked the Otago Hospital Board for direct representation; however, although the board was anxious to help, it could not do so under the existing circumstances. Because of such difficulties and the low level of morale, the appointment of a new dean was delayed in 1968 in order to allow the university to look at the school's problems and the development of its future role. In 1967 Professor R.V. Christie was invited by the council of the University of Otago to report on the medical school.[16] He recommended, among other things, that about four or five university representatives be appointed to the hospital board.

Christie's report led to a further expansion of staffing and the acceptance of major financial commitments, involving hospital board and university. Professor Christie considered an increase in the numbers of students, dealt with the problem of the lack of clinical material available in Dunedin, and surveyed the possibility of the establishment of

*In December 1961 the University of New Zealand was disbanded and its constituent university colleges were made universities in their own right—Otago (at Dunedin), Canterbury (at Christchurch), Victoria (at Wellington), and Auckland (at Auckland).

a second clinical school, either in Christchurch or in Wellington. It was decided that the student intake should be increased to 114 in 1969, to 150 in 1972, and by a further 50 to 200 in 1976. When it was agreed upon to increase the intake to 150, the University of Otago asked both the Canterbury and Wellington hospital boards to assist, and it was proposed that one-half of the fourth and fifth year students should receive their clinical training at the Christchurch hospitals and that sixth year students be shared between the Dunedin, Christchurch, and Wellington hospitals. The further expansion of the Otago intake to 200, however, required the agreement of the Wellington Hospital Board to establish a larger clinical school to take fourth and fifth as well as sixth year students; this was agreed upon.

The situation was complicated by the fact that at the end of 1964 the minister of education and the chariman of the University Grants Committee had given authority to proceed with the planning of a medical school in Auckland.[17] Auckland University College had first applied to establish a medical school in 1887, and the subject had been raised thereafter from time to time. In 1946 the senate of the then University of New Zealand established a committee to review medical education in New Zealand. That committee's report suggested that only the one medical school in Otago should continue. Undeterred, however, Auckland University College set up a steering committee on medical education in the late 1950s with Sir Douglas Robb, chancellor of the university, as chairman. This committee pressed for the provision of a second medical school and, with continuing pressure, planning approval was eventually granted in 1964. In the following year the post of dean was advertised, and in 1968 the first student was enrolled. The first class numbered 60, but by 1976 enrollment had increased to 130. In 1980 the intake was reduced to 110, and a further reduction to 100 was anticipated for 1981, as approved by the minister of health.

Meanwhile, in Wellington the question of a clinical school or a full medical school had become an issue, and Victoria University and the Wellington Hospital Board jointly commissioned a report on medical education in New Zealand and the need for a third medical school. The Department of Health at that time could foresee an additional output of graduates because of expansion of the two existing schools, so it is of interest that the University Grants Committee agreed that when a third full medical school was accepted as being necessary, it would recommend that it be established in Wellington. Since that report in the 1970s, however, the situation has changed drastically. The population has not increased at the rate that was anticipated; there has tended to be a net flow outwards of population; and there is a real fear that there will be a surplus of about 1,000 doctors by the mid-1980s. Because of this the intake of medical students was reduced 12½% in 1979 and a further 12½% in 1980. Increasing financial constraints prompted Otago University to commission a further report. Professor David Bates was asked to report on the most appropriate allocation in the 1980s of scarce and limited resources between the three divisions of the faculty of medicine and to advise on the most appropriate development of the faculty in light of the possible distribution of these resources.[18]

The report, which made a number of recommendations, was notable in its support for the continuance of the clinical schools at Wellington and Christchurch.

Admission and Selection

Applicants for medical school fall into two categories: school leavers and those who have undertaken tertiary education and obtained a degree. The former are in the majority.

Selection is made primarily on the results of a university bursary examination, and the competitiveness of entry requires that applicants have a very good A-pass bursary. The number who apply after taking a degree in another discipline is not large, and consequently, the competition is again very keen for the few places available. Although basic selection is made on academic performance, applicants may be required to attend for an interview. In Auckland there is a preference scheme for Polynesians. The average age of first year students is eighteen years.

Undergraduate Education

New Zealand's medical schools are within the university system. The basic programme is comprehensive and designed to lead the student steadily through theoretical training in the basic sciences to a growing clinical knowledge, experience, and responsibility at each stage of the course. Higher standards in special fields of medicine will result from postgraduate training programmes.

These principles still apply in the medical courses, but changing needs in health care and the greater knowledge now available have brought about important modifications. The courses at Otago, and particularly at Auckland, are now more flexible and are broader in their approach. The clear distinction between theory and practice is no longer so apparent, and students are involved at an early stage with people and the wider community. The increasing complexity of medical knowledge has led to a demand for more highly specialised training. This has developed rapidly through the Royal Colleges, which prescribe the training and experience required in the speciality before the appropriate qualifications are granted. No longer can a New Zealand doctor expect the basic qualifications to equip him or her adequately for the whole of working life; the concept of continuing education, whether or not a postgraduate qualification has been obtained, is now part of medical reality.

Figure 1 shows the pattern of the basic medical course. In Auckland there is a three-year human biology course leading to a degree, while the main examinations for the clinical years are at the end of the fifth year. There is no prescribed examination in the sixth year, but a satisfactory report on performance is required. After completing the medical course, a preregistration year of hospital board service is required by the Medical Council before the doctor is placed on the general register and is free to practice as an independent practitioner. Figure 1 shows six years in medical school ending in the MB,ChB, one preregistration year ending with registration with the Medical Council, and then a period of general professional training in a hospital, which may last from one to three years. The period for anyone specialising is usually three years, and thereafter recognition is required by the college or other controlling body that a candidate has fulfilled its requirements in gaining experience and advanced specialist training of five years. At this stage the person can apply to have his or her name placed on the specialist register kept by the Medical Council.

For the purpose of the payment of benefits, the Health Department also has a register of those they regard as specialists; however, these persons are not necessarily on the specialist register of the Medical Council.

Until recently there was no formal training in general practice and any doctor can practice as such who is on the register, including a person who, because of age or other reason, retires from any speciality, no matter what that might be. No postgraduate experience or qualifications are mandatory for general practitioners; concern over this prompted

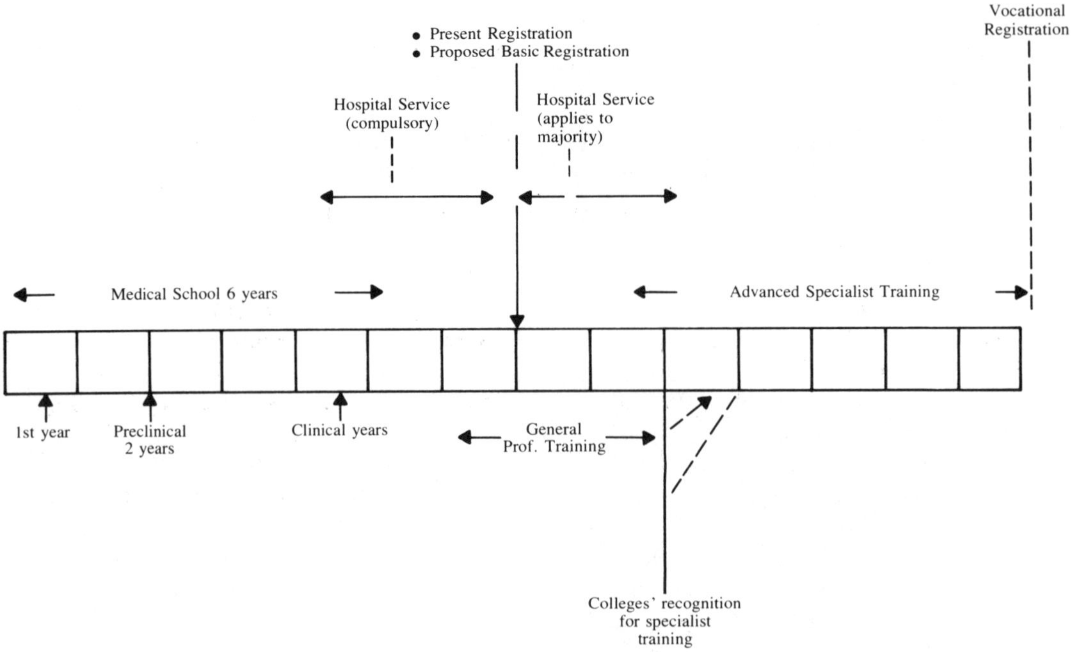

Figure 1 Medical school years with proposals for a basic and vocational register shown

officials to introduce a family medicine training programme in 1972. It began on a small scale in Southland and expanded, until now there are sixty trainees entering the programme annually. In 1977 it was proposed that this programme should come under the New Zealand Council for Postgraduate Medical Education; this body and the Royal New Zealand College of General Practitioners are now jointly responsible for the programme and enjoy strong government support.

Postgraduate Education: Degrees and Diplomas[19]

At Otago degrees include: Doctor of Medicine, Master of Surgery, Bachelor of Medical Science, and Master of Medical Science. Postgraduate diplomas include: Child Health, Child Psychiatry, Clinical Pathology, Clinical Pharmacology, Diagnostic Radiology, Health Services Evaluation, Industrial Health, Medical Information Science, Microbiology, Obstetrics, Psychology, Psychological Medicine, Public Health (discontinued 1981), and Community Health (1981). At Auckland degrees include: Master of Human Biology, Master of Medical Science, and Doctor of Philosophy. Postgraduate diplomas include: Obstetrics, Gynaecology and Obstetrics, Paediatrics, and Psychiatry.

Postgraduate Vocational Training

All medical graduates undertake one year's general apprenticeship before they obtain full registration. Further practical training is required if a career in one of the specific disciplines of medicine is envisaged. This training is undertaken as house surgeons and registrars in hospitals and in selected practices for general practice. The period involved ranges from two to six years.

Vocational training programmes have been established by the various colleges. These enable doctors who wish to become specialists to study for and sit college examinations while gaining practical experience and continuing their educations in approved appointments.

The first postgraduate course in New Zealand was held in 1911 in Dunedin. Only one person attended, but the full course was given as planned! The student graciously said that he had learned more than he had ever known before.[20] Following this was widespread activity in most centres of any size, and a number of postgraduate societies were formed. These were usually hospital based and sometimes formed under the wing of the Medical Association.

In 1943 the medical faculty at Otago decided to set up postgraduate committees in the parent faculty and in the branch faculties at Christchurch, Wellington, and Auckland. These committees met at the annual meetings of what was then the New Zealand branch of the British Medical Association. At one such meeting in 1947, it was agreed that postgraduate teaching fell more within the province of the medical faculty of the University of Otago than that of the British Medical Association; therefore; during the next ten years the postgraduate societies gradually began to recognise their regional responsibilities and extend their activities. In 1958, due to the efforts of Sir Douglas Robb, they combined to form the New Zealand Postgraduate Medical Federation, with eighteen members and three associate member societies. The federation was established to coordinate, aid, and develop the work of its member societies; its functions included disseminating information, arranging tours for lecturers, assisting medical education in the South Pacific, liaisoning with the Australian Federation, and helping with the visits of lecturers to the South Pacific.

In Auckland the postgraduate committee of the branch of the medical faculty changed its status in 1959 to become the Postgraduate Medical Committee in the University of Auckland. Although it receives no financial support from the university and continues to rely on money from other sources, such as the Auckland Postgraduate Society and the fees from courses, this committee represents a wide spectrum of medical interests and runs many comprehensive programmes and courses.

The Postgraduate School of Obstetrics and Gynaecology in Auckland is based at the National Women's Hospital and runs various courses, including one for New Zealand and overseas graduates that leads to the MRCOG qualification. It also runs short term refresher courses for general practitioners and weekend courses at provincial centres.

In 1966 an amendment to the Hospitals Act formalised an existing situation, and since then postgraduate medical education has been encouraged in all hospitals.

A steering group for the New Zealand Council for Postgraduate Medical Education was established in 1973 at the request of the New Zealand Medical Association and the New Zealand Postgraduate Medical Federation (representing the postgraduate societies); this provided a single national body covering all of those concerned with postgraduate medical education and enabled national policy to be discussed and advice to be given to the government on desirable developments in postgraduate training. This committee functioned in an informal capacity for about six years but became a statutory body in 1978 when the New Zealand Parliament passed the act to establish the New Zealand Council for Postgraduate Medical Education and to define its functions, powers, and duties. The delay was caused in part by the difficulty in deciding on the membership of the council, which eventually included representatives of almost every interest in postgraduate education in the health field, including hospital boards. The act divides the country into six regions with a director in each. All directors are members of the council, as is the director general of health, the chairman of the Medical Council, and the chairman of the New Zealand Postgraduate Medical Federation. Eight other persons are appointed by the governor-general on the advice of the minister of health, and there are representatives of the various colleges, the Medical Association, the New Zealand Registered Resident Medical Officer's Association, the University Grants Committee, and one (probably unhappy!) person who is not a medical practitioner. It is of interest that the directors in four regions, all of which have either a medical or a clinical school, are specified as the persons who, for the time being, are immediately responsible for postgraduate medical education in the faculties of medicine.

The functions of the council are to advise the minister on national needs in respect to the organisation and to the financing of postgraduate medical education; to initiate, coordinate, and support schemes for postgraduate medical education; to collect and disseminate information on postgraduate medical education; and to initiate, coordinate, and support research into evaluations of programmes for postgraduate medical education. The council also has statutory responsibility for administering the family medicine programme in close cooperation with the Royal New Zealand College of General Practitioners. Its budget is provided from the health vote—the funds voted to the Department of Health by Parliament in the annual estimates.

The universities have only recently become formally active in the field of vocational postgraduate training. The various Royal Colleges took the pioneering role in it and have remained there ever since with an established position, but with the formation in 1978 of the New Zealand Council of Postgraduate Medical Education as a statutory body with its own secretariat and with an organisation structure linked with the universities involved in medical training, the role of the Royal Colleges and the universities may well be reexamined in the future.

Finance for Medical Education

All fees for medical education are moderate by overseas standards and are heavily subsidised by the government. Students who are pursuing full-time courses and who have passed the University Bursary Examination, hold a scholarship, a Higher School Certificate, a Sixth Form Certificate or have passed the University Entrance Examination two years previously will receive a tertiary study grant. The period of tenure for medical students is five years, and an extension is normally available if an additional degree is sought. During their sixth year students receive a salary of approximately $6,000 to $7,000 from the hospital boards. Those qualifying for a tertiary study grant receive three-quarters of the cost of their tuition fees and an allowance of $23.00 per week throughout the academic year, a sum which may be increased in case of hardship.

There are also other allowances, such as the "A-Bursary" allowance. The student who so wishes may accept a medical bursary given by the Health Department, which is awarded to selected students undertaking the medical course. This bursary provides a $10.00 payment per week for the academic year, over and above the tertiary study grant, but recipients are required to sign a bond with the department. The bursary is paid for a period of up to five years. After full registration as a doctor and if the bursary has been paid for the full period, the doctor is required to give two years of service either in a hospital nominated by the Department of Health or as a general practitioner in a "special area." Bursaries are also available for certain postgraduate courses from the Department of Health or the hospital boards, but in these cases, again, the person is bonded for a stated period of time. Until recently most students were able to find work relatively easily during leave periods in order to supplement their income, but the changing economy will have bursaries relied upon more heavily.

Medical Research Council

Set up by the Medical Research Council Act 1950, the Medical Research Council is intended to initiate, foster, and support medical research; to furnish information, advice, and assistance to persons and organisations concerned with medical research; and to collect and disseminate scientific information and to publish appropriate reports. Research is widespread in the preclinical, clinical, and postgraduate fields, and increasing emphasis is being placed on social medicine, community health, and research into health services. Much work is being done in the South Pacific region.

The council keeps in close touch with research that is being carried out by private medical research foundations and societies such as the Cancer Society of New Zealand and the Regional Medical Research Foundations in Auckland, Wellington, North Canterbury, and Otago. It is staffed by about fifty full-time workers, and a further 200 to 300 are employed by other institutions under grants from the council. In addition, scholarships and fellowships are granted to selected graduates and undergraduates from the funds received from bequests and donations and the considerable financial support from the government.

CONTROL OF THE MEDICAL PROFESSION: THE MEDICAL COUNCIL

The Medical Council, which is the governing body of the medical profession in New Zealand, was established by the Medical Practitioners Act 1968 and comprises the director general of health, the deans of the faculties of medicine in the Universities of Otago and Auckland, and eight registered medical practitioners appointed on a representative basis.[21] The Medical Council is required to keep a register of doctors practising in New Zealand and to register a doctor only when satisfied as to his or her training. The intention is to protect the public from imposters, and the register therefore tells people that this doctor is approved by a council set up by the government for that purpose. If someone wishes to be registered, the council must be satisfied as to his or her training and experience; failing this, registration may be granted on a conditional basis. Such a person who is registered conditionally may practice and be trained only in an approved hospital, and the Medical Education Committee of the council exercises general supervision over the training, which is required.

The council is vested with certain disciplinary powers; it may, for example, remove the name of a doctor from the register for "disgraceful conduct." A right to appeal to the High Court is provided by the act, however.

In 1973 the Medical Council assumed responsibility for producing an official register of specialists. Anyone wishing to be recognised as a specialist must satisfy the council as to elegibility for entry into this register.

The Medical Practitioners Amendment Act 1979 came into force in 1980. It provides for more flexible supervision and control of medical graduates whose fitness to practice is in question because of mental or physical disability or whose professional conduct is the subject of disciplinary action. It also introduces, among other things, a residential qualification for overseas graduates. These two proposals aim at enabling the council to discharge its dual responsibility of keeping an effective register of those entitled to practice medicine in New Zealand and of ensuring adequate professional standards of skill. Before this amendment was passed, overseas graduates with suitable qualifications could register in New Zealand in absentia even though they perhaps had no intention of coming for many years, if ever, to New Zealand. The council was concerned that it had no power to enquire into the professional activities and standing of such practitioners, who might suddenly appear many years after their initial registration. A new residential qualification is designed to close this lacuna.

Currently there is widespread discussion about the replacement of the existing registers with a two-part basic and vocational register.[22,23] Following medical graduation from a New Zealand university and one year's required hospital experience, all doctors would be entered on the basic training section of the register. These doctors would not normally be recognised for independent practice but would be expected to work in an institution or in a group practice. The vocational part would include "all medical practitioners experienced and trained in their discipline within a named section," and only those in this section of the register would be recognised for independent practice in the discipline(s) in which they were registered.

Discipline within the profession is controlled by the Medical Council and by the Medical Practitioners' Disciplinary Committee, both statutory bodies. Divisional medical practitioners' disciplinary committees also play a part.

There has been considerable discussion recently about the restructuring of the Medical Council to bring about more open dialogue with the profession.

Admission of Medical Graduates From Other Countries

In order to practice medicine in New Zealand a doctor from overseas has to be eligible for registration by the Medical Council. There is usually no difficulty in registering if the applicant has already been registered in the United Kingdom by virtue of a degree, diploma, or other qualification granted in that country. Similarly, the holder of a medical degree from a recognised university in Australia and certain other places specified in the register would also be eligible. In the past, provided a doctor could be registered in New Zealand and had work to come to, permission to enter the country as a permanent migrant was seldom refused.

However, New Zealand now has a low fertility rate and a net outward migration that has brought the country to near-zero population growth. In addition, the late 1970s saw a marked increase in the number of students admitted to medical school. The result of these factors combined is that a surplus of doctors is forecast for the mid-1980s, a surplus which the country may be unwilling or even unable to afford. Mention has already been made of the reduction in student intake in 1980 and 1981 to remedy this difficult situation, but at that time it was also agreed that applications from overseas doctors to work in New Zealand would be reviewed by the Department of Health.

The current position on immigration is that doctors in training or wishing to work as resident medical officers are given temporary immigration permits. Permanent immigrants, whether specialists or general practitioners, are only supported if the applicant has assured employment in a recognised post for which there is no suitable NZ applicant.

NURSING[24]

Started in New Zealand in 1884, training for nurses was based on an apprentice-type system with a number of nursing schools being established and placed under the control of hospitals. The students were employees of the hospitals and learned "on the job." In the early 1970s it was recognised that, although there had been improvements in training, the great social and educational changes and the growing complexity of technology in health care were rendering this training obsolete. Certain fundamental changes in nursing education were required and implemented. A basic three-year registration programme, away from hospital schools and their service demands, was set up in technical institutions, and trainees were given full-time student status. The general public was slow to recognise the need for this change but now is gradually coming to accept it. In 1980, 17.8% of all students in three-year programmes were in technical institutions, and the number of nursing schools offering a three-year hospital course had been reduced to fifty. With the growing appreciation of the value of new training, there is no doubt that the number of hospital schools will decrease further in the future. At the post-basic level, an important development was the replacement of the diploma course for nurses by the establishment in 1973 of a nursing studies unit at Massey and Victoria universities and the introduction in certain technical institutes in 1978 of clinically orientated post-basic nursing courses. With these changes, there was steady expansion of community nursing services.

There were over 19,000 nurses in New Zealand in 1980 (the full-time equivalent of 15,000), and seven varieties of registered and enrolled nurses were covered by the term "qualified nurse." These were registered comprehensive nurse, general nurse, general and obstetric nurse, midwife, obstetric nurse, psychiatric nurse, and psychopaedic nurse. In addition, there are a number of unqualified people who give "nursing services." They include Karitane nurses, hospital aids or assistants, and hospital-based students, and number in excess of 6,000 (f.t.e. 5,000) for the first two and over 6,000 for the last. In total, over 31,000 men and women are employed to provide nursing services to a population of under 3,200,000—that is one nurse for every 98 people in the country, or in full-time equivalents one nurse to every 117.

The Nursing Council of New Zealand, established by the Nurses Act 1971, makes recommendations on (1) nursing programmes for examinations in relation to the minimum standard required for registration, (2) the conduct of examinations, (3) the granting of approval to schools of nursing (subject to ministerial concurrence), (4) the enrollment and registration of overseas nurses, and (5) the exercise of disciplinary powers. The Nurses Act 1977 repealed the 1971 act and its 1975 Amendment Act and, among other changes, removed the minimum age for sitting state examinations for all classes of students except those for enrollment, required male students to undertake the obstetric part of the general obstetric programme, and enabled males to undertake midwifery training.

The Nursing Education Review and Advisory Body, set up in June 1980, recently completed its first report and has accepted a proposal to establish a course of study for the Bachelor of Nursing at Victoria University, Wellington, and advised the minister accordingly.

New Zealand Nurses' Association

Membership of the New Zealand Nurses' Association is now more than 17,000. It is organised locally and nationally and is highly politicised. There are 57 branches and many special interest sections such as mental health, education, and nursing research.

The major drive is to improve the professional status of nurses, and in 1968 the association formed the Nursing Education & Research Foundation to provide funding for scholarships and workshops and to invite overseas speakers to visit New Zealand.

OTHER HEALTH PRACTITIONERS

Physiotherapists. Physiotherapists are employed in both private and public hospitals and are available to the community. They receive their training in technical institutes and are controlled by the New Zealand Physiotherapy Board, constituted under the Physiotherapy Act 1949. This board controls the state examination and registration of candidates, the issue of a special license, and the conduct of physiotherapists registered under the act. A state benefit is payable for the services of a physiotherapist.

Occupational Therapists. The Central Institute of Technology, situated near Wellington, conducts a three-year course of training, and clinical experience is obtained in different hospitals. Students who successfully complete the course are awarded a diploma in occupational therapy and are registered by the Occupational Therapy Board, which is constituted under the Occupational Therapy Act 1949.

Dietitians. A person holding a degree of Bachelor of Home Sciences or a diploma in home science from the University of Otago is required to do a training period of twelve months in a hospital training school. The Dietitians Board, constituted under the Dietitians Act 1950, is responsible for the training, examination, and registration of people wishing to practice dietetics.

Pharmacists. Pharmacy education requires a minimum of three years' attendance at the School of Pharmacy at the Central Institute of Technology, following which the diploma in pharmacy is granted; there is also a four-year degree course at the University of Otago. Graduates from both courses are required to gain twelve months' preregistration experience before they are eligible for registration as a pharmacist. There is a pharmaceutical benefit, and most drugs prescribed by a doctor are available to patients free of any cost.

Chiropodists. There is an increasing demand for the services of chiropodists. Some are employed in hospitals but most are in private practice. No health benefit is paid for their services. In 1970 a three-year training course, leading to a diploma in chiropody, was introduced at the Central Institute of Technology. Since 1976 the chiropody school has extended its activities to include post-basic courses for registered chiropodists. Registration has been a requirement since 1968.

Chiropractors. The role of the chiropractor has been the subject of much controversy over recent years. In 1960 an act was passed providing for their registration, this act being the legislative responsibility of the Department of Justice. A revised and updated bill was introduced into the House of Representatives on 22 September 1981, which transfers responsibility to the Department of Health and brings it more into line with other registration acts administered by that department. The bill makes provision for a reconstructed board and stipulates in greater detail the educational qualifications required for chiropractors. While chiropractors are registered in New Zealand, the scope of their practice is not easy to define. There is at present no subsidisation of their services under the government health benefit scheme, and the majority of their patients are private ones. However, provision does exist for some payment from the Accident Compensation Corporation.

NURSING HOME AND COMMUNITY HEALTH AGENCIES

Nursing care is provided in the home by hospital board community nurses, who give general nursing, and by certain hospital nurses who are specialised in such fields as oncology and paediatrics. These nursing services are regarded as an extension of the hospital into the community as part of the extramural hospital services mentioned previously. This closer hospital board involvement in community matters was accelerated by the injection of "beer and tobacco money," so called because the government levied an additional tax on tobacco and alcohol and distributed the money raised thereby to community health projects through local committees comprising senior district health office and hospital board staff. A prerequisite was that agreement on priorities should be reached before distributtion, the aim being to encourage both planning between the two major publicly funded bodies and innovative, nonrecurring projects. The latter aim has been only partially successful.

There has been a great increase in the number of homes for the elderly, and religious organisations have been very active there, aided by government loans and grants and the daily patient benefit.

There is also much interest and development in the care of the terminally ill, and private, public, and voluntary organisations are all cooperating in providing hospices for those patients.

HEALTH COSTS AND HEALTH INSURANCE

Health Costs

The subject of health costs has been touched on in preceding sections. The impact of high inflation and the adverse economic situation in New Zealand are adding to the cost of high technology and increasing the problem caused by the high expectations that more and more people have of modern medicine. In 1979–80 public health expenditure alone totalled $1157.8 million, a per capita cost of $371. Almost 70% was spent for hospital services; a modest 2.5% went for the traditional public health expenditure. It seems well nigh impossible to reverse this imbalance to take account of current views on community care and of the staggering toll of self-inflicted disease. This total, of course, does not take into account the financial contribution made by individuals towards their own private care, either directly or through health insurance payments, nor does it consider the money disbursed through the Accident Compensation Corporation.

Mention was also made earlier of the government's determination to contain costs and ensure a more equitable distribution of funds to hospital boards, and of its desire to restructure health services and establish a new type of health board.

Health Insurance

In 1961 a group of businessmen and surgeons set up an incorporated insurance scheme in Auckland to assist patients with the cost of surgical operations in private hospitals. The Southern Cross Medical Care Society was aided by the introduction (in 1967) of government tax incentives to industry for such insurance and now has a membership of 654,225—over 20% of the total population of New Zealand. Members are scattered throughout the country, and the society covers them not only for private hospital expenses and surgeons' fees but also for out-of-hospital services such as those given by general practitioners, specialists, and physiotherapists.

There are two other insurance organisations which together cover another 250,000 people, so that private health insurance is one of the most active areas of economic growth in the country. The usual arrangement is that after payment of the government benefit, the society is responsible for 80% of the balance and the patient the remaining 20%. In 1980, 28% of the population was estimated to be covered by private health insurance.

PUBLIC HEALTH

The public health is safe-guarded in New Zealand by a mixture of public, voluntary, and private care involving state, regional, and local authorities, and much of this has already been considered in earlier sections.

Central government stimulates, encourages, and provides financial and other incentives, in addition to rendering certain services itself. In the end, however, the government through the minister of health accepts final responsibility for most of the functions affecting the health of the community.

Public Health Services

Public health services encompass environmental, occupational, and family (including infant, preschool, and school medical and dental) health services as well as communicable diseases and quarantine, food and nutrition, and health education.

The major responsibility rests directly with the Department of Health through the Bureau of Public Health and Environmental Protection and the district health offices; it is, however, shared with general practitioners and with local territorial authorities, regional bodies such as the regional and united councils, regional water boards, and voluntary organisations such as the Plunket Society and the Intellectually Handicapped Children's Society.

The Department of Health is responsible to its minister and has a head office in Wellington, six specialised units, and eighteen district offices.

The structure of the head office is shown in appendix 1. The Bureau of Public Health & Environmental Protection is controlled by a deputy director-general of health and has two directors, one of whom, through an environmental section, deals with noise control, air pollution, and environmental engineering, and through an occupational health and toxicology section, deals with toxicology, occupational health, and aviation and transport medicine. This person also has sections that deal with health inspection and food control. The other director controls family health services; nutrition; community nursing; community psychiatric services; hearing problems and audiology; and alcohol, smoking, and drug abuse.

The six specialised units are described below. Only the first four are in the Bureau of Public Health and Environmental Protection, but the other two work closely with that bureau's staff.

The National Health Institute in Wellington is a national centre for the scientific study of public health problems. It has diagnostic and reference laboratories for microbiology and biology and an epidemiological section. Its services are used by medical officers of health, by public hospitals and private laboratories, and by general practitioners in New Zealand and in the South Pacific. The institute provides a national reference centre for such conditions as salmonellosis and leptospirosis and is the WHO Influenza Reference Laboratory and an International Centre for bacteriophage typing of staphylococci and salmonellae.

The National Radiation Laboratory in Christchurch provides the services, administrative and technical, required by legislation for the protection of workers and for the import or export or transport of radioactive material. It provides a monitoring service for both natural and man-made radioactivity and undertakes research in support of these functions.

The National Audiology Centre in Auckland provides referral audiology services, undertakes the training of audio-vision testers, is responsible for monitoring the work being done in respect to noise and deafness in industry, and initiates and undertakes its own research. In addition, it calibrates and repairs electronic audiological equipment and evaluates hearing aids and ear protection devices. Its services are used by district health officers, local authorities, and various consultant specialists.

The Health Education and Information Unit has recently been expanded and developed.

It is responsible for promoting healthy living, providing information to health workers and health services, and stimulating and educating workers in the health services.

The Management Services and Research Unit produces quantitative data for health services and advises management on how to improve its decision making. It has conducted a number of surveys on the use of health services and disability within the community, but its main preoccupation at the moment is the problem of manpower.

The National Health Statistics Centre publishes health statistics and reports on mortality, mental health, cancer, and hospital management annually; it publishes its "Trends in Health" every two years. The centre provides statistics for the World Health Organisation and works closely with it, and since 1975 has been involved in a survey concerning congenital malformation.

Health Districts

Each of the eighteen health districts is controlled by a medical officer of health who is a specialist in community medicine. The districts vary by size and population; some are rural in character, some urban, and others are a mixture of both. The work undertaken by the staff varies according to the nature of the area, the demands of an industrial city, for example, being very different from those of a rural community. To carry out the statutory duties, doctors, nurses, inspectors of health, and specialised technicians are employed. See appendix 2 for the structure of a district health office.

The Department of Health works closely with other governmental departments but also with private industry, the Accident Compensation Corporation, and voluntary societies towards the prevention of accidents, the development of first aid services, the prevention of occupational disease, the control of toxic substances, the safe use of agricultural chemicals, and the control of air pollution. The medical officer of health has wide statutory responsibilities and considerable independence if he or she wishes to use it. The medical officer carries out the policy of the head office but can also act as an innovator within general, broad guidelines. He or she also works with a wide range of other departments such as Social Welfare, where day care centres and child abuse are concerned; with the Justice Department in connection with the health of prisoners; and with local bodies such as harbour boards where there may be harbour pollution or problems existing with shipping. Mention has already been made that local territorial bodies are responsible for refuse collection and disposal, sewerage, water supply, housing inspection, and licensing of food premises; however, where infection occurs, the local health inspectors have direct responsibility to the medical officer of health, not to the local authority.

Departmental inspectors of the Health and Labour departments, public health nurses, industrial medical officers and nurses, and audio-visual testers all work in factories. Although some medical and nursing staff are employed by private industry, they have responsibility for the factory environment not only to the Labour Department but also to the medical officer of health, who in turn can, if necessary, obtain the help of a highly specialised team consisting of an industrial medical officer, an industrial nurse, and a technician. There are three such teams, one each in the central, northern, and southern areas of the country. Similarly, there are two regional groups for noise control, at Auckland and Christchurch, and four regional air pollution expert groups.

Communicable Diseases and Quarantine

The medical officer of health is responsible for the control of communicable diseases and for maintaining in the area high levels of immunity against certain diseases. This is done by carrying out new programmes of immunisation when these are introduced by the department, by providing free vaccine to general practitioners who are encouraged to participate in established programmes, and by educating the general public. The medical officer is also required from time to time to evaluate the level of immunity in the community. Medical officers of health are also responsible for quarantine arrangements for aircraft and shipping to prevent the introduction and spread of quarantinable disease from overseas.

Food and Nutrition

Food and nutrition standards are high in New Zealand, and labelling, packaging, storage, and the sale of poisons are all controlled by legislation.

Family Health

Of all babies after discharge from the hospital, 86% are supervised by the Plunket Nurses. Where a baby is not being supervised by the Plunket Society, the responsibility is taken by a public health nurse. The historical development of these two nursing services was such that until relatively recent years almost all Maori infants and children were supervised by public health nurses and the majority of European ones by Plunket nurses. Determined attempts have been made for these two services to work more closely, but the Plunket Society, being politically and socially very powerful, values its independence. Further, there are fundamental differences between the two groups in their approach to child care. Plunket nurses supervise children up to the age of five years only, while public health nurses have responsibility for infants not supervised by the society, children in kindergartens and child care centres (that is, children in groups up to five years), primary and secondary school children, in addition to certain families in their areas. Doctors employed by the Department of Health work with Plunket and public health nurses, and act as coordinators. A trial scheme to facilitate closer work between the two groups was recently introduced in South Auckland.

Audiovision testers, working under the supervision of professional staff, test the hearing of preschool and school children and also that of workers in industry.

The general practitioner is also involved in the care of the infant. He or she notifies the department after the birth and provides certain details about the child and its condition. The government pays for an examination of the baby after its birth, before it leaves the hospital, and again before it reaches twelve weeks of age. There is a special benefit paid for a further examination at one year.

A public health nurse is responsible for the health of the families in a geographical area, and in recent years there has been a determined attempt to station the nurse at a base in the working area. Decentralisation from the district office to such a local area is now more frequent and has been linked with an attempt to place hospital board community nurses in the same centres and to encourage Plunket nurses to work as part of the team. Another development has been the grouping together of public health nurses, which has enabled junior staff to have the support of more senior nurses and has allowed for more continuity of service to their areas—a problem in the past because of changes of staff and shortages caused by staff ceiling policies in the state services.

Dental Care

New Zealand is justifiably proud of its dental services for children. Because of the high incidence of dental caries, New Zealand pioneered the use of auxilliaries known as dental nurses. These nurses receive two years' training and are then based at small clinics sited in school grounds, where they take responsibility for the dental care (prophylaxis and treatment) of the children at the school. Back-up support is provided by a qualified dentist, who supervises a large geographical area but is readily available for consultation and advice. Allied to education and to the fluoridation of water suplies, the preventive dental health programme resulted in the government being able in 1980 to close the dental nurses' schools in Auckland and Christchurch, leaving the Wellington school to service all of New Zealand. Adolescents enroll with private dentists, and a dental benefit on a fee-for-service basis is paid to these private contractors. Treatment is paid for by the government until the age of sixteen is reached, but if the young person is dependent on his or her parents, it continues until eighteen. A condition of being enrolled in the adolescent scheme is that the dental repair work of the child should be up-to-date.

Control of Drugs

The medical officer of health is the registrar of poisons; another important member of this team is the pharmacist, who is concerned with the control of drugs and poisons, their storage, and the granting of licenses. Problems with drug control are becoming as apparent in New Zealand as elsewhere; there is a growing use and abuse of drugs, including alcohol, by the young.

Current life style hazards such as smoking, alcohol comsumption, and traffic accidents have resulted both in the further development of the health education and information unit and in increased activity in every health district.

Appendix 3 shows diagrammatically the connection of the health minister with the director general of health, the health districts, the hospital boards, the territorial local authorities, and the Board of Health.

CONCLUSION

New Zealand has a mixture of public, private, and voluntary health services. In the 1940s there was clear evidence that the majority of the people wanted a "free" health service; however, realisations that there is no limit to the demand for "health" services and that high-cost technology and existing economic constraints do not mix are forcing the acceptances that what is "free" should go to those who are in need and that many of the major life style problems should be dealt with by the individual or by society. The great difficulty, however, is to define need in terms of priorities. Is it, for instance, the purpose of high-cost technology to prolong the life of those who are already aged, or is it to assist those with most of their life ahead of them?

The value system in New Zealand is such that the response has been a pragmatic one, an expansion of private insurance and an encouragement of the use of private hospitals at the same time that demands for high standards of care in public hospitals have increased. The result has been a movement towards the acceptance of equity but away from the traditional approach to equality. If the health services are regarded as a continuum with private at one end and public at the other, New Zealand has come very close to a public or state system but with a strong movement towards the private, and with a residual flexibility for considerable movement in either direction. The ruling political party did not change at the recent general election, and the health policies of the government inevitably place increased emphasis on the private end of the continuum.

New Zealand has invested considerable resources in hospitals, and these continue to absorb a great disproportion of health resources. Hospital boards will find in the future that their funding will be allocated on a more equitable basis, so that some will have to introduce cuts in expenditure as well as accept very limited, if any, growth. They will therefore have to plan in a way that was not required in the past, when there was an open-ended financial commitment by the government.

The emphasis on the development of training for health administrators, the formation of the New Zealand College of Community Health and of the Institute of Health Administrators, and the possibility of a major reorganisation in the health field may result in some adjustment to the balance of money and may enable more to go into the community. It is unlikely, though, that the existing standard of hospital care and treatment will be reduced in any way. Whether or not it can be improved is very problematical.

At present a woman in New Zealand can have a baby without incurring any health costs and the baby will have free nursing and community health surveillance throughout school life. In the event of sickness, however, a proportion of the general practitioner's fees will have to be paid depending on the age of the child. If a specialist is required and the patient wishes to see a particular specialist privately, then a proportion of the specialist's fee will again have to be paid by the patient; otherwise, a free service will be available at the nearest outpatient department of the public hospital. If the illness is acute and requires hospitalisation, there will be no delay in obtaining admission to a public hospital free of charge. If a private hospital is used and no health insurance is held, then 50% or so of the costs will be paid by the patient. All of this is within a complex system of social benefits. Some are universal and on a flat rate, such as the children's benefit and the superannuation benefit for those over sixty years of age, while others are selective or income-related, such as in accident compensation payments, or selective or means-tested as for sickness, domestic, and unemployment benefits. All of these payments enable people to have a wider choice as to which health service they wish to use. Some years ago this was very real, but changing economic circumstances and the reduction in money available for health purposes make the choices rather more limited than in the past.

Appendix 1 The structure of the head office of the Department of Health

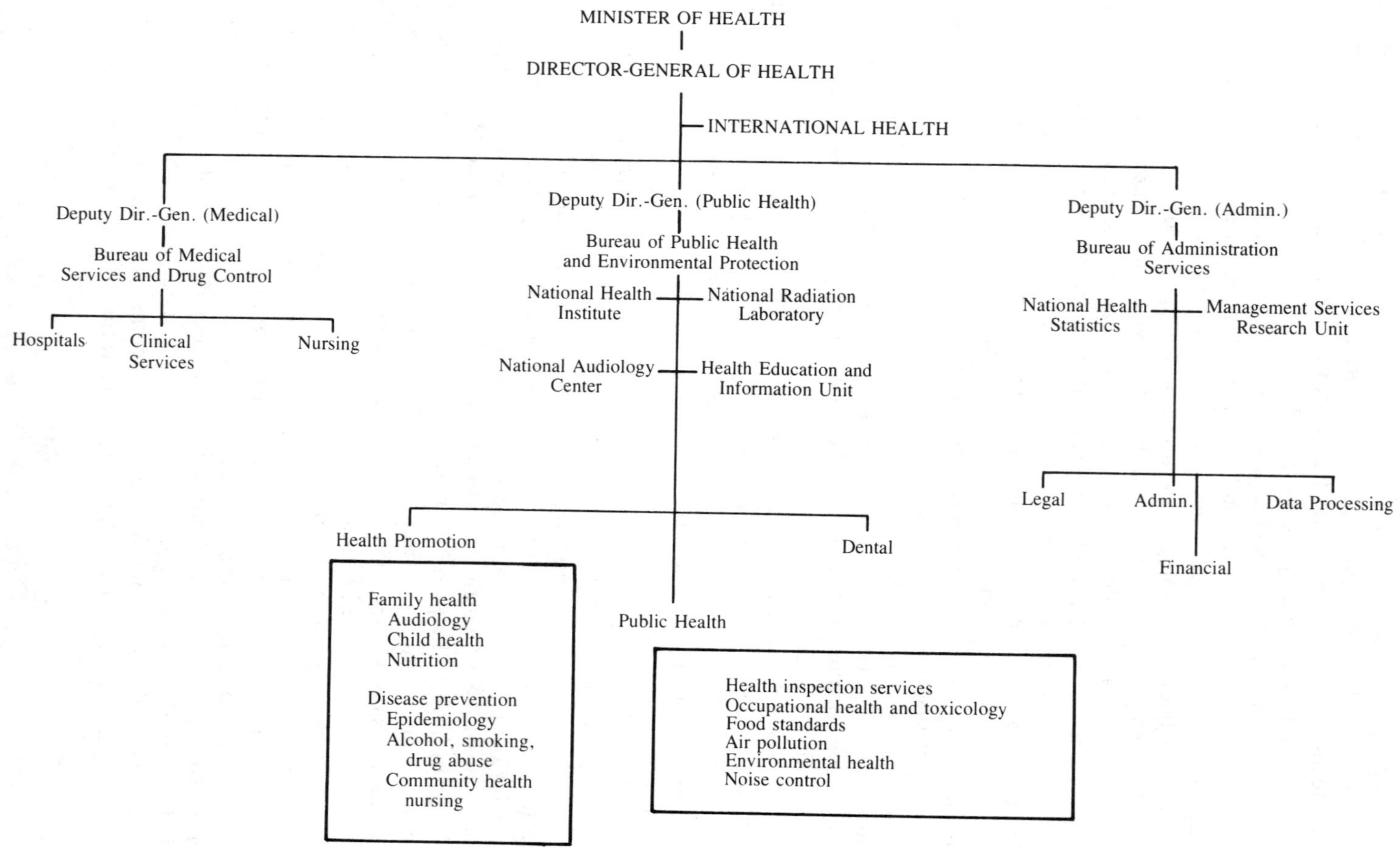

Appendix 2 The structure of a district health office, Department of Health

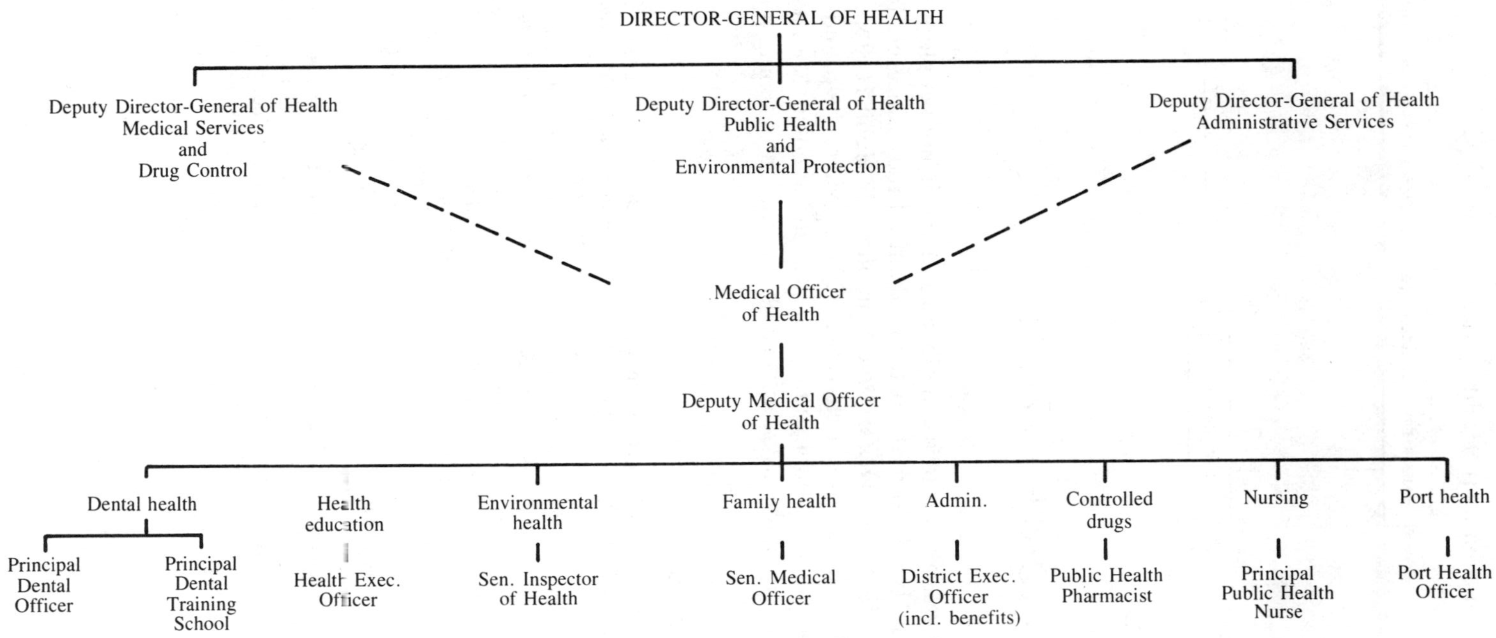

Appendix 3 Organisation chart: Health services

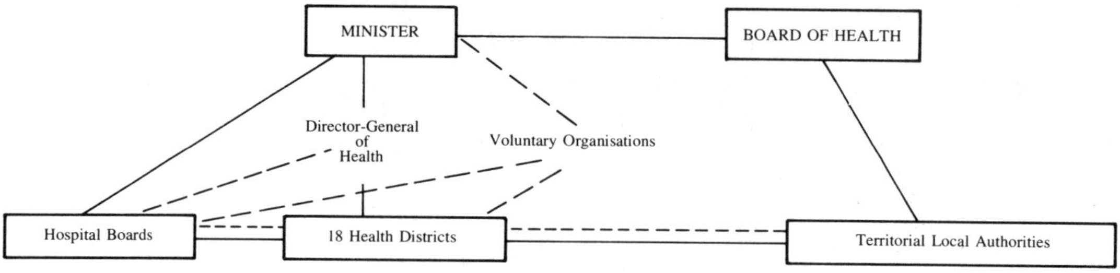

ACKNOWLEDGMENTS

Space does not permit me to list the names of the many people who have supplied me with information, but I do wish to thank them all most sincerely for their assistance. I must, however, single out Dr. George Salmond, Mr. John Hyslop, and the staff of the Management Services & Research Unit, without whose help and support this chapter would never have been completed. I am also indebted to Miss Pat Stanton, who, in addition to her many other tasks, undertook the burden of typing the manuscript for me.

References and Sources

1. Department of Statistics verbal communication, based on Department of Statistics Information Service 81/120, 29 May 1981.

2. Department of Health, *A Review of Hospital and Related Services in New Zealand* (Wellington: Govt. Printer N.Z, 1969), p. 9.

3. Advisory Committee on Medical Manpower, *Report to the Minister of Health on Medical Manpower Requirements,* May 1979, p. 26.

4. G. Parry, *Otago Medical School, 1875–1957* (Medical School, University of Otago, 1975).

5. Advisory Committee on Medical Manpower, *Report to the Minister of Health on Medical Manpower Requirements,* May 1979.

6. Management Services & Research Unit, Department of Health, unpublished data, 1982.

7. *New Zealand Medical Association Handbook, 1981–82.*

8. *New Zealand Medical Association News and Views,* 18 December 1981–420, p. 6.

9. Wellington Health Services Advisory Committee, *Appendix to the Report: Primary Health Care Shadow Service Development Group,* July 1981, p. 6.

10. Advisory Committee on Medical Manpower, *General Practice Manpower in New Zealand,* July 1981.

11. "Allocations to Hospital Boards, 1981/82," *New Zealand Medical Journal,* 25 May 1981, p. 342.

12. Department of Health, *Health in New Zealand, Information on Health Services, 1980–81* (Wellington: Govt. Printer).

13. Department of Health, National Health Statistics Centre, *New Zealand Health Statistics Report,* Hospital Management Data, 1980, Part I, ISSN 0110–1900.

14. Department of Health, *Health in New Zealand, Information on Health Services, 1980–81* (Wellington: Govt. Printer).

15. G. Parry, *Otago Medical School, 1875–1957.*

16. R.V. Christie, *The Report on the Medical School: University of Otago 1968.*

17. University of Auckland, *Faculty of Medicine & Human Biology Handbook* (University of Auckland School of Medicine, 1980).

18. D.V. Bates, *Report on the University of Otago Medical School,* October 1981.

19. University calendars, Otago 1981 and Wellington 1980.

20. J.P.S. Jamieson, "The Late Professor Champtaloup," *New Zealand Journal* 51:424 (1952).

21. *New Zealand Medical Association Handbook, 1981–82,* pp. 231–33.

22. H. Gowland, "Medical Registration in the Future: a Basic and a Vocational Register?" *New Zealand Medical Journal* 92:18–21 (1980).

23. Medical Council of New Zealand, "Medical

Registration, Basic and Vocational Register: Statement From the Medical Council," *New Zealand Medical Journal* 94:351–3 (1981).

24. Department of Health, *The Nursing Workforce in New Zealand, 1980* (Wellington: Management Services & Research Unit, 1981).

Bibliography

Department of Statistics. *New Zealand Official Year Book, 1980.* Wellington: Government Printer.

Government of New Zealand. *A Health Service For New Zealand.* Wellington: Government Printer, 1974.

Kennedy, D.P., ed. *Health in the 1970s.* Christchurch: Peryer Ltd., 1970.

Maternity Services Committee, Board of Health. *Maternity Services in New Zealand.* Wellington: Government Printer, 1976.

University Grants Committee. *Annual Report, 1970.* Wellington: Government Printer.

University of Auckland. *Postgraduate Medical Education in Auckland, 1964.* University of Auckland.

University of Otago. *Report on Medical Education in New Zealand and the Need For a 3rd Medical School.* University of Otago, 1975.

Table 1 Estimated New Zealand population by age, race, and sex, as at 31 December 1980

					%			
	Non-Maoris		Maoris[a]		Non-Maoris		Maoris	
Age	Male	Female	Male	Female	Male	Female	Male	Female
All ages	1,425,000	1,435,300	145,000	143,200	100	100	100	100
Under 5	113,620	109,650	16,980	16,180	8	8	12	11
5 to 9	131,590	126,500	20,350	19,720	9	9	14	14
10 to 14	134,340	127,530	20,560	19,810	9	9	14	14
15 to 19	141,600	134,020	20,400	19,820	10	9	14	14
20 to 24	121,430	115,240	15,170	14,770	9	8	10	10
25 to 34	214,820	216,190	20,240	20,320	15	15	14	14
35 to 44	165,160	161,700	13,400	13,840	12	11	9	10
45 to 54	148,120	140,150	9,400	9,530	10	10	6	7
55 to 64	126,650	132,450	5,140	5,390	9	9	4	4
65 and over	127,660	171,920	3,340	3,740	9	12	2	3
Median age	28.3	29.8	18.6	19.0				

SOURCE: *Monthly Abstract of Statistics* (Wellington: Department of Statistics, Aug. 1981), p. 10: table 1.05.

[a]Persons of one-half or more New Zealand Maori origin.

Table 2a Live births, birth rates, and fertility rates, New Zealand

Year	Births	Birth Rate	Fertility Rate
1978	51,029	16.31	75.1[a]
1979	52,279	16.73	76.2[b]
1980	50,542	16.14	73.0[c]

SOURCE: *Monthly Abstract of Statistics* (Wellington: Department of Statistics, Aug. 1981), p. 12: table 3.01.

NOTES: Birth rates per 1,000 population. Fertility rates per 1,000 women aged 15 to 44 years.

[a]Figure based on estimated mean age distribution of women for year ending 31 December 1978.
[b]Figure based on estimated mean age distribution of women for year ending 31 December 1979.
[c]Figure based on estimated mean age distribution of women for year ending 31 December 1980. Figure is provisional.

Table 2b Life expectancy at birth for 1975 through 1977, New Zealand

	Male	Female
Non-Maori	69.37	75.88
Maori	63.35	67.75
Total population	69.01	75.45

SOURCE: *New Zealand Official Yearbook, 1980* (Wellington: Department of Statistics, 1980), pp. 968–71.

Table 3 Infant mortality rates by age and ethnic group, selected years, New Zealand

	Total			Non-Maori			Maori		
Year	Under 1 Year	28 Days to 11 Months	Under 28 Days	Under 1 Year	28 Days to 11 Months	Under 28 Days	Under 1 Year	28 Days to 11 Months	Under 28 Days
1950	27.6	9.8	17.8	22.7	6.1	16.6	69.7	41.3	28.4
1960	22.6	7.8	14.8	19.7	5.2	14.5	44.5	27.3	17.3
1965	19.6	7.4	12.1	18.0	6.0	12.0	30.1	17.3	12.9
1970	16.8	6.4	10.3	15.1	5.4	9.8	27.5	13.5	13.9
1975	16.0	6.3	9.7	15.4	5.9	9.5	20.5	9.3	11.1
1976	14.0	6.1	7.9	13.0	5.4	7.5	22.0	11.4	10.7
1977	14.2	6.2	8.1	13.0	5.5	7.6	22.4	11.4	11.1
1978	13.8	6.4	7.4	13.2	6.0	7.2	17.9	9.0	9.0
1979[a]	12.8	5.9	6.9	—	—	—	—	—	—
1980[a]	12.9	7.0	5.9	—	—	—	—	—	—

SOURCES: NHSC Department of Health, *Mortality and Demographic Data 1978; News Sheet,* September 1981, National Health Statistics Centre.

NOTE: Rates per 1,000 live births.

[a]Provisional.

Table 4 Infant mortality rates by selected causes, selected years, New Zealand

Cause of Death	ICD Code	1965	1970	1971	1972	1973	1974	1975	1976	1977	1978
Total under 1 year		19.6	16.8	16.6	15.6	16.2	15.6	16.0	14.0	14.2	13.8
Certain gastrointestinal diseases	008,009,561	0.6	0.5	0.4	0.4	0.3	0.2	0.3	0.2	0.2	0.4
Influenza, pneumonia, bronchitis	466, 470–74 480–86 490, 491	3.2	2.9	2.5	1.9	1.9	2.1	2.0	1.9	1.8	1.6
Congenital anomalies	740–759	3.7	3.6	3.2	3.1	3.5	3.8	3.8	3.4	3.4	3.1
Birth injuries	764–768 771, 772	1.6	1.0	1.3	0.9	0.7	0.7	0.8	0.6	0.6	0.2
Asphyxia of newborn unspecified	776.0.4.9	2.5	0.6	0.7	0.6	0.6	0.5	0.7	0.4	0.4	0.7
Immaturity unqualified	777 769.4	2.2	1.3	1.4	0.9	0.9	1.0	1.0	1.0	1.1	0.9
All other causes		5.7	6.8	7.1	7.8	8.3	7.3	7.5	6.6	6.8	6.9

SOURCE: *Mortality and Demographic Data* (Wellington: National Health Statistics Centre, selected years).

NOTE: Rates per 1,000 live births.

Table 5 Death rates for the leading causes of death, New Zealand

Cause of Death	ICD Code	1968 Rank	1968 Death Rate	1968 % of Total Deaths	1977 Rank	1977 Death Rate	1977 % of Total Deaths	1978 Rank	1978 Death Rate	1978 % of Total Deaths
All causes			888.5	100		830.2	100		788.6	100
Diseases of heart	410–429	1	294.8	33.2	1	265.0	31.9	1	248.8	31.6
Malignant neoplasms	140–207	2	147.8	16.6	2	167.8	20.2	2	166.5	21.1
Cerebrovascular diseases	430–438	3	113.0	12.7	3	101.1	12.2	3	95.7	12.1
Bronchitis, emphysema, asthma	490–493	6	33.4	3.8	4	40.7	4.9	4	38.6	4.9
Influenza and pneumonia	470–486	4	51.2	5.8	5	31.1	3.8	5	35.0	4.4
Accidents (excluding suicide and motor vehicle)	800–999	5	33.7	3.8	6	30.9	3.7	6	27.1	3.4
Diseases of the arteries	440–448	7	22.9	2.6	8	21.5	2.6	7	22.7	2.9
Motor vehicle accidents	810–827	9	20.3	2.3	7	28.5	3.4	8	22.3	2.8
Diabetes mellitus	250	10	12.2	1.4	9	13.6	1.6	9	10.9	1.4
Suicide	950–959	12	9.6	1.1	10	11.7	1.4	10	10.3	1.3
Congenital anomalies	740–759	11	10.4	1.2	11	9.3	1.1	11	8.1	1.0
Certain causes of mortality in early infancy	760–779	8	20.7	2.3	12	8.7	1.0	12	7.3	0.9
All other causes			118.5	13.3		100.1	12.1		95.4	12.1

SOURCE: *Mortality and Demographic Data* (Wellington: National Health Statistics Centre, selected years).

NOTE: Rates per 100,000 mean population for year.

Table 6 Most frequent operative (surgical) procedures in public and private hospitals, 1979, New Zealand

ICD Code	Operative Procedure	Number	Rate Per 1,000 Population[a]
690	Dilation and curettage (uterus)	15,155	4.7
663 and 664	Ligation and division of fallopian tubes	6,948	2.2
200	Myringotomy	6,632	2.1
282	Tonsillectomy with adenoidectomy	6,404	2.0
530	Repair inguinofemoral hernia	6,023	1.9
470	Appendectomy	5,414	1.7
884	Local excision/destruction of skin and subcutaneous tissue	4,671	1.5
984	Immobilisation, reduction (closed) of fracture	4,641	1.5
683	Total abdominal hysterectomy	4,507	1.4
384	Ligation and stripping of varicose veins	4,432	1.4
281	Tonsillectomy (without adenoidectomy)	3,462	1.1
792	Open reduction with internal fixation	3,458	1.1

SOURCE: *Hospital and Selected Morbidity Data* (Wellington: National Health Statistics Centre, 1979): tables 12 and 14.

[a]Mean population year ended 31 December 1979

Table 7 Most frequent medical (nonsurgical) reasons for admission to hospitals, public and private, 1979, New Zealand

ICD Code	Reason for Admission	Number	Rate Per 1,000 Population	Average Length of Stay (Days)
493	Asthma	8,175	2.6	5.6
410	Acute myocardial infarction	5,950	1.9	14.9
427	Symptomatic heart disease	5,137	1.6	33.9
412	Chronic ischaemic heart disease	3,862	1.2	20.0
436	Acute ill-defined cerebrovascular disease	3,817	1.2	90.1
009	Diarrhoeal disease	3,769	1.2	6.4
250	Diabetes mellitus	3,523	1.1	26.3
491	Chronic bronchitis	3,166	1.0	24.0
481	Pneumococcal pneumonia	2,351	0.7	12.2
300	Neuroses	2,339	0.7	14.9
466	Acute bronchitis and bronchiolitis	2,148	0.7	6.6
794	Senility with psychosis	2,115	0.7	184.7

SOURCE: *Hospital and Selected Morbidity Data* (Wellington: National Health Statistics Centre, 1979), pp. 13–31, 105–18: tables 2 and 13.

Table 8 Estimated number and rate per 100,000 population of persons active in health occupations, New Zealand

Occupation	Number		Rate Per 100,000 Population	
	1976	1980	1976	1980
Medical practitioners	4,050	4,880	130	154
Dentists	1,070	1,140	34	36
Registered nurses	17,980	19,200	575	607
Optometrists, dispensing opticians	280	280	9	9
Pharmacists	2,200	2,250	70	71
Chiropodists	170	160	5	5
Physiotherapists	840	1,010	27	32
Dietitians	160	190	5	6
Biomedical technologists	—	385	—	12
Occupational therapists	310	380	10	12
Dental assistants	110	110	4	3
Dental technicians	330	310	11	10
Dispensing assistants	800	800	26	25
Medical laboratory technologists	640	730	20	23
Medical laboratory assistants	750	900	24	28
Nurse students (hospital based)	6,960	6,050	222	191
Nurse aids, orderlies	4,860	6,330	155	200
Radiographers (medical)	500	530	16	17
School dental nurses	1,390	1,350	44	43
Social workers (medical)	320	490	10	15
Total health sector workforce	68,000	73,000	2,176	2,310

SOURCE: Management Services and Research Unit, Department of Health, unpublished material.

Table 9 Operational medical schools, medical students, by sex, and graduates by sex, 1980, New Zealand

	Number
Medical schools	2
Total medical students	1,493
Women medical students	508 (34%)
Total medical graduates	233
Women medical graduates	77 (33%)

SOURCE: Management Services and Research Unit, Department of Health, unpublished material.

Table 10a Physicians, population, and physician/population ratios, selected years, New Zealand

Year	Physicians[a] Male	Female	Total	Total Population[b]	Physicians Per 100,000 Population	Population Per Physician
1956	2075	187	2262	2,174,062	104	961
1961	2374	199	2573	2,414,984	106	939
1966	2607	231	2838	2,676,919	106	943
1971	2799	281	3080	2,862,631	108	929
1976	3528	520	4048	3,129,383	129	773
1980	4082	799	4881	3,148,500	155	645

SOURCE: Management Services and Research Unit, Department of Health, unpublished material.

[a]1956–71 census population data; *Medical Council Annual Survey,* 1976-1980.
[b]1956–76 census populations; for 1980, *Monthly Abstract of Statistics,* (Aug. 1981), page 10.

Table 10b Physicians by category/specialty, New Zealand

Category/Specialty	1973	1977	1980
Resident medical officers			
House surgeons	658	897	569
Registrars			561
Medical officers of special scale	[a]	[a]	149
Primary medical care			
General practice	1,352	1,651	1,823
Other	14	26	54
Anaesthetics (s)[b]	114	167	155
Basic medical science (s)	[a]	[a]	26
Community medicine (s)[c]	114	126	113
Dermatology (s)	25	27	30
Diagnostic radiology (s)	91	104	101
Internal medicine (s)	242	302	304[d]
Obstetrics and gynaecology (s)	101	131	125
Oncology (radiotherapy) (s)	11	20	20
Ophthalmology (s)	59	69	69
Otolaryngology (s)	43	51	49
Paediatrics and child health (s)	50	71	76
Pathology (s)	104	125	117
Psychiatry (s)	122	139	129
Surgery (s)	271	307	337[d]
Venereology (s)	2	3	6
Other	71	41	68
Total	3,444	4,257	4,881

SOURCE: Management Services and Research Unit, Department of Health, unpublished data.

[a]Figures included elsewhere.
[b](s) indicates specialty.
[c]"Community medicine" means medicine in reference to populations, as in epidemiology, medical administration, and preventive medicine.
[d]Subspecialty list for 1980 as follows:

Internal Medicine	
General medicine	119
Cardiology	42
Clinical haematology	4
Clinical immunology	2
Clinical pharmacology	4
Endocrinology	14
Gastroenterology	20
Geriatric medicine	14
Intensive care	1
Nephrology	12
Neurology	22
Nuclear medicine	4
Physical medicine	7
Respiratory medicine	20
Rheumatology	19
Total	304

Surgery	
General surgery	186
Cardiothoracic surgery	15
Neurosurgery	8
Orthopaedic surgery	85
Plastic surgery	16
Urology	27
Total	337

Tables 11 and 12 Information not available.

Table 13a Hospitals, beds, admissions, average daily census, and percentage occupancy by type of hospital, year ended 31 March 1980, New Zealand

Type of Hospitals[a]	Hospitals	Beds	Admissions	Average Daily Census	Occupancy (%)
Total New Zealand	333	31,766	470,742	23,909	75.3
Total public hospitals	170	26,602	406,456	20,337	76.4
General	77	14,853	352,229	10,565	71.1
Maternity	53	1,379	37,868	717	52.0
Psychiatric/psychopaedic	16	8,412	10,248	7,269	86.4
Long-term geriatric	24	1,958	7,111	1,786	91.2
Total private hospitals	163	5,164	64,286[b]	3,572[b]	69.2
General	69	2,366	—	—	—
Maternity	5	29	—	—	—
Psychiatric/psychopaedic	1	11	—	—	—
Long-term geriatric	88	2,758	—	—	—

SOURCES: *Hospital Management Data,* 1980, part 1, (Wellington: National Health Statistics Centre): tables 2 and 4; *Private Hospital Discharges and Deaths, 1979,* (Wellington, National Health Statistics Centre, January 1981).

[a]Classified according to major use.
[b]Year ended 31 December 1979.

Table 13b Surgical operations and procedures, public and private hospitals, 1979, New Zealand

WHO Classification		Public Hospitals			Private Hospitals			Total		
		Male	Female	Total	Male	Female	Total	Male	Female	Total
010–999	Total all operations	84,059	104,423	188,482	24,502	30,270	54,772	108,561	134,693	243,254
101–059	The nervous system	1,791	1,630	3,421	447	673	1,120	2,238	2,303	4,541
060–079	The endocrine system	137	502	639	43	179	222	180	681	861
080–169	The eyes	3,596	3,453	7,049	926	1,253	2,179	4,522	4,706	9,228
180–209	The ears	2,999	2,473	5,472	2,262	1,841	4,103	5,261	4,314	9,575
210–299	Nose, mouth, pharynx	7,779	6,968	14,765	4,223	4,271	8,494	12,002	11,257	23,259
300–349	Respiratory system	693	303	996	21	22	43	714	325	1,039
350–399	Cardiovascular system	2,916	2,919	5,835	693	1,227	1,920	3,609	4,146	7,755
400–419	Hemic and lymphatic systems	443	357	800	50	62	112	493	419	912
420–549	Digestive system	13,955	11,748	25,703	3,646	2,474	6,120	17,601	14,222	31,823
550–599	Urinary tract	2,429	1,540	3,969	442	535	977	2,871	2,075	4,946
600–649	Male genital organs	6,485	13	6,498	4,633	3	4,636	11,118	16	11,134
650–719	Female genital organs	—	31,074	31,074	—	9,053	9,053	—	40,127	40,127
720–759	Obstetric operations	—	4,211	4,211	—	639	639	—	4,850	4,850
760–859	Musculoskeletal system	12,271	8,950	21,221	3,774	2,717	6,491	16,045	11,667	27,712
860–879	The breast	144	2,592	2,736	60	1,192	1,252	204	3,784	3,988
880–909	Skin and subcutaneous tissue	7,889	5,581	13,470	1,635	1,929	3,564	9,524	7,510	17,034
910–999	Ancillary surgical procedures	20,532	20,091	40,623	1,647	2,200	3,847	22,179	22,291	44,470

SOURCE: *Hospital and Selected Morbidity Data* (Wellington: National Health Statistics Centre, 1979): tables 12 and 14.

Table 14 Public and private hospitals: ownership or sponsorship as at 31 March 1980, New Zealand

Ownership/Sponsorship	Hospitals
Public ownership	170
Church or other nonprofit ownership	73
For-profit ownership	90
Total	333

SOURCE (for private hospitals): Department of Health, Division of Hospitals.

Table 15 Old people's homes and old people's home beds, at 31 March 1980 and 31 March 1981, New Zealand

	1980		1981	
Homes	Homes	Beds	Homes	Beds
Total	411	11,880	434	12,036
Religious and welfare	170	7,681	174	7,671
Private	208	3,223	227	3,389
Hospital board	33	976	33	976

SOURCE: Department of Health, Division of Hospitals.

NOTE: Table includes all old people's homes run by hospital boards, excludes all licensed geriatric hospital beds and independent flats operated by religious and welfare organisations.

Table 16 Average cost of public hospital care per inpatient bed-day, New Zealand

	1978–79	1979–80	% Change
Total expenditure (in millions $NZ)	556.1	646.1	16.2
Inpatient bed-days (in millions)	7.79	7.64	−2.0
Average cost per bed-day ($)	71.36	84.58	18.5

SOURCE: *Hospital Management Data* (Wellington: National Health Statistics Centre, 1980).

Table 17 National health expenditure (aggregate, per capita, percentage of Gross National Produce), year ending 31 March, New Zealand

	1925	1949	1961	1969	1974	1975	1976	1977	1978	1979	1980
National health expenditure ($M)[a]	7.0	44.4	125.4	234.9	488.6	596.4	731.5	840.4	987.0	—	—
Public	3.0	34.6	100.9	185.1	397.0	491.4	605.7	700.4	824.0	1,004.0	1,157.8
Private	4.0	9.8	24.5	49.8	91.6	105.0	125.8	140.0	163.0	—	—
Expenditure per capita ($)	5	24	53	85	164	196	236	269	315	—	—
Public	2	19	42	67	133	161	195	224	263	321	371
Private	3	5	11	18	31	35	41	45	52	—	—
Public expenditure as % of GNP	—	3.5	3.8	4.3	4.4	4.9	5.4	5.2	5.5	5.9	5.7
Population (M)[b]	1.360	1.844	2.388	2.760	2.987	3.047	3.098	3.121	3.129	3.129	3.125
GNP ($M)[b]	—	988	2,650	4,355	9,109	9,947	11,319	13,530	14,880	17,083	20,441
Annual % change											
National health expenditure	—	8.0	9.0	8.2	15.8	22.1	22.7	14.9	17.4	—	—
Public	—	10.7	9.3	7.9	16.5	23.8	23.3	15.6	17.6	21.8	15.3
Private	—	3.8	7.9	9.3	13.0	14.6	19.8	11.3	16.4	—	—
Population	—	1.3	2.2	1.8	1.6	2.0	1.7	0.7	0.3	0.0	−0.1
GNP	—	—	8.6	6.4	15.9	9.2	13.8	19.5	10.0	14.8	19.7

[a]A.G. Smith and P.M. Tatchell, *Health Expenditure in New Zealand—Trends and Growth Patterns,* Special Report No. 53 (Wellington: Department of Health, 1979). Public health expenditure has been modified by recent research.

[b]*New Zealand Official Yearbook, 1980* (Wellington: Department of Statistics): *Monthly Abstract of Statistics* (Wellington: Department of Statistics, Oct. 1981).

Table 18 Health expenditure by type of expenditure and source of funds (aggregate, percentage, and per capita), New Zealand

Type of Expenditure, 1973–74	Public	Private: Direct	Private: Insurance	Private: Other	Total	Total $ Per Capita
Expenditure ($M)						
Hospital services	277.7	13.3	5.8	1.1	297.9	99.73
Public	265.4	—	2.5	—	267.9	89.69
Private	12.3	13.3	3.3	1.1	30.0	10.04
General medical	21.6	14.8	0.3	—	36.7	12.30
Specialist medical	11.1	10.4	1.9	—	23.4	7.84
Dental services	10.0	18.5	—	—	28.5	9.54
Medicaments	45.6	24.4	—	—	69.9	23.41
Public health	10.2	—	—	0.8	11.0	3.68
Teaching	17.3	—	—	—	17.3	5.80
Research	3.4	—	—	0.5	3.8	1.28
Total	397.0	81.4	7.9	2.3	488.6	163.58
Percentage distribution						
Hospital services	69.9	16.4	72.6	45.9	61.0	
Private	66.8	—	31.5	—	54.8	
Public	3.1	16.4	41.1	45.9	6.2	
General medical	5.5	18.2	3.4	—	7.5	
Specialist medical	2.8	12.8	24.0	—	4.8	
Dental services	2.5	22.7	—	—	5.8	
Medicaments	11.5	29.9	—	—	14.3	
Public health	2.6	—	—	33.8	2.2	
Teaching	4.4	—	—	—	3.5	
Research	0.8	—	—	20.3	0.8	
Total	100	100	100	100	100	

Type of Expenditure, 1978–80, Public Only	1978–79 $M	1978–79 $ Per Capita	1978–79 %	1979–80 $M	1979–80 $ Per Capita	1979–80 %
Hospital services	697.0	223	69.4	804.9	258	69.5
Public	662.9	212	66.0	761.8	244	65.8
Private	34.1	11	3.4	43.1	14	3.7
General medical	72.1	23	7.2	79.0	25	6.8
Specialist medical	24.5	8	2.4	26.3	8.5	2.3
Dental services	21.8	7	2.2	28.5	9	2.5
Medicaments	115.5	37	11.5	134.5	43	11.6
Public health	25.6	8	2.5	29.4	9.5	2.5
Teaching	39.7	12.5	4.0	44.7	14.5	3.9
Research	8.0	2.5	0.8	10.6	3.5	0.9
Total	1,004.0	321	100	1,157.8	371	100

SOURCES: A.G. Smith and P.M. Tatchell, *Health Expenditure in New Zealand—Trends and Growth Patterns,* special report no. 53 (Wellington: Department of Health, 1979) and subsequent research.

Table 19 Information not available.

Table 20 New Zealand population covered by private health insurance, selected years

	1960	1965	1970	1975	1979	1980
% of population	2	3	9	18	26	28

SOURCE: Estimated from annual reports of major private health insurance schemes. Includes corporate membership.

Health Services in Sweden

Edgar Borgenhammar

INTRODUCTION

The Swedes, like people in other countries, place a high value on health and medical care. The health services are an important facet of the welfare state. There are reasons to believe that Swedes have access to as high quality of medical care as people do anywhere. Studies show that the health services system is highly regarded among Swedes, and that rising costs, tax financed, so far have not worried the population very much.

In 1975 personal interviews were performed on priorities with a representative selection of the population between the ages of eighteen and seventy. Among twenty-nine areas suggested for potential increase in use of the nation's total revenues, medical and dental care came first, followed by care for the elderly. This ranking of priorities was the same for all social groups (Tarschys 1975). A similar study from 1981 illustrates that 85% of the respondents considered higher taxes to be acceptable provided they were used for better care for the elderly. Seven out of ten preferred higher taxes to deteriorated medical care (Hälso- och sjukvården 1981).

Economic constraints will contain expansion of health services for the future. Efforts will have to concentrate on making better use of available resources. There is political unanimity on the need for restructuring the health services, although professional interests often aim at conservation and expansion of the present structure.

A Complex System

As is any other such system, the Swedish health service system is very complex. It serves a population of 8.3 million people (1982), spread over about 450,000 km^2. The population density is one of the lowest in Europe (18.4 per km^2). About 90% of the inhabitants live in the southern half of the country; eight out of ten live in towns and villages; about 20% have their homes in the three largest towns and their immediate environments. Less than 20% of the population is under fifteen years, and more than 16% is over sixty-five years

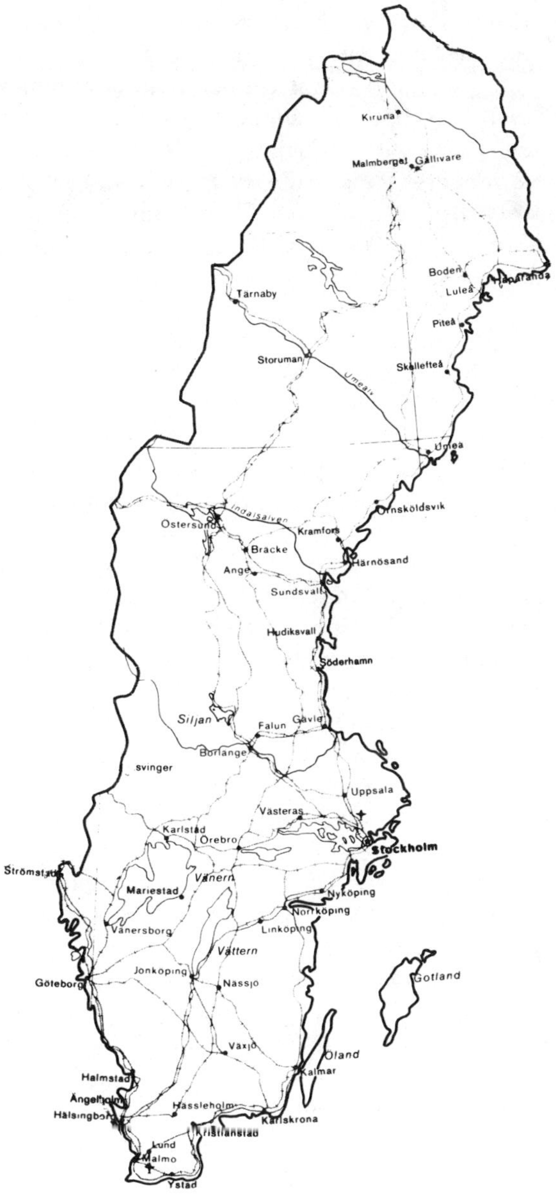

of age. About 10% of the population are immigrants, including naturalized Swedes. Most come from other Nordic countries. Emigration and immigration balance at about 30,000 a year.

Social and Political Context

Sweden is a constitutional parliamentary monarchy with a yet relatively homogenous population, most of whom are Lutheran Christians. Gross national income was 570 billion

Swedish kronor (Sw. kr.) in 1981, which means about 70,000 Sw.kr. per head. Sweden has enjoyed peace since the early nineteenth century, and the country considers itself neutral in relation to military disputes and is not connected to any military alliance. The official figures for unemployment are kept low: about 3% of the work force in 1981.

Health services delivery is regarded mainly as a task for the public sector. It is chiefly provided by local governments. Responsibility for medical care, inpatient as well as outpatient, rests with twenty-three county councils and three municipalities that are not part of the county council areas (Gothenburg, Malmö, and the island of Gotland).

The county councils were set up in 1863. Each council, as well as the municipalities, has the right to levy its own proportional income taxes. For 1982 the average county council tax was 12.89%, and the average municipal tax was 16.91% of income. To this is added state and church taxes. State income tax is progressive—its percentage increases with income. The state of Sweden also levies value-added taxes on all purchases. More than 66% of the GNP passes over public budgets: for consumption, investments, and transferrings. About one-third of the GNP is public consumption and investment—in municipal government, county councils, and state government. About 10% of the GNP is used for health services.

The county councils also operate the public dental service, which serves inhabitants through age sixteen (in some cases up to nineteen years of age) as well as providing about 50% of adult dental care, the rest being privately provided. County councils also care for the mentally retarded. Social welfare services are the responsibility of the municipalities, together with environmental hygiene.

The number of municipal governments has gradually been reduced, from about 2,500 in 1950 to 280 in 1982. Their activities include education, social welfare (particularly care for children and the elderly), fire prevention, and various cultural and recreational activities.

Private health care exists as a supplement to public health care. About 5% of the physicians are in private practice, mainly in the big cities; they take care of 15 to 20% of all ambulatory visits to physicians. About 50% of the dentists are in private practice. There is a limited number of private medical institutions to care for inpatients; most are small nursing homes for long-term care.

The number of full-time private practitioners decreased by 25% from 1975 to 1980; however, part-time private practitioners increased by 50% during the same period. This means that publicly employed physicians practice privately in off-duty hours.

On the average, the county councils have about 250,000 inhabitants. County council members are elected, every third year, on political lines.

THE ORGANIZATION OF MEDICAL CARE

The health services law of 1982 emphasizes the significance of preventive efforts, directed toward the community at large. It is the duty of the county councils to aim at health promotion as well as to find factors behind diseases. The councils have to provide health services that fulfill certain quality requirements. Ambulance services are part of the public health care system. The aim of the health services system is good health for the entire population and equity in services.

Health care services should be easy to reach and should be based on respect for the patient's integrity. As far as possible, treatment and care should be planned in cooperation with the patient, who should also be given information about his or her health condition and about what alternative methods of treatment are available.

It is the county council's duty to build a purposeful organization and to have sufficient cooperation with other public and private organizations in the society. The councils also must cooperate among themselves on health care issues. The law requires the councils to provide the personnel which are necessary to provide good care; it also gives a wide scope for the councils to choose their own organizational structure. One physician should carry the responsibility as chief of medical services in a hospital, and one of the district physicians should have the corresponding medical responsibility for activities outside of hospitals. Often, a health services district in a county includes hospitals as well as primary care institutions, just as in England.

Ministry of Health and Social Affairs

General plans and policy for health services are drawn up by the ministry of health and social affairs, in cooperation with the Parliament of Sweden. A permanent committee for national health planning is connected to the ministry. This committee studies the uses of public health resources and aims at coordination of plans.

Even if the county councils do depend on central government decisions—for example, for obtaining about 15% of their income—there is a strong tendency among them to flag for their independence. Attempts to govern from Stockholm are rejected wherever possible.

The National Board of Health and Welfare

The National Board of Health and Welfare has a supervisory function in relation to both public and private medical services institutions. The board is also responsible for stimulating the planning of health services at the national level and is involved in the establishment of new public service positions for physicians and in the inspection of medical care activities.

From the late 1960s there has been a strong tendency to let the National Board of Health and Welfare play a core role in Swedish health policy. The ministry has now taken back part of the initiative, even if most of the changes during the last few years have meant more power to the county councils.

The Association of County Councils

The Association of County Councils is the interest organization for the owners of hospitals and health services institutions. It represents the employers in negotiations with unions for physicians, nurses, aides, and many other groups. The association assembles statistics on the personnel situation, services, etc., and also negotiates with the Department of Finance regarding the economic scope for health services in the future. The functions, besides negotiations, are strictly advisory.

The National Institute for Planning and Rationalization of Health Services

The National Institute for Planning and Rationalization of Health Services is jointly operated by the state of Sweden and the Association of County Councils. It investigates planning norms, gives advice, and provides standardized principles for medical equipment and facilities. It has an outstanding information service that is highly valued by international students.

The County Councils

In each county council there is a health services board, and under it there generally are health districts for hospitals and health services. In most cases a district is headed by a director, and when he is not a medical doctor, a chief physician assists with advice in medical matters. It is rare that the director has a medical background. In many cases, nursing is represented in the district management group.

Different from England, there are no centralized directives regarding how medical care in a county should be organized. Consequently, there are great varieties of structures among counties; however, over time certain patterns can be observed. As an example, one-third of the county councils have, or have had, "bloc sector" organization, somewhat like the English "cogwheel committees," which serves a coordinative function. A chief of service is expected to coordinate related medical services across hospital borders. There generally is one separate "bloc sector" each for surgical specialties, internal medicine, psychiatry, primary care, long-term care (now mainly seen as part of primary care), and laboratory services. There are examples where dental care is included in the function of the health services board in the county councils, but in most cases there is a special dental board that runs its own services organization.

A law from 1977 requires negotiation with representatives from the unions before decisions are made for any major changes such as new investments, the annual or long-term budget, and employment of managers. Swedish unions are influential, and a high percentage of the employees are unionized—including physicians, managers, and nurses.

Some developments during later years with respect to influence are outlined in chart 1.

DEVELOPMENT OF THE HEALTH SYSTEM

A historic overview of the Swedish health services system goes back to 830 A.D., when Ansgar, a monk from the Benedictine cloister of Corbie in France, began to preach Christianity to savage Swedes. Although use of precipices and placement of unwanted babies in forests did not come to an end at that time, Christianity did mean a new set of ethics, where compassion and care for sick and weak human beings were given a wider scope than before. At the middle of the fifteenth century about twenty hospitals for the old and poor sick were available in connection with monasteries.

The Reformation, introduced by King Gustav Vasa in 1527, meant that most of the

Chart 1 Tendencies regarding the power structure

State institutions versus county councils and municipalities	"Framework laws" limit the authority of central state institutions to control county councils and municipalities.
Central versus local units in county councils and municipalities	During the 1960s and 1970s, central units increased their influence. During the early 1980s there has been a tendency toward more local influence, within a given economic frame.
Experts versus lay people	Increasing specialization, professionalization, and bureaucratization mean more power to experts and less to lay people.
Specialists versus generalists	Specialists tend to be involved increasingly in problem solving. As a result, the interest in general questions decreases, as does the influence of generalists.
Full-time versus part-time politicians	Full-time politicians have greater possibilities to influence decisions than other politicians have.
Union versus members	More and more persons work full time for unions as "ombudsmen." There is a risk that unions, which have to care for consequence and continuity, work instrumentally, while the members take a different and more situational approach.
Men versus women	Influential positions in political congregations, in management, and in unions are mostly held by men, though a change is coming.
Traditional versus new activities	The major part of the budget is prolongation of previous activities. Reevaluation means a risk of conflicts, and there is a limited scope for new activities.
Small versus principal issues	Routine issues tend to occupy most of the time, leaving only limited scope for principal issues.

property of the church was confiscated. The operation of hospitals became more difficult as many monks and priests left Sweden. Within a few decades, the hospitals were practically eradicated. In medieval times, superstition and fear were dominating, and there was not very much to battle it from scientific quarters. The last "witch" was burned in 1704, and it was not until 1979 that homosexuality was removed from the official list of diseases.

The first state-employed provincial doctors were introduced at the end of the seventeenth century. An important task of the doctors was to check the spread of venereal diseases, which limited the fighting ability of the soldiers. The first "modern" hospital, the Royal Serafimer Hospital in Stockholm, opened in 1752 with eight beds "for Sweden and Finland." The first local hospital was built in Växjö in 1762. During the 1780s, hospitals for epidemic diseases were set up. By 1809 there were twenty small asylums and about the same number of small hospitals. As Blanpain (1978, 195) points out "Swedish hospitals were initially established and financed by the government in reaction to an epidemic of venereal disease at the beginning of the nineteenth century."

When the county councils were established in 1863, hospitals were only one of several activities they were intended to handle. Others were education, traffic, and promotion of vocations. Within a few decades, however, 80% of the budget was spent on hospitals, a figure which still remains. It was not until 1963 that the previously state-controlled provincial (or district) doctors were organizationally taken over by county council administration. Formerly state owned, the Karolinska Hospital in Stockholm was taken over by the county council of Stockholm in 1982. This means that most health services now are county council managed.

The general health insurance dates back to 1955. Before that date, however, hospitalization had been almost free of cost to the individual patient; the county council tax covered the major part of the costs. The most important change in the reform of 1955 was the introduction of a daily allowance for all working people in case of illness.

The health insurance scheme is compulsory for everyone who lives and works in Sweden. It provides protection against loss of income due to illness, injury, disability, or childbirth. It is financed to about 85% by employers' contributions and to 15% by state grants. There are twenty-six local social insurance offices of the National Social Insurance Board. The board pays part of the costs of ambulatory services, outpatient services in hospitals, and consultation for inpatient treatment; half of the cost, up to a certain amount, for dental treatment, and three-quarters of the costs above that amount. Drugs and travelling expenses are also covered above a certain minimum "self-risk."

Sickness benefits under the health insurance scheme amount to about 90% of normal income, up to a fixed maximum income. Parental benefit, payable in the case of the birth or adoption of a child, enables either parent to be off of work for a total of twelve months. In the 1950s the proportion of the GNP that went into health and medical services was below 4%. Behind the growth to the present 10% level are such factors as the expansion of regional and central hospitals and long-term care hospitals. The increases in medical services costs have been faster than the growth of the GNP, though slow growth rates for both have been observed in later years. From 1963 to 1969 the GNP rose on the average by 4.1% annually, while medical services costs rose an average of 7.1%. From 1970 to 1979 the GNP showed an average increase of 2%, while a 3.9% annual growth was seen in medical services costs.

The Hospital System

The region hospital plan of 1958 had French ancestry. In France a plan was put forth at the beginning of the 1950s that divided the country into twenty-three health service regions. The main purpose of the change was to facilitate the planning of medical specialties. On a voluntary basis, Sweden was divided into seven regions with about one million inhabitants each, for the highly specialized types of care. In 1982 there were six regions with nine region hospitals, most of which are affiliated with medical schools and also serve as research and teaching hospitals. The director general of the National Board of Health and Welfare (1952–67), Dr. Arthur Engel, is known as the father of the regional hospital system.

Central hospitals for between 200,000 and 300,000 inhabitants have a somewhat lower degree of specialization, and they often have more than 1,000 beds. Smaller acute hospitals, the district county hospitals, serve 60,000 to 90,000 inhabitants and have four or more specialties.

A most remarkable growth characterizes long-term care. More than 50,000 beds are available, most of which have been added during a twenty-year period.

There still remain several big psychiatric hospitals in Sweden. Remnants of time past, they mirror an out-of-date philosophy. The closure of mental care beds has been considerably slower than planned. In many cases the mental hospital is the big "industry" in a city, and strong union and municipal protest is aired when closure is being discussed. Of 30,000 hospitalized mental care patients, more than 10,000 are estimated to be there more or less "unnecessarily."

The fact that Swedish health services are so heavily hospital based has to do with professional attitudes toward the "Höjer plan," presented by Dr. Axel Höjer when he was director general of the National Board of Health and Welfare in 1948. He proposed expansions of both local health centers and physician education. Reactions from physicians were vividly negative at that time. Instead, a period of great hospital construction started, and Höjer was replaced in 1952 by a more hospital-inclined physician, Dr. Arthur Engel.

The strong tendency toward concentration to a limited number of units should be observed as a significant trend in Swedish health policy. The number of acute hospitals is relatively small. The size in number of beds, in square meters, and in personnel is remarkably large by international standards. Equipment also holds a very high technical level. In 1980, out of the 99 hospitals for mainly acute care, at least 44 had more than 600 beds. In 1960 the corresponding figures had only 19 of 108 hospitals with more than 600 beds.

The number of single-handed surgeries decreased form 590 in 1970 to 200 in 1980. At the same time, the number of health centers for two or more physicians rose from 170 to 530. Despite this health center growth, no less than 3 out of 4 new positions for physicians have gone to acute hospital care from 1970 to 1977.

The Seven Kronor Reform

In 1970 the Seven Kronor Reform introduced two important changes in the Swedish health system. The first marked a fixed salary and fixed working hours for physicians in public service; the second set a fixed amount, at that time seven Swedish kronor, for a physician's visit, inclusive of laboratory and X-ray tests. The amount has increased over time and is thirty kronor in 1982. Since 1970, no person who is employed in public health is allowed to receive any direct compensation for inpatient or outpatient services. Private beds were removed from hospitals in 1959.

A Process of Changes

In 1963 a ceiling of fifteen kronor was set for patients on charges for drugs acquired in one transaction by a single prescription. The amount is forty kronor in 1982. The wholesale and retail drug business was largely nationalized in 1971. A dental insurance was introduced in 1974 with reimbursement of, in most cases, 50% of the fee for a visit to a private dentist.

Remuneration from the general health insurance for visits to a private physician was regulated in 1975 in such a way that the cost for the patient is just slightly higher than to a publicly employed physician. A private physician who is connected to the system is allowed to take no more than 3,000 patients during a six-month period.

Students of the Swedish health services system sometimes find it remarkable that it is possible to enter the system as a patient not only at the district physician level but also at the hospital specialist level. Another remarkable facet is the long waiting time for seeing a physician in a nonacute case. In most cases acute patients do go to emergency units at hospitals. The number of patients that a district physician takes per day is by international standards very low, often fourteen to eighteen patients. Most are making repeated visits. The number of assisting personnel is relatively high, and the extremely generous space in health centers surprises many foreign visitors.

After the seven kronor reform, the decrease in "productivity" of physicians per hour has accelerated. The decrease in "health services productivity," gauged by the insufficient measures that are available, is estimated to about 3% per year per working hour.

The accessibility of a district physician is connected not only to the patient flow; it also has to do with how work is organized, that is, how much of a doctor's working hours is devoted to patients. It has been observed that "administration" is a growing part of the Swedish physicians' working days.

Before 1970 the district physician was available more or less around the clock. Today, working hours are regulated according to collective bargaining, which also regulates compensation for work on nonoffice hours. Work of this type is compensated by as much as 200% in free time, that is, for night and holiday hours. Compensation can partly be made by means of money; though this is not very attractive due to high marginal taxes. The effect of compensation on quality of care has been pointed out as critical, particularly by surgeons. The generous compensation in free time for duty work ventures international comparisons. However, the system also makes continuity of care to the same physician more difficult for the patient. The case illustrates a dilemma. There is a tendency for the employee, and not the patient, to come first.

BASIC PRINCIPLES FOR PLANNING

The equity principle is a basic principle of health services planning in Sweden. Everyone should be given equal care whenever possible, and it is the need for medical care, not the patient's financial resources, which should be the entrance ticket to the system. Planning is a core concept in Swedish health services. The current plans have the following aims:

First, an increase in primary care visits should take place because of the organization of more outpatient facilities in local districts. The number of ambulatory visits to physicians is relatively low—less than three per year and per Swede on the average. On top of this, there is about one additional public health related visit to district nurses, physiotherapists, and other health personnel.

A primary care district has 5,000 to 50,000 inhabitants. District health personnel assume primary responsibility for the health of the population in their area. Each district has one or more local health care centers, and in many cases there is a nursing home as well for long-stay patients. At a health center, not only district physicians but also district nurses and district midwives serve. Many times there are also physiotherapists and social workers, the latter group belonging to the municipal social services. The school health services examine the health of school children on a regular basis. Special industrial health services cater to about 50% of the total work force at places of employment, such as factories. It is intended that this figure should increase.

Second, more and more resources will be devoted to long-term care in day care centers, nursing homes, and special long-term-care hospitals. The remarkably high proportion of elderly people is seen as an indication of the need. Recently, more emphasis has been given to home care, which is more in concord with what the patients themselves wish.

Third, an unchanged number of beds in acute somatic care is the official planning norm. However, the number of personnel has increased considerably and is likely to continue to grow, even if it will be at a slower rate.

In 1982 an evening newspaper made a headline of the fact that during the last ten years, 121,000 additional persons had been employed while only 1,000 new beds had been added. There are many reasons behind this. Specialization has gone farther, and at present there are no less than 43 official medical specialties in Sweden. The number of subspecialties is several hundred. The more specialized health care is, generally the higher is the number of needed personnel.

An estimation (Calltorp 1982) of the number of physicians with complete specialist training gives the following figures for 1985:

General practice	2,551
Anesthesiology	527
Pediatrics	619
Dermatology	166
Internal medicine	721
Infectious diseases	158
Lung diseases	119
Long-term care	517
Other internal medicine specialties	203
General surgery	713
Orthopedic surgery	334
Urologic surgery	89
Other surgical specialties	535
Gynecology	591
Neurology	104
General psychiatry	845
Child psychiatry	207
X-ray	586
Oncology	129
Eye diseases	305
Ear, nose, throat	353
Medical rehabilitation	106
Community medicine	28
Other specialties	256
Total	11,001

A fourth aim is a reduced number of beds in psychiatric care. Estimations state that more than one-third of the number of beds ought to be closed; however, the process of closure and reduction is as difficult in Sweden as in many other countries. There is a tendency to organize districts with a limited catchment area and a kaleidoscope of professions besides the psychiatrist to serve the population, largely on an outpatient basis. General central hospitals also have special psychiatric wards, and long-term psychiatric care is being integrated with somatic long-term care.

Fifth, closer links should be formed between the municipality's social service, which caters to the well old person, and health services for the sick ones, which are run by the county councils. So far, efforts seem to have had less effect than had been hoped for. Some of the observable outcomes are a joint location of health centers and social service centers, and coinciding borders for catchment areas. It is hoped that this will facilitate planning.

As a final goal, emphasis on preventive measures aims at eliminating or limiting medical and social risks in the society and in the occupational as well as traffic environment. More effort will be directed toward the health aspects of alcohol, smoking, drug abuse, exercise, and food. In Sweden, as in many other countries, alcohol, smoking and unhealthy food habits (too much fat, sugar, and salt) cater to a considerable part of diseases.

MEDICAL EDUCATION AND PERSONNEL

The fact that the Swedish health delivery system is rapidly changing is observed in the health sector's personnel structures. In 1960 there were about 115,000 persons employed; in 1977, 320,000 people; and in 1982 about 370,000 persons—approximately 7.5% of all employees in Sweden. This rapid growth is partly due to shorter working hours (at present 40 hours or 38 hours for shift personnel). There are about 300,000 full-time equivalents in the 370,000 figure.

Shortage of trained personnel has been a constant concern. The debate over the situation regarding physicians has been especially serious, in addition to talk about shortages of physiotherapists and of certain categories of nurses. The personnel situation has improved gradually, and a surplus of certain personnel groups is likely to be observed from 1985.

Medical Doctors

Training of medical doctors takes place at six medical schools, which are part of universities. They are located in Uppsala, Lund, Stockholm, Gothenburg, Umeå, and Linköping. For teaching purposes, a still greater number of hospitals are used. About 1,030 medical students are accepted every year. Admission is restricted, and many more apply than can be accepted every year. In the application process, points are given not only for performance in previous education but for work practice as well, the latter more highly graded than ten years ago. This has meant an increase in the average age of students. In 1982 a maximum age limit of forty-five years was decided upon for persons who start their medical studies.

The basic study program requires 5½ years, which is divided into preclinical, preparatory, and clinical periods. After receiving a degree as physician, the medical student must complete a 21-month period of general internship in order to obtain a license to practice. After that starts 4 to 5½ years of postgraduate training, which gives qualifications as specialist or general practitioner.

The National Board of Health and Welfare allocates so-called blocks to county councils for postgraduate training in concord with a physician distribution program that is outlined by the health planning committee of the ministry of health and social affairs. A system of further education for physicians has been set up in order to ensure that knowledge is maintained to a certain level.

How realistic are fears that there will be a surplus of medical doctors in the future? The Swedish Medical Association claims that there will be a surplus within the next few years and that, consequently, it would be wise to cut the number of students. However, the National Board of Health and Welfare argues that this is not very likely to occur within the next decades.

Nurses

There are several routes whereby a student can undergo nursing education and be registered by the National Board of Health and Welfare as a qualified nurse in Sweden. A direct nursing education is one possibility; this comprises 105 credits. For persons who have completed the two-year nursing line at an upper secondary school, a short-term nursing training is another option, and it gives 63 to 73 credits. A third, similar possibility is open for mental nurses with a training of 40 to 60 weeks, as well as for those who have 40 weeks of practical nurse training. All three routes offer qualifications as registered nurses.

The nursing and care sector of higher education includes the following state-sponsored general programs, besides the medical line with 220 credits and nursing: the pharmacy line with 160 credits, the logopedic line with 120 credits, the dispenser line with 100 credits, the physiotherapy line with 100 credits, and the dental line with 180 credits. There is also a municipal higher education system that includes the following programs for the nursing and care sector. The occupational therapy line with 120 credits, the audio-technology line with 80 credits, the medical laboratory technologist line for X-ray diagnostics and radiotherapy with 100 credits, the medical technologist line for ophthalmology with 80 credits, the medical technologist line with 100 credits, the social service line with 60 to 100 credits, and the dental hygienist line with 40 credits.

WHERE IS THE SYSTEM GOING?

In an analysis of the shaping of the Swedish health system, Carder and Klingeberg (1980, 146) state:

> While the expansion of the hospital sector provided Sweden with some of the finest facilities, it also created many problems. Expected to fulfil most health

care functions, the hospital sector developed into a "resource magnet"—monopolising investments, personnel, technology, and patients at the expense of other health care delivery subsystems. Hospital inpatient care is the most expensive type of health care. For these reasons, alternatives to inpatient care became important to the county councils. In tandem with an emphasis on alternative delivery modes outside the hospital, the predominant inpatient orientation of the hospitals began to change. After 1959, hospitals were required to maintain outpatient departments for the treatment of ambulatory patients.

At present, about 50% of all ambulatory physician visits take place at outpatient clinics in hospitals; 30 to 35% are to district physicians, 15 to 20% to private physicians. The remarkably weak primary care has been observed in several studies regarding health services in Sweden. For example, Stephen (1979, 158–59) says:

> A career in primary care is thought to indicate failure, and those who seek it are branded as "non successes." Such comments are common to many countries, but apply particularly to Sweden. In about 1963, when the new law concerning primary care gave the responsibility to the county councils, it was beginning to be realised by a few physicians and administrators that a fundamental mistake had been made, but the vast majority of the general public and politicians, although they sensed that something was wrong, still remained convinced by the image of a scientific, hospital-oriented medicine. In fact, as recently as 1970, Sweden's answer to the organisation of modern health was started—the building of a 1,400-bedded hospital in Stockholm. It is of course now realised that this ultimate folly of health care planning—a form of medical madness—can never solve the real health needs of the people, nor can any nation, even one as prosperous as Sweden, afford to build and staff such a hospital. Nor indeed can any country afford the dubious luxury of organising primary care through the hospital service.

Even as late as 1982, several Swedish counties had plans to build big new hospitals. The desire to create work possibilities in an unemployment situation seems to be a major reason for starting projects of this kind. Generally, the new hospitals are intended to replace older ones.

Can the development of health services be more rational? How far is it possible to come by means of planning? Anderson (1972, 202) compares the United States, England, and Sweden, and concludes:

> The concept of planning itself needs critical examination. Its successful application does not necessarily depend on the level of skills and sophistication. The problem is: do we know what we are doing when we plan in relation to resources, structures, and goals? My reluctant skepticism toward rational planning and structuring of services lies in our inability to set up specifications with any degree of precision; hence, I tend toward "loose" systems. England never thought she could afford such a system even if she were able to conceive of one; Sweden has been doing so for a long time. In the United States, a "loose" system is congenial, but now it may be regarded as too wasteful. England continues to want one gatekeeper—the general practitioner or a health center—and one central source of funds. Sweden wants a specified range of

gatekeepers and several sources of funds. The United States seems to be moving to the Swedish pattern, one that Sweden arrived at intuitively: diversity of funds and options in entering the system.

Will "Health for all by the year 2000" be read as "Medical services for all by the year 2000"? or even as "Patients for all by the year 2000"?

Four Models

Looking toward the future, one can expect a number of partly competing, partly supplementary models for health policy. (1) The *bio-mechanistic disease model* has long been the most influential one. Here, illness is regarded as a malfunction of cells or organs, and planning mainly emphasizes hospitals. (2) During the last decades, the emotional factors behind many an illness have been observed and debated. Some even argue that psychosocial factors can be found behind a majority of somatic diseases. The *psycho-dynamic "trouble" model* emphasizes the importance of conflicts in human health status. (3) A still broader perspective is emphasized in the *holistic environmental model.* Here, knowledge from sociology, ecology, and other sciences is used to widen the horizon, and planning deals with the society at large. (4) In the *active health enhancement model* individuals and groups are seen as active decision makers. Core concerns are the promotion of health and the prevention of diseases, and the stimulation of responsibility for a more enlightened life style. Efforts are directed at what various interest groups can do in order to improve the quality of life. Planning here deals with health in its broadest sense (see chart 2).

In the future there must be a certain balance between the four models. So far, the first model seems to have been given too many resources and too much interest. Attention now has to turn to the other three models as well, provided that we want results from our efforts in the health field.

THE NORDIC COUNTRIES

If we widen the scope to the four other Nordic countries—Denmark, Finland, Iceland, and Norway—we find that all have similarities with respect to population structure, cultural traditions, and social and economic conditions. The view regarding how a welfare state should function also has many similarities.

On the international scene, the Nordic countries are considered to have a relatively uniform system of health services. However, as one looks closer, a number of differences appear.

The five countries have a total of about 22 million inhabitants. Increases in population during the 1970s were minor. In 1981 Denmark had a population of 5.1 million, Finland 4.8 million, Iceland 0.2 million, and Norway 4.1 million. The age group of 65 years or older is relatively greatest in Sweden, with about 16%, and this is expected to grow to 17.5% by 1990. In Norway the corresponding figures are 14.4 % versus 15.2%, in Denmark 14.2% versus 15.2%, in Finland 11.7% versus 13%, and in Iceland 9.7% versus

Chart 2 Four competing models for health policy and hypotheses regarding what characterizes them

	The Bio-Mechanistic Disease Model	The Psycho-Dynamic "Trouble" Model	The Holistic Environmental Model	The Active Health Enhancement Model
Goal	Treat diseases, diminish suffering	Understand and act on psychosomatic problems	Ameliorate risks in the environment	Promote health-oriented action
Direction	Clinical, curative	Behavior analysis	Cost-benefit analytic	Promotion of change
Work method	Instrumental	Situational	Holistic	Insight creating
Research method	Positivistic	Hermeneutic	System analytic	Action oriented
Organization model	Hierarchic, type "locomotive and train"	Less hierarchic, type "convoy"	Interactive	Cooperative
Disease model	Malfunction of cells or organs	Conflicts	Environment problems	Life style problems
Planning orientation	Hospitals	Health services	Society	Health
Time horizon	Present time	Past time	Future	Present time and future
Model of belief	Science and proven experience	Practice and ideology	Probabilities	Insight and knowledge
Field of work	Big institutions	Institutions of various sizes	Society	Informal and formal groups and individuals
Ideal of care	Specialization	Moderate specialization	Optimation	Self-care
Focus	Introvert	Relatively closed	Extrovert	Relatively open
Relations	Technically correct	Emotionally carrying	Informative	Motivation creating
Common concepts	"We must . . ."	"Let us look at . . ."	"By and large . . ."	"You can . . ."

10.7%. The percentage of the GNP spent on public health care services were in 1978: Sweden 10%, Norway 9.3%, Denmark 7.9%, Iceland 7.6%, and Finland 6.1%.

Denmark

Denmark has fourteen county councils, excluding the two cities of Copenhagen and Frederiksberg, which function as both municipal authorities and county councils. Since 1970, responsibilities have gradually been transferred from central government to local authorities. Under the health insurances system, the individual may choose which of the two health insurance groups he will belong to. Of the total population, 95% belong to group 1, meaning that once a year they choose a general practitioner within a specified geographic area, for tax-financed primary health care. For tax-financed specialist care, the general practitioner must issue a referral. Those who choose the second group are free to decide on a general practitioner and a specialist, but health services are not entirely tax financed in this group; the physician decides how much the patient should pay. In addition to what the patient pays, the physician receives an amount from the county council that administers health insurance. Half of the private practitioner's salary is, as a rule, based on the number of patients registered in group 1. The other part of his income is based on performance, depending mainly on the number of visits.

The state of Denmark contributes to a considerable extent to the financing of health services. The basis is "objective criteria" for need in the various county councils, such as population in certain age brackets, and hospital days. About 40% of health services costs are paid for in this way by the state.

Finland

Finland has no county councils; instead, 464 local municipalities provide hospital and health care. To compensate, the municipalities organize health care of different types in close cooperation. The Public Health Act from 1972 puts strong emphasis on primary care and prevention.

On the average, more than 50% of the financing is provided from the state of Finland. The contribution depends on how wealthy a certain municipality is. Characteristic for Finland is the strong influence from Helsinki over the developments in health care. A five-year plan determines how much personnel of different kinds should be employed, as well as the investments. Over the last few years Finland has succeeded at decreasing the proportion of the GNP that goes into health care, probably largely thanks to the strong ambition to deemphasize hospital care to the benefit of local health services.

Iceland

The Icelandic health insurance system is financed to 85% by the state. Most of the remaining 15% is paid by local municipalities. As this system of financing is also used for investments, one finds remarkably spacious health centers also in remote areas in Iceland.

About one-half of the population lives in Reykjavik; thus, health services naturally have their focus there. Iceland has its own medical university, and a relatively high percentage of the youngsters turn to medicine. The Icelandic Medical Association has a very strong position and has been able to protect its interests in spite of what seems to be a surplus of physicians.

Norway

About 50% of hospital running costs are paid by the state of Norway to the eighteen county councils and the city of Oslo, which administer the main health services. From 1981 a "framework budget," based on "objective criteria," replaced detailed budget regulations for the county councils.

The state of Norway is responsible for publicly employed district medical officers, but local authorities provide premises and equipment. The larger part of general practice is done by private practitioners, who are also used by local authorities in preventive medicine and school health services. It has been proposed that the local municipalities take over district physicians, and this reform is likely to take place within the next few years.

The 1970s saw a strong emphasis on hospital building thanks to generous state support. On the whole, however, Norway, like Finland and Denmark, focuses on local physicians as a core in health services.

Sweden

In the Nordic family, Sweden is the country that publishes most on the subject of long-range health planning. However, when it comes to results, Sweden lags far behind Finland, which has a more authoritarian tradition and places a stronger emphasis on national plans.

About 70% of health services costs are financed by the proportional county council tax, which varies between counties. The state of Sweden finances the major part of what remains, either by tax equalization support or other kinds of contributions. Patient fees cover a more or less symbolic amount. As in many other countries, discussions take place regarding how much should be paid directly by the patient at the time of consumption of health services. The change in 1976 from a social democratic to a nonsocialist government, or the turn back to social democratic administration in 1982, has not meant any major changes in health policy.

Nordic Cooperation

The five Nordic countries have harmonized their labor market, which means that health personnel as well as others can work in any Nordic country if they find it suitable and get a job. Another example of Nordic cooperation is the Nordic School of Public Health in Göteborg, which is responsible for higher education for physicians, administrators, nurses, and others in leading positions. The school was formed in 1953 and got its present structure under the Nordic Council of Ministers in 1978.

Literature Cited

Anderson, O.W. 1972. *Health care: Can there be equity? The United States, Sweden, and England.* New York: Wiley.

Blanpain, Jan, et al. 1978. *National health insurance and health resources.* Cambridge: Harvard University Press.

Calltorp, J. 1982. Växande överskott på specialister. *Läkartidningen* 36: 3019–20.

Carder, M., and B. Klingeberg. 1980. Towards a salaried medical profession: how "Swedish" was the seven crowns reform? In *The shaping of the Swedish health system,* ed. A.J. Heidenheimer and N. Elvander. London: Croom Helm.

Hälso- och sjukvården i en begränsad ekonomi. 1981. Stockholm: Spri/Landstingsförbundet.

Stephen, W.J. 1979. *An analysis of primary medical care. An international study.* Cambridge: Cambridge University Press.

Tarschys, D., ed. 1975. *Offentlig sektor i tillväxt.* Stockholm: Studieförbundet Näringsliv och Samhälle.

Statistical tables for Sweden are grouped with the data for the other Nordic countries and appear at the end of the chapter on Denmark.—ED.

Health Services in the Union of Soviet Socialist Republics

Norma K. Raffel

INTRODUCTION

The Union of Soviet Socialist Republics is the largest country in the world, occupying one-sixth of the earth's land surface. It stretches from the Pacific Ocean across northern Asia through eastern Europe to the Baltic Sea, covering an area of approximately 8.6 million square miles. There are extremes of climate ranging from the frigid temperatures of the Arctic to the stifling heat of the desert. The population in 1981 was 267.7 million and included over 100 distinct national groups. The Slavs, who live mainly in the republics of Russia, the Ukraine, and Belorussia, are by far the largest group. Although many languages are spoken, Russian is the official language of the country.

The USSR is a federation of fifteen Union republics. Within four of the Union republics, major national groups are subdivided into autonomous Soviet socialist republics and autonomous regions.* The largest Union republic is the Russian Federal Socialist Republic, which contains 42% of the population (139 million) and 76% of the territory of the USSR. Within the Russian republic are sixteen autonomous republics. The Ukraine republic is the next largest in population, with 50 million people. The other republics each have populations of 16 million or less. Approximately 63% of the Soviet people live in cities or towns and 37% in rural areas, many of which are sparsely populated.

Each republic is divided into oblasts (regions), and each oblast into rayons (districts). The population of an oblast ranges from half a million to several million. The population of a rayon ranges from a few thousand in rural areas to half a million in a city like Moscow. This organizational structure is used for health as well as other administrative purposes. In the *health* organization, each rayon is divided into uchastocks (community units serviced by a physician). In urban areas there are four types of uchastocks: those covering an adult population of about 2,000, those covering a child population of 800 to 1,000, obstetrical and gynecological uchastocks, and industrial uchastocks covering about 2,000 workers at a particular factory or group of factories.[1]

*An *autonomous* republic is subordinate to a *Union* republic, which, in turn, is subordinate to the *All-Union* Republic. The All-Union Republic is synonymous with the Union of Soviet Socialist Republics.

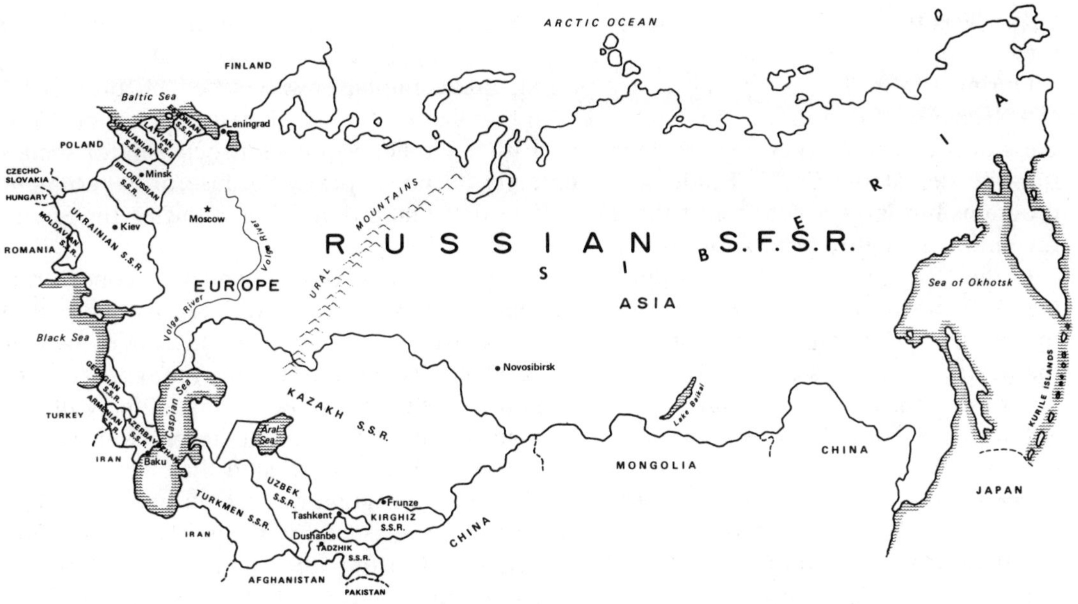

Uchastocks were first established in 1864 as part of the modernization of Russia by Alexander II and are thought to be the first attempt in the world to organize health services on a large scale.[2] This regionalization of health services was to provide primary care in the uchastocks and was directed mainly to the large rural population which at that time was inundated with infectious diseases (for example, typhoid fever, cholera, and smallpox). However, it was difficult to provide medical services to the rural populations. Despite generous incentives offered by the authorities, only 13% of the physicians in pre-Soviet Russia practiced in rural areas where 82% of the people lived. The rest practiced in cities, largely in private practice. According to Lidov, in 1913 there was approximately one doctor for 5,700 people in the entire country, but only one doctor for 26,200 people in the rural areas. There were 1.3 inpatient beds for 1,000 people overall, but only 1 bed for 4,400 in rural areas. Further, Russia lagged behind the rest of Europe in sanitary conditions: in 1912, as an example, there were 13 million cases of infectious diseases registered in the country.[3]

It is not surprising, therefore, that one of the primary concerns of the new Soviet government following the 1917 revolution was the health of its people—particularly the working people. As the new leader V.I. Lenin said, "The primary productive force of human society as a whole is the worker, the working people. If they survive, we shall save and restore everything."[4]

The Soviet health system did not take shape immediately. A considerable period of time elapsed from the moment its fundamental principles and tasks were proclaimed until they were actually being implemented.[5] A health department was established on the first day the Soviets assumed power in October 1917, but the fundamental political document that determined the basic principles and process of implementation of the Soviet health system (as well as other social and economic reforms)—the Program of the Russian Communist Party—was not adopted until 1919. As Navarro notes, the initial effort was on "enlarging and redistributing the numbers and types of resources. More and better distribution was the motto."[6] More doctors were produced, but it was still difficult to persuade them to work in rural areas.

During the early postrevolutionary period, great emphasis was placed on preventive care because of continuing epidemics. Lenin highlighted the problem at the second Congress of Medical Workers by proclaiming, "Either the lice will defeat socialism, or socialism will defeat the lice."[7] Epidemics eventually declined, partly because of government programs but largely because of the increase in the standard of living following the Soviet revolution at the end of World War I.

In the 1920s, when Stalin introduced a major change in economic policy by concentrating on the development of heavy industry, health services were more intensively directed toward the industrial effort. Since there was a shortage of manpower, the major task of the health service system was thus to boost productivity by reducing the time lost at work due to disability, and to ensure that workers took sick leave only when genuinely ill. To attain this, the number of sanitary-epidemiological units at industrial enterprises increased rapidly. These units supervised the safety of the workers and treated their illnesses. As women workers in industry increased, a special health program was established for maternal and child health. At the same time, polyclinics existed for the adult nonworking population of the community. (Polyclinics originated in the 1880s and combined outpatient primary medical care with specialist services for a variety of illnesses.) These three types of health service, operating with almost no coordination, exist in the current health system. The Soviet health system thus did not develop a comprehensive service at the outset; rather, it developed incrementally in response to specific needs as they arose.

An important document in the development of Soviet health care is *Fundamental Principles of Health Legislation of the Union of Soviet Socialist Republics and Union Republics,* which was adopted by the Supreme Soviet in 1969.[8] It defines the current rights and obligations of state agencies, public organizations, and citizens in the field of health. Article 4 states, "Citizens of the USSR shall be entitled to free and professional medical assistance readily available to all. It shall be provided by public health establishments administered by the state." The principles of health organization, the jurisdiction, authority, and administrative responsibilities of the state and Union republics are also defined, and there are sections on medical and pharmaceutical practice, sanitary and epidemic control, medical services, maternal and child health, treatment at sanatoria, special medical examinations, medications, and artificial limbs.

The system of Soviet health services is thus based on the principle that the health of the people is the responsibility of the government. Therefore, the Soviet or All-Union minister of health is ultimately responsible for all the medical and health activities of the fifteen Union republics. The minister of health is a member of the Council of Ministers of the USSR; the ministers are appointed by the Supreme Soviet of the USSR—the highest level of government. The minister of health directs the health services of the entire country through the ministries of health and the Union republics (see chart 1). The minister of health of a Union republic, in turn, administers the health services within the republic with guidance from the republic's council of ministers. This administration is exercised through local health authorities, agencies, institutions, and organizations directly subordinate to it, as well through some ministries of health of autonomous republics where they exist. At each level of the health organization there is a corresponding level of the political organization to which it is responsible (for example, ministry of health of a Union republic is supervised by the republic's council of ministers). Thus, health authorities at each level are responsible to two authorities—the appropriate local level governing body in general matters and the superior level health agency in departmental matters. This dual

Chart 1 Structure of health services in USSR

Political Supervision	Administrative Responsibility	Population Covered
USSR Supreme Soviet		
USSR Council of Ministers	USSR Ministry of Health	268 million
Republic Council of Ministers	Republic Ministry of Health	Up to 139 million[a]
Executive Committee, Oblast Soviet of Workers Deputies	Oblast Department of Health (regional)	1.5 million[b]
Executive Committee, Rayon Soviet of Workers Deputies	Rayon Department of Health (district)	40,000 to 150,000
	Uchastocks	About 4,000
	Feldsher-Midwife Post (in rural areas)	700 to 3,800

[a]All but 2 republics have populations of 16 million or less.
[b]Autonomous republics have a ministry of health similar to oblast Department of Health.

responsibility facilitates taking into account both national interests and local needs, and is similar to situations found in the United States and other countries where the local health agency is responsible both to local elected or appointed officials and to state health departments.

Health services in the USSR, like the economy and other social services, are developed on the basis of long-term, five-year, and annual plans. The planning process begins at the local level (that is, uchastock hospitals), which forwards its requirements to the next level (rayon hospitals), which incorporates the local requirements in its requirements and conveys them to the next level, until the requirements for the entire republic are gathered at the republic ministry of health. The needs of the republic are submitted to the central planning agency of the republic, approved by the republic council of ministers, and then they go the the USSR ministry of health and to Gosplan, which is the agency responsible for all aspects of planning and allocation of resources—namely, industry, agriculture, housing, education, health, etc. Finally, the plan is approved by the Council of Ministers of the USSR and the Supreme Soviet. The health needs are considered in relation to other areas of national need when determining priorities and the allocation of funds. The five-year health plan gives overall direction and sets priorities. The USSR ministry of health also sets "norms" and standards (for example, number of beds serving population, number of doctors serving various population groups, number of hospitals for population, etc.). The republics plan facilities and services in accordance with established norms and the budget that is allocated by the All-Union (USSR) ministry of health. When planning, the republic takes into account the needs of the republic and local areas, and may supplement the All-Union budget allocation by grants of money from industry or trade unions. By using supplementary funds, there is some flexibility for obtaining equipment and indeed even facilities which exceed the norms.

In urban areas the core of primary medical care is the polyclinic. The polyclinics are sometimes situated in conjunction with hospitals, but most are located away from the hospital site. There are separate polyclinics for adults, children, and industrial workers; there are separate clinics for maternity and gynecological cases, called women's consultation clinics. The area served by a polyclinic is divided into uchastocks, each of which is serviced by an uchastock physician. Uchastock physicians see patients at their polyclinic offices during the morning and make home visits during the afternoon. Important parts of their work are health education and "dispensarization"—which is the active follow-up of healthy population groups having similar physiological characteristics or similar working conditions, and of persons suffering from certain diseases. The purpose of this activity is to improve the health and increase the lifespan of the dispensarized. Uchastock physicians are usually the patients' first contact in the health system. They may treat patients, refer them to a variety of specialist teams (internal medicine, surgery, urology, oncology, infectious diseases, etc.—the number of specialities varies with the size of the polyclinic), or send them to a hospital.

As mentioned previously, health care for workers at large industrial enterprises is usually provided by separate polyclinics and hospitals. These medical health units are located at large industrial enterprises where there are more than 4,000 workers, and at chemical, coal mining, and oil refining enterprises with more than 2,000 workers.[9] Often family members of the workers are also treated. Workers who do not have such medical units at their places of work use the polyclinic in their communities. An industrial enterprise may have its own hospital or combine resources with another enterprise to build one. The medical facilities at the enterprises usually have sanatoria—prophylactoria located at or near the place of work to help improve the health of the workers (without interrupting their work) by using physiotherapy, mineral waters, pine and paraffin and other baths, mud therapy, and "oxygen cocktails."

The main function of the industrial medical health units is to reduce sick leave illnesses by providing high-level specialized care to workers, improving working conditions that affect the health of the worker, and preventing work-related accidents and disease. One mechanism for reducing accidents and illnesses is to set up "shop health posts" in various departments of the enterprise. These posts are supervised by the physicians in the medical health unit but are usually staffed by feldshers (see section on paramedical personnel). These posts carry out preventive activities, monitor working conditions that affect health and safety, and give primary care in case of accidents, poisoning, and sudden illness.

Another task of the industrial medical health unit is preventive health screening and dispensarization. In 1980 it was estimated that 60 to 70% of all industrial workers in the Soviet Union were under dispensarization.[10]

The health facilities at industrial enterprises are under the supervision of the republic ministry of health and they must consult with the ministry when planning additional structures or purchasing large, expensive pieces of equipment, and follow norms established by the All-Union ministry. The republic ministry of health pays the salaries of all health personnel, but the enterprise may offer bonuses to attract highly qualified people. The enterprises pay for buildings and equipment, which generally results in superior facilities. If workers must be admitted to hospitals that serve the general public, they are given priority. The quality of medical care at industrial enterprises substantiates the statement that "Priority in providing medicare to industrial workers, especially in the leading branches of industry, construction, and transport, was and remains one of the main tasks of the Soviet health services."[11]

The health care of the rural population is provided for by an organization that is similar to the urban organization but special because of the vast areas covered. The first point of contact with the health care system in rural areas is usually the feldsher-midwife post. Most villages and collective farms have such a post, which is staffed by paramedical personnel—a feldsher and a midwife, or one person combining both roles—who are supervised by a physician from the rural uchastock hospital. The tasks of the feldsher-midwife post are to provide first aid, treat minor illnesses, carry out immunization programs, improve sanitation and hygiene, and conduct a dispensarization program. There is an emphasis on preventive measures and home visits are frequent. Depending on the distance and travel conditions, there may be a few beds at the post for inpatient care. The population served by a feldsher-midwife post is 700 to 3,000, depending on the size of the village and the distance to other health facilities. It is planned eventually to replace feldshers with physicians for clinical activities, to combine some posts, and to close the small inpatient units.

Serious or complicated illnesses encountered at the feldsher-midwife posts can be treated by visiting physicians or the sick persons can be sent to the local hospital that has a basic staff. The rural (uchastock) hospital works closely with the rayon hospital, which has a variety of specialists available for consultation. Difficult cases are sent to the rayon hospital and unusual cases to the oblast hospital, which has a full range of specialties.

In addition to the above, the ministry of health administers the Fourth Administration (sometimes known as the Fourth Department), which caters to high government and Soviet party officials. It has grown from a Moscow-only service to a nationwide service with elite medical facilities located in each republic. There are also a number of Soviet medical facilities that are not under the supervision or control of the ministry of health; these serve special population groups and provide a higher level of care than is found in the public sector. Among these are facilities operated by the ministries of foreign trade, finance, railroads, higher and intermediate education, foreign affairs, the aviation industry, and the Academy of Sciences. The ministry of defense, merchant marine, civil aviation, the KGB, and the MVD maintain their own complete systems of medical care. Facilities and systems operated apart from the ministry of health are not considered in this chapter.

MEDICAL PRACTICE

The two most striking features of medical practice in the Soviet Union are the large physician to population ratio and the high degree of physician specialization.

There has been a dramatic increase in the number of physicians over the years, so that in 1980 there were 995,600 physicians, or 374 physicians for each 100,000 persons—more than any other developed country except Israel, and close to the ideal ratio of 382 per 100,000 established by the USSR ministry of health in 1973. It is estimated that nearly one-third of the world's physicians are in the Soviet Union.[12] The ratio varies among the republics from 234 per 100,000 in the Tajik republic to 467 per 100,000 in the Georgian republic.

The distribution of physicians among the republics, and between the urban and rural areas, is a continuing problem. Neither the assignment of physicians to areas of need upon completion of their medical studies, nor the incentives offered (higher pay, better living conditions, automobiles, early retirement, etc.) have significantly changed the situation. Many new physicians are able to evade being assigned to rural areas, and those who cannot often do not remain in rural areas once their compulsory service is completed. The disadvantages of living in remote regions—trying to practice modern medicine with the facilities in those areas—and the decrease in opportunities to advance have not been offset by any inducements yet offered.

Although not forbidden, private practice is actively discouraged, so virtually all medical practice is under the aegis of the state. However, Ryan and others report that "tipping," or unofficial payment, is rather common for services provided ostensibly under the state scheme.[13] A 1982 report by the Communist party's powerful Central Committee intimated that medical workers sometimes accepted bribes.[14] Physicians are paid a salary according to experience, specialization, and nature of work with funds provided by the republic ministry of health from All-Union ministry of health allocations. However, industrial enterprises often give bonuses of up to 40% of the physician's pay, and some establishments pay physicians an extra month's salary. There is a wide range of remuneration and prestige among physicians—the highest for those in academic medicine and the lowest for uchastock physicians. The *average* salary is 2,000 to 2,500 rubles a year, close to that of an engineer.

Some physicians in the Soviet Union, especially those in academic medicine and research, devote all available time to professional activities; however, most Soviet physicians work 6 to 7 hours a day, 5 days a week, with occasional weekend and little, if any, night duty.

The average primary care physician in a polyclinic or industrial medical unit usually spends the morning seeing patients at the clinic office, most of the afternoon making home visits, some time on health education and dispensarization programs, and considerable time filling out medical documents. One study reported that on the average, a physician in the clinic spends 2.4 minutes interviewing a patient, 2.9 minutes examining the patient, 1.8 minutes giving advice, and 4.5 minutes on medical documentation.[15] It is not known whether the amount of time the physician spends on each patient follows the official guidelines specifying how many patients should be seen each hour at the polyclinic and on home visits.

Uchastock physicians at polyclinics are assigned about 2,000 adults in their uchastock. This physician serves only adults. Children and women needing obstetrical or gynecological treatment in the same geographic area are assigned to special clinics. As mentioned earlier, the uchastock, or primary care, physicians treat minor health problems, refer patients to specialists at the clinic, and send patients to the hospital. Even when polyclinics and hospitals are located at the same site, physicians almost always work exclusively in one or the other.

Specialization is a key feature of Soviet medicine. It is based on the premise that "the new requirements of Soviet public health and the modern level of medical science demand that the main form of medical aid to the population be specialized medical assistance. The doctor of today must be a specialist in one of the medical professions."[16] The increased emphasis on specialization has resulted in a significant decrease in the number of "doctors of general practice." There are fifty-one official medical specialties (see chart 2); the last

Chart 2 Nomenclature of medical specialists and territorial level of their employment

		Level of Employment		
	Specialty	Rural Medical Sector	Institutions of a Rural District	Remaining Institutions
1	General physician	+	+	+
2	Cardiorheumatologist		+	+
3	Gastroenterologist			+
4	Nephrologist			+
5	Endocrinologist		+	+
6	Hematologist			+
7	Specialist in infectious diseases	+	+	+
8	Dietician		+	+
9	Physiotherapist		+	+
10	Specialist in curative physical culture and sport		+	+
11	General physician in clinical physiology (electrocardiography and functional diagnosis)		+	+
12	Surgeon	+	+	+
13	Pediatric surgeon		+	+
14	Traumatologist-orthopedist		+	+
15	Urologist		+	+
16	Neurosurgeon			+
17	Anesthesiologist-reanimationist		+	+
18	Cardiovascular surgeon			+
19	Thoracic surgeon			+
20	Oncologist		+	+
21	Oncological surgeon		+	+
22	Oncological gynecologist		+	+
23	Oncological otorhinolaryngologist		+	+
24	Oncological radiologist		+	+
25	Stomatologist	+	+	+
26	Stomatological surgeon			+
27	Stomatological orthopedist		+	+
28	Obstetrician-gynecologist	+	+	+
29	Pediatrician	+	+	+
30	Radiologist	+	+	+
31	Ophthalmologist		+	+
32	Pediatric ophthalmologist			+
33	Otorhinolaryngologist		+	+
34	Specialist in tuberculosis		+	+
35	Neuropathologist		+	+
36	Psychiatrist		+	+
37	Dermato-venereologist		+	+
38	Pathologist-anatomist		+	+
39	Toxicologist			+
40	Laboratory specialist		+	+
41	Forensic-medical specialist		+	+
42	Specialist in general hygiene		+	+
43	Specialist in communal hygiene		+	+
44	Specialist in occupational hygiene		+	+
45	Specialist in food hygiene		+	+
46	Specialist in the hygiene of children and adolescents		+	+
47	Specialist in radiation hygiene			+

Chart 2 *Continued*

	Specialty	Level of Employment: Rural Medical Sector	Institutions of a Rural District	Remaining Institutions
48	Epidemiologist (disinfectionist, parasitologist)		+	+
49	Bacteriologist (virologist)		+	+
50	Social hygienist-administrator (health administrator, statistician, specialist in methods of instruction, specialist in sanitary education)		+	+
51	Doctor of general practice	+	+	+

SOURCE: G.A. Popov, *Problemi vrachebnikh kadrov,* pp. 55–56, as reported by Ryan.

NOTE: Specialists in gastroenterology, nephrology, hematology, neurosurgery, cardiovascular surgery, thoracic surgery, dental surgery (maxillary-facial surgery) can be appointed only to the inpatient sections of hospitals or to the consultative polyclinics of regional (territorial) and republican hospitals.

is the doctor of general practice. Specialization begins upon entrance to the medical institute when the future physician chooses among the separate and distinct programs of curative medicine (internal medicine), pediatrics, environmental medicine, and stomatology. (Soviet statistics include stomatologists in the number of physicians and doctors. They represent 10 to 12% of the total physician population. Stomatologists are a kind of dental specialist, are different from dentists who do more routine work and are considered middle-level health workers.) The further specialization that occurs as medical training continues is described in the section on medical education.

Some Soviet health officials are concerned that the amount of specialization may be adversely affecting the quality of medical care and increasing the number of physicians required. G.A. Popov, a prominent health economist, said: "We have so many specialists already that no one is taking charge of the entire patient. We are duplicating services and many persons are being shuttled from one specialist to another. . . . All of these many contacts . . . make our system very inefficient and unnecessarily expensive."[17] As a result of specialization and the resulting compartmentalization of medical practice, a family can be attending four or more different clinics at the same time. For example, a woman may attend a polyclinic for a digestive complaint and a women's consultation clinic for a gynecological problem, may take children fifteen years or younger to a pediatric clinic, while her husband attends a clinic at his place of work. There is little, if any, coordination among these separate establishments. Another problem of increased specialization is that, as the number of specialists required in different areas fluctuates, physicians in one specialty may be required to practice in another.

There are various commissions and councils of physicians to advise on new methods of treatment and to ensure that uniform standards of medical care are provided at medical establishments, but physicians do not have an organizational structure through which they can influence medical policies. They belong to the Union of Medical Workers, which represents all medical workers and acts primarily as an adjunct to the Communist party and the government of the USSR.[18]

The point of entry into the health care system for most people living in cities and towns is the polyclinic or the medical health unit at the place of employment. There they are either treated by physicians or admitted to the hospital. Those who are unable to go to the polyclinic, particularly the very young and old, will be visited by a physician in their homes. In rural areas, if there is not a polyclinic nearby, the usual point of entry into the health care system is the feldsher-midwife post, where the patient is treated for minor illnesses, seen by visiting specialists, or admitted to the hospital if necessary. Although it is discouraged, patients can seek admission to the hospital without first consulting physicians at the polyclinic, industrial medical unit, or rural health post.

In large cities there are a series of first-aid stations located in places, such as major subway stations, where there are large numbers of people. These stations are staffed by a feldsher and a nurse who give first aid and, when necessary, call an ambulance.

An impressive feature of the Soviet health care system is the emergency medical service, or the *Skoraya.* It is organized separately from the polyclinic or hospital, and provides emergency medical care at the site of an emergency in cases such as accidents (burns, fractures, wounds, poisoning) or sudden life-threatening situations (heart attacks, respiratory difficulties, loss of consciousness, etc.), as well as transporting the patient to the hospital.

The emergency care system can be activated by dialing 03 on the telephone in any place in the Soviet Union. In cities, the call is received at a central station and is relayed to a substation, which dispatches an ambulance. Each ambulance has a team consisting of a physician, a feldsher, and a driver. There are special ambulances for accidents and cardiac, neurologic, pediatric, and obstetric emergencies. These ambulances have special equipment and special teams. A regular ambulance team can summon one of the special ambulances if necessary. Ambulances have a radio-telephone system and medical equipment, although random observation of regular ambulances in three Soviet cities revealed little, if any, equipment. Ambulances are mentioned as one of the shortcomings to be dealt with in the report issued by the Central Committee of the Communist party as reported in *Pravda* in August 1982. The physicians and feldshers in the Skoraya receive about two months of specialized training. Because a physician is part of the emergency team, the patient can be diagnosed and treated on the spot at a more sophisticated level than can be done by paramedical personnel. Also, the physician can decide whether to leave the patient at home and may contact the uchastock physician rather than admit to the hospital, which happens the majority of the time. Hospitals are obliged to take patients brought in by the Skoraya regardless of the availability of beds.

In rural areas, the emergency service is based at the local hospital. When the distances involved are great, airplanes, helicopters, motor boats, and cross-country vehicles are used.

HOSPITALS

As a consequence of the heavy destruction during World War II, there has been a massive increase in the number of hospitals and hospital beds in the Soviet Union, so that in 1980 there were 22,323 medical institutions providing inpatient care with a total of 3,324,200 beds. This represents 12.1 beds per 1,000 population, which exceeds similar figures for most industrialized countries with the exceptions of Norway, Sweden, and Finland. As with other health facilities, there is considerable variation among the republics, ranging from 8.34 per 1,000 in the Armenian republic to 13.68 in the Latvian republic. As in other countries, the urban areas are better served than rural areas.

The Soviet health system is very hospital centered. In part, this is a result of the high degree of specialization and the absence of general practitioners or family physicians. Under these circumstances, Ryan maintains that "out-patient specialists can hardly avoid a presumption that more sophisticated and effective treatment is available in hospital and as a consequence are all the more prepared to relinquish clinical responsibility to colleagues ranking at a higher level of medical technology."[19] This results in a high rate of hospitalization for illnesses which could be satisfactorily treated on an outpatient basis.

Administratively, the health services are dominated by hospitals. The major financial resources for Soviet health care are allocated to them. They not only treat the sick but are responsible for training medical personnel and for medical research. At the district (rayon) level, the chief physician who coordinates outpatient services is also the head of the district hospital as well as of all uchastock hospitals in that district. This administration, however, operates—as does the entire system—under norms and standards set by the All-Union ministry of health, which include such things as the amount of linen needed per bed and the workload of physicians in each specialty. To prevent the hospital from draining resources from polyclinics, the latter were physically and clinically separated.

Hospitals in the Soviet Union fit into the regional system of health services. At the lowest level is the uchastock hospital with 35 to 100 beds serving a population of about 4,000, located largely in the rural areas. Depending on the size and location, these hospitals have from two to six staff physicians, of whom one is usually a surgeon. When patients need more specialized attention, they are referred to the rayon (district) or oblast (regional) hospitals. The trend is to increase the number of beds in uchastock hospitals to about 100 in order to provide a more adequate number of specialists. Even so, many people in areas close to cities prefer to go directly to the city hospitals for more skilled medical care. In some remote areas there are inpatient units of 5 or more beds, but with the improvement in roads and transportation, these are being either closed or combined.

The next level of hospital is the rayon, or district, hospital, with 100 to 300 beds serving a population of 40,000 to 150,000. These hospitals have fourteen to sixteen specialties, and most of their patients are referred from the uchastock hospitals.

The next higher level of hospital is the oblast, or regional, hospital, with 600 to 1,200 beds serving a population of 1 to 5 million. These hospitals have a full range of specialties. Large cities may function as a single oblast. Currently, few hospitals are built with more than 1,000 beds, the rationale being to reduce management difficulties.

Besides these adult general medical and surgical hospitals, there are separate hospitals at industrial enterprises, specialized hospitals for children, obstetrics, as well as oncological hospitals, psychiatric and psychoneurological hospitals, tuberculosis hospitals, and infectious disease hospitals. In addition, there are All-Union specialized centers that serve all republics, such as the All-Union Scientific Cardiological Center with an inpatient department of 1,400 beds, and the All-Union Oncological Scientific Center with a 1,000 bed inpatient department.

Most often the physicians in the outpatient units refer patients to the lower level hospital and they are then transferred to a higher level if necessary. However, patients can be admitted to any level that can provide the required services. If a diagnosis is made at the polyclinic, patients can be admitted directly to specialized hospitals (e.g., oncological hospitals). People can seek direct admission to hospitals without going to outpatient units, but this is discouraged.

There is a very high rate of hospitalization. The number of persons admitted per year to hospitals continues to increase, reaching 22.1 for each 100 persons in urban areas and 23.6 for each 100 persons in rural areas in 1980.[20] As mentioned before, Soviet physicians tend to admit patients for conditions that are often treated on an ambulatory basis in other countries. For example, Stephen reports that "it appears to be a routine policy that many children under two years of age who are seen with a fever are admitted to hospital."[21]

Other factors that contribute to increased hospital admission are overcrowded living conditions and the lack of persons to care for the ill at home due to the large number of women in the paid labor force (about 85%).

The average length of stay in Soviet hospitals is about eighteen days. Patients are sometimes admitted four or five days before surgery.[22] In contrast to many other countries, the length of stay continues to increase rather than decrease.

The average occupancy of beds in urban areas in 1980 was 339 days per year, for a 93% occupancy rate; this is high when compared to many developed countries. The occupancy rate is the most often mentioned index of efficiency.[23] If it is of prime importance to keep the occupancy rate high, it is understandable that the average length of stay remains high. It has been suggested that extended hospital stays are caused by overloaded diagnostic departments and laboratories, and bottlenecks in operating theatres and treatment departments due to the shortage of machinery, anesthetics, suture material, and/or staff. There is, of course, no incentive to speed up the process: the patient receives adequate social security benefits, and the hospitals' average day costs per patient decrease rapidly following surgery, thus enabling a hospital to cope more easily with a tight budget linked to bed days.

According to Ryan, the USSR minister of health stated in 1968 that "hospitalization is not always provided in good time, especially for patients suffering from chronic diseases." Smith reports that nonemergency surgery dealing with chronic conditions often requires a waiting period of several months and even years at very prestigious institutions.[24] Nevertheless, in 1982 physicians at hospitals visited by the author claimed the longest waiting period to be one week—and that would be for elective surgery. It would be interesting to know how such a high occupancy rate can be maintained with practically no waiting lists for admissions.

Ryan reports that Soviet officials, concerned since the late 1960s that there be a more efficient use of hospital beds, stress that a reduction in the average duration of stay and an increase in annual average occupancy rate of a hospital bed would enable more patients to be hospitalized. Convalescence and rehabilitation units have been established to enable more efficient use of hospital beds. Also, some effort has been made to reduce hospital admissions by performing diagnostic tests on an outpatient rather than inpatient basis, and to improve the diagnostic capability of polyclinics.

Despite this, however, at the institutional level there appears to be little concern among physicians for reducing the length of hospital stay or controlling hospital costs.

Hospital services, like other health services, are free of charge at time of use. There is often a shortage of drugs, and disposable equipment is not available. High technology equipment is also frequently reported to be in short supply.

Hospital wards were observed to have a minimum of four beds, but typically more, and beds were sometimes placed in halls. There are virtually no private rooms and no "pay" rooms in the hospitals. However, there are "closed" hospitals and polyclinics known as the "Fourth Department" in the ministry of health, which provide superior hospital accommodations and care to certain elite people such as party members.[25] A very limited number of fee-for-service polyclinics have been reported to exist in a number of cities for general citizen convenience; the fees, however, do not go to the physicians.[26]

Sanatoria

There is heavy emphasis in Soviet medicine on the prevention of disease and health maintenance. It goes beyond the control of infectious diseases and the establishment of environmental standards, to the screening of populations at risk (dispensarization) and the provision of sanatoria and health resorts. The sanatoria are cooperative ventures between the ministry of health and the trade union organizations, and are considered an important aspect of the Soviet health system. They are based on the premise that some forms of disease can be effectively treated by removing patients from the daily stresses of life and treating them with rest, exercise, good diet, mineral or mud baths, heat treatments, massage, etc. Trade unions usually have their own or shared sanatoria where workers may go for three weeks for such illnesses as high blood pressure, diabetes, heart disease, ulcers, arthritis, and "stress." Some seem to have no specific medical problems but go for rest and relaxation. Each facility has a full-time medical staff, and each patient has an individual program to follow. Many sanatoria are located in resort areas on the Baltic, Black, or Caspian seas. Although theoretically open to all workers, it is reported that the sanatoria and health resorts are used as a reward for superior performance by workers. Although the trade union organizations sometimes meet the entire cost, the worker often must pay a portion, usually about 30%. There are also specialized local children's sanatoria.

In 1980 there were 13,141 sanatoria and rest and recreation establishments with 2,138,000 beds in which 40,040,000 people were treated.

MEDICAL EDUCATION

Scientific medicine was introduced to Russia during the reign of Peter the Great, the first medical school being established in 1706. It placed great emphasis on anatomy, following the European approach in which medicine was perceived as an intervention to repair parts of the body and achieve a balance between its fluids and solids.[27] The number of physicians grew from 10,000 in 1864 to 23,000 in 1913, and their training continued to follow the European approach to medicine.[28] By 1913 there were seventeen higher medical schools in all of Russia which graduated about 900 physicians each year.[29]

After the Soviet Revolution, measures were immediately taken to increase the number of physicians, and medical education continued to follow the traditional European model. Between 1918 and 1922, sixteen higher medical schools were established to train physicians, and by 1928 the number of physicians grew to 63,162.[30] Also, the years required for an adequate medical education were increased from three to four, while preventive medicine and hygiene were added as disciplines.[31]

According to Navarro, the sex and class of medical students changed radically at that time. As a result of the Soviet Revolution, universities and medical schools admitted both sexes as well as all classes and races of people who had been discriminated against previously. Preference was given to peasants, members of the working class, and women. Before the revolution women had accounted for less than 10% of all medical students and they could attend only special medical schools. In order to increase the number of physicians from the working class, special schools were established so that workers with at least three years of industrial employment could study to meet the entrance requirements of medical schools while continuing their employment.

The continuing need to increase the number of physicians and to improve their skills caused the Soviet government to reorganize the training of physicians in 1930. Physicians were required to be trained at medical establishments where specialized training as a general practitioner, pediatrician, health officer, or stomatologist was introduced. Medical faculties of universities were reorganized into separate medical institutes, and the post-graduate training of physicians was transferred from the system of public education to the People's Commissariat of Health. The number of physicians continued to grow, so that by 1940, Soviet medical establishments graduated 16,400. Also, between 1930 and 1940 the number of medical institutes grew from forty to seventy-two; these institutes were located at all of the Union republics.

In 1938 basic medical education was divided into three main specialties: general medicine, maternal and child care, and sanitation and hygiene. Training in these specialties started at the beginning of medical training. According to Navarro, this specialization was largely to meet the needs of industrialization to give preferential treatment to workers in leading branches of industry.

Between the 1930s and the 1940s the length of medical training increased to six years, after which the graduates were assigned their first clinical post. In 1968 a year of internship in large regional or city hospitals was added before students could take the state examination and be assigned a post.

Currently, the training of higher medical personnel in the USSR is conducted at eighty-three medical institutes and at nine university medical departments. Higher medical personnel include physicians, pharmacists, and stomatologists. There are five basic tracks in higher medical education: (1) the medical faculty (department), which includes internal medicine, surgery, obstetrics, and gynecology; (2) the pediatric faculty; (3) the stomatologic faculty (dentistry); (4) the sanitary medicine and social hygiene faculty (public health); (5) the pharmacologic faculty. Very few medical institutes have all five faculties; most have three or less. There is also a medical biological faculty at some institutes to train research scientists, but the number of students in this group in 1980 was quite small—about 1,000 for the entire country. In 1980 there were 34,426 students receiving higher medical training at medical institutes, of which 83% (28,426) were training to be physicians. The other 17% were studying stomatology, pharmacology, and medical biological sciences.

All of the higher medical education institutions follow a standard curriculum, which has been established by the USSR ministry of health with the cooperation of the USSR ministry of higher and special secondary education. The training of physicians (whether in the medical, pediatric, sanitary, or dental faculty) is essentially the same in the first two years, when they receive general biological and sociopolitical training.[32] Students study anatomy, histology, biology, chemistry, physics, physiology, and foreign languages, as well as history of the Communist party, political economy, and philosophy. Beginning in the third year, the curriculum differs for each of the faculties, so that the general courses—pathological anatomy, pathological physiology, microbiology, pharmacology, principles of internal diseases, and surgery—have a different emphasis depending on the faculty. For example, in the pediatrics faculty considerable time is devoted to age-group physiology, pathology of children, and children's diseases. In the sanitary-hygiene department clinical subjects are taught, but much less than in the medical faculty, and the main attention is devoted to pathogenesis and etiology of diseases and the effect of environment on public health. During the fourth and fifth years, students become further acquainted with the medical specialties within their track, observe patients, and work as low-level assistants. Students in the medical faculty work as nurses in hospitals during the summers. In the sixth year there is further specialization within the broad specialty. For example, students in the medical faculty can specialize in general medicine or surgery or obstetrics and gynecology, while students in the pediatric faculty can choose pediatrics, infectious diseases, or pediatric surgery. During the one-year internship, the new physicians may continue in their previous specialties or work in a narrow specialty for which they have suitable training. For example, a physician who specialized in surgery during the sixth year could intern in urology or ophthalmology. This specialization in physician training was explained in 1968 by the minister of health as being necessary because "it is impossible to conceive that only a single doctor with a broad background could fully guarantee highly qualified care for patients suffering from a variety of illnesses which are frequently complicated to diagnose and treat."

At the end of the sixth year of medical education, each student takes an oral examination given by a team of physicians from the ministry of health, other medical institutes, and professors from the student's own medical institute. The examination lasts about thirty minutes for each student and includes the observation and diagnosis of patients. Very few students fail because poor students usually drop out by the fourth year. Upon successfully completing the examination, the student receives a diploma and proceeds to a one-year internship. Interns are distributed to large regional or city hospitals in different parts of the country, according to the country's need and each graduate's situation and desires. In situations where a woman is married or has a child under one year old, or if a man has invalid parents, they are not required to take internships away from home. Internships are usually in the areas where the new physician will serve his or her three years of compulsory service; this service is considered payment to society for the medical training received.

Persons completing a general secondary education of ten years, and who are not more than thirty-five years old, may apply for admission to one of the medical institutions that trains physicians. Acceptance depends upon competitive examinations that include a written examination in the Russian language—or the language used in teaching in the republic in which the institution is located—and oral examinations in physics, chemistry, and biology. Secondary school grades are considered as well as the grade in the "significant subject of the year"—biology, chemistry, or physics, depending on the kinds of physicians that are needed. There are three to five applicants for each space. Priority is sometimes given to persons who have advanced from nurse to feldsher, or to nurses who have served in oncological hospitals.

The student is not charged for tuition for higher medical training. Approximately 85% of the students receive state stipends, the state taking into consideration their grades and "their material status."[33] Textbooks are inexpensive, and most out-of-town students can be accommodated in dormitories.

Even though the physician to population ratio is close to the ideal determined by the ministry of health, and it exceeds the ratio of virtually all other developed countries, there is no indication in talks with health officials and medical educators that the number of physicians being trained will be significantly decreased.

Advanced Medical Training and Continuing Medical Education

There are seventeen separate institutes and forty different faculties for the advanced training of physicians. During 1980 more than 119,000 physicians participated in some form of advanced training. Almost all physicians provide three to five years of service before they receive advanced training. Occasionally, a very bright graduate can begin advanced training in research and teaching careers immediately after the internship, or after the sixth year if he or she studies in the basic medical sciences.

Physicians wishing to pursue a career in medical research or teaching are admitted to the program based on the results of oral examinations in their area of interest, one foreign language, and political philosophy; acceptance is also determined by the needs of country as seen by the USSR ministry of health. The admission to programs is regulated by the All-Union Council on Science and Technology, which selects a preceptor and approves the study plan. Students take advanced courses (sometimes at universities), seminars, and foreign language training, and are assigned readings in political philosophy. At the end of the first year, they are examined on the topics covered in the entrance examinations but on a more advanced level. Students also must prepare and defend a thesis based on their research. The program is usually completed in three years, after which they are awarded a certificate as a Candidate in Medical Sciences. Students then obtain a teaching post and/or continue research training for an additional five to seven years, prepare and defend another thesis, and then are eligible for the degree of Doctor of Medical Science—the most prestigious award physicians can obtain. There are approximately six Candidates in Medical Science for each Doctor of Medical Science.

In the clinical area, many physicians improve their skills and further specialize by spending two years in a large hospital, where they spend most of their time working in their specialty field and some time working in related services. During their training period, physicians receive some formal instruction and have considerable responsibility for patient care.

Another avenue for advanced training is provided by the two- to four-month courses offered by advanced training institutes. Students may study at the institute for the entire time, combine correspondence study with study at the institute, or attend courses in their local area taught by faculty from advanced training institutes who travel to various parts of the country and conduct courses in conjunction with correspondence study. Physicians interested in studying at an institute for advanced training submit a letter of application along with the endorsement of the chief of the hospital. The ministry of health decides which physicians are accepted, but there are also a number of discretionary spaces (20% at one institute). All expenses for the advanced training of physicians are paid by the ministry of health. It is the policy that physicians should receive advanced training every five years.

Few foreigners are permitted to practice medicine in the Soviet Union. Those who do must be permanent citizens and have been trained in Soviet institutions. Legislation on this point is explicit.

WOMEN IN SOVIET MEDICINE

Much attention has been focused on the large number of women physicians in the Soviet Union as compared to other countries. After the Soviet Revolution, the number of women physicians increased dramatically. It is interesting to note that this change parallels the greater emphasis on industrialization. During this period, an engineer had more prestige and received higher awards than did a physician. Partly because men were needed in heavy industry and partly because of a continuing drop in the status of medicine, women were actively encouraged to take up medicine.[34] Women were the last to join the labor force, and during this period of a worker shortage, they participated in virtually all sectors; they predominated, however, in those sectors that enjoyed less prestige, for example, health services. As Navarro bluntly stated, "The second-rate workers—women—were to perform the second-rate jobs."[35]

Between 1928 and 1934, the percentage of women doctors increased from 52 to 75%, reaching a peak immediately after World War II, when 76% of the physicians were women. It is unlikely that the impressive increase in medical services could have occurred in the period of great manpower shortages without a great influx of women into the profession.

Since then the percentage of women physicians has been slowly declining; in 1980 approximately 70% were women. Recent classes at medical institutes are about 40% women and 50% men. In 1970 a U.S. report on Soviet medical care maintained that "many administrators and faculty members stated the ideal ratio could be 30% women and 70% men, since women have difficulty raising families while doing professional work."[36] This is a curious statement given the facts that the majority of Soviet physicians work about six to seven hours a day in a five-day week and the number of children has decreased to one or two per family. At any rate, the number of women training to be physicians is decreasing. Ryan reports that the passing grade for admission to medical institutes is lower for men.[37] Physicians are now, according to medical administrators, becoming more "fashionable" (prestigious), and the salary of a physician approaches that of an engineer.

The prestige and rewards of the physicians vary, with Doctors of Medical Science near the top, and primary care physicians at the bottom. It is not surprising, then, to note that although women are present at all levels of medical hierarchy, the large majority (about 90%) are in primary care, fewer are in tertiary care (30 to 40% in surgery), and fewer yet are in important policy-making positions at the republic and All-Union levels.

MIDDLE MEDICAL WORKERS (PARAMEDICAL PERSONNEL)

Middle medical workers in the Soviet Union play a vital role in the fields of environmental health, prevention of disease, and treatment of patients. There are eight categories of workers trained at the middle medical level: nurses, midwives, feldshers, sanitarian-feldshers, feldsher-laborants, dental doctors, dental technicians, and pharmacists. In 1980 there were 2,789,900 middle medical workers, or 105 for each 10,000 persons. The ratio of middle medical workers to population has steadily increased (87 per 10,000 in 1970, 98 in 1975).

Depending upon the category, their training varies from one year and ten months to two years and six months for students with a complete secondary education of ten years. Students are accepted with eight years of schooling (except for candidates for dental doctor), and the training program is extended for one more year to include a "general education cycle," which includes Russian language, literature, physics, chemistry, social sciences, foreign language, and, in national republics, the national language.

The middle medical workers are trained at *secondary* medical schools which are separate from the medical institutes and university medical departments where physicians are trained. In 1980 a total of 426,006 students were being trained as middle medical workers at medical schools. These schools are somewhat evenly distributed throughout the Soviet Union. The USSR ministry of health provides overall supervision of middle medical education. The curricula are developed by the USSR ministry of health and endorsed by the USSR ministry of higher and special secondary education, and are uniform throughout the country. The administrators and teachers at middle medical schools are mostly physicians rather than experienced nurses, midwives, or feldshers, although certain practical techniques such as patient care might be taught by skilled middle medical workers.

Admission to the secondary medical schools is based on competitive examinations at the school selected. Applicants must be less than thirty years old and have at least eight years of general schooling. Those with eight years of school must pass a written examination in the Russian language and an oral mathematics examination. Those with ten years of schooling must pass written examinations in the Russian lanuage and literature and an oral chemistry examination.

Nurses comprise almost one-half of the middle medical workers (48.9%). Their length of training is one year and ten months for students with ten years of schooling, and two years and ten months for those with eight years. Students with only eight years of schooling must take general education courses. All nursing students take general medical courses—biology, anatomy, physiology, microbiology, pharmacology, hygiene, public health organization, and Latin. They also study special subjects such as care of patients; internal diseases; surgery; children's diseases; obstetrics and gynecology; infectious diseases; epidemiology; eye, ear, nose, and throat diseases; physiotherapy; massage; curative physical culture; typing and shorthand. More than one-half of the time devoted to special subjects is set aside for practical training. The student must pass a standard All-Union examination on internal, surgical, and children's diseases, and the care of patients with those diseases in order to be awarded a certificate of graduation from their school and for certification as "nurse." In some instances, untrained personnel, such as elevator operators, receive the same pay as nurses. There is a "small shortage of nurses," according to health officials interviewed in 1982.

The next largest group of middle medical workers (about 22%) is the feldsher. This type of medical worker is unique to the Soviet Union and dates back to the eighteenth century when Peter the Great introduced the feldsher concept, derived from the Swedish and German army field surgeons. The role of the feldsher has been broadened and enhanced over the years, and today this worker is quite active in Soviet health care, especially in the vast rural areas of the Soviet Union. In 1982 there were 90,000 first-post feldshers.[38]

The length of training for feldshers is two years and six months for students with a ten-year general education and three years and six months for those with an eight-year general education—a year longer than nurse training. Those with eight years of schooling must take one year of general education. All students take the general medical courses that cover the same subjects as the nurses' general medical courses. The course names in the special subjects are also the same, but for feldsher training there are more hours devoted to classroom, practical, and laboratory instruction. In addition, there are twenty weeks of practical experience in hospitals: one week as a sanitarian, four weeks providing patient care and learning medical technology, five weeks functioning as a nurse, and ten weeks of practical experience in regional or district hospitals in a specialty area. Students choosing to become a feldsher-midwife would take more classes and practical work in obstetrics and gynecology; those students choosing to become a feldsher-sanitarian would have increased class and practical work in epidemiology, infectious and parasitic diseases, hygiene of food service, and community living. The curriculum for feldshers, like that of all middle medical workers, is prepared by the USSR ministry of health and is used throughout the country. Oral examinations are required for graduation and certification.

Feldshers are able to perform a variety of services in the health system. They can:

> (1) Head a feldsher-midwife post where they render pre-doctor services—provide ambulatory care, service patients in their homes, implement preventive programs, and give emergency medical care for acute diseases and accidents. The feldsher-midwife post is located on the outskirts of an uchastock area, in villages close to the people. They are usually staffed by a feldsher and a midwife (or one person qualified as a feldsher-midwife) and an auxilliary worker. These posts are under the supervision of the uchastock physician who visits regularly.
>
> (2) Work in the medical health units at industrial enterprises. In this setting, feldshers work in the "shop health-stations," which are satellite stations located directly in shops. These feldshers are able to provide independent emergency care, get patients quickly into the medical care system if necessary, check that workers take care of minor injuries and illnesses, administer recurrent injections or treatments, and observe the environmental health program of the shop, noting adverse conditions. Feldshers at industrial sites do not make even simple diagnoses of illness but send workers with sickness complaints to the physician at the clinic. Feldshers are responsible to a single physician at the clinic who, in turn, is medically responsible for workers in that shop.
>
> (3) Work on ambulances in the emergency medical service. Here feldshers are part of the ambulance team, which is composed of a physician, at least one specially-trained feldsher, and a driver.
>
> (4) Staff health stations in critical areas where people tend to congregate such as subway stations, worksites, or transportation routes. Here feldshers have two basic functions: to administer emergency care and to activate the medical care system by requesting medical help or transportation when needed.

In the urban areas the feldsher's role is one of assisting physicians in specific areas—in the emergency medical service, at industrial enterprises, and at health stations. However, feldshers do not work in polyclinics or hospitals where medical care is provided by physicians and nurses.

It is in the rural areas that feldshers play a significant and more independent role in medical care. At the feldsher-midwife posts, feldshers, in the absence of physicians, administer initial medical care: for example, diagnose and treat simple illnesses, perform basic medical procedures (e.g., removing foreign bodies, setting uncomplicated dislocation, opening abscesses), write prescriptions, and prepare medicines. They are also important in improving the health standards of the villages, reporting acute infectious diseases, and implementing the dispensarization programs. Feldshers spend a significant portion of their time visiting patients in their homes.

Although there is a policy to decrease the number of feldsher-midwife posts and replace them with units staffed by physicians, the amount of outpatient aid administered by feldshers continues to increase.

Experienced feldshers can temporarily substitute for physicians in a clinic or small hospital (up to ten beds) if a physician is available for consultation. They can also temporarily manage a rural medical district or substitute for the physician of the district.

Unlike nurses, feldshers can (in the absence of a physician) give medical advice, deliver babies, and write prescriptions. Feldsher's salaries are 10 to 15% higher than that of nurses (for example, feldshers earned about 125 rubles a month in 1982, nurses about 110). Over 90% of the rural feldshers are women, but only about 60% of those working with the emergency medical service are female.

NURSING HOME AND COMMUNITY HEALTH ACTIVITIES

The Soviet Union, like other industrialized countries, is experiencing an increase in the number and percentage of its elderly population. The percentage of elderly varies with the geographical area, being high in the European part and low in the Asian part of the country. This increase is especially marked in a number of rural areas and is the result of the division of families, with adult children migrating to urban areas leaving aged parents, many of whom must live alone. However, in the Soviet Union there is a legal obligation for children to care for aged parents. Many more women than men live alone due to the higher survival rate of women and their higher frequency of loss of spouse by death. These trends increasingly call for specialized social and medical services for the elderly.

According to Chebotarev and Sachuk, the medical care system is not able to meet the increasing needs of the elderly.[39] They report that 25% of all visits to clinics and 50% of home visits by physicians are made to persons over fifty years old, and that the hospitalization rate for persons sixty or more years old is almost three times as high as for the total population. They also report that most geriatric patients are hospitalized in general hospitals. Senile persons needing institutionalization are placed in special sections of mental hospitals.

In the Soviet Union, as in many other countries, the goal is for the elderly to remain in their own homes as long as possible. In fact, most of the elderly do live in their own homes or are cared for by families. Remaining in their homes is undoubtedly facilitated by the home visits of physicians. However, there is a growing number of elderly who need constant care or help in daily living and are unable to rely on relatives. Information on this segment of the population is hard to obtain. Inquiries about long-term care or nursing homes for the elderly are invariably redirected by Soviet officials to discussions about the value of *babushkas* caring for their grandchildren while both parents work or about biomedical research of the aging process.

There are "houses for the elderly," which resemble boarding houses for those who cannot or do not wish to live in their own homes or with relatives. They are under the supervision of the ministry of social affairs, which works with the ministry of health; physicians employed by these establishments are paid by the ministry of social affairs. There is a shortage of houses for the elderly, and the conditions among them vary greatly. However, their numbers are expanding and there is an effort to raise the living standards and medical care in these facilities.[40]

In some areas older persons living alone are supervised by nearby houses for the elderly, but this service cannot cover all of those who need it.[41] Also for the elderly are Red Cross nurses, volunteers, and domestic and training institutions to deliver food and hot meals to the home, assist in household tasks, and provide other types of assistance.

HEALTH COSTS

Health care must be paid for. In the Soviet system, the cost is derived primarily from the revenues collected by the government. This form of collective prepayment enables the government to provide health care to all persons free at the time of use. Although most of the health care costs are met by the Soviet government with funds allocated to the All-Union ministry of health by the Council of Ministers and the Supreme Soviet, additional funds are obtained from industrial enterprises, collective farms, or other public bodies. One source estimated this amount at about 20%. Funds from the USSR ministry of health cover most of the operating expenditures of the health sector and most of the capital investments for medical and advanced training institutes. Capital investments for other health establishments are raised in the republics.

The annual expenditures on health protection have steadily increased in both absolute and per capita figures. The total expenditures for health and physical culture from the state budget and other sources rose from 11.8 billion rubles in 1970 to 18.9 billion in 1980, of which the state provided about 78%.[42] The amount allocated for physical culture is less than 1% of the health budget. While the increase is impressive and is responsible for impressive improvements in the health care of the people, it is significant to note that expenditures for health have not risen relative to the national wealth over a period of more than twenty years. Health expenditures remains at about 4% of the total national income. (National income or national material product, rather than gross national product, is used in the Soviet Union.) This is a lower percentage than the comparable share of gross national product in most industrialized countries.[43]

Data were not available on the breakdown of recent health budgets. However, Ryan gives a breakdown on the expenditures in major categories of republic budgets in 1970.[44] At that time salaries accounted for 53.9%, food 10.6%, drugs and dressings 8.4%, and equipment and appliances 2.2%. The state gives a block of money to each republic to be used for social services (for example, health, education, pensions) and for the republic to allocate among the categories. Within the health budget, it is difficult at lower levels to transfer money from one category to another without authorization from a higher level.

There are some health service charges to the patient. The most noted is the charge for the medicine for outpatients (inpatients receive medicines free of charge). Certain groups of outpatients—such as those with tuberculosis, venereal disease, dysentery, leprosy, diabetes, cancer, schizophrenia, and epilepsy, and children under one year old—are exempt from drug charges. Charges vary with the medicine. Prostheses—eyeglasses, dental, orthopedic—are paid for by the patient, except that orthopedic prostheses are supplied free to children and adolescents and all types are provided free to invalids of World War II and those on "personal" pensions (pension given for valued service to the state).

There is some private practice in the Soviet Union, but it is not done openly because of heavy taxation on such income (up to 90%), and unspecified "administrative penalties."

Treatment for venereal diseases or abortions are common types of conditions for which people, particularly those in large cities, seek private physicians. There are also state-provided paying polyclinics and nursing homes in some large cities where patients have a choice of doctor and are able to obtain second opinions. The fee payments do not, however, go to the practitioner. Patients attending these facilities believe that there are shorter waiting times, better quality of care, and greater anonymity for persons with venereal disease. There was no evidence in discussions with health administrators that containing costs was a priority issue.

Although little is mentioned officially about the desirability of budget increases, it is obvious to an observer that greater financial resources would enable health facilities to obtain more up-to-date equipment and items that are not now available, and to modernize the buildings, many of which are very old. The physicians have not had a salary increase between 1978 and 1982 because of financial limitations.

It should be noted that the ministry of railways and the ministry of internal affairs maintain and pay for their own health systems while the ministry of defense provides health care to all military personnel. It is not clear whether or not these costs are included in the published expenditures for health in the state budget.

PUBLIC HEALTH

The sanitary-epidemiological services of the ministries of health of the USSR and of the republics are the basis of public health in the USSR. They are largely concerned with environmental sanitation and the control of communicable diseases. The basic operating unit is the Sanitary-Epidemiological Station. By 1976 there were about 4,800 of these stations, with 4,250 bacteriology, 179 virology, and 877 sanitary and hygiene laboratories.[45] The Sanitary-Epidemiological Service is directed and operated by specialized physicians called sanitarian-physicians. They are trained in one of the five tracks selected by students who enter the medical institutes which train physicians. Feldshers who specialize as sanitarian-feldshers play an important role in carrying out the instructions of the sanitarian-physician.

The rights and duties of the Sanitary-Epidemiological Service are embodied in the *Fundamental Principles of the Health Legislation of the Union of Soviet Socialist Republics and the Union Republics* and the *Statute of the State Sanitary Inspection of the USSR.* These documents extend the supervisory and implementation process of the service to prevent and reduce pollution of soil, water, and air, improve living and working conditions, and control infectious diseases. The service also monitors the use of new chemical substances in foods, growth stimulants in animals and farm products used as food, and chemical agents used to protect plants. In addition, the ministry of health must approve specifications for new types of raw materials, food products, manufactured goods, packaging materials, and building and synthetic materials, and see that the proper standards are observed in the construction and reconstruction of buildings. The state has established standards for the permissible levels of noise, vibration, ionizing radiation, etc. in industrial shops. The enforcement of a safe, healthy working environment is a major task of the Sanitary-Epidemiological Service.

In each of the republics there is a head Sanitary-Epidemiological Station and usually a station at the rayon level. Each Sanitary-Epidemiological Station has three main departments: a laboratory for bacteriological and chemical analyses, a department of epidemic control, and the department of disinfection.[46]

Recommendations from the Sanitary-Epidemiological Service have the force of law. For example, if a construction project does not meet the specifications set by the service, in the extreme a letter can be sent to the bank to cut off the supply of money and discontinue the project. A problem not settled at the local level goes to higher levels and may even go as far as the deputy minister in charge of sanitary epidemiological services for the USSR, who makes the final decisions.

CONCLUSION

The provision of medical care that is accessible to virtually the entire population is a phenomenal achievement of which the Soviet Union is justly proud. This is especially remarkable considering the vast and variable territory to be serviced, and the havoc which resulted from both the Soviet Revolution and World War II. Its success is largely due to the high priority accorded health by the Soviet government and strong centralized control of the health system. However, the centralized control is not as rigid as it at first appears. Although the USSR ministry exerts enormous control through the budget and the norms and standards to which medical establishments must adhere, there is some flexibility at the lower levels because implementation of the annual and five-year health plans can take the local needs into consideration; there are also opportunities to raise additional funds for health purposes.

Although there is still a significant variation in medical care among the republics and between urban and rural areas, the disparities have steadily decreased. The quality of care is roughly proportional to the general development of the area. Overall, the dramatic increase in the number of physicians and hospital beds has given the Soviet Union a greater ratio of physicians to population than any other developed country except Israel and a ratio of hospital beds to population that exceeds most other industrialized nations. The emphasis appears, however, to be more on the quantity of health care than on the quality. This has resulted in a basic level of health care for the population rather than modern equipment, methods, and high technology.

One of the highest priorities of the Soviet health system is the provision of medical care to industrial workers because of the commitment of the Soviet government to massive industrialization as a means of development. This has resulted in medical health units at large industrial enterprises that have superior facilities and medical care. Another high priority is the health care for the workforce of the future—the children. This is demonstrated by the large proportion of physicians who receive separate undergraduate training in pediatrics and by the extensive child health program.

Students of the Soviet health system have found it difficult to evaluate health services because of government censorship, the unavailability of basic data in certain areas, the reluctance of persons working in the health system to provide objective information, and the restrictions placed on foreign observers. Therefore, it is perhaps appropriate to begin with the assessment of the late premier of the Soviet Union, L.I. Brezhnev, who reported,

"The work of polyclinics, prophylactic centers, and out-patient clinics, which serve 80% of all sick people, should be substantially improved. Regretfully, in some places they have lagged behind the potentialities of medicine, there is a shortage of personnel, especially of middle and junior level, the equipment is obsolete, and modern medicine is in short supply. Plans for the construction of hospitals and health building centers fall behind schedule."[47]

In the book published in Moscow by Lidov, Stochik, and Tserkovny, the unresolved problems of practicing up-to-date medicine and the shortage of drugs and added optical items, medical technology, sanitary and specialized transport are cited.[48] The authors refer to "organizing work," improving efficiency, and "effective" control over the full use of financial means and resources as a means of improving both inpatient and outpatient establishments.[49] They also are concerned that the construction of health facilities are behind schedule and that the quality of construction is poor—an observation made by numerous foreign visitors. Improvement of rural health care, particularly the introduction of specialized medicine into the rural areas, is another concern of the Soviet health system, according to the Lidov group.

In 1982 the Central Committee of the Communist party issued a report on the Soviet health system that also listed such "shortcomings" as shortages of medicine, of modern medical equipment and ambulances, and of clinics and hospitals. One of the main charges was that there were too many instances of medical workers "violating their official duties" and of "inattentive and heartless attitudes" among some medical workers. An interdepartmental council under the USSR ministry of health has been established to study these problems.[50]

Still, little is seen or heard of their problems by those outside the system—discussions of the pros and cons of continued production of physicians, the specialization of physicians, the value of dispensarization, the frequency of well-person examinations and tests, modification in duties of nurses and feldshers, or other topics that might alter the course of health services. It appears that a system has been set in motion that is resistent to modification or innovation.

One of the issues prompting speculation is the desirability of continuing to produce a large number of physicians when there is a physician to population ratio considered close to ideal by the Soviet government. Can the physicians' skills be more efficiently utilized by assigning some of the less professional tasks (paper work, activities related to social work, notifying patients to keep dispensarization appointments) to middle medical personnel?

In an age when the pattern is changing from acute, life-threatening diseases to chronic, refractory, often multiple degenerative problems of middle and old age, there seems to be an unqualified acceptance of a highly specialized practice of medicine. While other countries are reassessing the need for a generalist or family practitioner to assess the present-day medical needs of the entire family or balance the treatment of several types of pathology in one individual, there is little debate over the effect of fragmentation or its impact on the future delivery of Soviet health services.

The dispensarization programs for the active follow-up of population groups with certain diseases or similar physiological characteristics or working conditions consumes an important part of the health resources. The number of persons in dispensarization programs continues to increase, and the goal is to have the entire population under dispensarization; however, there is little critical evaluation to see if this enormous effort is justified by the results.

The great emphasis on preventive health care in the Soviet Union was an important advance in health care. It was geared to the nineteenth-century type of illnesses—acute, life-threatening infectious diseases that necessitated a rather narrow range of preventive activities. The twentieth-century pattern of chronic diseases signals a need to go beyond the traditional immunization programs, screening programs, and health check-ups and to expand programs related to the environment, diet, life-styles, and personal habits (alcohol and smoking) of the population if preventive medicine is to remain a cornerstone in the health care system.

Also consuming health resources are procedures with questionable benefits such as the twice yearly Papanicolaou smear, yearly mammograms for women over forty, routine electrocardiograms for some groups of workers. A physician doing routine electrocardiograms responded that the results were not worth the time, money, and effort invested, but he would not deal with my question of whether or not the tests should be discontinued.

The Soviet Union, with one of the highest hospital bed to population ratios of industrialized nations, is continuing to increase the number of beds. It is planning to add 364,000 hospital beds between 1981 and 1985.[51] The admission rate for Soviet hospitals is very high when compared to other industrialized countries, and it continues to climb. Also, the average duration of stay in Soviet hospitals is already high and continues to increase, while in some other industrialized countries it has been decreasing. A fundamental evaluation of these trends in hospital use could be helpful in assessing the health system.

For more than twenty years the allocation of the total national income to health has remained at about the same level (4%) while many other countries have increased the percentage of their national wealth spent on health care. The increase in those countries was probably influenced by consumer pressure for optimum quality care, a pressure not evident in Soviet society.

The difficulty in presenting a balanced presentation of the Soviet health system is illustrated in the following situation. There has been much interest recently in the upward trend in infant mortality rates in the Soviet Union. This is interesting because the infant mortality rate is generally recognized as one of the basic indicators of the level of health care and because the Soviet increase differs from the trend in most other industrialized nations. Many reasons have been postulated for this increase. After 1974 the Soviet Union stopped reporting infant mortality rates. When inquiring about the availability of data since 1974, the All-Union first deputy minister of health replied that a government has a right not to publish whatever it chooses, that there is a tendency for the infant mortality to decrease, that they wished the rate was lower but they are satisfied with the present level. "This," he said, "is all I can tell you about it."[52]

Another measure of health conditions and services is life expectancy, but the last official figures were published in the early 1970s.

In summary, the Soviet Union has succeeded in providing a vast, diverse country with access to a basic level of health care. The number of medical personnel and health facilities has increased dramatically. This was accomplished in a relatively short period of time, despite the destruction of war and revolution, by the implementation of a highly centralized national health plan that is part of a total national plan for development. There has been little evidence of a basic evaluation of the health services as the task shifts from basic needs to improving the quality of medical care. The challenge is whether the immense organizational structure providing health care will become increasingly bureaucratic, rigid, and cumbersome, causing the level of health care to stagnate, or whether it will allow enough innovation and flexibility to use its resources efficiently and effectively to increase the quality of health care for its people.

Notes

1. G.A. Popov, *Principles of Health Planning in the USSR* (Geneva: World Health Organization, 1971), p. 52.

2. Henry Sigerist, *Medicine & Health in the Soviet Union* (New York: Citadel Press, 1947), p. 15.

3. I.P. Lidov, A.M. Stochik, and G.S. Tserkovny, *Soviet Public Health and the Organization of Primary Health Care for the Population of the USSR* (Moscow: Mir Publishers, 1978), pp. 51–53.

4. V.I. Lenin, *Collected Works* (Moscow: Progress Publishers, 1965), 29: 364. Quoted in Lidov et al., p. 54.

5. Lidov et al., p. 50.

6. Vicente Navarro, *Social Security and Medicine in the USSR* (Lexington, Mass.: D.C. Heath Company, 1977), p. 18.

7. Lenin, 30: 185.

8. Supreme Soviet of the USSR, *Fundamental Principles of Health Legislation of the USSR,* 1969. Translated and published by the John E. Fogarty International Center for Advanced Study in the Health Sciences, National Institute of Health, DHHS, Bethesda, Maryland, 1971. Also translated in Lidov et. al.

9. N.A. Shikhova, *The Organization of Medical Care to Industrial Workers* (Moscow: USSR Ministry of Health, 1980), p. 3.

10. Ibid., p. 16.

11. Ibid., p. 1.

12. Lidov et al., p. 137.

13. Michael Ryan, *The Organization of Soviet Medical Care* (Oxford: Basil Blackwell, 1978), p. 32. See also William A. Knaus, *Inside Russian Medicine* (New York: Everest House, 1981), p. 327, and Vic George and Nick Manning, *Socialism, Social Welfare and the Soviet Union* (London: Routledge and Kegan Paul, 1980), p. 122.

14. "In the CPSU Central Committee and the USSR Council of Ministers," *Pravda,* 26 August 1982, p. 1.

15. Ryan, pp. 86–87.

16. V.N. Varankin, *Principles and Organization of the Training of Medical Personnel in the USSR* (Moscow: USSR Ministry of Health, 1976), p. 12.

17. Knaus, p. 336.

18. Ryan, p. 67.

19. Ibid., p. 109.

20. "Health Care in the USSR in the Tenth Five-Year Plan," *Institute of Medical and Technical Information* (Moscow: All-Union Institute of Scientific Research, USSR Ministry of Health, 1981), table 43.

21. W.J. Stephen, *An Analysis of Primary Medical Care* (Cambridge: At the University Press, 1979), p. 173.

22. Personal interview.

23. Ryan, p. 106.

24. Ibid., p. 105, and Hedrick Smith, *The Russians* (New York: Quadrangle/New York Time Books, 1976), p. 74.

25. George and Manning, p. 124.

26. Knaus, p. 331.

27. Navarro, p. 11.

28. George and Manning, p. 107.

29. Lidov et al., p. 53.

30. Navarro, p. 25.

31. Ibid., p. 47.

32. Varankin, p. 7.

33. Ibid., p. 3.

34. George and Manning, p. 110.

35. Navarro, p. 48.

36. *Medical Care in the USSR* (Washington: Department of Health, Education, and Welfare, 1970), p. 35.

37. Ryan, p. 42.

38. Personal interview.

39. Dimitri F. Chebotarev and Nina N. Sachuk, "Union of Soviet Socialist Republics," in *International Handbook on Aging,* ed. Erdman Palmore (Westport: Greenwood Press, 1980), p. 408.

40. Ibid., p. 410.

41. Ibid., p. 409.

42. "Health Care in the USSR in the Tenth Five-Year Plan," tables 16 and 17.

43. Milton Roemer, *Comparative National Policies on Health Care* (New York and Basel: Marcel Dekker, 1977), p. 226.

44. Ryan, p. 27.

45. Lidov et al., p. 101.

46. *Medical Care in the USSR,* p. 27.

47. *Report to the Central Committee of the CPSU to the XXVI Congress of the Communist Party of the Soviet Union and the Immediate Tasks of the Party in Home and Foreign Policy* (Moscow: Novosti Press, 1981), p. 81.

48. Lidov et al., pp. 104–5.

49. Ibid.

50. "In the CPSU Central Committee and the USSR Council of Ministers," *Pravda,* 26 August 1982, p. 1.

51. Lidov et al., p. 106.

52. Personal interview, Moscow, 5 May 1982.

Table 1 USSR population by age and sex, 1980

Age (Years)	Number (Millions) Male	Number (Millions) Female	% Male	% Female
All ages	123.8	141.4	100.0	100.0
Under 5	12.0	11.5	9.7	8.1
5 to 9	10.6	10.4	8.6	7.4
10 to 14	10.3	10.0	8.3	7.1
15 to 19	12.4	12.0	10.0	8.5
20 to 24	12.5	12.2	10.1	8.6
25 to 34	19.4	19.1	15.7	13.5
35 to 44	16.3	17.5	13.2	12.4
45 to 54	15.3	18.2	12.4	12.9
55 to 64	6.9	12.3	5.8	8.7
65 and over	7.7	18.1	6.2	12.8

Source: U.S. Bureau of the Census, *Population Projections by Age and Sex for the Republics and Major Economic Regions of the USSR, 1970–2000,* ser. 91, no. 26 (Washington: GPO, 1979), table 3.

Note: All figures are estimated.

Table 2 Live births, birth rates, and fertility rates, USSR

Year	Births (Millions)	Birth Rate (Births Per 1,000 Population)	Fertility Rate
1950	—	26.7	—
1960	—	24.9	2.8
1970	4.205	17.4	2.5
1980	4.840	18.3	2.3

Sources: "Health Care in the USSR in the Tenth Five-Year Plan," table 3; *Population Bulletin* 37, no. 3 (Washington, D.C.: Population Reference Bureau, 1982).

Table 3 Infant mortality rates (per 1,000 live births), USSR

Year	1960	1965	1970	1971	1972	1973	1974	1975	1980
Rate	35.3	27.2	24.7	22.9	24.7	26.4	27.9	—	—

Sources: Official Soviet figures as reported in Christopher Davis and Murray Feshback, *Rising Infant Mortality in the USSR in the 1970s,* International Population Reports, ser. P-94, no. 74 (Washington: Bureau of Census, 1980), p. 3, table 2.

Note: The Soviets define infant mortality differently from most all other countries. They exclude live-born infants who die within seven days of birth when they are less than 28 weeks gestation, less than 1,000 grams in weight, and less than 35 centimeters in length. Since most other countries count these deaths in calculating their infant mortality rates, the Soviet practice leads to an understatement of the infant mortality in the USSR.

Table 4 Information not available.

Table 5 Death rates (per 100,000 population) by cause, USSR

	1960		1970		1980	
Cause of Death	Rate	% of Total Deaths	Rate	% of Total Deaths	Rate	% of Total Deaths
All causes	713.4	100.0	822.4	100.0	1,033.3	100.0
Heart disease	247.3	34.7	384.7	46.8	542.8	52.5
Cancer	115.5	16.2	127.2	15.5	140.0	13.6
Other	350.6	49.1	310.5	37.8	350.5	33.9

SOURCES: John Dutton, Jr., "Changes in Soviet Mortality Patterns, 1959–77," *Population and Development Review* 5, no. 2 (June 1979): 279; and "Vestnik Statistiki," no. 11, November 1981, as reported in *Population Bulletin* 37, no. 3 (Washington, D.C.: Population Reference Bureau, 1982).

Table 6 and 7 Occupancy of hospital beds and length of stay in the institutions of the system of the ministry of public health of the USSR, 1980

	In the Urban Setting		In the Rural Setting	
	Average Occupancy of Beds (Days)	Average Stay (Days)	Average Occupancy of Beds (Days)	Average Stay (Days)
All beds	328	17.6	311	14.5
Therapeutic	343	19.4	338	16.5
Endocrinological				
For adults	341	22.9	—	—
For children	274	23.1	—	—
Contagious				
For adults	295	14.7	282	15.4
For children	276	15.5	311	15.4
Surgical			327	12.9
For adults	335	13.5	—	—
For children	307	10.4	—	—
Neurosurgical				
For adults	338	20.1	—	—
For children	283	19.0	—	—
Traumatological			327	16.8
For adults	348	19.0	—	—
For children	308	16.1	—	—
Urological				
For adults	339	16.7	—	—
For children	—	—	—	—
Oncological				
For adults	332	27.6	—	—
For children	323	24.8	—	—
For pregnancy and childbirth (except pathology of pregnancy)	270	9.3	231	9.1

Pathology of pregnancy	303	12.2	—	—
Gynecological (except beds occupied for state-authorized abortions)	336	7.7	311	6.9
Tuberculosis				
For adults	317	81.3	273	87.2
For children	302	102.0	254	108.6
Neurological			332	19.1
For adults	343	21.4	—	—
For children	301	25.3	—	—
Ophthalmological			295	16.5
For adults	339	17.3	—	—
For children	301	16.3	—	—
Otolaryngological				
For adults	333	11.2	—	—
For children	301	9.7	—	—
Dermo-venereological				
For adults	334	21.6	—	—
For children	279	26.9	—	—
Radiological and x-ray	346	38.3	—	—
Pediatrics	229	15.0	298	12.4

SOURCE: "Health Care in the USSR in the Tenth Five-Year Plan," table 45.

NOTE: Exact data requested for tables 6 and 7 not available.

Table 8 Health care workers, USSR

Year	Total	Physicians[a]	Middle Medical Workers (Feldshers, Nurses, etc.)
		Numbers in Thousands	
1965	2,246.0	554.2	1,691.8
1970	2,791.4	668.4	2,123.0
1975	3,349.2	834.1	2,515.1
1980	3,785.5	995.6	2,789.9
		Percentage Distribution	
1965	100	32.7	67.3
1970	100	31.5	68.5
1975	100	33.2	66.8
1980	100	35.7	64.3
		Rate Per 100,000 Population	
1965	—	239 (212.7)[b]	728
1970	115.5	274 (243.9)	871
1975	132.2	326 (290.1)	984
1980	143.1	374 (332.9)	1,048

Source: "Health Care in the USSR in the Tenth Five-Year Plan," tables 19 and 20.

[a]Official Soviet statistics include two types of dentists in the number of physicians. Dentists are estimated to be 10 to 12% of the total number of physicians.

[b]Estimated number of physicians excluding dentists, computed dentists being 11% of physician population.

Table 9 Information not available.

Table 10 See table 8.

Table 11 Information not available; see chart 2 in text for list of specialties.

Table 12 Information not available.

Table 13a Hospitals in the USSR, 1980

Type of Inpatient Establishment	Number of Inpatient Establishments
Total	22,323[a]
Regional hospitals	178
City/town hospitals	3,742
Central district and district hospitals of rural areas	3,781
Local hospitals	8,918
Dispensaries, inpatient	2,179
Maternity homes	630
Mental and neuropsychiatric hospitals	480
Other hospital institutions	2,415
District children's hospitals	92
Children's hospitals (noninfectious diseases)	796
Other	1,527

SOURCE: "Health Care in the USSR in the Tenth Five-Year Plan," tables 30 and 33.

[a]These hospitals had a total of 3.324 million beds and represent all Soviet institutions, not just those that fall under the USSR ministry of health.

Table 13b Average occupancy of hospital beds in the institutions of the system of the ministry of public health of the USSR, 1980

	Occupancy of Beds (Days) Per Year			
	Urban Setting		Rural Setting	
		% Occupancy		% Occupancy
Regional, territorial, and republic hospitals (except children's hospitals)	339	92.9		
Regional, territorial, and republic children's hospitals	309	84.5		
Town/city hospitals	329	90.1		
Central district hospitals	325	89.0	315	86.3
District hospitals	329	90.1	309	84.7
Local hospitals			313	85.8
Hospitals for contagious diseases				
For adults	272	74.5		
For children	261	71.5		
Hospitals for tuberculosis				
For adults	306	83.8	274	75.1
For children	307	84.1	—	—
Children's hospitals (not for contagious diseases)	289	79.2	294	80.5
Maternity hospitals	289	79.2	302	82.7
Dispensaries				
Antituberculosis	322	88.2	282	77.3
Oncological	348	95.3		
Derma-venereological	334	91.5	338	92.6

SOURCE: "Health Care in the USSR in the Tenth Five-Year Plan," table 44.

Tables 14 through 20 Information either not applicable or not available.

Health Services in the United States of America

Marshall W. Raffel

INTRODUCTION

The U.S. health system is complex, serving over 227 million people. Most of these people reside in a land mass stretching 3,000 miles from east to west and 2,100 miles from north to south. Approximately 1.37 million of the 227 million people live in the noncontiguous states of Hawaii and Alaska.* Except for some 1.42 million native Americans (American Indians and Eskimos), all of the American people came to this land from other parts of the world, and they continue to come. The country is more diverse than most countries in terms of the national, cultural, racial, and religious origins of its peoples.

Essential to any understanding of the U.S. health system is an appreciation for the social and political context within which services are delivered. The United States is a federal republic, created originally by thirteen former British colonies along the eastern seaboard of the North American continent. Upon securing their independence from Great Britain, the former colonies individually faced the question of whether each should be a sovereign nation or whether they should band together in some form of union for the common defense and to handle disputes between them. A union was agreed upon, but because each of the thirteen former colonies had unique features relating to its population—religious and economic differences, differing political styles, and size—agreement was not easy. Their first attempted union under the Articles of Confederation was not terribly successful, and after a few years representatives from the former colonies met in Philadelphia to seek certain revisions. Instead, they drew up a new proposed constitution establishing a stronger federal or national government, but one with clearly specified powers, with all other powers (including the unspecified powers relating to health and education) reserved either for the individual state governments or for the people. In 1789 the new constitution was ratified by the necessary number of states, and the United States

*Not included are the citizens of the Commonwealth of Puerto Rico, the Virgin Islands, and Guam who are American citizens but not of one of the 50 states.

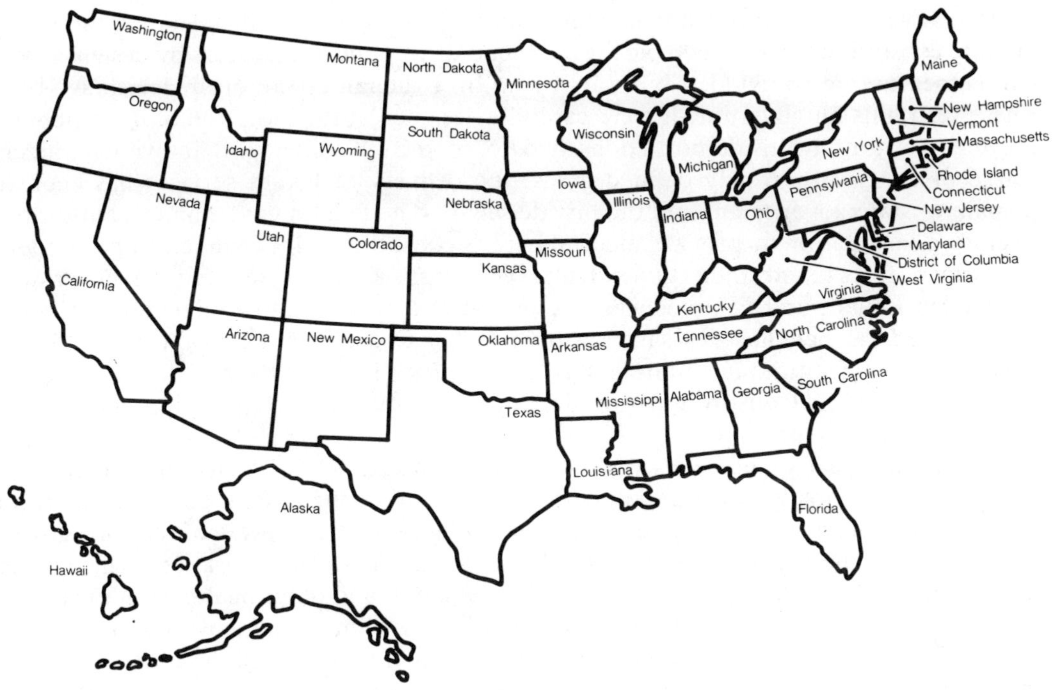

of America was formed. The original written constitution, with subsequent amendments, is still the supreme law of the land.

This federal system of government served the country well, for as the population moved westward to the Pacific Ocean and new states were formed, it allowed considerable room for decentralized development in terms of innovation and of adapting to their sometimes unique circumstances of the land and its population.

The individual states, as they were admitted to the union, each had a written constitution with clearly defined powers. Each state adopts its own laws, raises taxes, and provides a variety of services all within the scope of powers granted under the state constitution. Throughout history there has been a continuing state of tension between the states (both individually and collectively) and the federal government. Except for the Civil War in the mid-nineteenth century, the state of tension has been restrained. Disagreements have found expression in the federal legislative debates in the Congress of the United States, in litigation in the federal courts, and in elections. The tension is not unlike the tension that exists in most countries between central and regional or local governments. The principle difference is that in the United States there are written inviolate rules governing those relationships.

The American system of government is not parliamentary in form. The executive—the president, or the governor in the state government—is elected independently of the legislative body, and does not serve in the legislative body. The legislative body—the Congress in the federal government and the state legislature in each of the states—is limited in its authority by both the written constitution and the power of the executive to veto or reject legislative acts. Constitutional constraints can only be overcome by amending the federal or state constitution, which is typically a difficult or complicated process by design. Executive vetoes can be overridden but only by an overwhelming vote of the legislative body. These restraints on government were carefully designed at the inception of the republic to prevent rash or ill-considered actions and to protect the liberty of individual citizens. Except in some narrowly defined areas, the delivery of health services has been the domain of state government and the private sector. The federal government's authority to operate a hospital or to provide medical care is constitutionally confined to personnel in the armed forces and their dependents, veterans, wards of the federal government (American Indians and Eskimos who live on native lands), and to a relatively small cadre of other federal beneficiaries such as those in the Coast Guard and the Public Health Service. The constitutional limitation is not explicit since the word "health" does not appear in the U.S. Constitution; the limitation is rather by interpretation and resulting tradition or precedent.

The development of hospitals, medical schools, health departments, and other health agencies is thus mostly beyond the operational control of the federal government. Licensure of health practitioners and hospitals falls within the police powers of the state governments, as does the provision of most public health services. The operation of most hospitals and the provision of most medical, nursing, dental, and other health care for the bulk of the citizens are by institutions and practitioners licensed by state government but performing their work independently of government. Later, I shall describe some of the modifications that have occured in this model that governs the structure of health care in the United States.

Since the end of the Second World War, American society has experienced aggressive federal government action in a variety of health, education, and social service areas. Federal officials and members of the Congress have, from time to time, called for major changes in the health delivery system. In considering their views, and in seeking an understanding of federal actions—such as the support of medical education, health care for the aged, national health insurance, etc.—one should bear in mind that federal action comes mainly from the constitutional authority of the Congress to levy taxes and to provide tax monies for the general welfare. This has meant that federal action to influence the development and operation of health services is limited to the provision of monies to state and local governments and to the private sector, to do things in areas and in ways the federal authority wishes. In return for federal tax monies, agencies outside the direct control of the federal government are able to develop and provide services that are believed to be needed. The federal government's direction is limited to the provision of monies for use in line with specific legislation and the regulations that flow from the legislation. This is a powerful tool for influence by the federal government, and it has been used to encourage and facilitate the development of needed services and facilities. But, if a state government or a hospital in the private sector chooses not to use the offered or available federal money, then they are free of federal constraints and may do more or less as they wish.

A second constitutional basis for health action by the federal government is its authority to regulate foreign and interstate commerce. Over the years this has led to federal activity relating to the importation, transportation, and sale of foods and drugs and to a wide variety of environmental health activities that cut across state lines.

MEDICAL PRACTICE

There were approximately 450,000 active physicians in the United States in 1980.* About 10% of these physicians were women and about 19% were graduates of foreign medical schools. It should be noted that Canadian medical graduates are not classified as foreign medical graduates due to the marked similarities in the medical education processes of the two countries.

The ratio of physicians to population has been growing steadily over the years: in 1950 it stood at 149 physicians per 100,000 population; it now stands close to 200 physicians per 100,000 population, and it is projected that by 1985 the ratio will fall well over 210. This projected ratio assumes a decline in the flow of foreign medical graduates to the United States. Most authorities seem to agree that the nation will soon have a surplus of physicians, as evidenced by some competition for patients and by improved geographic dispersion.

While most physicians hold the MD degree, about 4% are DOs—doctors of osteopathy. The osteopathic school of medicine, which evolved during the late nineteenth century, believes in the value of manipulative procedures in addition to the usual methods used by MDs. While there was intense rivalry between the MDs and DOs, they are now for all practical purposes equal, and both can be fully licensed to practice medicine and surgery in all of the states.

Most physicians are in the *solo practice of medicine,* that is, they practice by themselves. Most are, moreover, paid a fee for-service. This mode of practice and method of payment are not without their critics.

The chief criticism of solo practice is that the physician practices in an unchallenged setting wherein he or she is not accountable to peers for either comprehensiveness or quality of care. In such settings, critics will note, sloppy and inappropriate care can too easily develop. Critics also typically go on to say that the quality of care in group or hospital-based practice is superior to that provided in solo practice. These beliefs are held by many who are not in solo practice, but data to support their assertions are sparse. To the extent there is foundation for these criticisms, they are being undermined by the almost universal requirement by state medical associations, medical specialty boards, or state government licensing authorities that all physicans participate on a regular basis in approved continuing medical education study. Moreover, some specialties—including family practice—are in the process of recertifying their members periodically by examination.

Critics of fee-for-service claim that this method of payment encourages a physician to provide more services than are necessary. Abuses of Medicare and Medicaid, government-financed insurance programs to pay for health care for the aged and the poor, lend some support to these criticisms, but how widespread these abuses are, no one really knows. It is generally agreed within professional circles that physicians are not as sensitive to cost implications as they might be due to the ways in which they were trained, and some believe that this accounts for most—but admittedly not all—of the excess visits and services.

*A *physician* in the United States is any licensed medical doctor, whereas in some countries *physician* is a term applied only to specialists in internal medicine. In the United States the specialist in internal medicine is an *internist;* the internist, being a licensed practitioner, is also a *physician.* It might also be noted that figures cited are approximate but reasonably accurate. The figures are also often deceptive because of the counting process: AMA data normally excludes DOs (doctors of osteopathy); sometimes the figures cited exclude inactive physicians, those overseas, and those in the military and other federal services—though sometimes not.

An increasing number of physicians—approximately 25%—are practicing in group settings. Most of the physicians in group practice are in small groups of from three to five physicians. Some of the groups are single specialty groups, and some limit their practices to general practice. The larger groups tend to be multispecialty. Most medical groups charge their patients a fee-for-service, but how the physican is paid varies from salary, to fee-for-service, to a percentage of the group's income. In a slowly growing number of the larger groups, the groups are contracting with a population group, usually an employee group, to provide comprehensive health services in return for regular payments whether the enrolled person uses the service or not—hence, no fee-for-service. Such groups are known as Health Maintenance Organizations (HMOs) because of their emphasis on prevention.

An increasing number—but still comparatively small in number—of physicians are entering hospital-based practice. Here, too, the method for paying the physician varies, but most are either salaried or salary plus a percentage of the income generated by each physician. Some of the hospital-based physicians provide routine primary care as part of the general hospital's ambulatory care effort in family medicine. We might note at this juncture that most acute hospital care is provided in hospitals by private physicians who charge their patients for care, although some of the larger hospitals—mostly medical school or other teaching hospitals—have a large number of salaried full-time physicians who either provide all of the care or provide some of the care with private physicians also taking care of patients. Hospital-based pathologists, radiologists, and anesthesiologists, common to most hospitals—teaching and nonteaching—may be salaried, paid on a fee-for-service basis, or on a salary plus percentage of the generated patient income. Emergency room physicians, common to a growing number of hospitals, tend to be paid in a similar manner.

Most phyicians will belong to their local (county or city) and state medical society or association. Whether they join the national organization—the American Medical Association (AMA) or the American Osteopathic Association (AOA)—will depend on whether or not their state medical society requires it (some do), whether they agree with the policies of the national association, and whether their other society memberships (typically, specialty societies) make the added membership worthwhile. Approximately 50% of the MDs in the nation belong to the AMA, 78% of the DOs to the AOA.

Generally, solo practice physicians have developed relationships with other physicians for coverage when away. While such coverage is considered a legal obligation, the need for it is lessened as general hospitals establish full-time medically staffed emergency rooms. Group practice physicians have a built-in system of professional coverage, and the patient may benefit from the covering physician's access to the patient's medical record, which would typically not be the case in solo practice. In larger communities, solo practice physicians often locate their offices in medical office buildings, which frequently facilitates consultation and access to radiologic and laboratory services.

Of the 272,000 active office-based, federal goverment-employed, and nonfederal physicians in 1980, an AMA census found them distributed among the major specialties as follows:

Specialty	
Total	272,000
General practice	48,020
General surgery	22,426
Internal medicine	40,617
Obstetrics-gynecology	19,513

Ophthalmology	10,603
Orthopedics	10,728
Radiology	7,802
Psychiatry	16,004
Anethesiology	11,338
Pediatrics	17,517
Other	67,432

It should be noted that this breakdown does not include some 104,512 active physicians who are in hospital-based practice (including 62,042 residents), the 12,209 in administration, the 15,377 in research, the 7,942 in teaching, or the 2,876 in other professional activities. Comparable data for the osteopaths (17,100) is not available.

The average American physician in 1980 worked 49.6 hours per week, seeing an average of 112 patients. Unlike physicians in most other countries, the typical office-based physician sees patients both in office and in hospital. What type of service the office-based physician is permitted to render his or her patients in the hospital, is defined by the hospital. In a very rural community hospital a family physician might be allowed to do general surgery, whereas in an urban hospital the same family physician would not be permitted to do surgery and the medical care services permitted might also be circumscribed. As might be expected, there is a spirited professional controversy between the surgical and family practice specialty organizations about the appropriateness of family practitioner performance of surgery.

The average net annual income of U.S. physicians for 1982 was reported by the AMA to be approximately $93,000. There were variations by specialty (see table 12) and there are also age group variations, the younger physicians earning on the average 20% less than those at the peak of their earning power. All of these income figures are net income subject to federal, state, and local income taxes; professional expenses have already been deducted.

Physician income figures are terribly deceptive, and like figures on hours worked per week need to be treated with caution. A $93,000 average income based on a 50-hour work week could be viewed as a $67,000 per year for 40 hours per week, with time and half payment for the remaining ten hours per week overtime. Also, the typical solo practice physician may not enjoy some of the nontaxable income benefits that usually fall to medical and nonmedical people in salaried employment: employer contributions to life insurance, retirement, and health insurance programs are typically given to salaried persons and are considered nontaxable income and yet may be valued at 25 to 30% of the salary paid to the employed person. Nonetheless, it is fair to say that physicians are among the highest income earners in the country. Incomes above $250,000 per year are not uncommon, particularly among some specialties, and there is growing public concern as to the social acceptability of such high incomes. In view of the fact that the cost of their medical education was heavily subsidized, this social concern is particularly understandable.

Primary Care Physicians

A primary care physician in the United States is defined as one who provides an individual or family with continuing health surveillance, along with needed acute and chronic care for which he or she is qualified to provide, with referral service to specialists as appropriate. General and family practitioners fall within this definition, as do pediatricians, internists, obstetricians and gynecologists, although not everyone will agree on OB-GYN.

In many countries, specialists rarely provide primary care. In those countries, pediatricians and internists serve primarily as consultants, devoting their time almost exclusively to the practice of their specialty. In the United States and a few other countries, however, most of these two specialties have evolved into primary care practice; most pediatricians and most internists provide primary care. Relatively few devote their time solely to practice of the specialty. This needs to be qualified in that the pediatrician typically limits his or her clientele to a certain age group; the internist usually will not handle some things that a family practitioner might handle such as obstetrics and pediatric problems. This is true also with obstetrics and gynecology, which has evolved largely as a primary care specialty but in this instance not for general care, but rather for categorical care for obstetrics and/or gynecological problems, with female patients going directly to the OB-GYN specialist without referral.

However, the generally accepted definition of a primary care physician leaves much to be desired. Other specialties handle a considerable amount of routine primary care which in other settings might be handled by a family practitioner or other health professionals. In this regard we should note the tendency of many people to self-diagnose and self-refer to a specialist—psychiatrist, surgeon, dermatologist, orthopedist—when in fact the family practitioner or other primary care medical specialist might well be able to handle the problem. Also notewothy is the frequent use of ophthalmologists and dermatologists when optometrists and podiatrists (both of whom are not medically qualified) might well suffice. In addition, the specialties of public health and general preventive medicine do a considerable amount of primary prevention, which reduces, to some extent, the need for primary care.

However one chooses to define primary care physicians, rural areas have considerable difficulty in recruiting and retaining them. This had led the government to pressure the medical establishment to emphasize family practice more vigorously in its training of young physicians. In recent years, because of government pressures, increased output of physicians from medical schools, and a number of other factors, the supply of primary care physicians seems to be expanding, and many areas are receiving increased physician services, though retention in very rural areas is still a problem.

Inner cities have also reported shortages of physicians. The problem here is somewhat different from that of rural areas. To some extent hospital outpatient and emergency departments have always handled considerable amounts of care of the poor. With the advent of Medicaid (a jointly funded program by the federal and state governments) the poor no longer had to rely on hospital charity but were entitled to private physician care. However, there were never enough physicians in the cities to cope with the volume. There was, moreover, some decreased availability due to physician movement to the suburbs, following their paying patients. There was a private physician shortage, particularly in primary care, but the hospitals continued to provide services. Recruitment efforts of new physicians to the inner cities were compromised by urban congestion, crime, high living costs, and the availability of all goods and services in the suburbs as well as paying patients who would pay what the physician charged and not just what the government programs paid.

One significant step to address the problem of physician distribution in primary care has been undertaken by the federal government: assignment of recently licensed physicians to rural and inner city areas as part of a loan forgiveness (repayment) scheme for those who borrowed federally appropriated monies to finance their medical education. This has generally enabled some communities to secure physicians usually for two to four years until the loan is repaid by service. Many physicians, however, leave these communities upon completion of the loan repayment service. Continuation of this federal program is doubtful in view of the growing supply of physicians.

Patient Access to Care

When a person in the United States desires some kind of health care, the typical route is to call for an appointment with a primary care physician. It will vary from physician to physician as to how long the patient must wait for the appointment: it may be that very day, the next day, or the next week. Usually the wait depends on the appointment schedule of the physician and the patient's perceived sense of urgency. Most physicians will see a patient the same day or the next day if the patient is actually ill. If the patient simply wants a routine physical examination, the wait for an appointment may be a week or longer. House calls by family physicians are rare.

Emergency care can usually be secured promptly with the physician, although an increasing number of patients are seeking emergency care at the emergency rooms of acute general hospitals. More and more hospitals are maintaining 24-hour emergency room service staffed by physicians.

If the primary care physician's patient requires a specialty service (such as laboratory or x-ray) that the physician does not provide as part of his or her practice, the patient is referred for that service. The service may be provided by a private laboratory or by a private practicing pathologist, radiologist, or other provider of the desired service. On the other hand, the service might be secured from the nearby general hospital. The fee the patient pays for that service may or may not be covered by the patient's health insurance policy.

If the patient of the primary care physician requires specialty consultation, the patient is also referred and pays a fee to the specialist for that consultation.

If the patient requires hospitalization, the patient is typically admitted to the nearest acute hospital and treated.

HOSPITALS

General Hospitals

Most hospital care in the United States is provided in nongovernmental hospitals by private physicians who admit their office patients, personally provide or supervise hospital care, and determine when to discharge the patient. The admitting physician may be a family practitioner, another type of primary care physician, or a specialist to whom the patient was referred by the family physician or to whom the patient went directly without referral. Patients in the United States have significant amounts of freedom to select the physician of their choice and to select the hospital in which care will be provided. The principal constraint here is whether or not the physician of choice has the privilege of admitting patients to the hospital of the patient's choice. If the patient's physician does not have admitting privileges at the chosen hospital, the physician can refer the patient to another physician who has admitting privileges or the patient can seek a consultation on his or her own initiative with an appropriate physician. This is not a difficult or complicated process for the patient who wishes to exercise his right of choice. But in practice most patients choose the hospital recommended by the physician who says hospital care is needed.

As in all countries, there are large and small acute general hospitals, the size generally determined by the population being served by the hospital and whether or not it is a hospital to which more complicated cases are referred. There is no formal classificiation of hospitals as in many countries, but the economics of running a hospital and maintenance of high quality care have more or less given the United States a pattern of regionalization without the formal structure.

Acute general hospitals in the United States have been started and run by various church groups, public-spirited citizens and benefactors in a community, individual or groups of physicians, investors, universities, and government. While most hospitals are nonprofit (not-for-profit), there is a small group of hospitals that are profit-making operations, owned by one or more physicians or by a group of lay investors. The for-profit hospitals are referred to as private hospitals, proprietary hospitals, or as investor-owned hospitals. It should be noted that the word *private* when referring to general hospitals differs from the use of the word in other countries where *private* means nongovernmental. In the United States this nongovernmental meaning of *private* applies to mental hospitals, but when applied to general hospitals it means for-profit. Nongovernmental hospitals in the United States which are nonprofit are mostly referred to as community hospitals, church-sponsored hospitals, or voluntary hospitals.

The community hospital is, like the church-sponsored hospital, a charitable institution, and is not required to pay taxes on its property or its income. It is *voluntary* because the development and financial backing of the institution is done voluntarily by citizens without governmental coercion. Responsibility for a community general hospital rests with a board of trustees, members of which are elected. Trustees receive no pay for their services as trustees; are responsible for determining the policies of the institution, for the hiring of senior administrators, and for the appointment of physicians to the medical staff; act as trustees for the assets which it holds in trust for the community.

Election methods for trustees vary. Some boards are highly restrictive, and almost self-perpetuating. In many cases the trustees are elected by voting members of the hospital corporation, voting members typically securing the privilege of the ballot by having contributed to the hospital. The hospital's charter will define the manner of election. Though the electorate may be nonrepresentative of the total community because the eligible voters may be nonrepresentative (trustees tend to be drawn from the business, banking, industrial, and professional leaders in the community), the general view is that the trustees are nonetheless trustees for the total community served by the hospital.

The reliance upon community business, industrial, and professional leaders on hospital boards has long-standing historical roots. These people were the very ones who could provide leadership in raising funds to support the hospital, and in a great many cases they underwrote hospital deficits with personal checks. Though the latter practice has declined sharply, these community leaders still tend to dominate the boards because of their ability to exercise influence on behalf of the hospital, because of their valued entrepreneurial skills that are engaged in hospital work without cost to the hospital, and because these people are in positions where they can readily allocate some of their working time to hospital activities.

A community general hospital, like most other general hospitals, may also be a teaching hospital. Teaching hospitals are defined by the presence in the hospital of an approved residency program for the training of medically qualified specialists. The presence of nursing or other health professional training programs in a hospital does not control its designation as a teaching hospital.

It might be noted that historically most teaching hospitals were either public general hospitals for the poor, or other types of general hospitals with a large number of indigent patients. These indigent patients were the ones on whom the medical students, interns, and residents learned. The patients, in a sense, paid for their care by allowing their bodies to be used for medical training purposes. The poor frequently resented this form of payment, and they often looked upon the hospital as the place where "they" experimented on patients. It was, in part, this perception by the poor which contributed to the development (in 1966) of Medicaid, under which all people were entitled to private care, but by that time teaching hospital practice had changed and all patients—paying as well as indigent—were teaching patients.

Government general hospitals are of many types. The federal government owns and operates general hospitals for clientele for whom it is responsibile. Specifically, the federal government, through the Department of Defense, has a large number of Army, Navy, and Air Force hospitals. While some of these hospitals specialize, most are general hospitals. The Veterans Administration (VA) also has a large number of hospitals throughout the country to care for veterans with service-connected disabilities, as well as nonservice-connected disabilities when the veteran cannot afford private care. Some of its hospitals are psychiatric, but most are general with strong rehabilitation medicine services. The Department of Health and Human Services (formerly, DHEW or HEW) has approximately fifty hospitals on various Indian reservations. General hospital services are also provided by the United States Department of Justice for inmates of federal prisons.

State government general hospitals are of three types. The first is the hospital owned and operated by the state as part of the state university medical school operations. These hospitals are more or less under the control of the university medical school. The second type of state general hospital is part of the state penal system. The third type is found in some states—general hospitals to serve poorer sections of the state. Pennsylvania, for example, has a number of state general hospitals serving communities like a community general hospital—that is, with paying patients—except that the governing board is politically appointed, some staff change with changes in the state administration, and the hospital budget is based on state appropriations. Not all states with such hospitals are, however, as patronage oriented.

County and city government general hospitals exist in many parts of the country. In the large urban areas these tend to be indigent hospitals, although since the advent of Medicare and Medicaid and the growth of private health insurance some of the predominantly indigent hospitals are beginning to take private patients. The governance of these hospitals by local government will vary from the highly political to the highly professional, depending on the style or pattern of political practice in that area. In the larger cities these are frequently teaching hospitals and also hospitals with strong medical school ties. Some famous hospitals in this group are Bellevue in New York, Cook County in Chicago, DC General in Washington, Boston City Hospital, and Baltimore City Hospitals.

One other type of governmental general hospital is one established by a special governmental hospital district or authority. Like school districts, these special governmental authorities typically have certain taxing powers as well as the authority to establish and run the hospital. These hospitals tend to be similar to community general hospitals.

University general hospitals are controlled by most—but not all—university medical schools. As noted earlier, state government universities usually have *de facto* control of the university medical school hospital although ultimate ownership is by the state government. Nongovernmental medical schools control their hospitals in similar ways except that ultimate control may rest with the university board of trustees. There are, of course, many variations and gradations vis-a-vis ownership and control. Some medical schools do not have their own hospitals but rely instead on affiliated institutions. Tradition, along with the affiliation agreements, may give the medical school considerable control of the institution even though it does not own or manage it.

The investor-owned hospitals are somewhat controversial. To appreciate the controversy, one needs to recognize that they labor still under the shadow cast by the many proprietary hospitals existing before the national hospital accreditation program began in 1952, a shadow cast as a result of many questions concerning quality of care in proprietary hospitals in terms of the qualifications of the doctors and nurses and the appropriateness of their services, the cleanliness and overall safety of the facilities, etc. The situation is different today in that most of the hospitals are accredited by the Joint Commission on Accreditation of Hospitals (JCAH) and are further monitored by state government licensing authorities and the Professional Standards Review Organizations (PSROs). There are no data to support the assertion that quality or efficiency of care is below the average standard of the other general hospitals.

The investor-owned hospitals contend that it is possible to provide quality care, with efficiency, at costs comparable to or below those of other general hospitals, and make a profit as well. The nonprofit hospitals contend, on the other hand, that the proprietary hospitals tend to be small and are thus able to handle the relatively simple cases, leaving the more complicated and more expensive kinds of care to the nonprofit institutions. This, the nonprofits argue, forces their average costs up. The proprietary hospitals, they continue, make a profit on the easy cases which "profit" in the nonprofit hospitals would be an off-set against the more expensive cases.

The answers in this debate are not available. It is true that 53.2% of the 1,045 investor-owned hospitals have less than 100 beds, and 84.2% less than 200 beds. The economics of the health field dictate that these hospitals can only handle a limited range of cases, and cannot justify much very sophisticated equipment and services. However, a growing number of investor-owned hospitals are large, though they are concentrated in the southern part of the country. Some recent studies have suggested, however, that the greater efficiency of the investor-owned hospitals cannot be substantiated.

The description of general hospitals applies to both *allopathic* (MD) and *osteopathic* institutions. While the allopathic-oriented institutions predominate in this country, the same types of hospital control apply also to the hospitals that were established to serve osteopaths. The separation has historic roots—when neither would relate to the other school of medicine. But times have changed, and now DOs serve on the staffs of allopathic institutions and MDs on the staffs of osteopathic hospitals. In some communities, mergers of the institutions have taken place.

Private, Semiprivate, and Ward Beds

Most general hospital beds fall into one of the private, semiprivate, or ward categories. Private room beds are for only one patient and provide a maximum amount of privacy.

They cost more than semiprivate rooms, which have two or more beds in them. While some semiprivate rooms have more than two beds, the tendency is for them to have only two. Most health insurance coverage is for care in a semiprivate room with the patient paying an additional amount if he or she elects a private room. (Some health insurance policies will pay for private room care if the private room is medically necessary.) Ward beds, historically for charity cases, were usually in a large room with beds (sometimes as many as 100 or more) lined up on each side, and sometimes some placed in the middle of the ward. While some wards such as this may still exist, there is a tendency for these beds to be in smaller rooms of from five to eight beds. The use of the word *ward* is becoming obsolete in the charity sense because most patients are now covered by some form of health insurance or government program which enables them to secure private care.

The distribution in the number of beds between private, semiprivate, and ward will vary from hospital to hospital.

Special Hospitals

Sponsorship of special hospitals will vary from community to church to government to investor-owned to university.

Over the years a number of special type hospitals—maternity, women's, eye-ear-nose-throat (EENT), and children's—developed, all of which are declining in importance. The growing complexity of medical practice and the needed hospital support services that usually are very costly have forced many of these hospitals to merge with other hospitals. To the extent that they are able to survive alone, it is usually only by a strong affiliation with some other institution that is able to complement the services in the special hospital.

There are rehabilitation hospitals in most or all of the states, which serve to rehabilitate the chronically ill to a maximum level of functioning. Chronic disease hospitals are typically long-term care institutions, some for the terminally ill, some for rehabilitation, some simply homes for the aged.

State governments, and some local governments, have played a major role in provision of care for the mentally retarded (in institutions commonly known as *state schools and hospitals*) and the mentally ill (in state mental hospitals). As in most countries, these hospitals have tended to be large institutions in remote locations. In recent years state governments have been closing these facilities as the emphasis shifts to community mental health programs where the patients are treated in community programs and clinics, and in acute general hospitals for short-term (under thirty days) inpatient care when necessary. In many states the closing of state mental hospitals has not been matched by the development of adequate community services, in large measure because of poor planning and because these states failed to shift the money to local governments to enable them to afford the development of the new services. The state mental hospitals have frequently been underfinanced and understaffed. In recent years they have attracted to their staffs a large number of foreign medical graduates who were often only provisionally licensed to practice in the United States and who very frequently had language difficulties.

There are many private mental hospitals, both small and large. They are generally better staffed than the state hospitals and provide more prompt work-ups and active treatment programs for all patients. Unlike state hospitals, the private mental hospitals do not normally keep custodial patients.

Hospitals in General

One should bear in mind that the definitions which apply to the various hospitals in the United States—both special and general—are not rigid. All hospitals are, in sense, compromises on the concept of the total hospital. Not only do hospitals in each category differ from each other in scope of services, but they also differ in patient mix. Whereas a special hospital may exist in one community, in another community the same kind of hospital may be part of a broader based institution. Specialized hospitals sometimes developed because of the presence of a benefactor, sometimes because a physician had a unique therapeutic approach which could best or easily be handled separately. What is clear, however, is that rising costs and regulatory constraints, coupled with new technology and the interdependency of the various specialties, are dictating affiliation arrangements and mergers. Where hospitals have merged, the merger often retains the separate institutions but coordinated them through a single management system. This is called *multi-institutional management.*

Hospital Licensure and Accreditation

Hospitals are licensed to operate by state governments, and each state has it own requirements. Generally, the various states have focused their attention for licensure on hospital physical plants—fire safety, heating space allocations, sanitation, etc. Some states have moved beyond this, however, to licensure based on professional standards.

The application of professional standards comes principally from the accreditation process. The Joint Commission on Accreditation of Hospitals (JCAH)—sponsored by the American College of Physicians, American College of Surgeons, American Medical Association, American Dental Association, and American Hospital Association—will on application of a hospital inspect the institution against JCAH standards and, if it meets the standards, grant the hospital accreditation status. JCAH accreditation, while not compulsory, is the best measure there is for assurance to the public that a hospital meets high professional standards, as assurance of its ability to provide an environment for the provision of high quality care. Failure to receive accreditation means that most health insurance programs will not pay for care in that hospital. It also means that the hospital will have difficulty in recruiting medical staff, and if a teaching hospital, recruiting residents for training purposes.

The founding of JCAH in 1952 marked the formal development of a mechanism to monitor the quality of hospital care. Every three years the accreditation team from JCAH visits each institution. The team checks many items, but three clinical items might be noted in particular: inspection to make certain that patient charts (clinical records) are complete and up-to-date; checking on the work of the tissue committee—a committee of the hospital's physicians which meets regularly to review the pathology reports on all tissue removed by surgery to make certain that unnecessary and inappropriate surgery does not occur; and review of the work of the medical audit committee, which periodically reviews patient charts to assess the appropriateness and quality of medical care in the hospital. The JCAH review of this work is, of course, not the critical element; what is really important is that the physicians, nurses, and other staff in the hospital routinely examine the care they are providing in preparation for the visit of the JCAH team. This process of self-regulation has provided reasonable assurance that the care provided in JCAH-accredited hospitals is of high quality. (The JCAH also will accredit, after appropriate review, nursing homes, ambulatory surgical and health centers, group practices, and other health service organizations.)

When the review committee detects inappropriate care or incomplete charts, corrective steps are taken by the hospital to warn the deficient physician, to limit what the physician may do in the hospital, and to recommend to the board of trustees that privileges for the physician be withdrawn. While this peer review system has contributed greatly to improve the quality of care in hospitals, there remains a need to strengthen it.

To assist the hospital physicians in their self-regulatory work, two professionally sponsored computer organizations have been developed which receive from cooperating hospitals the medical abstacts on all hospitalized patients. The resulting compilation from all participating hospitals permits an individual hospital to compare its performance against similar type institutions in the country. Hospitals generally participate in only one of the two computer organizations; participation by a hospital is voluntary, and the hospital has to pay its share for support of the computer organization's work.

In 1972 Congress mandated that there be established throughout the country Professional Standards Review Organizations to assure that the institutional services paid for under a number of federally funded programs were medically necessary, appropriate in terms of duration and level of institutional care, and of good quality. Implicit in this, of course, was the belief that containment of costs would result. Costs were not contained, and in late 1982 new legislation was adopted to replace the PSROs by PROs (Professional Review Organizations) with a stronger mandate for cost control of federally financed care.

Alleged Hospital Abuse

Critics of the U.S. health care system frequently focus on the acute general hospital, citing a number of alleged ills and abuses. Unnecessary surgery, unnecessary admissions, prolonged hospital stays, hospital competition and duplication of services, and rising hospital costs are the more common items receiving considerable publicity.

No one really knows how much unnecessary surgery is performed. Physicians often disagree on the indications for surgery, and this is particularly an issue when elective surgery contributes only to the improved quality of life. When quality of life considerations enter, be it for an orthopedic impairment, menstrual discomfort, or cosmetic reasons, the patient will often also have some feelings about the desirability of surgery and in many instances may insist upon it. Most of the debates in the United States regarding unnecessary surgery revolve around bona fide disagreements among specialists as to the appropriate indications for surgery.

The extent to which unnecessary surgery stems from inappropriate diagnosis or avarice is probably slight, because the various peer review mechanisms (JCAH and PSRO reviews, tissue committees, residency training programs, family physician referrals, and occasional second opinions before surgery), as well as the risks of malpractice (negligence) law suits, serve as regulatory devices. Certainly such unnecessary surgery is less today than in years past and is becoming less of a problem as peer review mechanisms are strengthened. If one were to hazard a guess as to where to look for unnecessary surgery from innappropriate diagnosis or avarice, it would be where peer review mechanisms may be weakest—nonaccredited hospitals and some nonaccredited, free-standing (not hospital-based) surgical clinics and offices. This is not to say that this is where unnecessary surgery necessarily occurs, but rather that this is where the peer review checks may be weakest.

Unnecessary hospital admissions are also of concern, and here, too, data on the extent of this abuse are not extensive. Hospital administrators, faced with low occupancy, are often anxious for physicians to admit patients, and they are also pleased to have patients stay longer than necessary. Both circumstances generate needed income for the hospital. This is a particularly tempting kind of abuse since many hospitals have more beds than they can fill, and empty beds have a negative effect on the financial position of the institution. PSRO reviews are beginning to deal with this problem; however, the situation is complex because the decision to admit and to discharge is that of the physician, and physicians often disagree as to need for admission and as to readiness for discharge.

Hospital competition and duplication of services are frequent complaints. The critics who raise these points, however, are usually also those who lament the alleged absence of competition in the health field. It seems as though these persons are anxious for competition to see who can offer services at the lowest possible cost but not for competition which relates to improved services, which may increase costs. This issue usually arises over the advent of new technology that is very costly. Physicians and the hospitals in which they work often desire the latest technology. Because hospitals are good credit risks for borrowing money, and because most health insurance usually pays the institutions for cost (or close to cost) of care to their subscribers, and some even pay hospital charges, there has been little incentive for hospital administrators to exercise restraint on purchases and on their subsequent use for which charges are made. They wanted the best, regardless of cost. In fact, federal government policies during most of the 1960s encouraged the development of new services and the acquisition of new technology that would contribute to higher quality care. During the 1970s, however, the rising cost of health services caused the government, the insurance companies, and the industrial firms, which pay most of the insurance premiums, to look more critically on the wisdon of these expenditures. It is these groups, moreover, who complain the most about hospital abuse and who are pressuring for appropriate and effective controls.

Hospital Costs

The average American is not terribly concerned about the rising cost of hospital care, because most people do not pay for it directly. Most have health insurance that pays for most of the cost, and a large percentage of those without insurance have it provided or paid for by some government program. Concern, as has been noted, is principally by those who pay—government, employers who pay employee premiums, and the health insurance companies. Ultimately, the consumer does pay through increased taxes and the increased cost of consumer goods, but the consumer does not pay much attention to this and, hence, is not very concerned. Some steps being taken by government to contain costs are described in the next section; steps being taken by some insurance companies and employers are noted in the later section on "Health Costs and Health Insurance."

Costs of hospital care have risen enormously. In 1950, for example, the average cost of inpatient hospital care was approximately $15.62 per day, and the average cost of the entire hospital stay came to $126.52. By 1981 the average cost per day was $284.30, and the average cost for each hospital stay came to $2,160.70. These are national averages. There are wide differences from state to state and from hospital to hospital.

Three factors account for the rise in hospital costs and in health costs generally. The first is population. There are more people today than there were in 1950 (231 million versus 153 million). This population is, moreover, an aging population, requiring more, longer, and costlier types of care. The second factor is inflation. Everything costs more—drugs, linens, food, fuel, and personnel. Nearly one-half of a hospital's budget is consumed by its payroll, and, as a heavy employer of unskilled labor, when the federally mandated minimum wage goes up (at it did in 1978 by 12%), hospital labor costs jump accordingly. This is also true with food and fuel and other items. The third factor in hospital and health care costs increases is new technology and new services. As a result of scientific advances, we are able to do more things to help people than heretofore. But the price of new technology is high. Not only is the equipment expensive, but the personnel needed to operate it are also costly.

Hospitals are making some effort to contain costs, seeking ways through cooperative buying, central laundries, etc. to trim their costs. Rates in some states are controlled by state government rate review bodies. Securing a certificate of need (see next section) is slowing down expansion, if only because of the time delays in securing a certificate. High interest rates also serve to dampen hospital expansion because of the high cost of borrowing money.

However, many of the elements of hospital costs are beyond hospital control. Hospitals, in addition, argue that government programs designed to pay the cost of care frequently pay less than cost, and they argue increasingly that the burden of regulation—new demands for physical plant alterations, new services, new reporting—all add to the higher costs of care.

Hospital Cost Control Efforts

To deal with the explosion in hospital costs, a number of state governments adopted *certificate of need* (CON) legislation, which generally provided that, for capital expenditures in excess of $100,000, health facilities must secure a certificate of need from the state government. In 1974 Congress concluded that this was a good approach and mandated that all state governments adopt certificate of need laws as a condition for continued receipt of federal health funds and payments for care. Some health insurance companies also began to tie their payments for care in hospital to the institution having secured a certificate of need for service or care in any hospital capital improvement. In effect, both government and health insurance companies were saying: if you expand your services in excess of $100,000 (now $600,000 for construction, $400,000 for equipment, and $250,000 per year in operating costs for expanded services) without a certificate of need, we will not pay for use of that service. Hospitals have reacted defensively to this legislation, and many have found ways to circumvent these restrictions. Moreover, hospitals are trying to get this legislation repealed, and came very close to success in late 1982; they are also trying hard to get the dollar limits raised.

Some state governments have also begun to regulate hospital charges, and the federal government in 1983 adopted hospital cost control legislation to be phased in over the next four years for payments under Medicare—the program which pays for care of those over age sixty-five. This federal payment mechanism will pay hospitals on the basis of a Diagnosis Related Groups (DRG) schedule, fixed payments for hospital care based on diagnosis rather than on a retrospective cost basis—which is the present mode for payment. Many anticipate that the DRG method for paying for Medicare admissions will likely be extended to Medicaid—the program for financing hospital care of the poor on a shared federal/state basis—and also that some insurance companies will adopt this approach. (While some insurance companies pay hospitals on a retrospective cost basis, some pay hospital charges. Many—but not all—Blue Cross plans [the major nonprofit hospital insurance companies] pay a per diem amount based on the average costs of the hospital.) It is hoped that the DRG mechanism will discourage keeping patients in the hospital longer than necessary and force the hospitals to pressure physicians to be judicious in ordering expensive tests, drugs, etc. This new federal legislation allows, however, for an alternative to the DRG system of payments, which is a federally approved state government mechanism to control hospital costs. Some believe that this new legislation—for Diagnosis Related Groups payments, or federally acceptable state government controls—will accelerate the trend toward hospital consolidation, and also toward corporate restructuring—whereby nonprofit hospitals established profit-making units to offset the constraints and the anticipated less-than-full-cost payments imposed by the DRG system. These for-profit operations have already provided, to a rapidly growing number of hospitals, income to offset losses from bad debts and any less-than-full-cost payments by government and health insurance companies; they also offer needed revenue for capital acquisitions as well as a mechanism for circumventing some regulatory devices of government. The mechanisms for making money include office buildings for private physician offices, provision of ambulatory care services by salaried physicians in group practice, and health management and consulting services. The acquiescence of hospitals with this new DRG system seems predicated on two points: it could be worse and it can be manipulated. It might be noted that extension of the DRG system to contain physician charges is being advocated by a growing number of people who are concerned with their rise.

MEDICAL EDUCATION

A Historical Perspective

A person who has some medical problem and goes to any family physician in the community can be reasonably certain that in that encounter he or she will be dealt with by a well-trained professional who is competent to deal with the problem presented, or that the physician will be knowledgeable enough to know when to refer the patient to a specialist and will do so. Moreover, if one goes to a specialist, either by referral from a physician or without a referral, one can also be assured that the specialist is qualified to deal with that problem or will know enough to refer the patient to someone else if he or she cannot deal with the problem appropriately. This does not say that there are no incompetent physicians, that no mistakes are made, or that improvements cannot be made. It says, rather, that a person can go to a physician confident that he or she is competent.

It was not always this way. In colonial America there were no medical schools until 1765, when the College of Philadelphia (later the University of Pennsylvania) began to train physicians. Until that time, what few medical school-trained physicians we had were trained abroad, mostly in Britain. At the time of the Revolutionary War in 1776, it is estimated that we had only 3,500 medical practitioners in the colonies. Only 400 of these had any formal training; only about 200 had medical degrees. Most medical advice was given by physicians who were trained as apprentices to other physicians, who themselves may have been similarly trained.

In the early colonial period, medical advice was also given by lawyers, churchmen, and other learned people: having the ability to read, they could acquire some medical knowledge and use it for the benefit of those who had no alternative. It should be clear, however, that the medical services available were rather primitive.

Following the Revolutionary War, medical schools began to develop in many parts of the new country. Their initial development was sparked by physicians who were trained abroad either for their initial medical education or for later postgraduate training. Trained in European, and mainly British, centers, they returned to the United States at the forefront of their profession, certainly so far as the new nation was concerned. They were appalled by the level of practice in the United States; many began to offer special lecture series for further education of those physicians who had not gone abroad; and they continued to develop and affiliate with the new medical schools.

During the nineteenth century the number of medical schools proliferated, many at universities and colleges and many as independent financial ventures. The quality of the schools was mixed, as was the quality of the medical practice.

The better physicians, particularly—but not exclusively—those who received training overseas, worked for reform, for an upgrading of both the quality of education and medical practice. One step taken was through the formation of various types of medical societies and associations at local and state levels and, in 1847, at the national level with the formation of the American Medical Association (AMA). The AMA had as its primary goal the reform of medical education, and it worked continually toward that goal. Another step was in the establishment of medical journals, vehicles for the dissemination of new knowledge and the continuing education of physicians. The third step toward reform came in 1876 with the formation of the Association of American Medical Colleges (AAMC), a group which focused its efforts directly on the medical education process. Finally, toward the end of the nineteenth century, licensure of physicians and the testing of candidates for licensure finally became widespread. Like an amoeba, each of these steps made progress—one inching ahead in an area, yielding to stronger developments in another area, and renewing its progress at a later time.

By the end of the nineteenth century, the major reform efforts were focused in the work of the AMA. The *AMA Journal,* for example, began publishing in 1902 the failure rate of each school's graduates on state licensing exams. In 1904 the AMA created its Council on Medical Education, which wielded the weapons of public exposure, embarrassment, inspection, and rating of the various medical schools. The council was dominated by professors from some of the better medical schools. Its ratings of schools exerted pressure to upgrade the curricula, the faculties, and the other resources allocated to the training of physicians. The AAMC was also applying increased pressure on its member schools.

But there was a feeling within this self-reform movement that some confirmation of work being done was needed, confirmation by some outside body. The AMA's Council on Medical Education moved then in this direction, enlisting the support of the Carnegie Foundation for the Advancement of Teaching. The Carnegie Foundation was persuaded to undertake a study of medical education in the United States and Canada, commissioning one of its staff members, Abraham Flexner, to carry out this study but to work closely with the AMA on it.

Flexner visited 155 schools and wrote a report, *Medical Education in the United States and Canada,* which was published in 1910. It was a searing critique of medical education at that time. Where schools were simple business ventures, Flexner said so. Where schools were a disgrace, where they should close, he said so. Only three U.S. schools came through relatively unscathed—Johns Hopkins, Harvard, and Western Reserve. Flexner recommended that the number of schools be reduced from 155 to 31. Within ten years of the report's release, the number was down to 85 and the quality of these schools was vastly improved. The report gave a boost to the efforts of the AAMC, and it seized the advantage to strengthen its membership requirements. Foundation money began to pour into the better schools, and the reform of undergraduate medical education was largely complete. Subsequent changes have largely been a rounding off of rough edges such as the restructuring and formalization of the medical school accreditation process and the improvement in medical licensure testing and procedures.

Medical specialties evolved over time as physicians developed special interests and expertise in different parts or problems of the body. The distinctions between physician, surgeon, and apothecary were, of course, of long standing. Major new emphases began, however, during the nineteenth century as physicians began to recognize the ineffectiveness of bleeding and purging and of most drugs then in use, as they identified specific pathology in different systems and locations of the body, as anesthesia was discovered, and as new diagnostic instruments were developed. Physicians interested in some kind of specialty practice organized specialty societies. Over time they set standards for admission to their societies, and in the twentieth century these societies, along with the AMA, sponsored national certifying boards in the various specialties.

There are presently twenty primary specialty boards, each of which sets its own requirements for training and testing in order to become *board certified* or a *diplomate* in the specialty. In addition to these primary boards, there are a number of recognized subspecialties within some of the boards (for example, the subspecialty of gastroenterology within the specialty of internal medicine) and three conjoint boards that are sponsored by two or more existing primary boards (in this instance rather than directly by the AMA and appropriate specialty societies). The conjoint boards are Allergy and Immunology, Nuclear Medicine, and Emergency Medicine. A fourth conjoint board, Critical Care Medicine, is scheduled to become operational in 1984.

Undergraduate Medical Education

There were 136 fully accredited medical schools in the United States in 1981. An additional 4 schools held provisional accreditation—that is, they have admitted students and will probably be accredited after the first class graduates. About 78 of these are part of publicly owned universities; the rest are part of private universities. Of the 140 schools, 15 award the degree of doctor of osteopathy (DO); 125 award the degree of doctor of medicine (MD). There are also 2 accredited schools of basic medical sciences, offering the first two years leading to the MD degree, the students of which transfer to the four-year schools to complete their studies. One additional four-year school is being planned. Accreditation is granted the osteopathic schools, after review, by the American Osteopathic Association (AOA). Allopathic (MD) schools are granted accreditation by the Liaison Committee on Medical Education (LCME), which is a joint committee of the American

Medical Association's Council on Medical Education and the Association of American Medical Colleges. These self-appointed accrediting bodies performed a very necessary function. Since 1952, however, the legitimization of these nongovernmental accrediting bodies came with recognition as to their legitimacy by the U.S. Office of Education in the U.S. Department of Education. For all practical purposes, the allopathic and osteopathic schools are the same, and the graduates, upon passing the licensing examinations of the state governments in which they wish to practice, are granted a license to practice medicine and surgery. In the 1980–1981 academic year over 18,000 students began medical studies in the 140 accredited and provisionally accedited schools. In 1980, 16,714 physicians (15,667 MDs and 1,047 DOs) graduated from the medical schools.

The process of becoming a physician is a bit longer than in many other countries. The typical medical student has completed twelve years of primary and secondary basic education, and four years at a college or university, earning in the process a baccalaureate degree—most times a BS or BA. Students wishing to study medicine tend to major in (emphasize) scientific studies, although they are required to study in a variety of fields in order to secure what is hoped to be a well-rounded education. These medically inclined students are in what is commonly known as the premedical (pre med) period of study, and there is no assurance that they will be accepted by a medical school. In fact, only about 48% of those applying to study medicine are able to proceed along that path. Many others shift career interests before applying.

Admission to medical school is based on a number of factors: performance in premedical studies as indicated by grades, interviews with the medical school, recommendations from premedical faculty, and performance on the Medical College Admission Test (MCAT). The MCAT is an objective test taken by nearly all applicants, which tests students on verbal and quantitative abilities, general information, and science. Competition for admission to medical school is intense. Those who are not accepted often go on for graduate study in some other area, and some try again the following year. Because medicine is a high prestige and well-paying profession, a significant number of those who are not able to gain admission to U.S. medical schools have gone abroad to study.

Racial and sexual discrimination by medical schools was once a problem. The racial barriers are down completely, although two of the existing schools and one developing school have predominately black students. Discrimination against women was until only a few years ago quite pronounced, but this, too, has now fallen and about 30% of the entering medical school students are now female; the percentage continues to rise.

About 7% of the entering medical students do not have a university degree. They are mostly students in a small number of integrated medical-premedical programs which generally can be completed in six years. Most medical students, however, have a degree before they begin medical school. The medical school period (referred to as undergraduate medical education) usually lasts four years, covering thirty-six months of study. A few schools have permitted summer study so that the student might finish in three years, but this approach is losing what little popularity it had among medical educators.

Medical education is costly. Estimates vary from school to school. Without some kind of subsidy, only the wealthy can afford to be trained as physicians. And subsidies there are: federal and state government grants, research grants, scholarships, and loans. Subsidy also comes from monies received for the patient care provided by salaried faculty. It is estimated that 91% of the cost of educating a physician is subsidized, which in part accounts for the growing concern as to the propriety of some high physician incomes.

In 1980–81 the average U.S. medical school had general operating expenses of $33 million—this is just to run the educational process, and does not include any costs borne by the hospital side of its operations or research funded from outside sources. The high cost of medical education is a deterrent to the development of new schools. This is mentioned because it is often alleged that the AMA restricts the number of schools and the supply of physicians. There is simply no data to support that assertion. The control is the cost of starting and running a school. While the federal government provided considerable sums to support the development of new schools in the 1960s, in the 1970s and 1980s federal monies were not as plentiful.

Licensure of Medical Graduates

The issuance of a license to practice medicine comes under the police powers of the state government. In each state, provision has been made for a board to test and license medical school graduates. In some states there are two licensing boards, one for the MDs and one for the DOs. Originally, each state developed its own licensing examination and administered it to candidates who appeared before the state licensing board. As the population grew and moved about, the need for an exam which would be national in scope became apparent. Two objective type of exams are in use, and both are recognized by nearly all of the states. The first exam is the three-part, five-day National Board exam, each part usually taken by medical students at different stages in their educational process. This exam was developed by the National Board of Medical Examiners, a nongovernmental, voluntary agency established in 1915 for the purpose of developing a standard examination which could be used by the various state boards for licensure. The board was quite successful, but over the years some states began to structure their own tests using National Board questions, and some states were erratic in terms of setting the pass levels. This prompted the Federation of State Medical Boards to develop an examination, called FLEX, with questions drawn from the National Board pool of test questions and graded by the National Board. FLEX—a three-part, three-day objective examination—is now accepted by all states, and is taken upon completion of the medical education process; the test scores are recorded by the federation and reported to the state boards where the physician seeks licensure, the individual state boards setting their pass grades. One important difference with FLEX is that now there is a single exam with a centrally available score, which overcomes some of the variances introduced by some states under the National Board exam system. But a more important difference is that the National Board exam is taken in stages when the material is fresh in the student's mind.

One might ask whether a national licensing system might not now be appropriate. This is not likely to occur because of the deep-seated tradition of states' rights. Also, licensing of medical practitioners nationally would raise questions about other professionals who are licensed by the states. This is not a silly concern because the existence of state control originally facilitated the raising of standards in many areas: progressive states moved ahead and were not held back by those who were more conservative; the movement of individual states on their own initiatives persuaded others to do likewise. It is recognition of this that makes the yielding of states' rights to the federal authority controversial and difficult to bring about.

The need for national licensure is not critical, however, since nearly all states grant licenses on a reciprocal basis to American- and Canadian-trained physicians who are licensed in other states or in Canadian provinces. Reciprocity for foreign medical graduates who are licensed in one state varies: many states require reexamination; some individually review the applications.

Graduate Medical Education

Graduate medical education consists of a period of supervised training in an approved clinical setting following graduation from medical school.

The laws on licensure vary from state to state, and thus present a rather complicated picture. While nearly all medical graduates complete some form of graduate medical education, it is required by thiry-six states for licensure of American medical school graduates and by nearly all states for graduates of foreign medical schools. There are two types of graduate training: the internship (which typically lasts one year and is a basic requirement in thirty-six states for licensure) and the residency (which generally lasts three to five years, depending on the specialty).

Most physicians go through an internship. In its early form, the internship was a rotating one in which the intern rotated through the various clinical departments of the hospital, securing that extra bit of on-the-job supervised experience before going out into his or her own general practice. In some respects the rotating internship was less than satisfactory because the intern would be spending so little time in each department that the value of the experience was questionable. This was increasingly a concern as clinical departments expanded and specialties increased in number. As a consequence, the rotating internship began to evolve into an experience wherein the intern limited himself or herself to two or three clinical services. As specialties began to develop, so, too, did another type of intership, the straight intership, in which the intern specialized in one of four clinical areas: internal medicine, surgery, pediatrics, or pathology.

As more and more physicians went in for specialty training, and as family practice moved toward specialty status, the purpose and value of the internship was questioned. Over time a consensus seemed to emerge to the effect that the internship as a free standing educational opportunity was of dubious value in today's medical world, that the internship should be thought of as the first year of residency training. The AMA in its *Directory of Approved Residencies* no longer lists internships that are not tied to residency training programs. However, at the 1982 annual meeting of the AMA, concern was expressed that the tie of internships to residencies did not contribute to broad training. The debate continues.

Postgraduate or Continuing Medical Education

Keeping up-to-date has always been an important responsibility for all professional people. Physicians have sought to do this in a variety of ways. We have seen how the establishment of medical societies and of journals were important steps for the dissemination of knowledge, enabling a physician to acquire new knowledge and to refresh his or her memory about many clinical matters.

With the legitimate focus of the profession on improving the quality of undergraduate medical education, on the development of rigorous specialty training requirements, and on the improvement of the sites of specialty training programs, the matter of continuing education until recently received relatively little organized attention. Hospitals, of course, usually mandated that physicians on the staff attend the periodic medical staff meetings, where, among other things, there would be some continuing education activity, such as the presentation by the pathologist of some interesting case or the showing of a film on some medical topic by a representative of a pharmaceutical manufacturer. Like the exhibits and lectures at the annual meeting of the AMA or state medical society, attendence was spotty and the programs often left something to be desired. During the 1950s, beginning with the American Academy of General Practitioners (later, the American Academy of Family Physicians), an increasing number of organizations began to require that their members take a specified number of approved continuing education courses. Over the years, the trend accelerated. At least seventeen state medical societies now require continuing medical education for maintenance of membership. At least eighteen states demand it for renewing one's medical license. Some specialty boards are now also obliging their members to require this as part of the developing recertification process. Interestingly enough, the American Board of Family Practice, having as one of its sponsoring societies the pioneering American Academy of Family Physicians, was the first board to set a recertification exam. It might be noted that in 1970 the AMA House of Delegates urged all medical specialty boards to consider the desirability of periodic recertification. The response has not been enthusiastic.

When this movement first began, the value of many of the continuing education programs was questionable. The AMA began to move directly on this matter in 1961 by accrediting the continuing medical education programs. In 1975 the Liaison Committee on Continuing Medical Education was established for accrediting programs, with members drawn from the AMA and other organizations, now succeeded by the Accreditation Council for Continuing Medical Education.

Similar developments have occurred within the osteopathic movement.

Foreign Medical Graduates (FMGs)

The United States has always attracted graduates of foreign medical schools, who came for a variety of reasons—to escape wars, religious persecutions, and other repressions, as well as to seek new opportunities that frontiers frequently offer in terms of adventure, economic well-being, etc. In the eighteenth and ninteenth centuries, these physicians often provided a level of expertise very much needed in this land. Following the Second World War, we began to experience a new wave of physician immigration, graduates of European schools who sought to establish a new life in America mostly as a result of the dislocations caused by the war or of the economic chaos which reigned in the postwar period. As Europe was reconstructed, the flow of physicians waned. The stream from both Latin America and Canada also tapered off from the mid-1960s through 1972.

A new group of physicians began to come from Asia to the United States to establish new lives and to receive advanced training; under the guise of advanced training some came with a hope to stay. During the 1950s and 1960s the flow from Asia did not contribute much to the permanent physician supply in the United States because our immigration laws were weighted heavily against Asians and Africans. Changes in 1968 and 1970, however, opened the gates to immigration from all countries. Many physicians came from the Philippines (a former American colony), from newly found military allies (South Korea, Thailand, Iran, Taiwan), and from India. The United States welcomed them because they helped to fill the physician shortage which was just beginning to be felt as a result of a rapidly growing population, hospital expansions to meet population needs, and added expansions due to research and technological advances. Many, if not most, of these physicians came from medical schools relatively unknown to Americans, and many of the physicians—again, if not most—also had language difficulties. The unknown quality of the foreign schools raised legitimate questions about the adequacy of their student training and the competency of their graduates. The language barriers caused communication problems between doctor and patient as well as between the foreign medical graduate and his or her American colleagues.

To deal with the uncertainties of foreign training and with language problems, a special examination was developed by the Educational Council (now, Commission) for Foreign Medical Graduates (ECFMG), drawing questions from the National Board of Medical Examiners' pool of questions and an English language exam. The examination was administered in the United States and at overseas locations. It became a prerequisite for entering all American graduate medical education training programs. Requirements were tightened in 1976 and 1977, whereby foreign medical graduates who wished to enter the United States to practice or to undertake training were required to either pass parts I and II (but not part III) of the National Board exam or to pass an acceptable equivalent, which became the two-day Visa Qualifying Exam (VQE). The required examination on English language proficiency was continued. Those who pass the VQE and meet other procedural requirements are eligible for ECFMG certification based on the VQE results.

These requirements are just to get into the United States for advanced training. For licensure, foreign physicians must also take FLEX, and most states also require that the individual take one to three years of graduate medical training. In July 1984 the ECFMG and the VQE exams will be replaced by a single two-day Foreign Medical Graduate Examination in the Medical Sciences. FLEX will still be required for licensure.

NURSES AND PHYSICIAN ASSISTANTS

Nurses

The nursing profession is undergoing rapid change in terms of the educational and training programs for nurses as well as the things that nurses do.

Nursing began as a helping profession in America with training programs associated with general hospitals. The pattern which developed dominated the nursing field until after the Second World War: nurses were trained for three years in special schools associated with hospitals; upon successful completion of the course of study, the graduating student was awarded a diploma; upon passing the state licensing exam, the nurse became a registered nurse (RN). Most registered nurses today (approximately 70%) are graduates of hospital diploma schools of nursing. This percentage, however, is changing as diploma programs close due to costs and to professional pressures, and as the number of graduates from other types of nurse education programs rises.

Hospital diploma school programs commonly had a large nursing service component—that is, the training was heavily weighted in favor of on-the-job training rather than academic training. From the beginning, these programs served as a form of labor exploitation because so much of the student's time was spent on the wards nursing patients without compensation, save perhaps room and board. As these programs evolved, more and more adopted stronger academic components, and in some states the students took some of their courses at local colleges and universities.

During the First World War a number of university nursing programs developed which granted, instead of a diploma, a baccalaureate degree. Upon passing the same state licensing exam taken by the diploma school graduates, the baccalaureate graduate also became an RN. Baccalaureate programs have experienced a rapid rise, and these graduates now constitute over 15% of the total registered nurse population; however, because of the growth in baccalaureate programs, these graduates represent over 25% of the total number of nurses completing programs each year, and this percentage is rising.

A third type of nurse training program began to develop during the 1950s in community colleges. These programs lasted 2 to 2½ years, upon completion of which the student was granted an associate degree; upon passing the same state licensing exam as taken by the diploma school and college or university graduates, the student became a registered nurse. About 6% of all practicing RNs are associate degree students. Over 42% of the new RNs each year are now associate degree students.

There are, therefore, three basic pathways to becoming a registered nurse. Each has an academic component; each uses hospital facilities for clinical training. Each graduate becomes registered by taking a common state examination administered by the state board of nurse examiners. It is generally acknowledged that the clinical (on-the-ward) components of the diploma programs are of greater length than in the other types of programs; it is also agreed that the associate degree graduates frequently do not have sufficient clinical training and that this must be augmented by in-service training upon being hired by a hospital. There are, of course, great variations among programs, with strong and weak programs in each pathway. The baccalaureate approach is distinctive in that it alone has a public health nursing component. In addition, a baccalaureate degree (in nursing or some other field) is necessary if an RN wishes to pursue graduate training. There is considerable debate over the comparative operational competencies of the graduates from the different types of programs, and there have been attempts to categorize the programs. The data to support the various categorization attempts are far from conclusive because of the great variability among programs within each pathway and the variability on admission requirements by the programs.

However, there is clearly a movement on the part of nurse leaders to get the diploma schools to close because, the leaders believe, nurse training should be part of an educational system and should not be under the control of a hospital or of any other profession. Diploma schools are closing and, while professional pressures are operative, the cause is chiefly that of costs. The costs of diploma education can no longer be buried in general hospital costs and covered by health insurance and government payments.

Nursing Education Approval and Accreditation

Nursing programs—licensed practical nurse (see below), diploma, associate degree, and baccalaureate degree—must be approved by an agency of state government if graduates are to be permitted to take the licensing exam. The state board of nurse examiners is typically the agency in a state that handles this. The National League of Nursing (NLN) provides a mechanism for academic accreditation over and above the state approval process. RNs who are graduates from NLN-accredited programs will normally have their licenses endorsed by other states.

Clinical Specialists in Nursing

The complexity of the health field results largely from the growth of knowledge. We know more and more today, and health practitioners are able to do more. But, in nursing as in medicine, coping with this new knowledge has forced specialization. A nurse with a baccalaureate degree may undertake graduate study in a variety of clinical areas to develop the needed special competence—for teaching, for supervision, and for advanced practice. Most of these graduate programs were a formalization in an educational setting of developments that were occurring in practice, just as diploma and, later, baccalaureate educational programs were a formalization in an educational environment of what was being learned on the job on the hospital wards.

In addition to training in such clinical specialties as pediatrics, obstetrics, medical-surgical, public health, psychiatric, anesthesia, and midwifery nursing, there have developed a large number of specialized programs, including transcultural nursing and occupational health nursing, and a number of nurse practitioner nursing programs. Some nurse practitioner programs are geared to training nurses who will work on their own in private practice or as equals on a health care team; other programs are geared to training nurses to provide primary care in rural and other settings.

Graduate programs in nursing can be professionally accredited by the NLN. Approval of graduate programs is usually beyond the scope of state government authority. In addition to NLN accreditation, specialty subcomponents of a graduate program are sometimes also accredited by a nurse specialty body.

Students completing a university graduate program are usually awarded a graduate degree—a masters degree in science (MS) or in nursing (MSN).

Doctoral Programs in Nursing

A growing number of nurses are pursuing doctoral education. In 1980 the American Nurses' Association listed 4,108 nurses with some type of doctoral degree; considering that there were 1.6 million nurses in 1980, this number is small. Most of these doctorates are in fields other than nursing—sociology, psychology, higher education, etc.—principally because until very recently there were only a few nurse doctoral programs. For some time there was question as to whether there was sufficient knowledge to nursing to justify nurse doctorates, but nurse leaders seem to have answered this in the affirmative, and programs are developing. There is still no accrediting process for doctoral programs, but this will probably develop in time under the NLN umbrella.

American Nurses Association (ANA) and the National League for Nursing (NLN)

The ANA is a professional organization with a primary focus on nursing practice. It is broadly based and accredits the nursing continuing education programs. The NLN focuses principally on educational programs—from LPN, diploma, AD, baccalaureate, and advanced degrees. Some disagreement exists between the two groups as to ANA accreditation of continuing education programs.

Licensed Practical Nurse (LPN)

The LPN, or LVN (licensed vocational nurse in California and Texas), is prepared to provide a variety of nursing services to patients who are not acutely ill and to assist the registered nurse with those more seriously ill. The LPN is not an RN. The LPN licensing examination is different from the test administered to graduates of diploma, associate degree, and baccalaureate programs. The LPN curriculm is also different, lasting an average of twelve months. While some LPN programs are run by hospitals, community agencies, and community colleges, most are part of public vocational schools. Except in only one or two training programs, there is no upward mobility for an LPN in nursing unless the LPN starts in one of the other nursing programs from the beginning with no transfer credits. LPNs are assuming more and more duties in hospitals, duties formerly assigned to the RN.

In 1980 there were over 1.6 million RNs in the country—1 million diploma RNs, 308,600 associate degree RNs, 288,000 baccalaureate RNs, and some 82,000 RNs who went on for a master's or doctoral degree. The number of LPNs was somewhere between 550,000 and 600,000.

Physician Assistants

The physician assistant (PA) movement is a relatively recent phenomenon, beginning in the mid-1960s. Most PA programs were originally designed to capture hospital corpsmen or medics who were discharged from the armed forces. Since many of these people had formal training and usually a considerable amount of experience, it was believed that their talents could be effectively employed in civilian health care. As the military draft ended and the flow of returning corpsmen and medics tapered off, PA programs began to take people who had no previous health training. Some programs found, however, that many nurses wanted to expand their skills by becoming PAs.

The length of training in PA programs varies. Some lead to a baccalaureate degree and require four or five years. Many last twelve or fifteen months. Others are of much shorter duration. Some programs are highly specialized; others are geared to primary care.

The primary care programs have caught most of the attention because of their potential to make physicians more efficient by allowing them to delegate certain functions and because they offered the possibility for meeting the needs of underserved areas that had not been able to attract physicians.

The great variability among programs led to a PA certifying process administered by the National Commission on Certification of Physicians Assistants. The AMA was a major mover in the establishment of the commission. In addition, the AMA, in collaboration with various allied health organizations and medical specialty societies, moved to establish the Committee on Allied Health Education and Accreditation (CAHEA), which assumed from the AMA's Council on Medical Education the responsibility for accrediting allied health programs including PA programs, but no nurse programs.

NURSING HOMES AND COMMUNITY HEALTH AGENCIES

Nursing Homes

The nursing home, a type of long-term-care facility, represents one of our more difficult problems. Scandals erupt with fair regularity—in homes that cheat, physically abuse, and neglect patients, and provide inadequate medical and nursing care, and in homes that are fire traps. To make matters worse, we have an insufficient number of good nursing home beds to deal with the growing multitude of aged persons who need such care.

The roots of this problem lie in history. Nursing homes began as the county poorhouses (or almshouses) of the eighteenth and nineteenth centuries. Local governments established these institutions to care for the poor—to provide them with shelter, food, clothing, and with work to help pay the costs of their care. As might be expected, many, if not most, of these people were older and had no families to care for them, and, being older, many were also invalids. Over time these almshouses became the community dumps for all castoffs—not only the poor and the physically ill but also the mentally ill and mentally retarded and the alcoholics, because there were often no places for them to go except the local poorhouses. Generally, conditions in these homes were not good, for they had to get along on meager public appropriations and on charity. The public had little sense of identity with these institutions or the people in them: the inmates were poor and noncontributing to the general welfare, and many were transients without previous history of community contributions. Why reward them with ideal facilities? The politicians gave the almshouses the levels of support the electorates wanted—bare minimum.

Of course, periodically scandals erupted—as they do today—and public consciences were pricked. Over time the mentally ill and retarded were pulled out and sent to more appropriate institutions, mostly state, rather than local, administered. On the eastern shore of Maryland the conditions in county almshouses were so bad that the state set up a state-run chronic disease hospital to care for the infirm, in return for the closing of the county almshouses. Other states made improvements from time to time, and these county homes, as patients were reassigned, were left mainly with the aged poor and the physically disabled who did not need hospital care but who were unable to subsist without some form of health service support.

In recent decades the state governments began to regulate these homes along with all other nursing homes—church, fraternal, proprietary—inspecting them and setting standards for performance. But the touch of state regulation was generally applied lightly, for few states were prepared to close many of the county, voluntary, and proprietary homes because that would force the state to assume full responsibility.

As noted above, nursing homes developed under other sponsorships. Church groups and fraternal organizations started homes for care of their members. These were mainly homes for the aged, but they had to gradually develop supporting health services to meet the needs of their residents. These homes received strong support from their sponsoring bodies, not only direct financial aid but also much "In kind" support in terms of gifts of equipment, volunteer maintenance, and—where there were farms—harvesting services, as well as a variety of volunteer direct patient care services such as help in feeding patients, occupational and play therapy, and social visiting. It is widely acknowledged that the quality of service in church- and fraternal-sponsored homes is high, and one rarely finds in them the shortcomings often found today in local government nursing homes and in the proprietary nursing homes.

The private (for-profit or proprietary) nursing homes emerged as a force during the 1930s as a result of the Social Security Act of 1935, which provided welfare benefits for patients in nongovernmental institutions. The original exclusion of benefits for patients in public institutions (since repealed) apparently stemmed from congressional concern over conditions in county government poorhouses and a desire to have them closed.

However, many health professionals and civic leaders were concerned over the resulting rapid growth in the private nursing home sector, believing that high quality care could not be developed and maintained in many of the homes if the homes depended on income derived primarily from welfare recipients, for these homes not only had to provide the needed care but also leave enough profit to make the owner's investment of money worthwhile. Resulting scandals in the proprietary sector have borne out the fears of these people. Not only were the payments insufficient both to maintain quality care and to assure a reasonable return on the owner's investment, but also the very availability of large sums of money to pay for care in facilities which were in short supply proved to be an open invitation for the unscrupulous to enter the business.

Foreseeing these kinds of circumstances developing, health professionals and civic leaders attempted to encourage the development of nonprofit nursing homes. Congress responded by amending the 1946 Hill-Burton hospital construction act to make construction grants also available for public and nonprofit nursing homes, and some states also developed grant programs.

The distribution of nursing homes and beds between the public, proprietary, church and fraternal, and other nonprofit sponsorships shifts constantly, but the proprietary sector is clearly dominant, with over 70% of the beds, and over 75% of the homes. Growth in the public and nonprofit sectors is slow, and many factors affect this slow growth. For one, local governments are financially hard-pressed and are reluctant to extend their commitments in the nursing home area, for the population is aging, costs are rising, and insurance and government programs do not pay all of the costs—besides which, their length of benefit periods are limited and sometimes there are retroactive denials of payment. The fear is that local government will not only be saddled with the initial investment but also with the unmet costs and the costs forced by changing state requirements for state licensure and changing federal requirements for Medicare and Medicaid. Add to this the bureaucratic hassles and paper work that a nursing home has to put up with, and the motivation to launch an expanded effort often dissipates. Similar considerations affect the nonprofit sector. This then leaves the field open to the proprietary sector, in which one finds some very good homes and many bad.

The unmet need for nursing home beds has persisted for some years and is, in fact, becoming more critical. Along with the aging of our population comes an increased amount of chronic disease. As family units become smaller and all able persons are working, no one is at home to care for the older folks, thus further increasing the demand for facilities for care of the aged. The demand accelerated enormously with the implementation of Medicare and Medicaid, which paid for some of this care, and also with the rapid growth of catastrophic health insurance coverage in the private sector, which also paid for some (usually 80%) of this care. The demand also increased as government and health insurance companies sought to reduce the lengths of stay in acute hospitals by moving patients of all ages to a lesser level of care.

Two types of nursing homes should be mentioned because they provide a level of service which qualifies them for federal payments under Medicare and Medicaid: skilled nursing facilities and intermediate care facilities, the former providing the highest level of nursing care. Medicare provides payment for skilled nursing facility care only; Medicaid provides benefits in both kinds of facilities. Beyond these, there are other kinds of facilities that are called nursing homes, but their level of service and/or mix of patients do not qualify them for payment under the above programs.

Many general hospitals will also have skilled nursing facilities under their management, developed in part to provide more efficient use of their acute beds and sometimes as a justification for the building or retention of acute beds. Some hospitals are experimenting with "swing beds," which can handle acute cases one day and skilled nursing facility

(SNF) cases the next. This allows a hospital some flexibility and is a particularly inviting approach to a hospital with low occupancy; it is doubly inviting if there is a shortage of SNF beds in its area. Rather than close beds or keep them unoccupied, they can be used and be income-producing, but for a level of care less than acute general hospital care. If the hospital is pressed for acute beds at any time, it then has the option of converting the long-term care beds back to acute beds.

The process for elevating the quality of nursing homes, and of the care they provide, continues. Apart from the notorious homes that provide substandard care and abuse both the patients and the agencies which pay the bills, the process of reform and upgrading is still up-hill because of the rising number of people needing care, the increased recognition as to the new types of care needed, and the rising costs of care in a difficult economy.

Hospices and Care of the Terminally Ill

The hospice movement in the United States is a relatively recent development but is growing very rapidly. It takes on two basic forms: in some areas facilities for hospice care have developed where, in an institutional setting, a wide range of nursing and support services have become available to ease the final days of those who are incurably ill and dying; in other areas the hospice programs are community rather than institutionally based, providing a range of supportive services in the patient's home. In 1983 Congress approved payment for some hospice care under Medicare, and some insurance policies are likely to follow suit.

Ambulatory Care: Neighborhood and Primary Care Centers

Neighborhood health centers (NHCs) began to develop in the late 1960s, initially wtih funding from the Office of Economic Opportunity (OEO) and later from HEW. These centers were primarily to provide comprehensive ambulatory services for a defined population of poor people. The poor had always received large amounts of care from health departments, indigent hospitals, and, on charitable or government-financed bases, nongovernmental general hospitals. The larger hospitals, and particularly the medical school hospitals, had long histories in both inpatient and outpatient care of the poor. The outpatient care was often demeaning—impersonal, crowded surroundings and long waits on hard benches. The neighborhood health center was designed to overcome these demeaning features, not only by providing a broad range of primary and secondary ambulatory care services by salaried physicians and other health professionals but also by emphasizing prevention, having available a wide range of supporting nonmedical services, and providing these services in the neighborhoods where the people lived. Important, too, was the concept that the people served—the consumers—should be involved in the control of their centers.

Primary health care centers are like neighborhood health centers except that they serve all people, not just the poor, and they provide a more limited range of services and focus on primary care. Their physicians may be on salary or on a fee-for-service payment system. The number of primary care centers increased rapidly, particularly in underserved rural areas, but their further development and continued existence are threatened by sharp reductions in federal funding. Like the neighborhood health center, the primary care centers have major financial problems, and the rural centers also have difficulty attracting and retaining professional staffs. Many of these centers developed initially with support from one of several federal programs, support which augments local organizational efforts and local building of the facilities. The typical center will have two family practitioners and one dentist. The supporting services beyond nursing vary from center to center. Some will have visiting consultant services, some pharmacy services, some nutrition services, and some other services. The financial problems are varied. Some result from community over-building of the facility, incurring a debt which is difficult to pay off from center earnings. Some centers have overextended themselved in terms of the supporting services they provide. A steady flow of patients who pay a fee-for-service is also a problem: being rural, there is frequent turnover of the professional staffs; with each turnover the centers lose patients—people seeking older practitioners who are likely to stay around, even though the patients may have to travel greater distances. Some centers also report a drop in patients due to the unaccustomed high cost of care—the newer and younger doctors who practice in these centers generally practice a type of care which employs more tests than the old-time practitioners used. The patients sometimes reject this more advanced type of care, preferring to find an older practitioner who will not be as fancy and who relies upon clinical judgment instead of costly tests, consequently delivering care which will not be as costly. The long-term survival of many of these centers will depend not only on attaining financial stability but also on finding a way to attract and retain professional personnel.

Community Mental Health Centers

Following the Second World War, psychiatric theory began to shift more and more to notions of community care. The community psychiatry theories were greatly abetted by the advent of tranquilizing pills in the 1950s, for with tranquilizers the need to keep many patients in mental hospitals was obviated. The tranquilizers suppressed symptoms sufficiently that patients could be treated in the community. In many of the states during the 1950s, general hospitals, mental hospitals, health departments, and others began to experiment with new types of community-based ambulatory therapeutic programs, and success stories began to be heard with increased frequency. Some local health departments had a wide range of services—for psychiatric emergencies and both individual and group psychotherapy. Some hospitals and health departments established day hospitals where patients who lived at home could go during the day for psychiatric treatment; some also established night hospitals, where patients who lived and worked in the community could go after work for needed psychiatric care. New York State in 1954 enacted its Community Mental Health Services Act. Later, sufficient experience was at hand for the Congress to pass the Mental Retardation Facilities and Community Mental Health Center Construction Act of 1963.

The aim of the federal legislation, with subsequent amendments, was to stimulate, via grants of money, the development of comprehensive mental health services through community mental health centers. The centers were to be the focal point for development and coordination of services in their areas. Some services were provided by the centers; others were developed by appropriate agencies, often because of proddings by the centers; still other services, which had been operational long before the advent of the centers, were tied into the centers by formal and informal working agreements.

By the mid-1970s federal grant support began to taper off. By 1978, only continuation staffing grants were available. At the end of fiscal 1980, there were 781 centers supported by federal grants, serving about 55% of the nation's population. More than half of the centers were in poverty areas. The decline in federal monies and the concentration of centers in poverty areas highlight the major problem facing these centers: despite all the good they may do, financial problems are major and inevitably must affect the comprehensiveness of service, let alone the survival of the centers.

Home Health Agencies

Home health agencies operate under various names, with varying organizational ties and differing services. Generally, these agencies, whether independent, hospital-operated, or health department-managed, provide a variety of health and health-supporting services in patient homes. Some agencies, however, are single purpose, offering only one type of service—for example, meals-on-wheels. Financial support for these agencies vary. Medicare, Medicaid, and insurance companies pay for some services; government grants (now mostly state and local) pay for some; patients also pay; charity contributes.

A visiting nurse association (VNA) is one type of home health service where a nurse—usually one with public health training—visits a patient's home to provide some type of nursing service—perhaps to change a dressing, give an injection. Many of these VNAs will also provide physical and speech therapy services by qualified personnel.

Some home health agencies will supply health aids for the home, such as crutches, walkers, wheelchairs, and other equipment and appliances. Some will provide homemaker services—housecleaning, maintenance and repairs, cooking.

Meals-on-Wheels, common in most cities today, are where an agency supplies usually one hot meal a day to those confined to their homes. This is usually the noon meal, the assumption being that someone is at home in the morning and evening to provide the other meals. Many of these agencies use volunteers to deliver the meals, which are secured from various agencies—the hospital or the school kitchen being two common suppliers.

Ambulance and Emergency Medical Services

Ambulance services are provided by a variety of agencies. Funeral homes are frequently the source for this service, but it is also available, depending on the community, from the police or fire deparments, hospitals, volunteer groups, or private ambulance companies. Considerable effort has been made in recent years to train ambulance crews in dealing with the kinds of emergencies they are likely to encounter.

An increasing number of communities are served by radio-dispatched emergency medical service teams—specially trained paramedics who respond to emergencies in specially equipped ambulances. In many areas the service is secured by telephoning 911.

Clinical Laboratories

The physician may require a variety of laboratory analyses to facilitate his or her diagnosis and treatment. Some physicians have their own lab technicians to carry out whatever tests are desired. Some tests, however, are very complicated and require costly equipment. For these tests, as well as for some of the simpler tests, the physician without a lab technician and who does not do the tests himself or herself, may have an arrangement with the nearby hospital. Also, very often the physician may use a free-standing clinical laboratory run by a pathologist or by a registered medical technician. The physician may send the patient or the specimen to the lab. In rural settings, the doctors may have to mail the specimen to a lab, or the lab may arrange for periodic pick-ups of specimens.

Although there is state licensing of clinical laboratories and federal monitoring of those labs working across state lines, there has always been conern over the quality of laboratory analyses. Studies are occasionally completed which call into question the accuracy of some clinical lab results. This typically leads to improved surveillance of laboratories by the regulatory agencies.

Ambulatory Surgical Centers

In recent years there has been an upsurge in the amount of surgery performed on an ambulatory basis. Hospitals all over the country are experiencing a rise in the number of surgical cases on patients who come into the hospital and go home the same day—cases which previously had required at least an overnight stay in the hospital if not a two- or three-day stay. One can appreciate how this can affect a hospital's need for beds and its overall organization.

Many surgeons, however, have been accustomed to performing ambulatory surgery in their offices, the limit on what they did depending on the surgeon's facilities, support services, and self-imposed limits. One of the major limits was anesthesia. The surgeon commonly would employ a local but not a general anesthetic.

During the 1970s, a number of free-standing surgical centers were established in several parts of the country, the surgical center having more complete facilities, support services, anesthesia services, and, significantly, an augmented system (compared to the surgeon's office) for monitoring the quality of surgical practice. The number of centers is quite small but growing. It already appears, however, that a professional conflict is emerging over the desirability of independent centers over hospital-based centers.

Family Planning Centers

Family planning services are provided by local health departments, private physicians, some hospitals, and free-standing family planning centers (clinics). The latter are supported primarily by government grants and charity.

HEALTH COSTS AND HEALTH INSURANCE

The health sector in the United States—the physicians, nurses, optometrists, dentists, physiotherapists, and other health workers; the hospitals, nursing homes, health insurance companies, medical equipment manufacturers, pharmaceutical companies, government health workers, etc.—represent one of the largest economic sectors in the country, and accounted in 1981 for 9.8% of the Gross National Product, up from 9.4% in 1980. This growth of the health sector has risen considerably since 1929, and there has also been a marked rise in the public or governmental share of those costs. (Table 17 illustrates this.)

The rise in personal health care costs from 1965 through 1981 have been attributed to three main factors: a small amount (9%) has been attributed to population increase—more people needing service; 32% can be attributed to increased utilization brought about by new technology, improved case finding, and new knowledge; 59% is due to price rise, inflation—higher pay for employees in a labor intensive industry, and increased costs of such components as food, fuel, equipment, supplies, services, and construction. (see tables 18 and 19.)

Apart from the overall rise in the health sector's share of the GNP, a particularly sharp shift of the public's share of health expenditures can be noted in 1965 to 1970. This reflects the introduction of Medicare and Medicaid in 1966.

Medicare and Medicaid

Medicare is a insurance program for health care of the aged (over 65). It is financed mainly by the federal government out of social security tax monies, and also financed by the aged. The aged paid in 1982 for the first $260 of hospitalization, and a portion of the hospital costs after 60 days of hospital care—$65 per day in 1982. For skilled nursing facility care, the Medicare recipient must pay $32.50 per day after the first 20 days in a skilled nursing facility. For physician services, which are not part of the universal basic coverage, most Medicare recipients paid a monthly health insurance premium ($12.20 per month in 1982). However, physicians are free to charge whatever they wish for services. There are clearly shortcomings in Medicare. Many of the aged have taken out private health insurance to cover charges not taken care of by Medicare. The federal government's efforts to broaden Medicare coverage have been slowed by the cost implications resulting from the very rapid growth in health costs, exacerbated by the traditional method for paying hospitals at cost of care.

Medicaid is a federal/state-funded program covering the needy, regardless of age. The federal share of costs varies from state to state, depending on state need, with the federal share ranging from 50 to 78%. The benefits are not uniform from state to state, except that federal regulations require a basic minimum to qualify for federal funds—specifically, inpatient and outpatient hospital services; skilled nursing facility services; physician services; home health care; family planning services; and early and periodic screening, diagnosis, and treatment of eligible children under twenty-one years of age. Optional services, which only some states cover, include dental services, prescribed drugs, eyeglasses, and intermediate care facility services.

Medicaid is financed out of general revenues. Like Medicare, costs have risen sharply and are of growing concern to both state and federal governments. In an effort to slow the rate of expenditure growth, income eligibility levels are being tighted, and services covered and payments are both being reduced. Under Medicare more and more costs are being shifted for the patient to pay, and hospital payments are more tightly controlled. Both programs have been used fraudulently by some physicians, pharmacists, laboratories, and other providers.

People Covered by Health Insurance

Estimates vary as to the number of people covered by health insurance, the two principal estimates being from the U.S. Department of Health and Human Services and the Health Insurance Association of America (HIAA). The counting process is complicated by: duplication of coverage (for instance, husband and wife each covered through places of employment); Medicare beneficiaries who also elect to take out health insurance; the unknown number of dependents (estimates run from 5 to 7 million) covered under the Civilian Health and Medical Care Program for the Uniformed Services (CHAMPUS); Veterans Administration patients who are without health insurance because they are totally dependent on the VA system for care (also an unknown number); and long-term residents of state and local mental hospitals and prisons, many of whom are without insurance.

It would appear, however, that approximately 90 to 95% of the population is protected by health insurance or some government program, and the coverage for the more expensive services is quite complete (see table 19). It is for this reason that the covered person is not terribly concerned over the rising cost of health care. This does not say, however, that the existing health insurance policies are ideal. Many contain gaps, but many people would also argue that as a matter of public policy not all gaps should be filled.

Who are the uncovered? Some people have chosen not to secure coverage. Some are in small groups that have not been able to meet the group enrollment minimums of the health insurance companies. Some are the unemployed; some are between jobs or are not eligible on their new job until they have been employed for a certain period of time. Some are the poor who are too well off to be eligible for Medicaid but with not enough money to be able to afford the costs of health insurance. Some are probably the custodial patients and inmates in state, local, and federal hospitals and prisons.

Services Covered by Health Insurance

Of the total health expenditures for 1980 for *personal* health care (excluding expenditures for environmental and other public health activities, research, and construction), 67.6% of the $217,900 million was paid for by the third-party payments—insurance, industry, or government programs. That would leave the consumer to pay 32.4%, or $70,600 million. The significant cost items, however, are hospital care, physicians' services, drugs and drug sundries, and home care. Here third-party payments covered 90.9% of hospital care (some of the uncovered being cosmetic surgery—generally not covered, private room charges, and costs incurred by the uncovered [including many unemployed persons] and those who just joined and have not fulfilled any waiting periods); 62.7% of physicians' services (the uncovered portion being in two main categories: routine office medical care, which most health insurance policies do not cover and which many others feel should not be covered, and added charges by physicians who find the third-party allowances less than their perceived value of their services); and 58.1% of nursing home expenditures, including those not certified for payment by Medicare and Medicaid, but providing some level of nursing care.

Nearly all people in the United States are covered either by health insurance or by some government health program, but there is a need to extend coverage to those relatively small numbers not covered, to improve the benefits payments for nursing home care and for catastrophic or major medical illness, and to strengthen some of the inadequate policies—mostly nongroup policies—which are aggressively advertised.

Full payment of hospital care is within the country's grasp. Policies need some strengthening in this area though not very much since not all of the consumer-borne expenses cited earlier ought to be covered. However, much more needs to be done in other high cost areas, particularly for nursing home care and major medical coverage. The problem in extending coverage comes down, basically, to cost—who will pay, how payment will be made, and whether or not all charges should be covered. Should there be coverage for care in homes for the aged? Should all routine diagnostic tests—including high cost tests—be covered? Should all physician office visits be covered? Such questions are at the heart of the public debates in the United States as people wrestle with the question of national health insurance. Those who see a need for some consumer share in costs believe that rationing might best be done by the consumer rather than by a public system. The critical element is to have a system of consumer sharing in costs that contributes to judicious consumer choices but does not act as a deterrent to needed services or consumer preferences.

Complicating this picture is the economic crisis of the 1980s, reflected in unemployment, inflation, business down-turn, rising hospital and physician charges. As a consequence, health insurance coverage becomes less extensive due to failure of policies to keep pace with inflation, and many large employers seek ways to reduce their costs by reducing insurance benefits. A growing number of employers and insurance companies, particularly in California, are experimenting with *Preferred Provider* mechanisms whereby individual or groups of physicians agree to accept the insurance payments as full payment for services. This approach is particularly attractive where there is a large supply of physicians competing for patients. Patients will usually still be free to go to the physician of their choice, but if not a Preferred Provider, a lesser payment is sometimes made and, of course, that physician is free to set his or her own fees. Some consideration is also being given to employing the same approach as a way to contain hospital costs—an extension of, and variation on, the DRG system that the federal government has mandated for Medicare. Government programs—both Medicare and Medicaid—have likewise tended to shift the burden of costs back to the consumer. Many of the unemployed, moreover, have lost their health insurance coverage. The impact of this is not clearly reflected yet in the statistical data. If not a temporary aberration, it will certainly lead to pressure to control physician charges as well as hospital charges, and it will certainly rekindle the movement for a system of national health insurance.

PUBLIC HEALTH: STATE AND LOCAL

State Health Agencies

Administrative Organization of State Health Agencies

How a state government organizes its public health functions will vary from state to state. History, personalities, federal grant programs, and chance all play a role. The traditional public health functions include communicable disease control, maternal and child health services, environmental sanitation, health education, laboratory services, and vital statistics. Until recently these were placed administratively in state health or public health departments. In the last decade there has been a tendency in some states to remove some of the environmental health activities and place them in new environmental protection agencies. But a state government's health responsibilities (and being government health activities, they are appropriately public health activities) go far beyond these basic six functions. Not only have the basic functions spawned a large number of related program prevention activities far beyond the original range of services—such as cancer and chronic disease control, crippled children's services, nutrition services, and occupational health—but the states have also been responsible for care of the mentally ill and mentally retarded, and for professional and institutional licensure. Whether these latter functions are or are not located in the state's chief public health agency, the state health department, varies. Some states have all these activities in a single agency; some break them out into separate agencies. In any one state the organizational pattern may from time to time change as new problems arise and as new opportunities are seized. As might be expected, reorganizations within bureaucracies are resisted by some, favored by others.

Within any one state, where health agency functions are split, there may be a variety of administrative forms.

There are in the states three basic models. The first is the health agency headed by a board of health with policy or administrative functions over the agency. The board is usually appointed by the governor and approved by the state senate. Board members are typically nonsalaried, and where the boards have policy or administrative roles to play, physicians tend to be in the majority. In addition to overall direction of the agency, boards of health (including boards with only advisory functions) very frequently have authority to enforce public health laws by holding hearings on violations, hearing appeals on health officer actions, and by issuance of board orders for compliance. Board orders must be enforced by law enforcement agencies, although the recipient of a board of health order can, of course, appeal it in the state courts. Many boards either appoint key agency personnel or have a strong influence in their appointment. As one might expect, there have been good and bad, progressive as well as nonprogressive, boards of health. Some boards have been highly politicized by the types of people appointed to them; other boards have been highly professional with no partisan politics or political hacks. Advocates of policy boards argue that they provide not only good professional advice to the agency (which they could get, of course, from advisory boards equally as well) but also a buffer when the chief health officer must take unpopular stands on public health issues or when the political leaders want something done or not done for political reasons—such as closing their eyes to a problem, not rendering advice which might prove costly and therefore politically difficult for the elected official to deal with, or support for a budget cut. Critics of policy boards argue that they inhibit political accountability. How can a governor be held accountable if he or she must work through a board which the governor probably has inherited? This criticism has not always been persuasive, given the frequently held belief that many politicians will avoid accountability when the going gets tough if at all possible. Political escape acts have been common in the areas of mental health and mental retardation when poor conditions were publicized.

A second pattern for health agency governance is to have a gubernatorial-appointed secretary or commissioner of health. Like boards, this type of leadership can be good or bad, depending on the quality of the appointed official and the quality of the governor. If a governor avoids tough issues, if a governor tends to appoint incompetents or political hacks, then the board system might be preferred. But here the *if* is *if* a good board is inherited or appointed. If, on the other hand, there is an unprogressive board, then a strong governor with a competent secretary of health would be preferred. The political style of a state often dictates how well each of the systems work. There is a tendency in recent years to move away from policy boards to the cabinet system of government where the health agency head is the secretary of health. In at least one state where this occurred, it has lead to a marked deterioration in the quality of health programming. The cabinet approach allows for greater political management and fiscal control, which has clear political advantages but can also be professionally disadvantageous.

In recent years a number of states have sought to create umbrella organizations, bringing together under one secretary several human service agencies of state government. Where these super agencies have been created (frequently called a department of human resources), no set pattern exists as to which agencies are included, though health, mental health and retardation, education, and welfare are most common. Other agencies may also be included, such as corrections. The rationale for these super agencies stems from the fact that many of the clientele of one agency are frequently the clientele of one or more of the other agencies, and by placing these agencies under one authority, improved coordination would take place, resulting in more effective and more efficient services. While success stories abound for this approach, the "successes" are usually reported by those who created these super agencies or who benefited job-wise by their creation. There are considerable anecdotal data to suggest that, while the theory is true, the practice has in fact not been operationalized at the state levels due to the jealous guarding of prerogatives by the various bureaucracies: a health professional, for example, may be very supportive of new initiatives in education or corrections so long as it is not at the expense of the health budget.

Some public health programs are operated directly by a central department in state government (commonly, state mental health, and mental retardation hospitals; licensure of professional personnel, hospitals, nursing homes, and other health facilities). Some programs are decentralized to regional offices of the state agency, if regional organization is employed. More frequently, programs have a shared responsibility between state and local government health agencies. (It should be noted that, legally, local governments are creatures of the state government and thus subject to the constitutions and all laws of the state in which the local government exists.) Where this shared responsibility occurs, the state agency will typically set performance standards under which local programs will operate in return for the allocation of some state monies to supplement local government resources. State standards also often govern the operation of nongovernmental agencies; sometimes these standards must be met in order to be eligible for a license or for payment under some state-administered program.

Some programs for which there is shared responsibility will entail some state service along with complementary local services. Standards are usually minimal standards: if one proposes to provide a service, it must at least meet those standards. Standards are, in a sense, a floor below which a program is not considered acceptable.

The mix and the sophistication of programs and the population served by programs vary considerably from state to state, and from unit to unit within a state. Most states serve all the people through environmental health programs, assuring the quality and safety of the environment through a variety of program activities. These activities involve health agency inspections, citations on deficiencies, and board of health or police action if deficiencies are not corrected. Yet, while all states engage in environmental health activities, the degree and extent of activity varies.

Similarly, all states have some personal preventive service programs, particularly in areas relating to maternal and child health, school health, and immunizations. Moreover, most have program activities relating to crippled children's services with a variety of diagnostic and treatment services available. In some states, however, access can be a problem, particularly where the state may require referral from a private physician or where it makes access to the service difficult through a lack of public information about the service, infrequency of services, and remoteness of service. Some of these barriers are intentional, some accidental.

In a great many states, public health agency services have moved far beyond the traditional areas of environment, personal preventive, mental health, and mental retardation services, with the states, directly or through local public health agencies, providing many of the services that are provided by hospitals and private physicians in other states. Where this occurs, one often finds the public health agencies paying for care in general hospitals and hiring private physicians to provide special medical services, thus supplementing the more general services provided by the full-time physician staff. While most of the personal preventive and the medical care services are provided to the poorer people of the state, some programs are available to all citizens regardless of income status. This, again, will vary considerably from state to state.

Local Health Agencies

The pattern of local health department organization also varies from state to state. A few states have no local government health units; whatever services are available, are provided by the state. But most states have local government departments, and typically some of their monies come from state and federal coffers. In New England, local departments tend to be on a city or town basis, county government being weak or nonexistent. Southern local departments tend to be organized on a county basis. There are also in-between arrangements, as in Pennsylvania, where there is provision for county health departments (but very few in existence) but there are local government (sub-county, town, borough, etc.) units with largely environmental responsibilities, as well as regional state health department offices. Some parts of the country have metropolitan and other kinds of multijurisdictional departments—that is, multicounty or combined city-county departments. How much autonomy the local (county, town, city, or multijurisdictional) department has from the state authority will vary from state to state, and even within the state—depending on the extent of state support, the dynamism of the local health officer, the relative political strengths of the different local governments, as well as the administrative style of the state health agency leaders.

PUBLIC HEALTH: FEDERAL

The federal government was the source for 28.7% of all monies spent for health in 1980 (see table 17). The federal government paid for 41.5% of the total funds spent for hospital care, 31% of the total funds spent for nursing home care, and 20.2% of the total spent for physician services (see table 19). In terms of research the federal government accounts for 87% of the total expenditures (see table 18).

Citing expenditure statistics is an appropriate way to begin this discussion because although it provides some direct services, the federal government's chief role has been that of stimulating the development of new and improved services by provision of monies to buy the action it wanted to see developed. Indeed, except in some circumscribed areas, the federal government has no constitutional authority to provide direct health services for people, this being the domain of the states.

The Congressional Role in Health

For government to do anything requires money that must be raised by some form of taxation. The use of that money, as well as the raising of it, must have a legal base—somewhere in the U.S. Constitution there must be a clause which justifies a law and, in turn, an appropriation for government to do what it does. This applies to all areas of government activity. The U.S. Supreme Court is arbiter when otherwise unresolvable disputes arise as to whether or not the activity of the government is in accord with the authorities granted government by the Constitution.

The *Powers of Congress* part of the Constitution (Article 1, Section 8), provides authority to raise and support armies, to provide and maintain a navy, and to make all laws "necessary and proper" for carrying out those powers. One can quickly see how this justifies the allocation of monies for military and naval and air force hospitals and health services. It requires only a slight extension of logic to justify the Veterans Administration work in health—be it the building of a hospital or a clinic for treatment of veterans with service-connected disabilities or the support of medical education to assure an adequate supply of doctors so that there will be enough to meet the manpower needs of the VA system. Similarly, one can justify the new medical school for the armed forces in Bethesda, Maryland.

The Constitution also grants to Congress the power to regulate foreign and interstate commerce. This justifies much of the federal activity regarding regulation of foods, drugs, product and occupational safety, and some environmental health activities because they move in, or affect, interstate or foreign commerce. The power to control federal lands, along with the presidential power to make treaties (with the advice and consent of the Senate) are the sources of federal activity in providing health services for the Indians and Eskimos. Other direct service activities also rely on these clauses for legitimization. However, by far the greatest federal influence comes from the distribution of monies to the states, local governments, and nongovernmental agencies. Sometimes these grants of money can be justified as "necessary and proper" for carrying out the specific constitutional powers already cited. An even more significant basis for grant monies derives from the power of the Congress "to lay and collect taxes, duties, imports, and excises, to pay

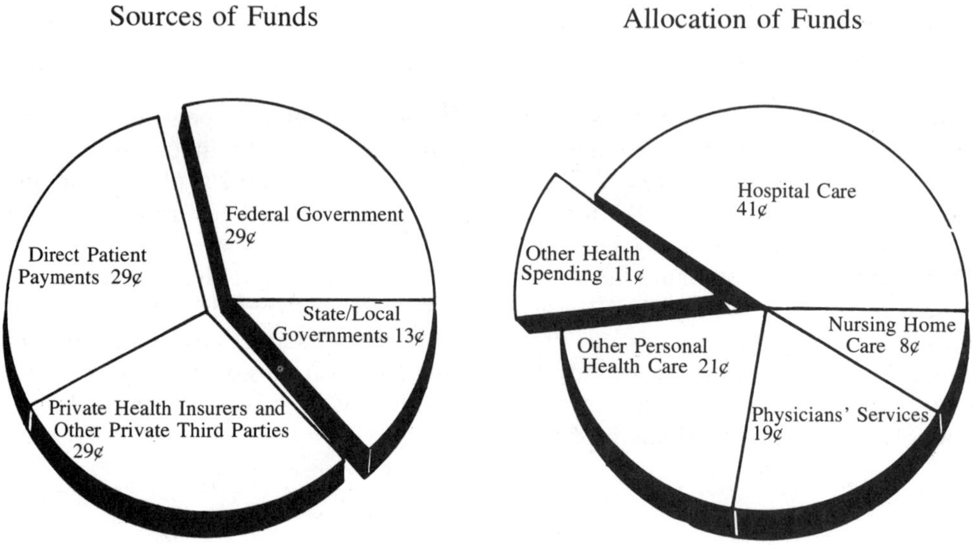

Figure 1 The nation's health dollar in 1981

the debts and provide for the common defenses and general welfare of the United States. . . ."

It is the "general welfare" clause that justified support for medical research, Medicare, Medicaid, health manpower training, health planning, etc. The power to make monies available for certain general welfare activities also permits the writing of regulations setting out the conditions which must be met in order to get the money. The regulations are applications of the law written by the administering agencies in the executive branch of government and are published in the *Federal Register,* a daily official publication of the U.S. Government. Since regulations have force of law, they must follow the intent of the Congress. Frequently, litigation revolves around whether or not a regulation has followed the intent of the Congress, and this the courts determine drawing not only upon the law itself, but also upon congressional committee reports that indicate the thinking of the Senate, the House, and sometimes of the conference committee on the bill as each reports it—the House committee report to the House of Representatives, the Senate committee report to the Senate, and the conference committee report to both houses of the Congress. The Conference Committee is an *ad hoc* group of representatives from the Senate and the House, convened to iron out or resolve different versions of similar bills, one passed by each house.

The Legislative Process

Any proposed law must begin by being introduced in the Senate or the House by one of the respective members. On introduction, it is assigned a number (for example, HR 1 or

S-9). To become law, a bill must be passed in identical form by both houses of the Congress and signed by the president of the United States. If the president vetoes the bill, it can become law without his signature if two-thirds of both houses vote to override his veto; if the president does not sign or veto the bill, it can still become law if after 10 days (Sundays excepted) no such action is taken. If during these ten days Congress adjourns, then the bill does not become law. The drafting of a bill may be done in the executive branch and given to a member of the Senate and/or House for introduction, or it may be drafted within the legislative branch and introduced by one or more members of the respective houses. Bills may also be drafted by individual citizens or groups and given to a willing member of Congress for introduction. In the United States the executive branch of government does not control the introduction, let alone flow, of legislation to the extent that it does in some parliamentary countries.

Upon introduction, a bill is referred to an appropriate committee for study and for report to the full house. The process in the Senate is very similar to that of the House of Representatives, and each goes through the entire process in considering a bill—each typically holds its own hearings on a bill and writes its own report. Neither body defers to the other on such matters.

Many bills die in committee. Some die in conference. More important bills usually have hearings whereby proponents and opponents of the bill may testify to give information to the committee which will help or influence the committee's thinking about the bill. With the benefit of this information and advice from its professional staff, a committee can then decide what action it wishes to take on the bill. It has a report prepared on the bill, which accompanies the bill to the full House or Senate. The report will explain what the bill is intended to do. Committee reports can be secured from the respective committees, as can published hearings.

The movement of a bill through the House or Senate is a complicated process, affected by the views of the committees handling a bill, the volume of business before the house, as well as political considerations of influential leaders, the administration, interest and pressure groups, and the views of individual members of the house.

The General Accounting Office

The General Accounting Office (GAO) is an agency of the Congress. Its job is, in part, to help the Congress monitor the performance of federal agencies, though it is much more than a bookkeeping operation: it conducts a large number of studies to determine how well the intent of law is being carried out in terms of program activities, effectiveness, and efficiency. As might be expected, its reports are often discomforting to agencies in the executive branch.

Health Responsibilities of the Executive Branch

There are a number of major federal agencies concerned with health services. Principal among these are the Department of Defense, Veterans Administration, Department of Labor, Environmental Protection Agency, and Department of Health and Human Services.

The Department of Defense administers a rather large network of health facilities to serve the armed forces. The Veterans Administration also runs a large network of hospitals (272 with 82,000 beds and ambulatory services) to treat veterans of the armed services who have service-connected (not necessarily war-related) disabilities as well as nonservice-connected disabilities for veterans who cannot afford private care. Some dependents of veterans are also entitled to care. In addition to hospitals, the VA has over 8,700 beds in 95 nursing homes, and provides or pays for services in a variety of other institutions. Since 1946 the VA has expanded greatly and affiliated many of its hospitals with medical schools around the country. Increased use of VA services is apparent as the aging World War II veterans reach retirement age and seek VA care because of shortcomings in the Medicare program.

The Department of Labor is responsible for the Occupational Safety and Health Administration (OSHA), which is playing an increasingly important role in establishing standards and regulations to govern the safety and health of the work environment and to carry out periodic inspections. The Environmental Protection Agency (EPA) is an independent regulatory agency for setting and enforcing standards and regulations governing the environment. Both the OSHA and the EPA frequently work through the environmental health authorities of state and local governments.

The principal public health agency, however, is the Department of Health and Human Services (DHSS or HHS). Its activities are varied. The Public Health Service (PHS) is one of the organizations within this large agency.

Public Health Service

The National Institutes of Health (NIH) is composed of eleven research institutes, a large research hospital, and the National Library of Medicine. Located just outside of Washington, D.C. in suburban Bethesda, Maryland, the NIH is a large complex where a considerable amount of basic and applied research in the health sciences is carried out. In addition to this intramural research, the various institutes administer a variety of research grant programs, using outside reviewers for grant proposals and awarding research grants after appropriate review to universities, research institutes, and hospitals both here and abroad. The institutes at NIH are the National Cancer Institute; National Institute on Aging; National Institute of Child Health and Human Development; National Institute of General Medical Sciences; National Heart, Lung, and Blood Institute; National Institute of Allergy and Infectious Diseases; National Institute of Dental Research; National Institute of Neurological and Communicative Disorders and Stroke; National Institute of Arthritis, Diabetes, and Digestive and Kidney Diseases; National Institute of Environmental Health Sciences; National Eye Institute.

The Alcohol, Drug Abuse, and Mental Health Administration (ADAMHA) like the NIH, carries out intramural research and provides funds for extra-mural research around the country. The National Institute of Mental Health within this agency has also supported the training of mental health professionals, and administers a psychiatric hospital in Washington.

The Food and Drug Administration (FDA) is a regulatory agency assuring the safety of foods, radiologic devices, and drugs and other biological products which move in interstate commerce.

The Centers for Disease Control (CDC), based in Atlanta, Georgia, maintains a number of laboratories for the study of infectious and communicable diseases, and provides training and technical assistance for state and local public health officials.

The Health Resources and Services Administration (HRSA) encompasses the Indian Health Service, which provides direct care to more than 500,000 American Indians and Alaskan natives through 48 hospitals, 81 health centers, and several hundred health stations and field clinics. The HRSA also runs a hospital for Hansen's disease and administers medical programs for the U.S. Coast Guard and the Federal Bureau of Prisons. Its units have also been active in assisting states and communities in developing emergency medical services and providing financial support for experimental innovative health delivery systems. It also administers the National Health Service Corps (NHSC), which assigns recent medical school graduates and other health professionals to rural and inner-city primary care centers—centers which are mostly community (not government) sponsored. Many of these assignees are serving in lieu of repayment for government educational loans.

The Bureau of Health Professions within the HRSA reviews grant applications for the training of various health workers. It has been historically a major resource for funds for medical, dental, nursing, public health administration, and other health professional academic programs.

Health Care Financing Administration

The Health Care Financing Administration (HCFA) is another major unit of the Department of Health and Human Services. It is not part of the Public Health Service. It has units that oversee the Medicare and Medicaid bureaus as well as the Bureau of Quality Assurance, which oversees the Professional Standards Review Organizations that have developed under federal funding.

The Office of the Secretary

In the Office of the Secretary of Health and Human Services there are a number of special units that serve a departmentwide function. Two are particularly noteworthy: the National Center for Health Statistics and the National Center for Health Services Research (NCHSR). The latter supports a limited number of research projects concerned with improving the delivery mechanism for health services.

International Health Activities

The Office of International Health (OIH) is within the office of the Secretary of Health and Human Services and is the principal health representative of the U.S. Government in the international arena. It works directly with foreign governments and with the World Health Organization (WHO). OIH has a particularly close relationship with the Agency for International Development (AID), which is the foreign aid arm of the State Department. AID is engaged in a wide variety of health projects overseas—financing some projects, sending consulting teams on other projects. The Fogarty International Center (FIC) is a part of NIH and serves as a base for the exchange of knowledge on biomedical research, medical education, research training, and health care. It works closely with biomedical scientists who visit the United States, arranges international conferences, and sponsors studies of foreign health systems and practices.

It should be emphasized once again that the principal role of the federal government is as a facilitator—facilitating the work of state and local governments; universities, including their medical and other professional schools; as well as a wide range of community health agencies. This facilitation comes mainly through the provision of grant monies to enable these agencies to perform activities for which they seek money. The federal influence is seen in the laws and regulations that govern the allocation of these funds.

A second item to note is that large federal agencies—like all large organizations—are always in the process of reorganization. However, though the names change and the organizational units shift, generally the same basic functions continue. The outsider simply has to look more closely to find them.

HEALTH PLANNING

New knowledge is offering new opportunities to treat what was previously untreatable—to prolong life, to save lives, to lessen disability and pain, and in general to improve the quality of life. That many of these new opportunities turn out to be enormously expensive is a matter of growing concern, considering that the health sector commands such a large and growing share of the Gross National Product. In recent years these opportunities and resulting costs have led to the development of a national health planning system.

The system is national in the sense that federal legislation provided resources to develop nationwide the type of planning effort that proved so successful on a voluntary or state government basis in a few of the states. Because the provision of most health care was a state government or nongovernmental function, health planning necessarily had to develop largely on a voluntary basis.

During the late 1930s and 1940s, hospitals in our larger cities voluntarily got together, collected data and talked about that data, negotiated differences, and agreed on planned, orderly development of facilities. No one forced the hospitals to get together; there was no law mandating it. It just seemed like the sensible thing to do. Similarly, professional groups—most notably, the American Medical Association and the American College of Surgeons—took it upon themselves early in this century (the AMA actually starting in the mid-nineteenth century) to bring about reform in terms of improving the quality of medical schools, medical practice, and hospitals. Each, along with others, planned to deal with some of the problems that they saw and that they thought they could do something about.

In Maryland in 1940 the state medical society persuaded the State Planning Commission to appoint a Committee on Medical Care to oversee the state's health needs and to make periodic recommendations in the form of health plans. Over some twenty-five years the Committee on Medical Care—working with private physicians, voluntary hospitals, medical school faculty, and cooperatively, with the Maryland State Health Department—developed pioneering plans that were implemented by the state government and led in the 1950s and 1960s to some of the most advanced public health programming in the nation.

The Maryland experience is cited because it illustrates vividly the base for most health planning in the United States today. Maryland's Committee on Medical Care represented a partnership between government and the nongovernmental sector. This planning recognized the democratic, nonelitist character of the society in which citizens get together and, in a dialogue with the state government, advise what needs to be done. The state government, in the process, was able to enlist on behalf of the government and the people it served an impressive array of professional and consumer talent.

Health planning in the United States has essentially been planning from the local community to the state and, if necessary, to the federal government. It operates on the principle that the best plans are ones that enjoy the support of those who must implement them, and the best way to secure that support is to get those people and agencies—in and out of government—to participate in the development of the plan.

In 1966 the U.S. Congress formalized the process it saw occurring in various parts of the country by providing funds for the development of state government and areawide (usually sub-state or metropolitan) comprehensive health planning agencies. Most of the areawide health planning agencies were voluntary (nongovernmental) agencies.

The development of these agencies—both state and areawide—was slow, and their achievements showed mixed results. Despite enthusiastic support at their inception, that support was eroded by 1974 when new federal legislation was adopted. The chief problem stemmed from the fact that, as the agencies were developing, the country entered into a period when resources for health sector allocation were more limited. State and federal governments were particularly concerned by the inflationary spiral of the 1970s because of the costs they had to pay. The health planning agencies thus began to be pressured by various government levels, including the legislative branches, to do something about rising health care costs; however, these agencies had little power because of the basic structure of the law, which prescribed the planning process as a partnership involving negotiation and compromise on the part of all parties. As costs rose, and pressures were applied to the agencies, some states took the initiative by the adoption of *certificate of need* legislation and the creation of hospital rate control bodies. In 1974 the Congress, in adopting new health planning legislation, mandated that all states adopt certificate of need legislation as a condition for receipt of federal funds under a variety of federal health programs; the Congress also strengthened the federal role by directing the secretary of health, education, and welfare (now secretary of health and human services) to develop standards governing the appropriate supply, distribution, and organization of health resources as part of the federal government's *National Guidelines for Health Planning*. This very strong move toward more federal control led to physician, hospital, medical school, and other health provider dissatisfaction. Implementation of the 1974 legislation also led to considerable litigation because for the first time the United States was moving toward a federally regulated health system.

Thus—while there was in each state government a State Health Planning and Development Agency with an advisory State Health Coordinating Council, and each state had one or more health systems agencies (HSAs), and each HSA had to develop a long-range health systems plan and annual implementation plan—the grass roots planning effort was severally constrained by central direction from the federal government. The congressional amendments to the legislation in late 1979 clouded the future development of this structure, since the Congress stated that the HSAs and the state agencies need no longer conform to national guidelines. How this will affect the health planning movement remains to be seen. Federal appropriations for these agencies were cut in the 1980s, and pending legislation in 1983 would eliminate all federal support for their work. Some HSAs have ceased to operate; others have continued to function with monies from state government and/or the private sector; some still receive federal monies at sharply reduced levels.

Though much of what occurs today under the aegis of the health planning agencies is a negation of the traditional mechanism for health planning on a partnership basis, it needs to be recognized that the rising cost of health care is posing serious financial problems for state governments and for the federal government. Critics of the current federal planning legislation, while acknowledging that the payment of health care costs at cost does not encourage provider economy or provider restraint, argue that the health industry is basically a victim of actions and pressures from government and the economy in general.

It is fair to say that there is considerable ferment and debate over the health planning legislation, the development of the health planning agencies, and the move to regulate the health industry in new and different ways.

CONCLUSION

The health system in the United States is complex. Sponsorship of agencies and facilities (hospitals, nursing homes, health centers, etc.) range from the investor owned to church to community to local government to state government to federal government. Most facilities and services are provided by the nongovernmental sector. Finance of the system also varies, with government responsible for only 43% of all health expenditures and 40.4% of all *personal* health care expenditures. (*Personal* health expenditures differ from the larger category of *all* health expenditures in that the former excludes expenditures for environmental and other public health activities, research, and construction.) There are also organizational and financial differences from state to state and between communities within a state, variations in structure, breadth of services, cost of services, lengths of hospital stay, and clinical patterns of practice.

To the person looking at the system for the first time, the system's complexity often appears as a nonsystem. It seems as confusing as the description by Ptolemy of the movement of heavenly bodies. However, looked at another way—as one would abandon the Ptolemaic perspective for that offered by Copernicus—the health system in the United States is quite orderly and works reasonably well. The perspective should not be from the outside looking in, but from that of the patient who needs health care.

After all, most people in the United States do have easy access to care. There are none of the surgical waiting lists that one finds in many countries. The quality of care is high, yet the never-satisfied health professionals in the United States are forever seeking ways to improve that which is already at a high level: criticism of existing practices and laments over the opportunities being missed are part of the strategy for bringing about change.

The quality of hospital care and medical practice in hospitals is subject to constant scrutiny, in large measure through professionally designed and accepted mechanisms for self-criticism, and changes are being instituted as required to strengthen this quality wherever possible. Medical practitioners are trained in schools and hospitals that also are assessed and inspected regularly. Graduates must pass rigorous objective examinations developed and administered by outside bodies, not by their medical schools. The quality of medical practice is further strengthened by the almost universal mandate for participation in approved continuing medical education programs, and strengthened as medical specialties are moving toward the periodic reexamination of their members. Nearly all new physicians, moreover, enter specialty training in one of many medical specialties (including family practice), which requires at least three years of supervised clinical training after medical school. Forces for improvement within the health sector are as vigorous as ever.

There still are some shortcomings. While physicians are moving into rural areas, retention is still a problem. There is an enormous need for upgrading nursing homes and their services. Mental health programs have made considerable progress, but financial resources for optimizing the opportunities are very limited. The cost of health care is high, and there are some excesses, but paying for this care does not greatly worry most Americans, with perhaps the exception of those over age sixty-five, to whom physician charges frequently exceed Medicare payments by significant amounts. Comparatively few people have no health insurance or protection—albeit limited—by some government program. The high cost of some illnesses, which is often publicized, is not a deep concern to most: very few face this kind of catastrophy, and approximately two-thirds of the people have some form of catastrophic (major medical) health insurance. Perhaps the greatest immediate need is to improve upon major medical insurance and to get all protected by it, and in particular to extend this type of protection to those over sixty-five years of age. A secondary need is to improve coverage for nursing home care. The concern over rising health costs is mostly a concern of (1) government, which must use tax monies to pay for 43% of all costs, (2) business and industrial leaders, whose firms pay the cost of most health insurance premiums (and must thus increase their prices to cover these costs), and (3) the health insurance companies, which are placed in the difficult position of constantly revising their premiums and trying to get business and industry to accept the increases. Their concerns, though real, do not in themselves prove the case that costs are too high. Indeed, many people believe that the nation can still afford to spend much more than it does.

The final test of the system, however, is the health of the American people. Here, the data are mixed. For conditions that rely on medical intervention, hospital practice, and traditional public health activities, the record is outstanding. Life expectancy is increasing. The infant mortality rate is decreasing and particularly so among the disadvantaged groups that have evidenced poor health in the past. Due to effective immunization programs, most of the serious communicable diseases no longer pose threats to communities. There are still problems in these areas among the new, large immigrant groups from poorer areas of the world. There is, moreover, the everpresent problem, as in all societies, of keeping the health education levels of the people high so that high health levels can be maintained.

Two areas of health concern needing much more attention are personal prevention and environmental health.

Americans eat too much and too many non-nutritious foods. They drink and smoke too much, drive recklessly, and exercise too little. Each of these contributes to illness and disease. Control is largely within the domain of the individual citizen, and this makes progress in these areas extremely difficult.

Remarkable progress has been made in the environmental area in terms of food safety and water quality control, but as new knowledge is acquired we sometimes find that what was once thought safe may not be safe. As new technology develops, we are also faced with new environmental hazards which need to be monitored and sometimes controlled. In both instances, of course, employment is often affected, and control costs can be significant, thus making implementation of controls sometimes difficult to secure.

On the balance, though more can be done and should be done to improve health and the quality of life in the United States, progress has been significant and it continues. The American people—complain as they will at times—are basically proud of the health system they have, proud with good cause.

For Further Study

American Hospital Association. *Hospital Statistics.* Chicago: American Hospital Association, annual.

American Medical Association. *American Medical News.* Chicago: American Medical Association, weekly.

———. *Socioeconomic Issues of Health.* Chicago: American Medical Association, annual.

American Medical Association, Council on Medical Education. *Medical Education in the United States.* Printed annually in *JAMA* (the journal of the American Medical Association).

Raffel, Marshall W. *The U.S. Health System: Origins and Functions,* New York: Wiley, 1980.

U.S. Government, Department of Health and Human Services (formerly, Health, Education, and Welfare). *Health Care Financing Review.* Washington D.C., quarterly.

———. *Health·United States.* Washington D.C., annual.

In addition to the above sources, there are a number of leading journals that regularly carry items relating to the organization and finance of health services in the United States, including research findings. Among these journals are : *Inquiry; Journal of Health Politics, Policy and Law; Hospitals; Journal of the American Public Health Association; Public Health Reports;* and *The New England Journal of Medicine.*

Table 1 United States population by age, race, and sex, 1980

	Number (Thousands)			
	White		Black and Other	
Age (Years)	Male	Female	Male	Female
All ages	91,670	96,671	12,516	13,972
Under 5	6,483	6,148	1,228	1,208
5 to 14	14,092	13,400	2,599	2,564
15 to 24	17,310	16,929	2,788	2,919
25 to 34	15,303	15,322	1,955	2,254
35 to 44	10,679	10,905	1,228	1,479
45 to 54	9,556	10,057	1,019	1,251
55 to 64	9,025	10,186	851	1,056
65 and over	9,220	13,724	846	1,240
Median age	30.0	32.6	23.6	26.2
Total population (all ages)	226,505			

SOURCE: Statistical Abstract of the United States.

NOTE: Population estimate for 1981: 231 million.

Table 2 Live births, birth rates, and fertility rates, United States

	Births	Birth Rate	Fertility Rate
1978	3,333,279	15.0	65.5
1979	3,494,398	15.6	67.2
1980	3,612,258	15.9	68.4

SOURCE: "Final Data from the National Center for Health Statistics," *Monthly Vital Statistics Report* 31, no. 8 (30 November 1982).

NOTES: Rates on an annual basis. Birth rates per 1,000 population and fertility rates per 1,000 women aged 15 to 44 years.

Table 3 Infant mortality rates by age and color, selected years, United States

	Total			White			All Other		
	Under 1 Year	28 Days to 11 Months	Under 28 Days	Under 1 Year	28 Days to 11 Months	Under 28 Days	Under 1 Year	28 Days to 11 Months	Under 28 Days
1950	29.2	8.7	20.5	26.8	7.4	19.4	44.5	16.9	27.5
1960	26.0	7.3	18.7	22.9	5.7	17.2	43.2	16.4	26.9
1965	24.7	7.0	17.7	21.5	5.4	16.1	40.3	14.9	25.4
1967	22.4	5.9	16.5	19.7	4.7	15.0	35.9	12.1	23.8
1969	20.9	5.3	15.6	18.4	4.2	14.2	32.9	10.4	22.5
1970	20.0	4.9	15.1	17.8	4.0	13.8	30.9	9.5	21.4
1971	19.1	4.9	14.2	17.1	4.0	13.0	28.5	8.9	19.6
1972	18.5	4.8	13.6	16.4	4.0	12.4	27.7	8.5	19.2
1973	17.7	4.8	13.0	15.8	3.9	11.8	26.2	8.3	17.9
1974	16.7	4.4	12.3	14.8	3.7	11.1	24.9	7.7	17.2
1975	16.1	4.5	11.6	14.2	3.8	10.4	24.2	7.5	16.8
1976	15.2	4.3	10.9	13.3	3.6	9.7	23.5	7.2	16.3
1977	14.1	4.2	9.9	12.3	3.7	8.7	21.7	6.5	14.7
1978	13.6	4.3	9.5	12.0	3.6	8.4	23.1	7.0	14.0
1979	13.1	4.2	8.9	11.4	3.3	7.7	21.8	6.9	12.9
1980	12.5	4.1	8.4	—	—	—	—	—	—
1981	11.9	3.9	8.1						
1982	11.4	3.7	7.7						

SOURCE: "Annual Summary for the United States," *Monthly Vital Statistics Report* 26:10 (7 December 1978); 27:9 (13 August 1979); 31:9 (17 December 1982); *Health · United States 1981;* and unpublished data.

NOTES: For 1978, based on a 10% sample of deaths; for 1972, based on a 50% sample of deaths; for 1980 and 1981, data is provisional; for 1982, data is for 12 months ending May 1982 but does not include figures for Colorado, New Jersey, and Connecticut; for all other years based on final data. Rates per 1,000 live births in specified group.

Table 4 Infant mortality rates by selected causes, selected years, United States

Causes of Death	1960	1965	1970	1975	1979	1980(Est.)	1981(Est.)
Total, under 1 year	26.0	24.7	20.0	16.1	13.07	12.5	11.7
Congenital anomalies	3.6	3.6	3.0	2.7	2.6	2.5	2.4
Respiratory Distress Syndrome	—	—	—	—	1.6	1.4	1.2
Sudden Infant Death Syndrome	—	—	—	—	1.5	1.5	1.4
Immaturity, unqualified	4.6	3.8	2.3	1.4	1.0	1.1	1.0
Newborn affected by maternal complications of pregnancy	—	—	—	—	.5	—	—
Asphyxia of newborn unspecified	4.6	4.1	2.5	1.3	.4	.4	.4
Birth injuries	2.4	2.1	0.6	0.6	.3	.3	.2
Influenza and pneumonia	3.1	2.9	1.7	0.7	.3	.3	.2
Accidents and adverse affects	—	—	—	—	.3	—	—
Infection specific to perinatal period	—	—	—	—	.3	—	—
All other causes	7.8	8.3	9.8	9.4	4.3	—	—

SOURCE: "Annual Summary for the United States," *Monthly Vital Statistics Report* 17:5 (15 August 1969); 22:5 (27 June 1974); 23:5 (30 May 1975); 27:9 (13 August 1979); 31:9 (30 September 1982); 30:13 (20 December 1982) for 1980 and 1981 estimates.

NOTE: Rates per 1,000 live births.

Table 5 Death rates for 15 leading causes of death, selected years, United States

Cause of Death	1968 Rank	1968 Death Rate	1968 % of Total Deaths	1977 Rank	1977 Death Rate	1977 % of Total Deaths	1978 Rank	1978 Death Rate	1978 % of Total Deaths	1979 Rank	1979 Death Rate	1979 % of Total Deaths	1981 (Est.) Rank	1981 (Est.) Death Rate	1981 (Est.) % of Total Deaths
All causes		967.9	100.0%		878.1	100.0%		883.4	100.0%		869.5	100.0%			
Diseases of heart	1	373.5	38.6	1	332.3	37.8	1	334.3	37.8	1	333.1	38.3	1	330.6	38.2
Malignant neoplasms	2	159.8	16.5	2	178.7	20.4	2	181.9	20.6	2	183.3	21.1	2	184.3	21.3
Cerebrovascular diseases	3	106.0	11.0	3	84.1	9.6	3	80.5	9.0	3	77.0	8.9	3	71.7	8.3
Accidents	4	57.6	6.0	4	47.7	5.4	4	48.4	5.5	4	47.8	5.5	4	44.5	5.1
Influenza and pneumonia	5	36.9	3.8	5	23.7	2.7	5	26.7	3.0	6	20.5	2.4	6	23.7	2.7
Diabetes mellitus	7	19.2	2.0	6	15.2	1.7	6	15.5	1.6	7	15.1	1.7	7	15.2	1.7
Cirrhosis of liver	10	14.6	1.5	7	14.3	1.6	7	13.8	1.6	8	13.5	1.6	8	12.9	1.5
Arteriosclerosis	8	16.8	1.7	8	13.3	1.5	8	13.3	1.5	9	13.1	1.5	9	12.5	1.4
Suicide	11	10.7	1.1	8	13.3	1.5	9	12.5	1.4	10	12.4	1.4	10	12.3	1.4
Certain causes of mortality in early infancy	6	22.0	2.3	10	10.8	1.2	10	10.1	1.1	11	10.7	1.2	12	9.2	1.1
Bronchitis, emphysema, and asthma	9	16.6	1.7	11	10.3	1.2	11	10.0	1.1	5	22.7	2.6	5	26.1	3.0
Homicide	13	7.4	0.8	12	9.2	1.0	12	9.4	1.1	12	10.2	1.2	11	10.7	1.2
Congenital anomalies	12	8.4	0.9	13	6.0	0.7	13	5.9	0.7	14	6.1	0.7	14	5.8	0.7
Nephritis and nephrosis	14	4.7	0.5	14	3.9	0.4	14	4.1	0.5	13	7.1	0.8	13	7.6	0.9
Septicemia	15	1.5	0.2	15	3.3	0.4	15	3.6	0.4	15	3.6	0.4	15	4.4	0.5
All other causes		112.3	11.6		111.9	12.7		113.8	12.9		93.3	10.7		94.9	10.9

SOURCE: "Annual Summary for the United States," *Monthly Vital Statistics Report* 26:24–25 (13 August 1979); 31:6 (30 September 1982); 30:13 (20 December 1982) for 1981 estimates.

NOTE: For 1978, based on a 10% sample of deaths; for all other years, based on final data. Rates per 100,000 population.

Table 6 Average length of stay for selected operative procedures, 1980, United States

Operation	Number of Procedures (Thousands)	Average Length of Stay (Days)
Dilation and curettage, diagnostic	813	3.3
Cesarean section	610	6.5
Hysterectomy	538	8.0
Reduction of fracture	522	10.8
Repair of inguinal hernia	497	4.8
Excision of lesion of skin and tissue	494	8.7
Low forceps operation with and without episiotomy	457	3.5
Extraction of lens	440	3.7
Biopsy	434	8.8
Cholecystectomy	423	10.9
Bilateral destruction or occlusion of fallopian tubes	383	2.9
Dilation and curettage after delivery or abortion	273	1.9
Prostatectomy	273	11.3
Appendectomy excluding incidental	267	5.6
Tonsillectomy with adenoidectomy	264	1.9
Cardiac catheterization	262	4.9
Operations on muscles, tendons, fascia, and bursa	248	4.2
Repair of current obstetric laceration	244	3.1
Tonsillectomy without adenoidectomy	185	2.3
Open heart operations	167	16.1

SOURCE: Division of Health Care Statistics, National Center for Health Statistics: unpublished data from the National Hospital Discharge Survey for 1980, as reported by the American College of Surgeons in its *Socio-Economic Factbook for Surgery 1982*.

NOTE: Number of procedures and average length of stay are for first-listed operations. Average length of stay may reflect days in the hospital for procedures in addition to the first-listed procedure. For example, average length of stay for biopsy may also include days in the hospital for subsequent operative procedures.

Table 7 Discharges and average length of stay for discharges with no procedures by selected first-listed diagnoses, 1981, United States

Diagnosis (ICD–9–CM codes)	Discharges With No Procedures (Thousands)	Average Length of Stay (Days)
Total (includes discharges for diagnoses not listed)	17,975	7.1
Pneumonia (480–486)	686	7.8
Cerebrovascular disease (430–438)	551	11.2
Diabetes mellitus (250)	522	8.1
Psychoses (290–299)	519	14.9
Alcohol dependence syndrome (303)	428	10.4
Asthma (493)	399	5.5
Acute myocardial infarction (410)	377	11.6
Coronary atherosclerosis (atherosclerotic heart disease) (414.0)	370	9.0
Congestive heart failure (428.0)	361	9.4
Cardiac dysrhythmias (427)	330	6.6
Disorders of the central nervous system (320–349)	277	8.6
Neuroses and personality disorders (300–301)	272	9.9
Essential hypertension (401)	263	5.8
Sprains and strains of back (including neck) (846–847)	254	7.1

SOURCE: Division of Health Care Statistics, National Center for Health Statistics: unpublished data from the National Hospital Discharge Survey for 1981.

NOTE: Discharges from short-stay, nonfederal hospitals. Excludes newborn infants.

Table 8 Estimated persons active in selected major health field occupations, 1980 and 1978, United States

		Rate Per 100,000 Population
1980		
Dentists	126,240	56.4
Optometrists	22,330	10.0
Pharmacists	144,260	63.3
Podiatrists	8,880	4.0
Registered nurses	1,678,000[a]	740.8
Veterinarians	36,000	16.1
1978		
Dieticians	28,000	
Physical therapists	30,000	
Medical records administrators	12,000	
Medical records technologists	68,000	
Medical Technologists	125,000	
Cytotechnologists	7,000	
Occupational therapists	15,000	
Speech pathologists/audiologists	36,000	

SOURCES: Figures for 1980 from U.S. Department of Health and Human Services, *Supply and Characteristics of Selected Health Personnel,* DHSS Pub. no. (HRA) 81–20; 1978 from U.S. Department of Health and Human Services, *A Report on Allied Health Personnel,* DHEW Pub. no. (HRA) 80–28.

[a] Figure from the American Nurses Association.

Table 9 Operational medical schools, medical students enrolled by sex, and medical school graduates by sex in 1979–80 and 1980–81, United States

	1979–80		1980–81	
	MD	DO	MD	DO
Medical schools	125	14	125	14
Total medical students	64,195	4,544	65,497	4,966
Women medical students	16,315 (25.4%)	837 (18.4%)	17,373 (26.5%)	901 (18.1%)
Total medical graduates	15,135	1,033	15,677	1,133
Women medical graduates	3,497 (23.1%)	192 (18.6%)	3,892 (24.8%)	228 (20.1%)

SOURCE: "Annual Report on Medical Education in the U.S. (1979–1980; 1980–1981)," *Journal of the American Medical Association,* 26 December 1980 and 25 December 1981. Data on osteopathic medicine from the American Osteopathic Association.

Table 10 Active physicians and physicians per population, selected years (including projections), United States

		Type of Physician		
	Total	Doctors of Medicine (MD)	Doctors of Osteopathy (DO)	Professionally Active Physicians Per 10,000 Population
1950	219,900	209,000	10,900	14.2
1960	259,500	247,300	12,200	14.2
1970	323,200	311,200	12,300	15.5
1975	378,600	364,500	14,100	17.4
1976	390,600	376,100	14,700	17.9
1977	395,200	380,200	15,400	17.9
1978	419,520	403,420	16,100	18.8
1979	433,550	416,680	16,870	19.3
1980	449,500	432,400	17,100	20.2
1985	523,900	502,000	21,900	22.5
1990	591,200	563,300	27,900	24.3
2000	704,700	665,700	39,000	27.1

SOURCE: *Health · United States, 1981* (Washington, D.C.: U.S. Department of Health and Human Services).

NOTES: Data are based on reporting by physicians and medical schools.

The population for selected years 1950 to 1980 includes residents in the 50 states and the District of Columbia, and civilians in Puerto Rico and other U.S. outlying areas; U.S. citizens in foreign countries; and the Armed Forces in the United States and abroad. For 1985 and 1990, the Series II projections of the total population from the U.S. Bureau of the Census are used. Estimation and projection methods used are from the Bureau of Health Professions. The numbers of MDs differ from American Medical Association figures because a variant proportion of the physicians not classified by specialty is allocated into the totals.

Table 11 Federal and nonfederal physicians by specialty and activity, 31 December 1980, United States

		Major Professional Activity							
		Patient Care				Other Professional Activity			
				Hospital-Based Practice					
Specialty	Total Physicians	Total	Office-Based Practice	Residents All Years	Full-Time Physician Staff	Medical Teaching	Adminis-tration	Research	Other
Total physicians	467,679	376,512	272,000	62,042	42,470	7,942	12,209	15,377	2,876
General practice	60,049	58,633	48,020	6,339	4,274	368	737	95	216
Medical specialties	125,755	109,543	76,090	21,980	11,473	3,194	3,171	9,365	482
Allergy	1,518	1,419	1,371		48	19	16	57	7
Cardiovascular disease	9,823	7,759	6,729		1,030	357	232	1,416	59
Dermatology	5,660	5,356	4,378	631	347	106	57	120	21
Gastroenterology	4,046	3,086	2,737		349	188	70	694	8
Internal medicine	71,531	62,959	40,617	16,160	6,182	1,460	1,869	4,967	276
Pediatrics	28,342	25,435	17,517	5,166	2,752	763	747	1,308	89
Pediatric allergy	461	395	362	8	25	14	4	47	1
Pediatric cardiology	559	466	331	15	120	55	29	108	1
Pulmonary disease	3,715	2,668	2,048		620	232	147	648	20
Surgical specialties	110,778	106,486	81,931	17,405	7,150	1,348	1,173	1,476	295
General surgery	34,034	32,587	22,426	7,525	2,636	365	495	494	93
Neurosurgery	3,341	3,198	2,468	473	275	45	29	62	7
Obstetrics/gynecology	26,305	25,261	19,513	4,133	1,615	361	365	255	63
Ophthalmology	12,974	12,448	10,603	1,309	536	131	66	296	33
Orthopedic surgery	13,996	13,596	10,728	2,050	818	172	61	119	48
Otolaryngology	6,553	6,333	5,266	712	355	91	55	60	14
Plastic surgery	2,980	2,873	2,438	263	172	47	11	42	7
Colon and rectal surgery	719	699	657	12	30	2	3	13	2
Thoracic surgery	2,133	1,976	1,604	165	207	37	49	64	7
Urological surgery	7,743	7,515	6,228	763	524	97	39	71	21

Table 11 *Continued*

Specialty	Total Physicians	Major Professional Activity							
		Patient Care				Other Professional Activity			
				Hospital-Based Practice					
		Total	Office-Based Practice	Residents All Years	Full-Time Physician Staff	Medical Teaching	Adminis-tration	Research	Other
Other specialties									
Anesthesiology	15,958	14,945	11,338	1,495	2,112	588	170	217	38
Dermatology	7,048	6,568	4,191	1,343	1,034	161	46	136	137
Neurology	5,685	4,776	3,253	898	625	247	100	519	43
Psychiatry	27,481	24,469	16,004	3,282	5,183	553	1,769	533	157
Public health	13,402	11,067	5,963	1,960	3,144	438	546	755	596
Physical medicine	2,146	1,927	1,014	252	661	39	117	45	18
Radiology	11,653	10,770	7,802	864	2,104	237	129	306	211
Other	34,961	27,328	16,394	6,224	4,710	769	4,251	1,930	683
Not classified	20,629								
Inactive	25,744								
Address Unknown	6,390								

SOURCE: *Physician Characteristics and Distribution,* 1981 ed., American Medical Association.

NOTE: Excluded from the above figures are 6,755 foreign physicians who are in the United States temporarily.

Table 12 Estimated annual medical practice income of physicians (MDs) by specialty before taxes, but excluding business- or practice- associated expenses, United States

	Income		
	1975	1981	Annual % Change
All physicians	$56,400	$93,000	8.7
By specialty			
Surgery	68,200	118,600	9.7
Anesthesiology	57,100	118,600	13.0
Radiology	75,200	116,900	7.6
Obstetrics/gynecology	63,300	110,800	9.8
Internal medicine	57,000	85,100	6.9
General or family practice	45,400	72,200	8.0
Psychiatry	44,800	70,600	7.9
Pediatrics	44,300	65,100	6.6
Other	54,900	86,700	7.9

SOURCE: *American Medical News,* American Medical Association, 1 October 1982.

NOTE: For 1982, the average net income rose by 7% to $99,500, but surgery rose 10%, radiology 17%, and anesthesiology 10.8%. (*SMS Report,* AMA, July 1983).

Table 13 Hospitals, beds, admissions, average daily census, and occupancy rate by type of hospital, United States

Type of Hospital	Hospitals		Beds (Thousands)		Admissions (Thousands)		Average Daily Census (Thousands)		Occupancy (%)		Average Length of Stay (Days)	
	1970	1980	1970	1980	1970	1980	1970	1980	1970	1980	1970	1980
Total	7,123	6,965	1,616	1,365	31,759	38,892	1,298	1,060	80.3	77.7	—	—
Federal	408	359	161	117	1,741	2,044	128	94	79.6	80.1	—	—
Nonfederal	6,715		1,455		30,018		1,170		80.4			
Psychiatric	519	534	527	215	598	566	447	183	84.8	85.2	—	—
Tuberculosis	101	11	20	2	36	8	12	1	61.8	67.0	—	—
Long-term general	236	157	60	39	132	76	49	33	82.0	85.9	—	—
Short-term general	5,859	5,904	848	992	29,252	36,198	662	748	78.0	75.4	8.2	7.6
Community hospitals	5,859	5,830[a]	848	988[a]	29,252	36,143[a]	662	747[a]	78.0	75.6[a]	8.2	7.6[b]
6–24 beds	397	259	7	5	241	165	4	2	55.7	46.8	—	5.3
25–49	1,327	1,029	48	37	1,655	1,274	30	20	63.6	57.4	—	5.8
50–99	1,490	1,462	105	105	3,669	3,704	74	68	70.7	64.2	—	6.7
100–199	1,275	1,370	177	193	6,414	7,156	134	138	75.8	71.4	—	7.1
200–299	592	715	142	172	5,148	6,590	114	133	80.3	77.4	—	7.4
300–399	356	412	121	139	4,348	5,360	99	111	82.3	79.7	—	7.6
400–499	190	266	83	118	2,915	4,402	70	96	84.3	81.2	—	7.9
500 or more	232	317	166	218	4,862	7,496	136	179	81.8	82.1	—	8.7

SOURCE: *Hospital Statistics,* 1981 ed., American Hospital Association.

NOTE: Figures may not add due to rounding.

[a]Deleted from this category are 74 short-term general hospitals that are part of other institutions whose facilities and services are available to the public; before 1972 these institutions (specifically, prison hospitals and college/university infirmaries) were included in the category of community hospitals. These 74 institutions tend to have a lower occupancy rate. The average length of stay column includes, however, these 74 institutions.

[b]Averages include the 74 short-term general hospitals that are part of other institutions.

Table 14 Hospitals by type of ownership or sponsorship and beds in each category, 1980, United States

Hospital Ownership or Sponsorship	Hospitals	Beds (in Thousands)
Federal	359	117
Nonfederal psychiatric	534	215
Nonfederal TB and other respiratory diseases	11	2
Nonfederal long-term care and other special hospitals	157	39
Total nonfederal short-term general hospitals	5,904	992
Nonprofit	3,339	693
For profit (investor owned)	730	87
State or local government	1,835	212
Total hospitals	6,965	
Total beds		1,364,516

SOURCE: *Hospital Statistics,* 1981 ed., American Hospital Assocation.

Table 15a Nursing homes, by certification status and type of ownership, 1978, United States

	Certification Status			
Type of Ownership	Skilled Care	Intermediate Care	Both Skilled and Intermediate Care	Not Certified and Unknown Certification
All types of ownership	7,411	4,670	3,134	6,641
Government	601	320	306	293
Federal	11	5	1	35
State and local	590	315	305	258
Proprietary	5,250	3,502	2,068	5,271
Nonprofit	1,560	848	760	1,077
Church	390	195	211	226
Other	1,170	653	549	851

SOURCE: Division of Health Resources Statistics, National Center for Health Statistics, U.S. Department of Health and Human Services, Washington, D.C.

Table 15b Nursing homes, by certification status and bed size, 1978, United States

Bed Size[a]	Certification Status			
	Skilled Care	Intermediate Care	Both Skilled and Intermediate Care	Not Certified and Unknown Certification
All bed sizes	7,411	4,670	3,134	6,641
3–9 beds	629	89	117	2,035
10–24 beds	359	356	72	1,946
25–49 beds	803	1,181	222	1,201
50–74 beds	1,160	1,339	404	622
75–99 beds	1,254	639	522	292
100–199 beds	2,558	948	1,389	427
200–299 beds	446	79	271	70
300–499 beds	154	27	99	30
500 beds or more	48	12	38	18

SOURCE: Division of Health Resources Statistics, National Center for Health Statistics, U.S. Department of Health and Human Services, Washington, D.C.

[a]Nursing homes with less than 3 beds are not included in the National Master Facility Inventory.

Table 16 Adjusted expenses per inpatient day in community hospitals, 1980–81, United States

Bed-size Category	Adjusted Expenses Per Inpatient Day		% Change
	1980	1981	
Total community hospitals	$245.12	$284.33	16.0
Bed-size category			
6–24 beds	203.49	244.44	20.1
25–49	197.14	230.54	16.9
50–99	190.98	223.44	17.0
100–199	215.16	249.57	16.0
200–299	239.17	276.13	15.5
300–399	247.86	288.45	16.4
400–499	263.01	303.62	15.4
500 or more	288.03	332.22	15.3

SOURCE: *Hospital Statistics,* 1982 ed., American Hospital Association.

Table 17 National health expenditures: aggregate and per capita amounts by major source of funds and as percentage of the Gross National Product, selected years, United States

	1980	1979	1975	1970	1969	1968	1967	1966	1965	1960	1950
National health expenditures (billions)	$247.2	$214.6	$132.7	$74.7	$65.7	$58.2	$51.3	$46.1	$41.7	$26.9	$12.7
As a percentage of the GNP	9.4%	8.9%	8.6%	7.5%	7.0%	6.7%	6.4%	6.1%	6.0%	5.3%	4.4%
Sources of funds											
Private expenditures	$143.0	$124.5	$76.5	$46.9	$40.8	$36.1	$32.4	$32.5	$30.9	$20.3	$9.2
Public expenditures	104.2	90.1	56.2	27.8	24.9	22.1	19.0	13.6	10.8	6.6	3.4
Federal expenditures	70.9	60.8	37.1	17.7	16.1	14.1	11.9	7.4	5.5	3.0	1.6
State/local expenditures	33.3	29.3	19.1	10.1	8.8	8.0	7.0	6.1	5.2	3.6	1.8
Per capita expenditures	$1,067.06	$936.92	$603.57	$357.90	$318.50	$284.97	$253.73	$230.29	$210.89	$146.30	$81.86
Sources of funds											
Private expenditures	617.10	543.61	348.08	224.68	197.78	176.82	159.98	162.47	156.32	110.20	59.62
Public expenditures	449.96	393.31	255.49	133.22	120.72	108.15	93.75	67.82	54.57	36.10	22.24
Federal expenditures	306.14	265.41	168.61	84.69	77.95	69.05	58.90	37.19	27.97	16.42	10.49
State/local expenditures	143.83	127.70	86.88	48.54	42.77	39.10	34.84	30.63	26.60	19.69	11.75
Percentage distribution of funds	100.0%	100.0%	100.0%	100.0%	100.0%	100.0%	100.0%	100.0%	100.0%	100.0%	100.0%
Private funds	57.8	58.0	57.7	62.8	62.1	62.0	63.1	70.6	74.1	75.3	72.8
Public funds	42.2	42.0	42.3	37.2	37.9	38.0	36.9	29.4	25.9	24.7	27.2
Federal funds	28.7	28.4	27.9	23.7	24.5	24.3	23.2	16.1	13.3	11.2	12.8
State/local funds	13.5	13.7	14.4	13.6	13.4	13.7	13.7	13.3	12.6	13.5	14.4

SOURCE: *Health Care Financing Review*, September 1981.

Table 18 National health expenditures by type of expenditure: aggregate and per capita amounts and percentage distribution by source of funds, 1980, United States

		Private					Public		
			Consumer						
Type of Expenditure	Total	Total	Total	Direct	Insurance	Other[a]	Total	Federal	State and Local
Total (in billions)	$247.2	$143.0	$135.5	$70.6	$64.9	$7.5	$104.2	$70.9	$33.3
Health services and supplies	235.6	138.7	135.5	70.6	64.9	3.2	96.9	65.7	31.3
Personal health care	217.9	131.5	128.7	70.6	58.1	2.9	86.4	62.5	23.9
Hospital care	99.6	45.3	44.1	9.1	35.0	1.2	54.2	41.3	12.9
Physicians' services	46.6	34.3	34.3	17.4	16.9	[b]	12.3	9.4	2.9
Dentists' services	15.9	15.3	15.3	12.0	3.3	—	.6	.3	.3
Other professional services	5.4	3.9	3.9	3.2	.7	.1	1.5	1.0	.4
Drugs and medical sundries	19.2	17.7	17.7	15.9	1.8	—	1.6	.8	.8
Eyeglasses and appliances	5.1	4.6	4.6	4.4	.2	—	.5	.4	.1
Nursing home care	20.7	9.0	8.8	8.7	.1	.1	11.8	6.4	5.3
Other health services	5.4	1.4	—	—	—	1.4	4.0	2.8	1.2
Prepayment and administration	10.4	7.2	6.8	—	6.8	.4	3.2	2.0	1.3
Government public health activities	7.3	—	—	—	—	—	7.3	1.2	6.1
Research and construction of medical facilities	11.6	4.3	—	—	—	4.3	7.3	5.3	2.0
Research[c]	5.4	.3	—	—	—	.3	5.1	4.7	.5
Construction	6.1	4.0	—	—	—	4.0	2.2	.6	1.6
Total per capita amount[d]	$1,067.06	$617.10	$584.71	$304.65	$280.06	$32.38	$449.96	$306.14	$143.84
Health services and supplies	1,017.10	598.64	584.71	304.65	280.06	13.93	418.46	283.41	135.05
Personal health care	940.62	567.67	555.30	304.65	250.65	12.36	372.96	269.91	103.05
Hospital care	429.80	195.70	190.37	39.12	151.24	5.33	234.10	178.32	55.79
Physicians' services	201.18	148.16	148.04	75.04	73.00	.12	53.03	40.64	12.38
Dentists' services	68.42	65.88	65.88	51.61	14.27	—	2.54	1.45	1.09
Other professional services	23.30	17.04	16.79	13.84	2.95	.25	6.26	4.50	1.76
Drugs and medical sundries	83.00	76.28	76.28	68.63	7.65	—	6.72	3.36	3.36
Eyeglasses and appliances	22.10	19.78	19.78	18.88	.89	—	2.32	1.94	.38
Nursing home care	89.46	38.17	38.17	37.53	.64	.54	50.75	27.70	23.06
Other health services	23.34	6.12	—	—	—	6.12	17.22	12.00	5.23
Prepayment and administration	44.93	30.97	29.41	—	29.41	1.56	13.96	8.43	5.53
Government public health activities	31.55	—	—	—	—	—	31.55	5.07	26.48
Research and construction of medical facilities	49.96	18.46	—	—	—	18.46	31.50	22.73	8.77
Research[c]	23.50	1.39	—	—	—	1.39	22.11	20.09	2.02
Construction	26.46	17.07	—	—	—	17.07	9.39	2.64	6.75

Total percentage distribution	100.0%	100.0%	100.0%	100.0%	100.0%	100.0%	100.0%	100.0%	100.0%
Health services and supplies	95.3	97.0	100.0	100.0	100.0	43.0	93.0	92.6	93.9
Personal health care	88.2	92.0	95.0	100.0	89.5	38.2	82.9	88.2	71.6
Hospital care	40.3	31.7	32.6	12.8	54.0	16.5	52.0	58.2	38.8
Physicians' services	18.9	24.0	25.3	24.6	26.1	.4	11.8	13.3	8.6
Dentists' services	6.4	10.7	11.3	16.9	5.1	—	.6	.5	.8
Other professional services	2.2	2.8	2.9	4.5	1.1	.8	1.4	1.5	1.2
Drugs and medical sundries	7.8	12.4	13.0	22.5	2.7	—	1.5	1.1	2.3
Eyeglasses and appliances	2.1	3.2	3.4	6.2	.3	—	.5	.6	.3
Nursing home care	8.4	6.3	6.5	12.3	.2	1.7	11.3	9.0	16.0
Other health services	2.2	1.0	—	—	—	18.9	3.8	3.9	3.6
Prepayment and administration	4.2	5.0	5.0	—	10.5	4.8	3.1	2.8	3.8
Government public health activities	3.0	—	—	—	—	—	7.0	1.7	18.4
Research and construction of medical facilities	4.7	3.0	—	—	—	57.0	7.0	7.4	6.1
Research[c]	2.2	.2	—	—	—	4.3	4.9	6.6	1.4
Construction	2.5	2.8	—	—	—	52.7	2.1	.9	4.7

SOURCE: *Health Care Financing Review*, September 1981.

[a]Spending by philanthropic organizations, industrial in-plant health services, and construction financed privately.

[b]Less than $100 million.

[c]Research and development expenditures of drug companies and other manufacturers and providers of medical equipment and supplies are excluded from "Research Expenditures" but are included in the expenditure class in which the product falls.

[d]Based on July 1 population estimates, which include the resident U.S. population and that of the outlying territories, plus federal military and civilian employees and their dependents overseas.

Table 19 Personal health care expenditures by source of funds and type of expenditure: Aggregate and per capita amount and percentage distribution, 1980, United States

Source of Payment	Total	Hospital Care	Physicians' Services	Dentists' Services	Other Professional Services	Drugs	Glasses	Nursing Home Care	Other Personal Health
Total (in billions)	$217.9	$99.6	$46.6	$15.9	$5.4	$19.2	$5.1	$20.7	$5.4
Direct payments	70.6	9.1	17.4	12.0	3.2	15.9	4.4	8.7	—
Third-party payments	147.3	90.5	29.2	3.9	2.2	3.3	.7	12.0	5.4
Private health insurance	58.1	35.0	16.9	3.3	.7	1.8	.2	.1	—
Philanthropy and industrial in-plant	2.9	1.2	—	—	.1	—	—	.1	1.4
Government	86.4	54.2	12.3	.6	1.5	1.6	.5	11.8	4.0
Federal	62.5	41.3	9.4	.3	1.0	.8	.4	6.4	2.8
Medicare[a]	35.6	26.3	7.7	—	.7	—	.4	.4	.1
Medicaid[b]	13.9	5.2	1.3	.3	.3	.7	—	5.7	.5
Other	13.0	9.8	.4	.1	—	—	.1	.4	2.2
State and local	23.9	12.9	2.9	.3	.4	.8	.1	5.3	1.2
Medicaid[b]	11.4	4.3	1.0	.2	.2	.6	—	4.7	.4
Other	12.4	8.6	1.8	—	.2	.2	.1	.7	.9
Total per capita amount[c]	$940.62	$429.80	$201.18	$68.42	$23.30	$83.00	$22.10	$89.46	$23.34
Direct payments	304.65	39.12	75.04	51.61	13.84	68.63	18.88	37.53	—
Third-party payments	635.97	390.68	126.15	16.82	9.47	14.37	3.21	51.93	23.34
Private health insurance	250.65	151.24	73.00	14.27	2.95	7.65	.89	.64	—
Philanthropy and industrial in-plant	12.36	5.33	.12	—	.25	—	—	.54	6.12
Government	372.96	234.10	53.03	2.54	6.26	6.72	2.32	50.75	17.22
Federal	269.91	178.32	40.64	1.45	4.50	3.36	1.94	27.70	12.00
Medicare[a]	153.76	113.44	33.44	—	2.99	—	1.56	1.69	.64
Medicaid[b]	59.96	22.46	5.44	1.13	1.29	3.18	—	24.46	2.00
Other	56.19	42.42	1.77	.32	.21	.19	.38	1.55	9.35
State and local	103.05	55.79	12.38	1.09	1.76	3.36	.38	23.06	5.23
Medicaid[b]	49.35	18.52	4.49	.93	1.07	2.62	—	20.17	1.55
Other	53.70	37.26	7.89	.16	.70	.74	.38	2.89	3.68

Total percentage distribution	100.0%	100.0%	100.0%	100.0%	100.0%	100.0%	100.0%	100.0%	100.0%
Direct payments	32.4	9.1	37.3	75.4	59.4	82.7	85.5	41.9	—
Third-party payments	67.6	90.9	62.7	24.6	40.6	17.3	14.5	58.1	100.0
Private health insurance	26.6	35.2	36.3	20.9	12.7	9.2	4.0	.7	—
Philanthropy and industrial in-plant	1.3	1.2	.1	—	1.1	—	—	.6	26.2
Government	39.6	54.5	26.4	3.7	26.9	8.1	10.5	56.7	73.8
Federal	28.7	41.5	20.2	2.1	19.3	4.1	8.8	31.0	51.4
Medicare[a]	16.3	26.4	16.6	—	12.8	—	7.1	1.9	2.7
Medicaid[b]	6.4	5.2	2.7	1.7	5.5	3.8	—	27.3	8.6
Other	6.0	9.9	.9	.5	.9	.2	1.7	1.7	40.1
State and local	11.0	13.0	6.2	1.6	7.6	4.0	1.7	25.8	22.4
Medicaid[b]	5.2	4.3	2.2	1.4	4.6	3.2	—	22.5	6.6
Other	5.7	8.7	3.9	.2	3.0	.9	1.7	3.2	15.8

SOURCE: *Health Care Financing Review*, September 1981.

[a]Total expenditures from trust funds for benefits; trust fund income includes premium payments paid by or on behalf of enrollees.

[b]Includes funds paid into Medicare trust funds by states under "buy-in" agreements to cover premiums for public assistance recipients and for persons who are medically indigent.

[c]Based on July 1 population estimates, which include the population of outlying territories and armed forces and federal civilian employees and their dependents overseas.

Table 20 Persons (in thousands) with private health insurance protection by type of coverage, United States

End of Year	Hospital Expense	Surgical Expense	Physician's Expense	Major Medical Expense	Disability Income Short-term	Disability Income Long-term	Dental Expense
1940	11,962	4,900	3,000		—	—	
1945	32,072	12,602	4,713		—	—	
1950	76,639	54,156	21,589		37,793	[a]	
1955	101,400	85,681	53,038	—	39,513	[a]	
1960	122,500	111,525	83,172	32,590	42,436	[a]	—
1965	138,671	130,530	109,560	69,666	46,927	4,514	—
1970	158,847	151,440	138,658	103,544	58,089	10,966	11,972
1975	177,980	168,895	161,854	134,092	62,971	18,396	30,246
1979	184,121	174,686	164,754	147,555	65,808	19,920	70,171[b]
1980	189,000	178,223	169,529	155,192	65,400	21,093	80,528[b]
1981							
Under 65	172,726	165,638	153,319	154,513	—	21,682	—
65 and over	15,614	11,260	10,625	3,189	—		—
Total	188,340	176,898	163,944	157,702	60,306	21,682	86,302[b]

Sources: Health Insurance Association of America, Blue Cross Association, Blue Shield Association, and the U.S. Department of Health and Human Services. All of the data is reported by the Health Insurance Association of America in its *Source Book of Health Insurance Data 1982–1983*.

Note: Some data are revised from previous years. For 1975 and later, data include the number of persons covered in Puerto Rico and other U.S. territories and possessions. The data refer to the net total of people protected, i.e., duplication among persons protected by more than one kind of insuring organization or more than one insurance company policy providing the same type of coverage has been eliminated.

[a]Included in "Short-term," with the possibility of some duplication of disability income coverage for these years.
[b]Estimate.

Dominant Issues: Costs and Values

Marshall W. Raffel

The health systems of the industrialized countries described in this book have all served their people well, and continue to do so. There is clear evidence in each of the countries of improved access to health services, quality of care, and health status. It is important to stress these achievements because in the debates and analyses of contemporary affairs, the focus on shortcomings often causes people to lose sight of what has already been accomplished. The critics are nonetheless important catalysts for further reform because each health system could further improve the health of its population.

These fourteen countries, however, share a problem common to all countries: limited resources. Not one has the resources to do all that can be done for its population's health and quality of life. Besides health services, there are other vital needs such as for food, clothing, housing, transport, defense, and a vast array of other goods and services, all of which compete with the health sector for a share of the limited resources. Each country has to strike a balance among the competing demands, a balance which is essential to maintain social stability. Equilibrium is threatened whenever one sector's uncompromising claim to the available resources threatens to deprive other sectors to an extent that is socially unacceptable.

The national defense debates in the United States in 1983 highlight this point. The economy was in recession and the expanding entitlement programs such as Social Security and Medicare were being curtailed, and other budgets and services throughout the society were being cut except in the defense sector, where the budgets were rising. The public debate in part revolved around one sector's proposed expansion while all other sectors were forced to cut back. The debate was spirited. As one White House spokesman put it: "The clash over resources comes down to a choice between the armed services and the old folks, or between free school lunches and troops in Korea."[1] The author who quoted the spokesman went on to say that "Social Security retirement benefits and Medicare together consume today as much of the budget as the armed services. These are the programs that old people have come to depend on; they feel they have a contract with the Government and it must be honored." He noted that these conflicting claims to the available resources "have to be massaged through the world of politics."

The health sector now poses special problems, for in all industrialized societies its claims for resources are increasing in dramatic fashion. In most instances the demands are not just for incremental increases, nor do they arise from whim or from promises which stand little likelihood of fulfillment. There are sound bases for most of these claims, which stem from research efforts that have contributed new knowledge, new technology, and new drugs for the treatment of disease. These tools accrue to the benefit of all segments of the population, and with an informed population, the demand to meet all societal needs is being made forcibly. The pressures are most acutely felt as a result of a rapidly aging population which has an increasing impact in the electoral processes of democratic society, a population whose demands and needs are increasingly supported by others either out of social conscience or out of recognition that they will also soon be in that age category.

Each of the countries described in this book is seeking ways to control the rising health care cost phenomenon. In the USSR and China the paucity of resources, coupled with the structure of their governments, permits a more controlled management of the cost issue. In the other countries, however, because of their affluence, the dispersion of both power and resource control among the levels of government and the private sectors, as well as the general population's awareness of recent medical advances, the societies have not been able to adopt a simple control mechanism. Rather, they have been forced into fine-tuning efforts or tinkering with the health cost phenomenon. The fine-tuning efforts that have taken place are described or alluded to by each of the authors.

AN OVERVIEW OF NATIONAL EFFORTS AT COST CONTAINMENT

Some countries—for example, Australia, Belgium, and, to some extent, the United States—have been paying hospitals less than cost, thus forcing them to scrutinize the work they are doing and presumably manage more efficiently. This practice is also implicit in some of the other countries in terms of hospital financing mechanisms. But, as Dewdney points out, in Australia greater efficiency on the part of hospitals is difficult to achieve, considering that their principal cost item—wages—is set by independent wage tribunals. This is, of course, a problem in most countries where employees negotiate wages through wage tribunals, unions, or under the threat of individual departures to higher paying jobs. In the United States the problem is exacerbated whenever, as a result of inflationary pressures, the Congress raises the minimum wage and the social security tax contribution rate. There are, also, other cost factors that are beyond hospital control, such as fuel, electricity, food, and telephones.

Australia has managed, to a limited extent, to control physician incomes by adjustments in the amounts the insurance schemes will pay for specific items of service. This has led to a state where physician incomes are not keeping pace with the cost of living (which is, of course, the lament of most other groups as well—in all societies). Eichhorn notes that Germany has also made adjustments in the schedule of medical benefits in order to encourage use of certain services and discourage use of others. In all countries except the United States there is strong governmental influence, if not direct control, on the amounts paid to physicians. The U.S. exception stems in large measure from a societal reluctance to impose controls in any sector. More will be said of this later.

Medical fraud was identified as a problem in Australia and the United States. This problem stems from the availability of large sums of money coupled with payments on an item-of-service basis. The ease of access to that pot of gold is an inducement to unprincipled behavior on the part of some, particularly so since cheating an impersonal agency is apparently thought less onerous than cheating an individual. The absence of significant direct patient payments to the physician also contributes to decreased judicious behavior on the physician's part in selecting appropriate treatment. How widespread fraud and injudicious prescribing are, no one knows, though it will become less of a problem as computers are used to monitor the practices for which payments are sought. Dewdney refers to computer monitoring of practices as a potential positive outcome from Australia's unsuccessful Medibank Mark I experiment. Canada is also monitoring medical practices with the aid of computers, and its efforts have apparently been very successful. Belgium also seems to have embarked on this system of surveillance. Limited U.S. moves in this direction have *thus far* largely been confined to government-financed care. Krasnik notes, however, the resistance of Danish physicians to the development of detailed information systems that may limit clinical freedom and medical influence. Although such monitoring may be unpleasant in the eyes of most physicians, it may be the only currently available alternative for minimizing the tendency toward fraud and for encouraging judicious physician prescribing of both drugs and tests.

In most countries, control of the supply of hospital beds has been an especially attractive means for trying to cope with the rising cost of health care. Since hospitals are the major cost component, the rationale seems to be that with fewer beds there will be waiting lists which will control the flow of hospital patients through the system, and that this will permit regulating the rate at which hospital costs are incurred. The resulting waiting periods would also encourage the use of alternative services. However, even without queues, governments are encouraging non-hospital care through a range of ambulatory and home care services, which will result, it is believed, in a reduced demand for hospital beds and, in turn, lower costs. This theory has yet to be proved. In both England and New Zealand the rationing of hospital beds has prompted a growing number of people to seek care in the private hospital sector, though the New Zealand government appears to be seeking ways to make this a less viable alternative. Private sector development in Denmark is also reported by Krasnik.

Quaethoven and Nys suggest that Belgium has shied away from direct bed reductions because of the adverse reaction that waiting lists would generate, and that Belgium has also found that control on the expansion of beds has not worked because of the ease by which controls can be circumvented. To a considerable degree, this failure of controls applies to the U.S. experience. Japan is not controlling bed supply, but, as Hashimoto notes, its hospitals are different in that they routinely handle both acute and chronic illnesses. The Japanese model in this regard is being tried in some U.S. hospitals as a way to prevent the closure of beds and to increase occupancy, turning an acute bed into a long-term-care bed if the former is not needed. This is known as the "swing bed" concept.

Along with hospital bed supply controls and a shift toward ambulatory care, a number of countries have sought to control health care costs by shifting the payment of some costs to the patients. The rationale is that this will discourage frivolous utilization by making the patient exercise better judgement in deciding whether or not to incur the costs. Belgium, China, France, the United States, Germany, and Sweden are among those countries that have gone this route with mixed, if any, results. The Hatchers note the Canadian experience in this matter: "Deterrent charges to patients when they are sick and need care have been tried on a limited scale in Canada, but have been ineffective as cost contraints, and politically unpopular." They further note what others have come to recognize (but have also not been able to deal with effectively to date)—that the main determinant of health costs is physician behavior. The unpopularity of deterrent charges, however, is also a manifestation of the fact that patient preferences are likely to be, in most countries, a powerful countervailing force to cost shifting.

HOSPITAL COSTS—PREVENTION AND AMBULATORY CARE

The data from most of the countries are clear: the hospital sector is the major consumer of health resources. Small wonder that most nations are beginning to place greater emphasis on prevention and on ambulatory care.

Prevention is certainly a partial long-range solution, except in such areas as accident prevention and communicable disease control, where the results are more immediate. Much of what constitutes prevention, however, depends on individual self-discipline in changing habits related to such things as exercise, diet, drinking, smoking, and rest—all difficult changes to achieve. Some prevention, of course, depends on environmental protection and control, and there has been much progress in this area. However, as we identify new hazards in areas we thought were safe, control measures are often difficult to formulate and impose: controls may be costly and may affect employment as well as the cost of products produced, which in turn may affect the company's competitive position in the domestic and world marketplaces. But preventive programs are also easily cuttable when monetary savings are necessary; Krasnik notes that this has occurred in Denmark, as it also has in the United States.

Another aspect of prevention which might be cited as possibly increasing health care costs, stems from the assertion that by preventive screening and check-ups, early diagnosis will be made and treatment will be less costly—to which one has to respond, *sometimes* or *maybe*. Many public health professionals maintain that the more one screens, the more one finds, and that this will increase costs. (I recall the budget director in one state government who, after more than several decades of experience, said: "I have never seen a health program that saved me money!") This is not to argue against screening, but rather to note that the argument for it on economic grounds may not be valid. Indeed, some of the declining influence of physicians in a number of countries may stem in part from the overly optimistic projections made as to the economic advantages to be derived from new health programs as the physicians sought to justify their requests for government support. A related factor in declining physician influence was cited to me by a Danish physician, who said, "The politicians don't like to hear that support for a new and costly program will save lives." Here, too, the medical profession in Denmark and elsewhere has often not been able to produce convincing evidence of success with new programs, which leaves the politicians skeptical of later requests for support of preventive and life-saving programs.

As noted earlier, ambulatory care as an alternative to institutional care is also receiving considerable emphasis in most industrialized countries as a means for reducing costs. It has, of course, always been part of all health systems. New and expanded ambulatory services, however, have been made feasible by therapeutic advances that permit more outpatient surgery, outpatient and home medical care, as well as initiating an array of expanded home health and social services.

There are some trade-offs to expansion in ambulatory care, among them the increased economic and social burdens sometimes placed upon the family, for increasingly in the industrialized societies both spouses work, living spaces are smaller, and apartment living is becoming more commonplace. The resulting problems are frequently exacerbated by the discharge of patients from hospitals and nursing homes before the needed ambulatory services are in place. Another challenge, which stems from the resort to ambulatory medical services, is that of quality control or quality assurance mechanisms to monitor those services. While most practitioners may be both competent and ethical, there is legitimate concern over those whose clinical judgement and skills deteriorate and over those who are unethical. Where the more complicated medical services are in the hospital—as inpatient or outpatient services—there is likely to be some institutional surveillance which serves, or could easily serve, as a quality assurance mechanism. The peer review committees in U.S. and Canadian hospitals illustrate how such monitoring could be handled in an inoffensive manner, although it needs to be said that the monitoring could be strengthened in many of their hospitals. However, this monitoring is absent in most non-hospital settings, which raises the question of the extent to which non-hospital ambulatory medical services—and, indeed, other ambulatory services as well—should be encouraged until there is some mechanism to assure both their necessity and their quality.

Ambulatory services, while seemingly cost effective, may not prove to be so in the long run. A recently released study by the General Accounting Office (GAO) in Washington found that the provision of ambulatory services did not reduce overall health care costs because expanded services were utilized by many who had not used such services previously, which confirms what many have thought—that is, if you offer services, they will be used even by those whom you did not predict would use the services.[2] Put another way, supply creates demand. Tiddens et al. state also that in the Netherlands, with the passage of the Exceptional Medical Expenses Act (AWBZ), many mentally deficient individuals who were cared for at home or in other nonhealth settings, suddenly appeared as health sector patients. In addition, the GAO found that expanded home health services did not decrease nursing home or hospital usage. The Belgian authors also report that expanded ambulatory and home services for the elderly have not had an impact on hospital care. More research is clearly needed. This is not meant to denigrate the value of expanded ambulatory, social, and home health services, for they can contribute much to improved quality of life. The English effort in this area is particularly noteworthy, though others have also made significant progress.

HOSPITAL COSTS—WAITING LISTS

Several countries have dealt with the cost problem by rationing services by queue, asking citizens for non-emergency hospital surgical care to get in line and wait their turn—the wait can sometimes take three or four years. In the interim, the citizen's quality of life is affected, some die from other causes, and others decide to live with the disability. Interestingly, Mackay reports that over 28% of the population of New Zealand elected to buy private health insurance, which is used primarily to avoid the surgical waiting list by going to a private hospital for surgery. The same pattern seems to be emerging in England and Denmark. Private hospitals in New Zealand have been relatively unregulated, but whether their easy use by citizens as a surgical alternative will persist, in light of the government's recent moves to force a balance between the public and private sectors, remains to be seen.

There have been reports of countries denying access to certain services because of age or work status. This would seem to be a variation on the queuing system, in that those who are not eligible are simply denied the opportunity to get in the queue. In some cases, such as renal dialysis and organ transplant, in the absence of clinical contraindications, denial of access constitutes an early sentence to death.

While denial of access in most countries seems to be based more on age and probable life years remaining, in the Soviet Union denial of access also appears to be based on the perceived value of the individual. The political elite, who are valued, are served by the Fourth Department; workers and future workers (children) receive more attentive care than other ordinary citizens. In many countries, including the Soviet Union, the problem is that the health sector is not allocated sufficient funds for it to give every person optimal care. In some instances this may be a temporary expedient until resources are shifted, facilities built, or personnel trained. In other instances, such as in the countries of eastern Europe, it may be due to the structure and operation of their economies, which do not give them sufficient convertable currency to purchase the drugs and technology from industrialized countries outside their economic orbit. (The health professional traveling in eastern Europe cannot help but be struck by the enormous pride taken by some clinicians in the scarce—to them—high technology equipment they have managed to acquire, particularly from western Europe and the United States, which is perceived as superior. But such equipment is in short supply. As one surgeon put it: "See may hands? I am an artist. I have to be because I do not have the tools to be otherwise.")

Where a country persists in denying access when it would be feasible to shift resources to provide access, certain ethical and moral questions arise and might well be asked of the decision makers. This will be discussed later.

Another issue relating to queueing and cost control surfaces in France and Belgium. Lacronique reports that prior authorization is necessary for any costly procedure or prolonged hospital stay. He notes, however, that problems sometimes arise because of the delays that occur in receiving authorization, and consequently, a new procedure is being tested that seems to allow for an approved length of stay which is related to the diagnosis. This appears to be somewhat like the U.S. experimental system to pay hospitals on the basis of a Diagnosis Related Groups (DRG) schedule. It is a cost control mechanism designed in part to encourage judicious clinical decisions by the physicians. In Belgium, Quaethoven and Nys report, except for emergency instances, prior authorization for admission to a hospital is necessary, though it is typically granted automatically. Prior authorizations in the United States are generally viewed as inappropriate, an interference in the doctor-patient relationship. As an alternative, an increasing number of insurance and government programs in the United States are requiring second surgical opinions as to the need for non-emergency surgery; if surgery is performed without a confirming second opinion, less than full payment may be provided.

HEALTH COSTS—PHYSICIAN INCOMES

In most countries, physicians enjoy high incomes. Of the countries included in this book, China and the USSR are exceptions. It is interesting to note, however, that in most of the other countries, charges to patients are controlled: through negotiated fee schedules; by the physicians being paid a salary or by capitation; by a very progressive tax system; by medical practitioner restraint in establishing fees, which (based on personal observation) seems to be at least partly the case in New Zealand for private practice physicians. This is all noteworthy because there is little control on physician charges in the United States and there is growing concern that an increasing number of physicians in fee-for-service practice lack restraint. This has become manifest as the gap widens between U.S. medical practitioner charges and the amounts allowed by third-party payers (health insurance firms and government programs). One explanation for fee inflation in the United States has been suggested by a number of U.S. and Canadian economists: it is the target-income hypothesis which holds, as Dyckman put it, that "physicians have a target level of income. And when demand for their services is insufficient to achieve that income level, they raise their fees to achieve it."[3] Others argue that more critical factors may be the provision of additional diagnostic and therapeutic services due to new knowledge and technology, the ability of people to secure access because of an increased ability to pay or to have the costs covered, and an aging population with its increased morbidity. Whatever the factors, it will be interesting to monitor this as the supply of physicians approaches a surplus and to see at what point physician charges begin to moderate because of competition for patients or at what point charges are deemed to have gone beyond socially tolerable limits. The latter event would, of course, force the United States to deal directly with the matter, perhaps by adapting one of the mechanisms employed in western Europe.

Allen reports a shortage of anesthesiologists and radiologists in England, and he cites the attractive opportunities abroad as a contributing factor. One has only to note the reported average annual incomes in the United States for such specialities in 1982. Those reported in the text are national averages, and incomes (after business expenses have been taken out, but before personal income taxes) well in excess of $250,000 per year are now common. Hesitancy to deal directly with the issue of physician charges and incomes in the United States stems, as noted earlier, from a societal reluctance to impose controls on any sector. But hesitancy is also understandable given the experiences of other countries. In Canada and France, for example, there have been strike actions. In Sweden, the Seven Kronor Reform prompted many Swedish physicians to opt out of medical practice or "to work the rules"—that is, to work the prescribed hours per week and no more. This contributed—at least temporarily—to a shortage of physicians. The obsession for the 40-hour work week by general practitioners was also apparent in my recent visit to Denmark. The Swedish problem apparently persists, for Borgenhammar indicates a continued deceleration in physician per hour productivity. Even in the Soviet Union, medical workers are charged with often violating their official duties and exhibiting inattentive and heartless attitudes. But as Tiddens et al. note, "Persistence by the medical profession, i.e., the specialists, and their supporters, in demanding extremely high incomes and complete autonomy, can hardly be allowed to continue." Some large business firms and health insurance companies in the United States are just beginning to deal directly with this by signing up physicians and physician groups as Preferred Providers, whereby the physicians agree to accept the insurance payments as full payment; if the patient goes to another physician a lesser payment may be given, and the physician may charge whatever he or she wishes. Where there is a surplus of physicians, this, it is hoped, will force a reduction in fees overall.

However, finding an appropriate balance between physician income desires and what is socially and politically acceptable is difficult; hence, incremental changes tend to be made. For example, Australia found it necessary to allow its hospital-based, salaried physicians an opportunity to augment their incomes from a modest private practice, modest being defined as an additional 20% income. A similar set-up exists in England, some of the private practice occurring in public hospital beds. Use of public hospital personnel and services for private practice has been controversial, and in England, at least, the major political parties have had strong differing views on this. France also found it necessary to allow limited private care in public hospitals, but is now phasing out this practice. In phasing it out, however, Lacronique reports it was necessary to compensate the physicians for the lost opportunities for augmented incomes. Many teaching hospitals in the United States also permit their salaried physicians an opportunity to supplement their incomes by limited private practice. In New Zealand most specialists in public hospitals still work on a part-time basis, thus permitting them to practice in private offices and private hospitals. In the Soviet Union unofficial payments are reported to be a common and expected practice, particularly for hospital care in many republics, though Knaus reports that in the Baltic republics of Estonia, Latvia, and Lithuania such "direct payments are considered in poor taste and are only infrequently made."[4]

Apart from those in China and the Soviet Union, the medical associations have been strong and effective in representing their constituencies, particularly on economic issues. Hashimoto notes, for example, that the Japan Medical Association is the most powerful medical group in the country, exerting considerable influence on national medical policies. Its power must undoubtedly be strengthened by the fact that about 90% of those in active practice belong to it. A similar situation exists in Germany, where membership in the general medical councils is compulsory. By contrast, both the Australian Medical Association and the American Medical Association have only about 50% of all physicians in their respective countries as members, but only in Australia has there developed another physician group with a national constituency to challenge the policy positions of the Australian Medical Association. Notwithstanding, both medical associations have been well organized and staunch defenders of their members' economic rights. The American group has been particularly active in political affairs, and its members heavy contributors to political campaigns.

Medical association militancy, however, can also be counterproductive in the long run. In both Germany and Denmark, for example, the influence of medical doctors is reportedly declining, and Dewdney notes the popularity in Australia of the Doctors' Reform Society, "nurtured by the media grateful for having a youthful telegenic opposition to the AMA establishment." In the United States the Federal Trade Commission has been taking steps to assure that the medical associations do not set fees, prohibit advertising, and otherwise restrain trade and competition.

The German mechanism for paying non-hospital-based physicians—by their own association of sickness fund physicians—may be of some interest for the United States and possibly also for other countries. As noted earlier, some physician incomes in the United States, which are based upon charges to patients, are exceeding what a growing number of people would hold as reasonable. In some states, moreover, it is not uncommon for physicians to bill Medicare (over age sixty-five) patients, appending a note to the bill stating that upon receipt of payment, the physician will then send the patient the necessary itemized bill which the patient can send to Medicare for reimbursement. Where the bills are sizeable, this can pose a cash-flow problem for the patient. Any attempt at government control in the United States would generate widespread physician opposition, although the problem exists mainly with a limited number of medical specialties. (The average income figures reported by the American Medical Association highlight some—but not all—of these specialties.) How to deal with such physician lack of restraint without incurring the adverse effects experienced by other countries is a dilemma. As we have seen, some attempts are being made to deal with this through the Preferred Provider movement. The German practice, however, would also seem to offer a possible approach for some countries. As Eichhorn notes, in Germany it is not government, nor the health insurance firms, but rather the physicians' own organization that has the immediate power over them. Peer pressure and peer control is possible and probably more acceptable than direct government control. What gives those associations power beyond peer pressure, however, is the fact that they are also publicly chartered and have certain legal responsibilities.

By contrast, the Blue Shield insurance plans in the United States, which cover physician costs, were initially sponsored by state and/or local medical associations, but they did not have the legal sanctions to back up their payment schemes. Because Blue Shield-participating physicians could easily refuse to accept Blue Shield payments as full payment for low-income patients, the plans became a mechanism only to help subscribers pay the bills; the plans failed to provide an effect control over physician charges. While all the medical societies had grievance committees to handle complaints from patients, these committees have not been very effective.

While medical association control or sponsorship of Blue Shield plans has largely disappeared, the German experience certainly suggest that a return to some form of medical association control offers interesting possibilities for the control of excessive charges to patients and overall cost containment. This would probably entail negotiation between medical associations and insurance companies, as in Germany. In the United States it would also require some modification of the federal antitrust laws since a medical association (state or national) would be a more powerful negotiating force than a small group of physicians in Preferred Provider organizations. This mechanism may be less threatening than the Preferred Provider approach and would certainly seem preferable to try before more drastic measures that the medical profession might find especially distasteful, if not intolerable. In fact, in the 1940s and 1950s the state of Maryland had a modified version of this. The state medical association leaders in the 1940s, fearing a national health system, decided to cut the ground from under that drive by proposing that the state government finance a program for health care of the indigent and medically indigent. While the state did not turn over the monies to a physician organization as in Germany, it secured on a continuing basis both physician and hospital advice regarding program policy and administration. The Maryland Medical Care Program worked extremely well until replaced in 1966 by Medicare and Medicaid; it succeeded because trust existed between medical leaders and state government officials, and also because there was a cadre of physician leaders who knew that unless they paved the way for medical behavior which was responsive to social needs, the medical profession's independence and ability to govern itself would ultimately be lost. The program in its impact and administration proved to be a case where what was good for the state and its citizens was good for the medical profession. It should, of course, be emphasized that the size of the United States and the cultural diversity of its population—including that of its medical practitioners—make effective policy positions difficult to attain and choices difficult to implement, except on a state-by-state basis.

It is interesting to note that a similar pattern may be developing within the Australian Medical Association, emanating from what Dewdney perceives as "a genuine concern among some of the Association's leaders for those broader issues." The American Medical Association has also initiated steps to join forces with hospital, insurance, dental, labor, and business groups to forge a national health policy, but whether it will address physician fees is doubtful.

The German experience of involving the various provider groups is also interesting. Rather than operate in exclusively an adversary environment, the provider groups are brought into the health planning process. By contrast, in the United States the federal initiatives since 1966 tried to keep the provider groups at arms length lest they overly influence the "objectivity" of the planning process. The U.S. experience has been a dismal failure and has alienated in the process most of the provider groups.

PHYSICIAN SURPLUSES AND FUTURE COSTS

Most of the countries included in this book are anticipating a surplus of physicians, if that surplus has not already arrived. Assessment of what constitutes a surplus is, of course, a rather complicated matter. Although physician unemployment is reported by a number of countries, this only proves an excess under the present allocation of resources to the health sector of the economy. The excess may entirely disappear if all access restraints are removed, if there is an optimal supply of facilities, and if all technological advances and treatment modalities are available for use.

Determining future supply is further complicated by the extent to which nurses and other health personnel are utilized. Another variable concerns the changing life styles of physicians in terms of the hours per week they choose to work. As noted earlier, Swedish reforms in 1970, and changes in Denmark, led to a significant reduction in the hours worked by primary care physicians. While U.S. data are not conclusive, from 1970 to 1980 American physicians worked 3.5% fewer hours per week. Whether this trend will continue is not known, but some observers believe that the physicians' desire for more leisure time will lead to a more regular and shorter average work week. The sharp rise in the number of female physicians may have bearing on this: indeed, Quaethoven and Nys report that in Belgium a shorter work week for female physicians is already evident. Still another factor in physician supply relates to the rapidly aging populations whose specific needs, coupled with advances in knowledge and technology, will create new needs and demands. Renal dialysis, hip replacements, and organ transplants are examples which already impact upon most nations as do advances in the treatment of cancer. An artificial heart is now emerging and will undoubtedly be improved to the point where it could be effectively used by significant numbers of people. Anticipating the consequent demand for additional physicians, nurses, supporting personnel, drugs, equipment, and hospital beds is mind boggling, for the advances in cancer diagnosis and therapy and in heart disease affect a significant segment of the population. The costs will be staggering, but public pressures to meet the demand will also be enormous. Tiddens et al. note Dutch manifestations of this where the population has become "less tolerant of all sorts of 'inconveniences.' . . ." Borgenhammer cites a Swedish study which concluded that 85% of the population would consider higher taxes acceptable if used for better care of the elderly, and that 70% would rather pay higher taxes than experience a deterioration of medical care. The growth of private health insurance in England, Denmark, and New Zealand also emphasizes this point, as does the difficulty of governments in a number of countries to persuade communities that they do not need a specific type of hospital or hospital service; consumers do not want to hear from authorities why access to some services should be less convenient for them than for others. Direct consumer pressures for sharing power seems particularly evident in Denmark.

NEW OPPORTUNITIES, NEW DEMANDS, AND SOME ETHICAL ISSUES

Heart disease and cancer are the leading causes of death in all fourteen countries. We have, however, crossed the threshold of major advances in both areas. Accompanying the aging populations with their chronic degenerative diseases, which will increase as we continue to make advances against heart disease and cancer, costs will continue to rise inexorably, as will the need for medical and other health workers, facilities, equipment, and drugs. We have noted that to date governments have sought to contain costs, to keep their economies in balance, by a number of mechanisms. It will be more difficult, however, for governments to maintain such a stance in the face of technological advances and new treatment methods, for as knowledge of these becomes widespread, there will be stronger citizen demands for access. Reassessment of societal priorities may well be at hand.

The queueing practice and denial of access to health care have been of special interest to many health professionals because of the ethical dilemmas they pose. Since these forms of rationing will be tempting more and more societies in the years ahead, it would be appropriate to note some of those dilemmas.

We might do this by citing two patients, both age fifty, who would benefit from hip replacement surgery. Because of the queue which may be dictated by a shortage of beds, surgeons, anesthesiologists, or nurses, let us assume that the patients must wait three years. The patients have identical incomes, but one (patient A) has not saved. He has used his money to travel, buy an expensive home, eat well—to live, in other words, from paycheck to paycheck. Patient B has lived more modestly and has saved money. Should B be permitted to use his savings to improve his quality of life sooner, not by moving ahead of A in the queue (which would not be equitable and would hence be inappropriate) but by avoiding the queue and securing the hip replacement in the private sector?

In this regard New Zealand offers an interesting point for reference. Let us assume that these two hypothetical cases and the accompanying circumstances described above occured in New Zealand.* Patient A would have to wait his turn on the queue and be

*For the sake of my New Zealand colleagues, let me note here that I have no idea what the surgical waiting list time is for hip replacement surgery in New Zealand, or indeed if there is even any delay in access for this procedure.

inconvenienced. His quality of life might be affected, but his life would not be threatened by this condition while he waited. Patient B, on the other hand, may decide to circumvent the public system and go to a private hospital to have the surgery performed immediately, thereby improving his quality of life and paying for that privilege either out-of-pocket or by having purchased private health insurance.

For many years this New Zealand competitive structure worked. Though not completely equalitarian, it enabled those who accumulated the resources to benefit from the fruits of their labor and their thrift. The private sector was not always appreciated by the public sector bureaucrats because it was partially subsidized by government and was competitive. However, the private sector was a constant challenge to the public sector, challenging it to do better lest the population shift to the private sector—which it did from time to time. In this regard, Allen quotes a recent Royal Commission view that "the private sector responds much more directly to patients' demands for services than the NHS and . . . provide[s] a useful pointer to areas where the NHS is deficient." In the current world economic crisis, however, Mackay notes that the New Zealand government seems to be trying to rationalize the allocation of the nation's resources by restraining public sector development, forcing it to consider what exists in the private sector. The competitive challenge will thus be less, and the environment will not be as conducive for maintaining—let alone strengthening—the process of raising standards and improving quality of care. But, public sector investments will be restrained. The implication for patients A and B could be significant: the waiting list queue for A may grow longer because B and those like him will now be on the same list, thus increasing the difficulty in access for both the As and Bs, and the pressure will increase for expansions in the private sector, thus shifting more costs to the As and Bs, who will find longer waiting lists less tolerable.

One might extend this example and line of reasoning beyond inconvenience and quality of life to a life or death situation. Suppose B is seventy years old and A is only fifty; both need renal dialysis, and renal transplants are not feasible. In a number of countries this service is or was rationed, including England and France during the early 1970s at least. In reporting this, Cooper notes that in Britain "available resources have to be severely rationed amongst potential gainers so that under ten percent of all cases and one percent of those over fifty-five years old, are likely to receive optimal treatment."[5] Similar rationing is practiced to some extent in all of the other countries. If, in this hypothetical case, access is denied seventy-year-old B on the basis of age, he is, in effect, sentenced to death because of society's unwillingness or inability to allocate the necessary resources—unless B has the money and/or insurance to secure private dialysis treatment in his own or in some other country.

Let us now view these examples on the basis of economic class. Suppose that A has a low income enabling him to live modestly but not save; B has a much higher income and is able to save. Both are the same age. Should B be able to secure private care for nonemergency surgery? This example, similar to that posed earlier on hip replacement, may not trouble some because the wait is not life threatening. But suppose the conditions of A and B were life threatening and government did not provide sufficient resources to take care of A and B. Should B be able to secure private care? If not, should B be permitted to fly to some other country for the life saving services? If B could secure care because he had the money, would this not then constitute a socially sanctioned two-class system? If it is a two-class system, who created it and for what reasons? It should be noted that allowing private services to be developed and used by people who have the money very conveniently decreases the pressure on government to reallocate the resources at its disposal. To what extent is such a two-class system just? If unjust to A, would a one-class system be unjust to B? It would, after all, be his life which is at stake, and the fruits of his labor and judicious behavior which he would propose to spend.

A related issue has arisen in England. Allen asserts that some feel the middle class is particularly well served by the NHS because it knows how to use the service better. Has the one-class NHS thus inadvertently become a two-class system?

Some rationing is of course necessitated by circumstances over which societies and their governments do not have control. It takes time, after new technology has been developed and proven, to manufacture sufficient equipment and train the personnel to operate it. In the interim some rationing has to take place. Here the ethical dilemma—if there is one—of being able to secure private care in one's own country or in another country is clearly different from the set of circumstances that exists when society or its government chooses not to allocate new resources. In the latter instance, is it just for both A and B to die because of government's unwillingness or inability to provide resources? Is it just to ask B to die because A does not have the money to save himself? If B secures private care and survives, is he to be blamed? or is the blame—if blame is to be assigned—government's?

These questions are not easily answered. Each case has special circumstances and there are dilemmas. There is a tendency on the part of many, however, to depersonalize these dilemmas as the only way to deal with the general problems, and yet in depersonalization we often lose sight of the impact on individual human beings. Moreover, in depersonalization the risk is that the focus will be so fixed on objective data, such as costs, that sight of value considerations will be lost. Indeed, one might well ask: has the health sector been forced to deal with health needs by rules which are set by nonhealth professionals and which deemphasize societal values to too great an extent? In the United States today, for example, it is fashionable for health sector people to use the language of business and economics—cost effectiveness, marketing of services, price competition, vendor payments, multi-institutional management, corporate structure, risk management, and the health industry (as though it were comparable to the automobile, banking, or airplane industries). It is businesslike language and it even speaks of health sector competition, though what is usually meant is price competition and not quality competition.

Cunningham addressed this in a recent issue of *Hospitals* when he asked, "What has become of the underlying, care-before-cost philosophy—the system of motivating beliefs and concepts that created our hospitals and guided their activities for so many years? Given all the pressures of inflation, regulation, competition, and now the determination of government, insurers, and employers to cut down the amounts they are spending for health care, how could the direction of our ideas and convictions have shifted so far so fast?"[6] He is concerned that the hospital has overreacted to the pressures and that "the danger now is that there could be a confusion of means and ends; acceptance of the methods of commerce could lead to acceptance of the values of commerce." He concluded that "there is time still to moderate the march on the market. . . ."

The health sector certainly is not an island; it must coordinate with other sectors in society. But in doing so, there is evidence to suggest that the health sector may be failing to maintain and emphasize adequately the value component of its claim for resources, for it is the value element that can assist society in making a more balanced choice in the allocation of resources.

In the ensuing debate, however, it should not be forgotten that as important as value considerations are, there is an economic aspect which is often lost sight of: the health sector is not a nonproductive consumer of resources, as critics often imply. In point of fact, the health sector in all countries makes a significant, positive contribution to national economies: as a major employer of both skilled and unskilled labor, its workers pay taxes and spend money, thus fueling their economies; as a heavy purchaser of supplies, drugs, and equipment, it generates employment in these firms, and it does likewise with the construction industry in the need for new buildings and for modernization of existing plants. One cannot help but observe the ease by which a new weapons system is sold, a weapons system that may never be used, whereas the health system still has difficulty in selling the need for new scanners, additional renal dialysis equipment, a quicker turn around time for hip replacements, more long-term-care beds, and the desperately needed community health and social services that would demonstratively improve health and the quality of life in general as well as contribute to the nation's economy.

I have tried to identify some of the major health systems issues which many countries share. There are other issues that the reader will certainly find of special interest, be they the cross national influences in the development of the systems of medical education, the rapidly developing interest in quality assurance and continuing medical education, the training and utilization of nurses, the relationships between central governments and their regional and/or local health authorities, or the many other items brought out by the various authors. It is hoped that these accounts will stimulate readers to explore in greater depth the health systems of different countries and, in particular, the further study of comparative health systems.

Notes

1. T.H. White, "Weinberger on the Ramparts," *The New York Times Magazine,* 6 February 1983, p. 19.
2. Comptroller General of the United States, *The Elderly Should Benefit From Expanded Home Health Care But Increasing These Services Will Not Insure Cost Reductions* (Washington: General Accounting Office, 1983).
3. Z.Y. Dyckman, *A Study of Physician's Fees* (Washington: The Council on Wage and Price Stability, 1978), p. ii.
4. William A. Knaus, *Inside Russian Medicine* (New York: Everest House, 1981), p. 136.
5. Michael H. Cooper, *Rationing Health Care* (London: Croom Helm, 1975), pp. 90f.
6. Robert M. Cunningham, Jr., "More Than a Business: Are Hospjtals Forgetting Their Basic Mission?" *Hospitals,* 16 January 1983, pp. 88–90.